1610 Questions:
Passage-based and 'discretes' structured like the real exam!

AFTER YOUR REVIEW

7 Full-length Practice Tests for the MCAT®

5 in the book and 2 online

Be a Hero, Share the Truth!

It's hard to accept, but studies show that false information disseminates faster than the truth. Some individuals and some companies have policies of fake posts, fake reviews and disseminating fake news. We don't have that policy, and as a result, we struggle to get authentic Amazon or other reviews. We don't want you to say something that you don't believe. But if you truly believe that this book represents an unusually helpful attempt to get you to your objective, please let someone know: Amazon, FB, Google, or anywhere in social media. Thanks! Oh, and a short dedication poem . . .

North and South
Love and Peace
Mom and Dad

MCAT-PREP.COM

Sean Pierre BSc MD • Thomas Pritchard BSc MD
Jeanne Tan Te • Rita W Meneses MA PhD • Bamboo Dong BSc PhD
Harvie Gallatiera (cover design, illustrations) • Gilbert Rafanan (typesetting)

Free Online Access Features* includes 2 different, full-length MCAT practice tests, answers and explanations to all 7 exams, discussion boards, as well as relevant, topical science videos for background information for many science questions.

*One year of continuous access for the original owner of this book using the enclosed online access card (appended to the inside cover of this book).

Be sure to register at www.MCAT-prep.com by clicking on Sign Up in the top right corner of the website. Once you login, click on the image of your book and follow directions. Please Note: benefits are for 1 year from the date of online registration, only for the original book owner, and are not transferable; unauthorized access and use outside the Terms of Use posted on MCAT-prep.com may result in account deletion; if you are not the original owner, you can purchase your virtual access card separately at MCAT-prep.com also by clicking on the image of the book.

Visit: The Gold Standard's Education Center at www.gold-standard.com.

ISBN: 978-1927338445

Address all inquiries, comments, or suggestions to the publisher. For Terms of Use go to: www.MCAT-prep.com.

RuveneCo Publishing
334 Cornelia Street # 559
Plattsburgh, New York 12901, learn@mcat-prep.com

Printed in China.

INTRODUCTION

Summary of this MCAT-prep.com 7 Full-length (FL) Exams' Book

Even as you read these words, someone is commenting online about a question that you may not see for days, weeks or months, and as a result, we are adding new explanations or images or video links so that when you get there, your learning experience will be even better. You'll never need to worry if there is a wrong answer in this book because there are no answers in this book! It's all online and every answer comes with a detailed explanation and a discussion area so you will have no doubt about what's right or wrong or why, and you'll never feel as though you are studying completely alone. This book is a living, learning experience.

Exam	Page
GS-1	GS1-1
GS-2	GS2-1
GS-3	GS3-1
GS-4	GS4-1
GS-5	GS5-1
GS-6, 7	online*
Answer documents	AK-1**
Science summaries	SS-1**

**using the access code on the back of your online access card after registering for a free account.*
***these pages at the back of this book are perforated to make it easier to pull out.*

Summary of your real MCAT Test and Schedule

Section	Topic	Questions	Time
Tutorial *(optional)*	-	-	10 minutes
1. Chemical and Physical Foundations of Biological Systems [Note: many students are surprised to see that about 1/3 of this section is BCM + BIO]	• Biochemistry (25%) • Biology (5%) • General Chemistry (30%) • Organic Chemistry (15%) • Physics (25%)	**59**	**95 minutes**
Break *(optional)*	-	-	10 minutes
2. Critical Analysis and Reasoning Skills (CARS) [Very similar to the 'old' MCAT Verbal Reasoning but no pure science passages.]	Non-sciences. All information necessary to answer the questions (MCQs) can be reasoned from the passages.	**53**	**90 minutes**
Mid-Exam/LUNCH Break *(optional)*	-	-	30 minutes
3. Biological and Biochemical Foundations of Living Systems [Some heavy research BCM/BIO passages mixed with 'old school' BIO passages]	• Biochemistry (25%) • Biology (65%) • General Chemistry (5%) • Organic Chemistry (5%)	**59**	**95 minutes**
Break *(optional)*	-	-	10 minutes
4. Psychological, Social, and Biological Foundations of Behavior [These MCQs are often knowledge based and so do not tend to use the same advanced reasoning skills as avg. MCQs from the other 3 sections.]	• Psychology (65%) • Sociology (30%) • Biology (5%)	**59**	**95 minutes**
Total Content Time	-	-	**6 hours, 15 minutes**
Total "Seated" Time (approx.)	-	-	**7 hours, 30 minutes**

Note: The total time does not include check-in time on arrival at the test center.

How is the real MCAT scored?

When you take the real MCAT, the AAMC will access your raw scores which are based on the number of correct answers in each section (note: there is no penalty for wrong answers). Your raw scores from each of the 4 sections of the MCAT will then be converted to scaled scores which are the only scores that interest medical school admissions committees. You will receive five scores for the MCAT: one for each of the four sections scored from a low of 118 to a high of 132, with a midpoint of 125; and one combined total score which will range from 472 to 528, with a midpoint of 500.

MCAT Scores

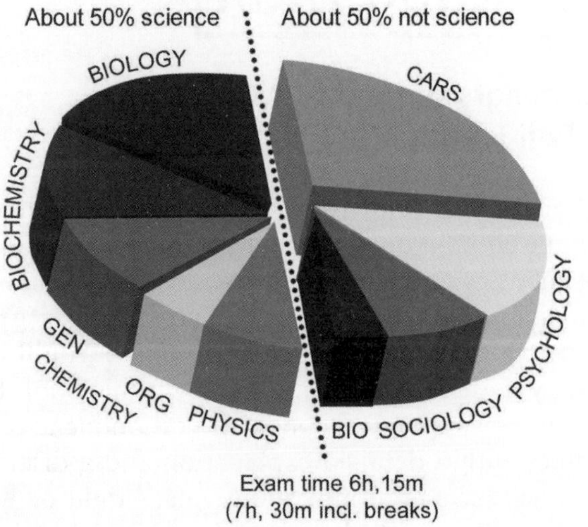

What is an average, good and high MCAT score?

Average, good and high MCAT scores are relative terms and, as such, are dependent on perspective, the cohort and the medical school to which you intend to apply. There is no pass or fail score for the MCAT, there are only scores that are acceptable for specific, individual medical schools. Consider consulting specific medical schools, or their websites or aamc.org, for past trends.

Please keep in mind that the percentile rank indicates your test performance relative to all the students who sat the same test on the same day. It records the percentage of students whose scores were lower than yours.

	Average score acceptable to some medical schools	**Average score acceptable to most medical schools**	**Average score acceptable to Ivy League medical schools**
Qualitatively	average MCAT score	good MCAT score	high MCAT score
Percentile* rank	50th percentile	80th percentile	95th percentile
Sectional MCAT score (max. = 132)	125	127**	129**
Total MCAT score (max. = 528)	500	508**	516**

Note: the expression "average score" does not have the same meaning as cutoff or minimum score. Rather it refers to the simple average of students accepted to medical school (historic and predicted averages). Having an acceptable MCAT score in no way guarantees medical school admissions since acceptance is also contingent on GPA and non-academic factors (i.e. personal statement and/or autobiographical material, letters of reference, and the medical school interview).

* percentile does not refer to the percent, which relates to the ratio of correct answers to the total number of questions. The percentile rank records the percentage of students whose scores were lower than yours. Percentile ranks are not used as medical school admissions criteria. Only the scaled score matters for medical school admissions.

** This assumes that current percentile rank predictions for the new MCAT remain stable.

Medical School Admissions Data Based on MCAT Scores for the 2017-2019 Admissions Cycles, AAMC Data (aggregated; n = 95,797)

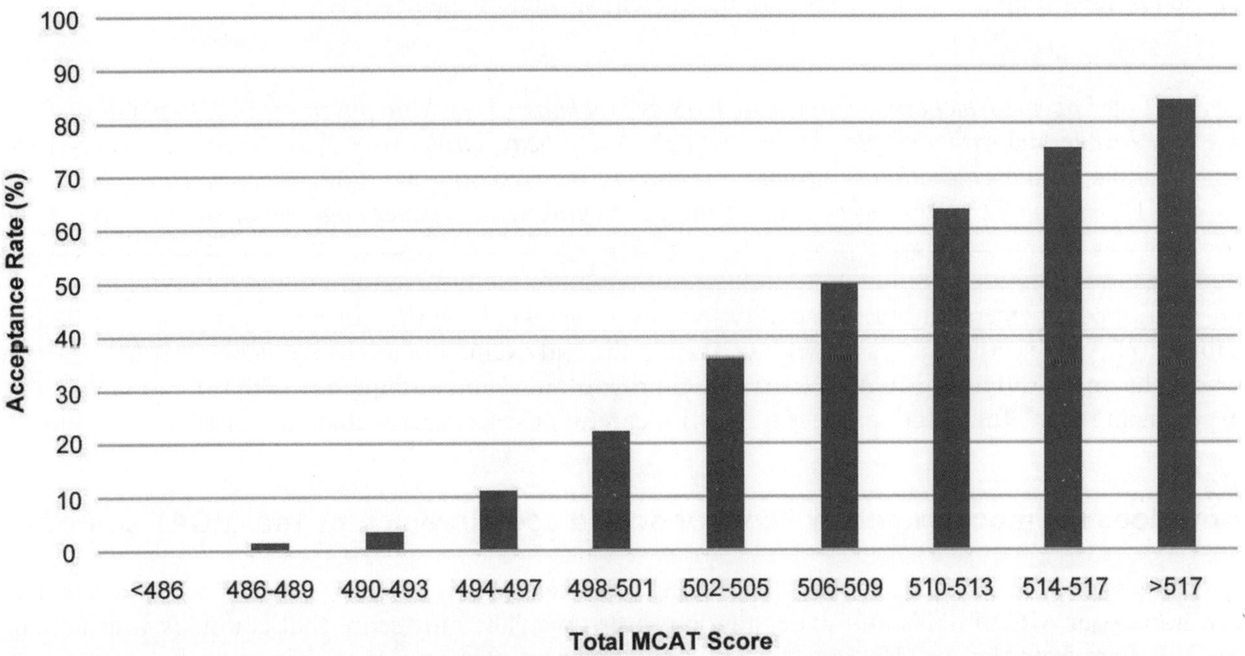

The higher rates of admissions with higher MCAT scores is nothing new. However, it is of value to note that a score of 500 has a rate of admissions just over 20% and lesser scores may still result in admissions. Conversely, an exceptional score (above 517) does not guarantee medical school admissions.

The MCAT-prep.com online MCAT Guide has a free medical school admissions calculator based on GPA and MCAT score.

Is it really important to try many mock exams?

Although there are some students who believe that 'more MCAT practice is better', perhaps a more realistic expression would be: 'more effective MCAT practice is better'. There is little value to have extra full-length MCAT practice tests if you don't have the time and motivation to use them as full-length practice (which should include a careful review of answers and explanations over 1-2 days per exam).

Frankly, re-taking mock exams is not usually an efficient use of time. However, taking brief, efficient notes from your MCAT practice test experience and reviewing all of those notes several times per week builds knowledge, reasoning and confidence moving forward. Choose the number of practice exams according to your needs, budget and schedule.

It's also important to note that no one company provides the perfect practice test experience. Of course, the AAMC - being the official MCAT organization - is best but other than that, there are as many opinions as learning styles. Most students with high, official MCAT scores have used a variety of reputable MCAT practice tests.

The MCAT can produce wildly different experiences and a significant amount of practice can help to mitigate the chance of a distressing experience. Here are some direct quotes from different student ID's on Reddit regarding their experience with the current version of the MCAT:

> *Holy Enzyme Kinetics!!! • barely any physics problems • Very little physics • wow, hi physics. :/ I wound up with multiple physics and calculation-heavy problems • Virtually no chemistry for me • heavy calculations. Aargh. • lots and lots of physics for me. • A LOT of biochemistry • +++ orgo • TONS of Orgo. • Very little orgo • entire scratch paper page full of calculations*

Of course, part perception but part reality: Not everyone will have the same exam experience whether subjectively or objectively assessed. In fact, during the real exam, you might be sitting next to someone who is having a different MCAT experience than you are. The consequence is that there is value in experiencing many full-length practice tests (with careful post-test review and very brief note-taking).

How does my mock exam raw score or scaled score predict my real MCAT score?

It's complicated. The simple answer is that taking practice exams followed by careful post-exam review can hone your MCAT skills and understanding over time. The only score that counts is your actual, MCAT score from the AAMC. Mock exam scores can have predictive power for some subgroups and not others – the predictability is uncertain because the AAMC is the only organization that has access to the ideal data sets.

There are literally thousands of threads in online MCAT forums with students analyzing the results from more than a dozen MCAT companies and, of course, no mock exam has perfect predictive value. By far, the most accurate would be the most recent released, scored MCAT practice tests by the AAMC.

The scales used by most commercial MCAT prep companies cannot compare to the accuracy of the AAMC's scored practice exams which can draw on specific item performance from within 70,000-90,000 students who take the MCAT in a given year. Thus all MCAT prep companies have some degree of statistical sampling error. This is complicated by the fact that inconsistencies do not affect all 'categories' of students. This fact alone creates tremendous misunderstandings in discussion forums.

And, it's much worse than that! Consider the AAMC's MCAT Sample Test, their very first full-length practice test with the current format which is not scored because the AAMC does not have enough data to score it accurately! Now think of all of the commercial companies with scored MCAT practice tests: none will have the quality of data that the AAMC has and yet the AAMC will not score that test!

The real purpose of practice is not to overly fixate on practice test scores, or comparisons between different scores obtained from different companies, but rather to follow your progress with reasoning and application through timed, full-length testing followed by a meticulous review of your exam experience.

The other take-home message: The AAMC's exams are a powerful component of your MCAT prep. Some students will still complain that their real MCAT exam experience was somehow dissimilar to their AAMC practice test. There are many reasons for this but it is most important to focus on the following: Using quality practice exams followed by a routine, comprehensive review will result in an improved MCAT score in the medium to long term.

Where are the answers and worked solutions?

Online!

As mentioned on the front cover and in this Introduction, your access is for 12 consecutive months. Your access period begins once you login to MCAT-prep.com and input your unique online access code from your online access card appended to the inside front cover of this book.

Where do I put my answers?

You can either just mark your exam paper directly, or for convenience, there are answer sheets at the back of this book (located after the 5 exams but before the science summaries). The answer sheets are perforated so you can tear them out to use for the 5 full-length exams in this book. Of course, you will be correcting your exam once you access the answers online and, thereafter, you can review the explanations and access discussion boards, and when available, videos for background information.

When you sign in to your MCAT-prep.com account and click on Tests in the top Menu, you will also be able to convert your raw scores to estimated scaled scores.

What do I do after completing a full-length MCAT practice test?

Score it, lick your wounds, and spend 1-2 days reviewing all questions while taking brief notes that only you would understand (practically hieroglyphics; notes that require you to think when you are reviewing them). We call these brief, personal summaries: 'Gold Notes'.

So here is our suggested routine:

1. Full-length MCAT practice test under strict, timed conditions; score your exam

2. Next day: Review mistakes, doubts and all solutions while adding to your Gold Notes

3. Consolidate: review all your Gold Notes and condense them further where possible

4. Repeat until you get beyond the score you need for your targeted medical school

Do these exams have any typographical errors?

Yes, definitely.

This is a first edition book.

Thus far, I have never read a medical or surgical textbook that did not have typographical errors, and more rarely, content errors. This is the nature of publishing. However, we can assure you that this book is more than 99% error free, and we have created an unusual 'bonus' of permitting students to interact with the authors by asking for clarification if the explanation was not clear enough, or if the student suspects an error. Each of the 1610 questions has a discussion board embedded in the explanation to ensure that no one is left in the dark about any question. Of course, please be respectful, we are on the same team!

Over the years, however, we have noticed that some students think that there are typos based on their own personal experiences not realizing that sometimes their professors or even their college textbooks may actually be the source of the issue. Science has some very specific rules that are often bent on campuses.

A small example: The Kelvin (capitalized) scale uses the kelvin (not capitalized as a unit and NOT a degree) as the SI unit of temperature. Unlike the kelvin, Celsius is capitalized and associated with 'degree' (just like Fahrenheit, F). And so, the absolute zero, 0 K (no degree), is equivalent to −273 °C; also note the degree symbol is not meant to be attached to the number (a common mistake) but rather to the letter C or F, but never K.

Aside from the dozens of such science rules, the AAMC has their own formatting 'rules' regarding capitalization after questions, continuation, periods after answer choices under certain circumstances, etc. These 'rules' do not always follow what a university professor may have for their multiple-choice exam but, of course, we follow the AAMC's rules as well as standard, official notation for sciences and social sciences (unless otherwise required for the question).

Why are the answers and explanations online?

There are 3 main reasons: It allows you to pay less for this book, it allows us to keep doing what we do, and it's better for the environment (we apologize in advance for putting this item third!).

For the last few years, one GS exam was priced at approximately $35 for one year of online access. You can imagine how much 7 mock exams would cost! We had to find a way to drastically reduce the unit cost despite the increased complexity of this book project . . . printing, online access codes, servers, technical support, etc.

The most expensive part of a book is the paper. If all 7 exams and detailed explanations were in this book, there would be 4 times more paper (over 2000 pages) and the price would be such that most students would never consider purchasing it. At the time of publishing, no company offers so many full-length MCAT practice tests associated with one publication.

When online, we can upkeep and change explanations and some questions in real time based on new trends. We can conduct continual editing, offer live chat most days of the week for access issues or technical problems, provide discussion boards for 1610 MCQs, and provide unlimited access to worked solutions during your access period despite the cost for servers. Those are your advantages.

The trade off for us is to minimize digital piracy. Incredibly almost all MCAT preparation companies that have ever offered more than 4 mock exams have ceased operations in part due to online sharing of their content.

Does MCAT-prep.com have practice test questions that are NOT on the AAMC's official topic list?

Yes, definitely.

'Madness' you say? Well, it's because the AAMC has had topics not on their official list appear, presumably, on real exams. Of course, we can only discuss what is already in the public realm, specifically, the AAMC's scored exams: scored because they contain, presumably, operational questions that have been used by students.

Once upon a time, the AAMC had pedigree analysis, alkane/alkene/alkyne chemistry, momentum and many other topics on their official MCAT syllabus but, once those topics were removed in 2015, most MCAT prep companies removed any questions that even hinted at those topics and some labeled companies including such questions as 'outdated' (some went so far as to call the "Gold Standard," the "Old Standard" ☹).

The AAMC's MCAT Practice Exam 3 (MPT3), based on real MCAT questions (and some students believe that MPT3 is the most accurate practice test representing the current exam) has a passage with clear pedigree analysis as underlined in the AAMC's explanation (MPT3 BB Passage 2, Questions 6-9). One pedigree in their first 3 scored exams means that you will see 2 pedigrees in the 5 exams in this book, while some other companies will not have any.

Understanding elimination reactions - also not on the official AAMC topic list since it is related to alkene chemistry - is required for the AAMC's MPT1, C/P Question 7 (again, specifically referenced in the AAMC's explanation and avoided by most MCAT prep companies). There are many more such examples but just to say that we have you covered. If the AAMC is asking that question type, we will find a way to get you ready for that and similar question types.

Please understand: We are not saying that all the other commercial MCAT prep companies have nothing to offer you. Many of these companies offer a different perspective and teach in a way that some may find helpful. Some day in the future, when you are preparing for your medical licensing exam, you will discover that there does not exist 1 single company that prepares you for your objective. Rather, a judicious combination of resources based on your personal learning style will optimize your exam performance. This lesson is also true for MCAT prep.

BTW, we did waste some paper . . . but we saved a forest!

At least 20 times in this book, we skipped a page in order to maximize the chance that when you are reading a passage, the questions will be on a page facing that passage to minimize the chance that you need to flip pages between the question and the passage. Of course, the system does not always work, but it usually does. However, the big picture is that we kept the number of pages at around 25% of what it would otherwise have been had we included the additional exams and all answers with explanations.

Surely, some students will say that our Introduction was a waste of paper (!!) but ya can't please everyone!

Sometimes, the most difficult MCAT question is the easy one.

MCAT companies will often try to avoid easy questions because someone will go online and say "too easy, what a joke!". However, the real MCAT will often have a few shockingly easy questions which may even take a good high school student aback. For example, what group in the periodic table a common atom may be, or do prokaryotes have a nucleus, or going from a few gas molecules to many, would that increase disorder? The AAMC is allowed to do that, but MCAT companies are wary.

But this also causes confusion for some students! After completing a complex passage with many layers, to get an easy question on the real MCAT .... is this a trap?

We try to follow the rhythm of the AAMC: Long complex passages, short straightforward ones, high-order reasoning skills, basic you-know-it-or-you-don't MCQs, questions where more than 80% get it right, and questions where more than 80% get it wrong.

Hey, what about "How to design an MCAT study schedule" and stuff like that?

MCAT-prep.com has a comprehensive, free MCAT Guide online. Introductory MCAT information, GPA and GAMSAT scores required across the US and Canada, a free medical school admissions' percent predictor, how to use MCAT practice tests, designing a personal study schedule, a detailed MCAT topic list, and much more: www.mcat-prep.com/what-is-the-mcat

The MCAT is challenging, get organized: www.mcat-prep.com/mcat-study-schedule

Any last words of wisdom?

> *Practice isn't the thing you do once you're good. It's the thing you do that makes you good.*
>
> — Malcolm Gladwell

It will not be easy at the very beginning. Your confidence will increase as you practice, review, learn, and practice again.

We hope to impart to you our excitement about the awesome beauty of learning, and of sharing the mental maneuvers of those who are still here, and others throughout history from Aristotle to Pythagoras, and from Freud to Newton.

Practice, review, learn, and practice again.

Let's begin.

Full-length MCAT Practice Test GS-1

Periodic Table of the Elements

You may consult this page anytime you wish during the following exam sections:

- Section I: Chemical and Physical Foundations of Biological Systems
- Section III: Biological and Biochemical Foundations of Living Systems

On the real exam, the computer-based shortcut to see the periodic table is Alt + T.

1 **H** 1.0																	2 **He** 4.0
3 **Li** 6.9	4 **Be** 9.0											5 **B** 10.8	6 **C** 12.0	7 **N** 14.0	8 **O** 16.0	9 **F** 19.0	10 **Ne** 20.2
11 **Na** 23.0	12 **Mg** 24.3											13 **Al** 27.0	14 **Si** 28.1	15 **P** 31.0	16 **S** 32.1	17 **Cl** 35.5	18 **Ar** 39.9
19 **K** 39.1	20 **Ca** 40.1	21 **Sc** 45.0	22 **Ti** 47.9	23 **V** 50.9	24 **Cr** 52.0	25 **Mn** 54.9	26 **Fe** 55.8	27 **Co** 58.9	28 **Ni** 58.7	29 **Cu** 63.5	30 **Zn** 65.4	31 **Ga** 69.7	32 **Ge** 72.6	33 **As** 74.9	34 **Se** 79.0	35 **Br** 79.9	36 **Kr** 83.8
37 **Rb** 85.5	38 **Sr** 87.6	39 **Y** 88.9	40 **Zr** 91.2	41 **Nb** 92.9	42 **Mo** 95.9	43 **Tc** (98)	44 **Ru** 101.1	45 **Rh** 102.9	46 **Pd** 106.4	47 **Ag** 107.9	48 **Cd** 112.4	49 **In** 114.8	50 **Sn** 118.7	51 **Sb** 121.8	52 **Te** 127.6	53 **I** 126.9	54 **Xe** 131.3
55 **Cs** 132.9	56 **Ba** 137.3	57 **La*** 138.9	72 **Hf** 178.5	73 **Ta** 180.9	74 **W** 183.9	75 **Re** 186.2	76 **Os** 190.2	77 **Ir** 192.2	78 **Pt** 195.1	79 **Au** 197.0	80 **Hg** 200.6	81 **Tl** 204.4	82 **Pb** 207.2	83 **Bi** 209.0	84 **Po** (209)	85 **At** (210)	86 **Rn** (222)
87 **Fr** (223)	88 **Ra** (226)	89 **Ac**** (227)	104 **Unq**** (261)	105 **Unp** (262)	106 **Unh** (263)	107 **Uns** (262)	108 **Uno** (265)	109 **Une** (267)									
			*	58 **Ce** 140.1	59 **Pr** 140.9	60 **Nd** 144.2	61 **Pm** (145)	62 **Sm** 150.4	63 **Eu** 152.0	64 **Gd** 157.3	65 **Tb** 158.9	66 **Dy** 162.5	67 **Ho** 164.9	68 **Er** 167.3	69 **Tm** 168.9	70 **Yb** 173.0	71 **Lu** 175.0
			**	90 **Th** 232.0	91 **Pa** (231)	92 **U** 238.0	93 **Np** (237)	94 **Pu** (244)	95 **Am** (243)	96 **Cm** (247)	97 **Bk** (247)	98 **Cf** (251)	99 **Es** (252)	100 **Fm** (257)	101 **Md** (258)	102 **No** (259)	103 **Lr** (260)

CANDIDATE'S NAME ______________________

RAW SCORE AND SCALED SCORE ______________________

GS-1 Section I: Chemical and Physical Foundations of Biological Systems

Questions: 1-59
Time: 95 minutes

INSTRUCTIONS: Of all the questions on this test, most are organized into groups preceded by a passage. After evaluating the passage, select the best answer to each question in the group. Fifteen questions are independent of any descriptive passage or each other. Similarly, select the best answer to these questions. If you are unsure of an answer, eliminate the alternatives that you know to be incorrect and select an answer from the remaining alternatives. To indicate your selection, use a pencil to blacken the corresponding circle next to the answer choice and/or you can use the answer document at the back of this book. No marks are deducted for wrong answers.

The computer-based real MCAT has an on-screen highlighter function and ~~STRIKEOUT~~ function. These tools help to spotlight text or assist in the process of elimination. You may use a yellow highlighter for this paper-based exam and/or a pen (or preferably a pencil to make it easier should you change your mind) to mark text. At the time of publishing, both highlighting and strikeout functions can be used for passages, questions and answer choices. You can also flag a question to review later should time remain.

For the real exam, you will be provided with a dry erase board which is a white laminated noteboard booklet accompanied by a fine point marker. The noteboard includes 9 graph-lined pages for you to write though you cannot erase. You can simulate the experience with a fine point marker on a noteboard or with 8" x 14" plain graph paper.

You may consult the periodic table at any point during the science subtests.

Please note: For the real MCAT, a small number of field-tested questions will remain unscored.

This practice test has been designed exclusively to test knowledge and thinking skills. This exam may contain hypothetical statements and/or express controversial ideas. Statements contained herein do not necessarily reflect the policy, position, or view of RuveneCo Inc. or MCAT-prep.com.

START EXAM ONLY WHEN TIMER IS READY.

Passage 1 (Questions 1–5)

Terpenes are major biosynthetic building blocks. Steroids, for example, are derivatives of the terpene squalene and the terpenoid lanosterol. The difference between terpenes and terpenoids is that terpenes are hydrocarbons, whereas terpenoids contain additional functional groups.

Terpenes are derived biosynthetically from units of isoprene, which has the molecular formula C_5H_8. Isoprene units can be linked together "head to tail" (i.e., from one end of the longest chain to the other end from another molecule) to form linear chains, or they may be arranged to form rings. The isoprene unit is thus one of nature's common building blocks.

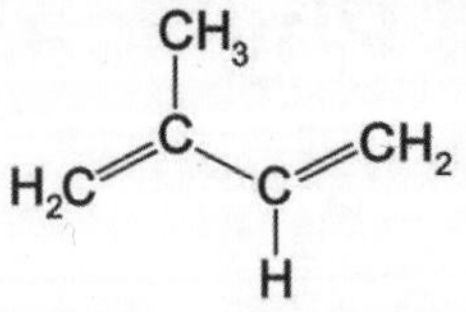

CH_3, H_2C, C, C, CH_2, H

Isoprene (methylbuta-1,3-diene, a hemiterpene)

Table 1 Classification of Terpenes

Terpenes	Isoprene units
Monoterpenes	2
Sesquiterpenes	3
Diterpenes	4
Sesterterpenes	5
Triterpenes	6
Carotenoids	8

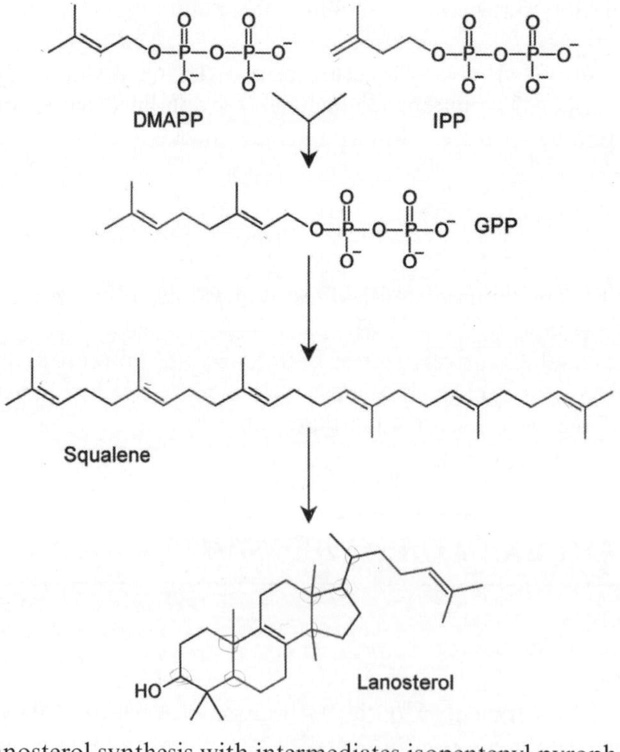

DMAPP

IPP

GPP

Squalene

HO

Lanosterol

Figure 1 Summary of lanosterol synthesis with intermediates isopentenyl pyrophosphate (IPP), dimethylallyl pyrophosphate (DMAPP), geranyl pyrophosphate (GPP), and squalene shown. Some intermediates are omitted.

Question 1

Consider the structure of geranylfarnesol.

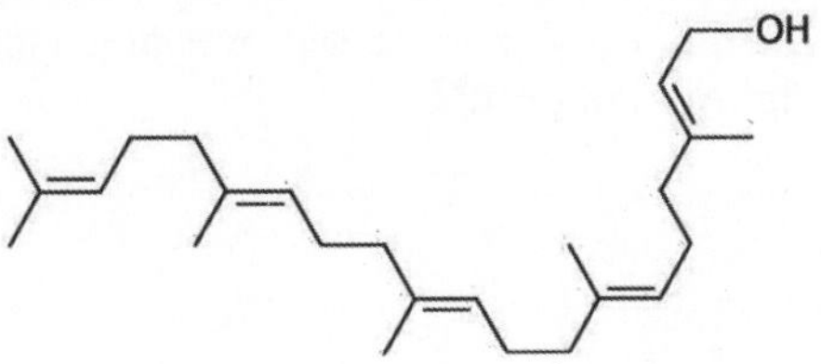

Geranylfarnesol is best classified, based on the number of carbon atoms in its structure, as which of the following?

- O **A.** Sesquiterpenoid
- O **B.** Diterpenoid
- O **C.** Sesterterpenoid
- O **D.** Triterpenoid

Question 2

Consider the following image.

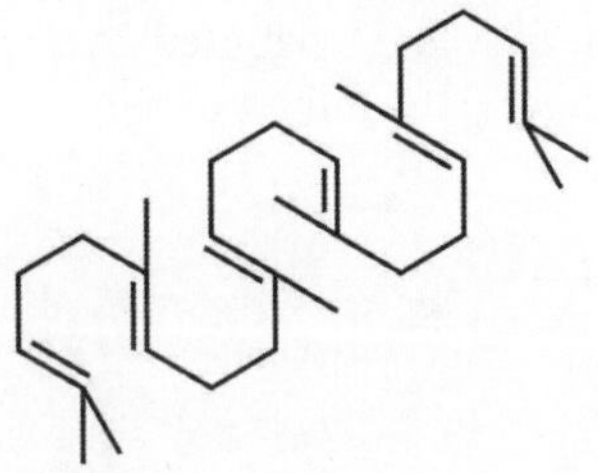

The molecule above is best categorized as:

- O **A.** a sesterterpene.
- O **B.** a steroid.
- O **C.** an all *Z* hydrocarbon.
- O **D.** squalene.

Question 3

From the pathway illustrated in Figure 1, which of the following could NOT have reasonably occurred?

- O **A.** The half reaction: NADPH + $H^+ \rightarrow NADP^+ + 2e^-$
- O **B.** Condensation reaction
- O **C.** Oxidation
- O **D.** All the above could have reasonably occurred.

Question 4

How many different stereoisomers of lanosterol are possible?

- O **A.** Fewer than 10
- O **B.** Between 10 and 50
- O **C.** Between 50 and 100
- O **D.** More than 100

Question 5

The pathway in Figure 1 occurs spontaneously:

- O **A.** as written.
- O **B.** only if coupled with a sufficiently exergonic reaction or series of reactions.
- O **C.** only if coupled with a sufficiently endergonic reaction or series of reactions.
- O **D.** in conditions that cannot be determined with the information provided.

Passage 2 (Questions 6–9)

The essential stages in the manufacture of H_2SO_3 involve the burning of sulfur or roasting of sulfide ores in air to produce SO_2. This is then mixed with air, purified, and passed over a vanadium catalyst (either VO_3^- or V_2O_5) at 450 degrees Celsius. Thus, the following reaction occurs.

Reaction I

$2SO_2(g) + O_2(g) \leftrightarrow 2SO_3(g)$ $\Delta H = -197\ \text{kJ mol}^{-1}$

If the SO_2 is very carefully dissolved in water, sulfurous acid (H_2SO_3) is obtained. The first proton of this acid ionizes as if from a strong acid, while the second ionizes as if from a weak acid.

Reaction II

$H_2SO_3 + H_2O \rightarrow H_3O^+ + HSO_3^-$

Reaction III

$HSO_3^- + H_2O \leftrightarrow H_3O^+ + SO_3^{2-}$ $K_a = 5.0 \times 10^{-6}$

The concentration of H_2SO_3 in antiseptic fluid was determined by titration with 0.10 M NaOH (strong base) as shown in Figure 1. Two equivalence points were determined using 30 ml and 60 ml of NaOH, respectively:

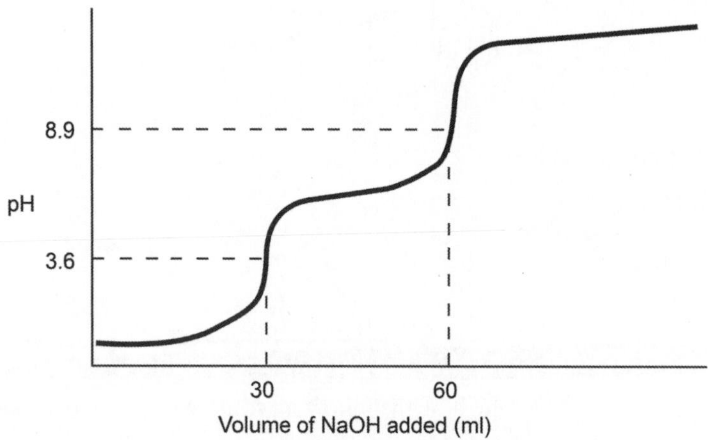

Figure 1

Question 6

What is the oxidation number of sulfur in sulfurous acid?

- ○ **A.** +3
- ○ **B.** +4
- ○ **C.** +5
- ○ **D.** +6

Question 7

What is the percent by mass of oxygen in sulfurous acid?

- ○ **A.** 31.9%
- ○ **B.** 19.7%
- ○ **C.** 39.0%
- ○ **D.** 58.5%

Question 8

Which of the following acid–base indicators is most suitable for the determination of the first equivalence point of the titration shown in Figure 1?

- o **A.** Cresol red (color change between pH = 0.2 and pH = 1.8)
- o **B.** p-Xylenol blue (color change between pH = 1.2 and pH = 2.8)
- o **C.** Bromophenol blue (color change between pH = 3.0 and pH = 4.6)
- o **D.** Bromocresol green (color change between pH = 3.8 and pH = 5.4)

Question 9

The antiseptic property of H_2SO_3 is due in part to its interaction with the bacterial cell wall as a Lewis acid. Thus, sulfurous acid:

- o **A.** is a proton donor.
- o **B.** accepts a pair of electrons.
- o **C.** reacts with NaOH.
- o **D.** possesses oxygen atoms.

The following questions are NOT based on a descriptive passage (Questions 10–13).

Question 10

Magnesium phosphate is a component of kidney stones (renal calculi). If completely dissociated, what would be the concentration of magnesium ions in a 0.1 M solution of magnesium phosphate?

- O **A.** 0.1 M
- O **B.** 0.4 M
- O **C.** 0.2 M
- O **D.** 0.3 M

Question 11

Nitric oxide (NO) is an important cellular signaling molecule involved in many physiological and pathological processes. It is a powerful vasodilator with a short half-life of a few seconds in blood. Which of the species in Table 1 is best suited to oxidize NO given that:

$HNO_2 + H^+ + e^- \leftrightarrow NO + H_2O$

$E° = +1.00$ V

Table 1

Electrochemical reaction	E° value (V)
$Ce^{4+} + e^- \leftrightarrow Ce^{3+}$	+1.695
$H_2O_2 + 2e^- \leftrightarrow 2OH^-$	+0.880
$MnO_4^- + e^- \leftrightarrow MnO_4^{2-}$	+0.564
$Cd^{2+} + 2e^- \leftrightarrow Cd$	-0.403

- O **A.** Ce^{4+}
- O **B.** Ce^{3+}
- O **C.** Cd^{2+}
- O **D.** Cd

Question 12

The ear canal (external auditory meatus) is a tube running from the outer ear to the middle ear. The adult human ear canal is analogous to a cylindrical pipeline about 24 mm long and closed at one end. Consider consecutive resonances occurring at two wavelengths. Which pair of values given below corresponds to the possible values of the two wavelengths in the adult ear canal?

$L = n\lambda/4$

L = length of cylinder

n = 1, 3, 5, 7 . . .

λ = wavelengths

- O **A.** 48 mm and 12 mm
- O **B.** 48 mm and 19.2 mm
- O **C.** 12 mm and 24 mm
- O **D.** 32 mm and 19.2 mm

Question 13

An important function of the pentose phosphate pathway is the generation of:

- O **A.** NAD^+, which is used for glycolysis.
- O **B.** NADH for the production of ATP via the electron transport chain.
- O **C.** NADP, which is a substrate in amino acid metabolism.
- O **D.** NADPH for fatty acid synthesis.

Note: This page is left blank so that the passage would be visible without turning pages while assessing the passage-based questions.

Passage 3 (Questions 14–18)

A defibrillator is a machine used in emergency situations to deliver a therapeutic dose of electrical current to the heart of a patient aiming to restore a regular heart rhythm. A capacitor is used by the defibrillator to store energy at thousands of volts. Conducting 'paddles' are placed on the patient's chest, the capacitor is discharged and a short pulse of current flows from one paddle to the other, having traversed the patient's heart.

The energy stored by a capacitor is given by

$$W = \frac{1}{2} QV$$

where Q is the charge in coulombs and V the voltage in volts.

The time constant for the discharging capacitor is measured in seconds and denoted by the Greek letter τ (tau),

$$\tau = R\,C$$

where R is the resistance in ohms, and C is the capacitance in farads.

The equation for a discharging a capacitor is

$$V = V_0(e^{-t/RC})$$

where V_0 is the original voltage, V is the voltage at any time t, and the number e (approximately equal to 2.718) is the mathematical constant that is the base of the natural logarithm.

Data from the defibrillator was used to construct Figure 1 and Figure 2.

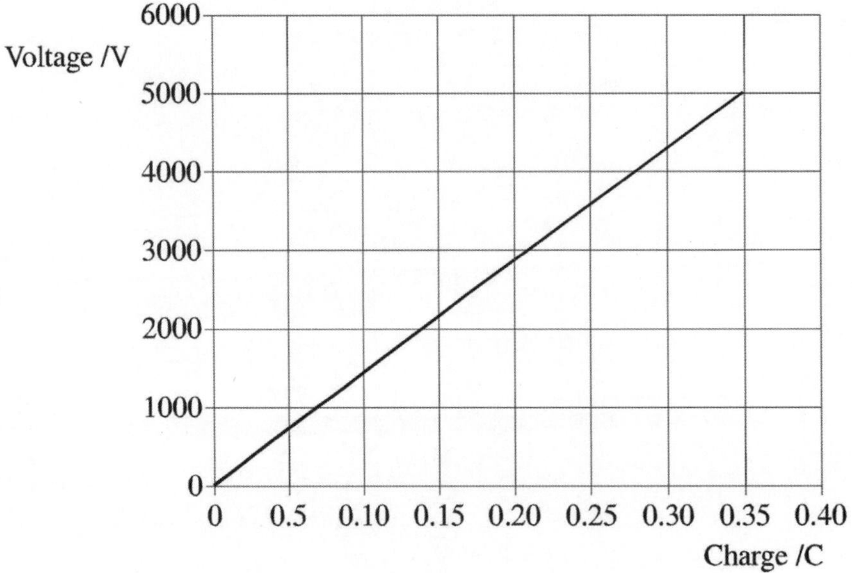

Figure 1 Voltage vs charge for a capacitor used in a defibrillator.

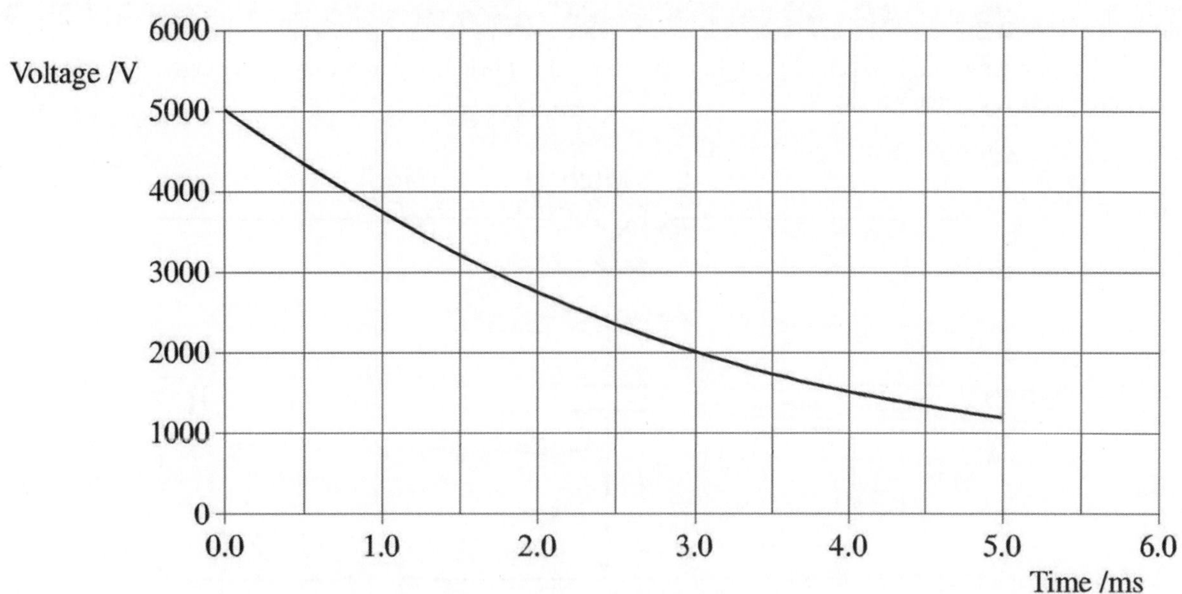

Figure 2 The variation in voltage with respect to time as the capacitor discharges across a patient's chest.

Question 14

Based on Figure 1, calculate the energy stored by the defibrillator's capacitor when charged to 5 kilovolts.

- ○ **A.** 438 J
- ○ **B.** 875 J
- ○ **C.** 1 750 J
- ○ **D.** 3 500 J

Question 15

Using the information provided, determine the time t in seconds consistent with the time constant τ for the defibrillator's discharging capacitor.

- ○ **A.** 1.3×10^{-3} s
- ○ **B.** 2.3×10^{-3} s
- ○ **C.** 3.3×10^{-3} s
- ○ **D.** 4.3×10^{-3} s

Question 16

The defibrillator has multiple settings. On one particular setting, the discharge lasts for 1.8 ms. Calculate the energy left in the defibrillator's capacitor after the 1.8 ms discharge.

- ○ **A.** 290 J
- ○ **B.** 580 J
- ○ **C.** 1450 J
- ○ **D.** 2900 J

Question 17

Consider the following simplified circuit diagram of a typical defibrillator. Note that current emanates from the larger terminal of the battery (cell).

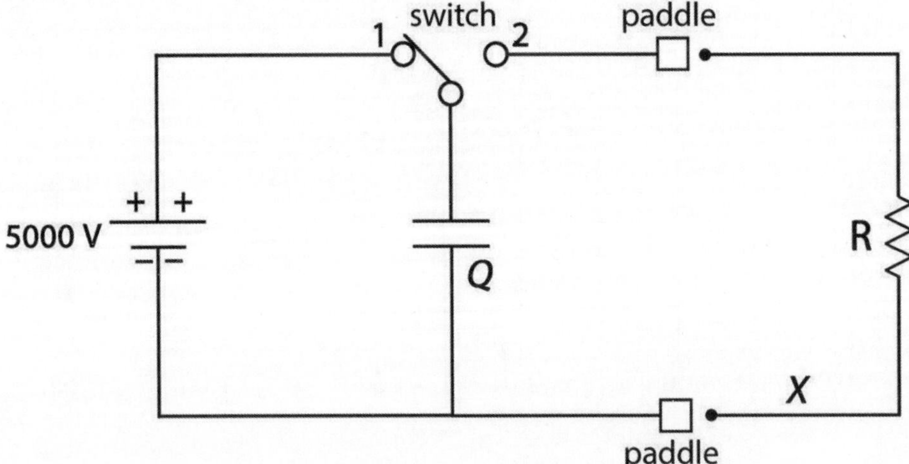

Which of the following is NOT likely to be consistent with the circuit diagram provided?

- O **A.** The defibrillator cannot discharge while the switch is in the position in the diagram.
- O **B.** When the patient is being defibrillated, current in the segment of wire X will be flowing towards the patient.
- O **C.** The plate Q of the capacitor in the center of the diagram has a negative charge.
- O **D.** The label R likely represents the patient's chest.

Question 18

In radioactive decay, the time constant is called the decay constant (λ) and it usually represents the time it takes for all but 37% of the atoms to decay. For this reason, as compared to the decay constant λ, half-life is:

- O **A.** shorter.
- O **B.** longer.
- O **C.** approximately the same.
- O **D.** impossible to determine without more data.

Note: This page is left blank so that the passage would be visible without turning pages while assessing the passage-based questions.

Passage 4 (Questions 19–22)

Kidney stones (renal lithiases) are small, hard mineral deposits that form inside kidneys. Kidney stones can affect any part of the urinary tract from kidneys to bladder. Often stones form when the urine becomes concentrated, allowing minerals to crystallize. Passing (i.e., eliminating through the natural path) kidney stones can be quite painful, usually only requiring pain medication and increased water intake, but sometimes other medications or shock waves are needed. On rare occasions stones become lodged in the urinary tract, requiring surgical intervention.

Calcium oxalate, a derivative of the diprotic oxalic acid, is the most common component in kidney stones. The following is the structure of oxalic acid.

HO–C(=O)–C(=O)–OH

The first pKa value for oxalic acid is 1.27, and the second pKa value is 4.28. The K_{sp} for calcium oxalate is 2.7×10^{-9}. Consider the following sequence of reactions:

$$(1)\ HOOCCOOH \leftrightarrow HOOCCOO^- + H^+$$

$$(2)\ HOOCCOO^- \leftrightarrow {}^-OOCCOO^- + H^+$$

$$(3)\ Ca^{++} + {}^-OOCCOO^-(aq) \leftrightarrow Ca(OOCCOO)(s)$$

Healthy kidneys can concentrate urine. This is accomplished in different ways, including the countercurrent multiplier function of the loop of Henle and the secretory function of the nephron. Consider the data in Table 1.

Table 1 Relative Concentration of Selected Solutes in Urine as Compared with Approximate Values in Plasma

	Plasma concentration (millimol/L)	Typical concentration in urine
urea	5.1	60x
ammonia	0.062	500x
sodium ions	140	6x
calcium ions	2.0	1.5x
creatinine	0.85	100x

Question 19

Based on the information provided, determine the minimum oxalate ion concentration in urine that would be required to form kidney stones.

- ○ **A.** 9.0×10^{-7} M
- ○ **B.** 9.0×10^{-4} M
- ○ **C.** 6.0×10^{-7} M
- ○ **D.** 6.0×10^{-4} M

Question 20

When the body's intake of calcium is low, in order to maintain homeostasis, there is an increased renal absorption of calcium. Based on the information provided, which of the following changes in urine is most consistent with a decrease in calcium intake in a person with kidney stones?

- O **A.** Decreased oxalate ions
- O **B.** Increased solubility product
- O **C.** Decreased pH
- O **D.** Increased pH

Question 21

Potassium citrate is a medication that can be used to treat gout. A side effect of potassium citrate is the alkalization of urine. Would calcium oxalate kidney stones be more or less likely to be produced in a person taking potassium citrate?

- O **A.** Less likely, because the increased hydroxide concentration will bind the protons producing water
- O **B.** Less likely, because the reaction is buffered by monohydrogen oxalate
- O **C.** More likely, because the increased pH will lead to increased oxalate ion concentration
- O **D.** More likely, because the conjugate base of oxalic acid is the oxalate ion

Question 22

Organic chelating agents have been used to bind calcium ions thereby dissolving calcium oxalate kidney stones. What can be inferred regarding the interaction between the chelating agent and the calcium ions?

- O **A.** The calcium ions bond ionically to the chelating agent.
- O **B.** The coordination of calcium ions is to carbon and hydrogen.
- O **C.** The binding is via coordinate covalent bonds.
- O **D.** The chelating agent must be a strong conjugate acid.

Passage 5 (Questions 23–26)

Protein kinases play a key role in the regulation of a variety of physiological processes, and their dysregulation has been implicated in many disease states including cancer, inflammation, diabetes, and immunological disorders. However, most protein kinases have similar structures in their active sites, and so the development of specific inhibitors is challenging. One method for promoting specificity is the synthesis of bivalent ligands (BLs), which was used recently to convert the promiscuous kinase inhibitor staurosporine into a potent BL for protein kinase A (PKA) by linking a small molecule to a cyclic peptide via a varying number of β-alanines in the polyethylene glycol (PEG) linker region (*see* Figure 1).

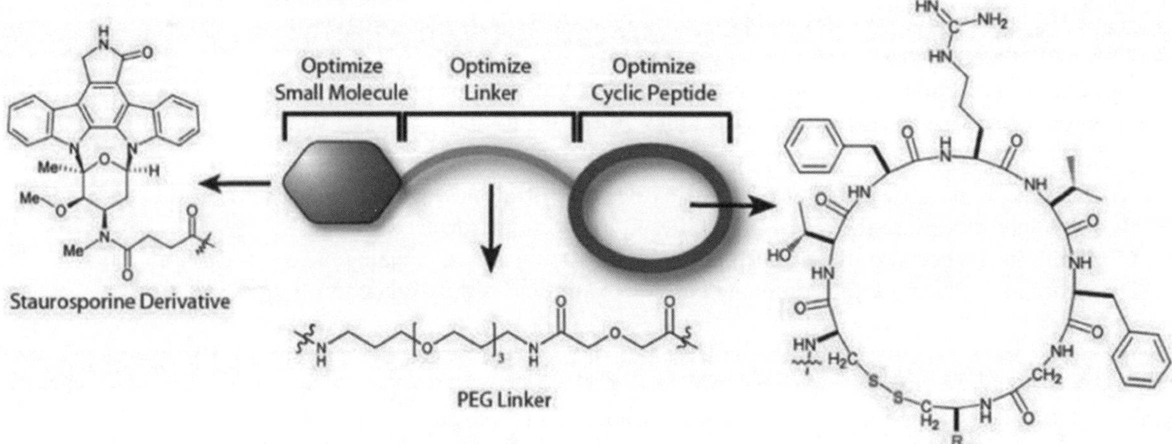

Figure 1 The strategy used to generate BLs of staurosporine

The optimal size of the linker region is complex, since short linkers prevent the simultaneous binding of both ligands, but longer linkers are costly entropically. To determine the optimal length of this region, compounds 2–5 were developed, which contain 3, 5, 7, and 9 β-alanines, respectively. The number of linkers has a significant effect on the ability of the BLs to inhibit PKA activity (*see* Figure 2).

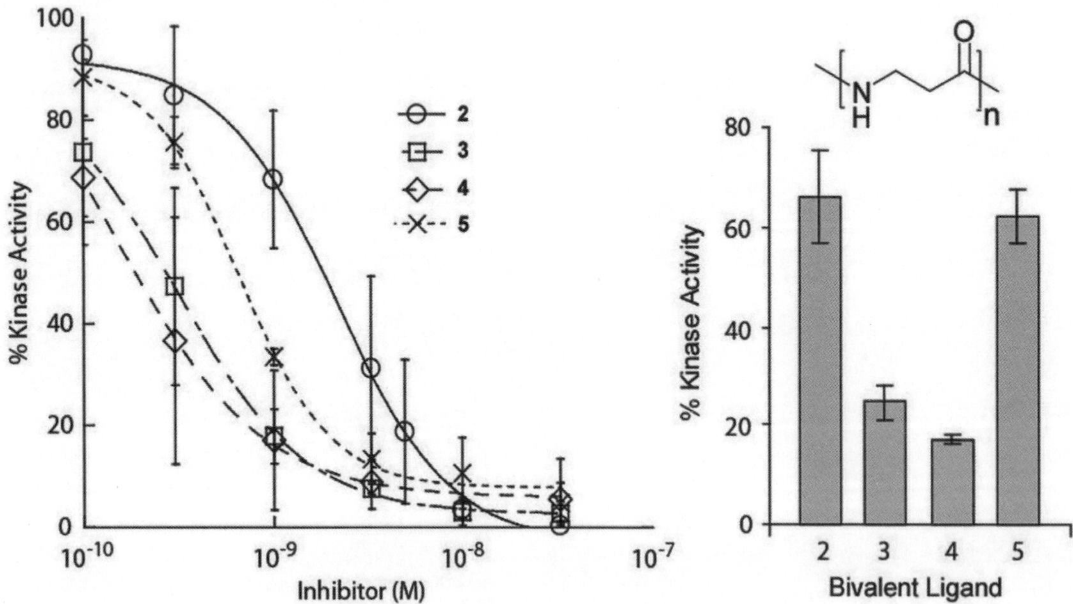

Figure 2 Optimization of the BL linker length

PKA kinase assays were performed using BLs with varying linker lengths (compounds 2–5) using 0.5 nM PKA. Full IC_{50} curves could not be obtained; therefore, the relative activity of 3.3 nM of each BL was determined.

The kinetics of parental BL and its K_i were then investigated by generating a Lineweaver–Burk plot to determine the mode of inhibition (*see* Figure 3).

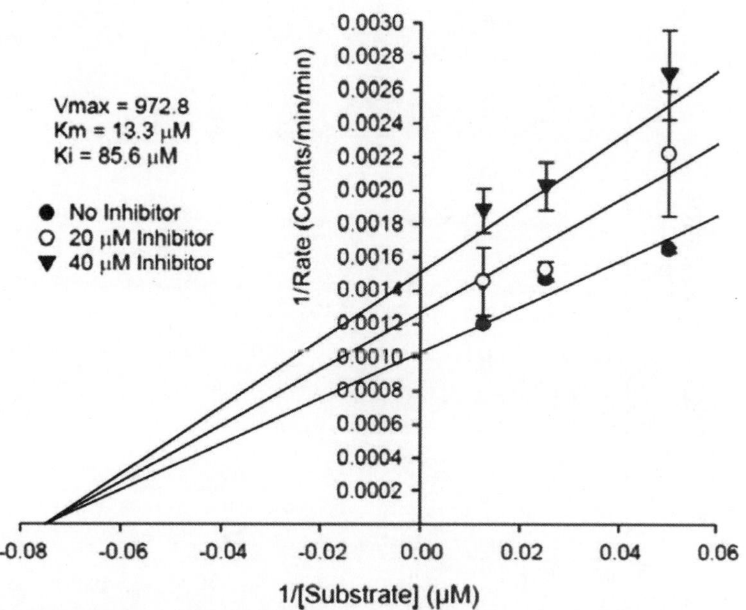

Figure 3 Lineweaver–Burk plot of the kinetics of BL

At the end of the experiment, further analyses were made to determine IC_{50}, the half-maximal inhibitory concentration.

Source: Adapted from nih.gov, PMC2749490.

Question 23

What is the optimal number of β-alanines required to achieve a potent PKA inhibitor?

- O **A.** 3
- O **B.** 5
- O **C.** 7
- O **D.** 9

Question 24

What is the method of inhibition of BL?

- O **A.** Mixed
- O **B.** Competitive
- O **C.** Noncompetitive
- O **D.** Uncompetitive

Question 25

BL binds to PKA both inside and outside the enzyme active site and inhibits the ATPase activity. The most important amino acid for the inhibitory activity is R9 (amino acid R at position 9 along the primary structure). Which of the following mutations is most likely to have the greatest effect on the inhibition of the interaction between PKA and BL?

- O **A.** R9H
- O **B.** R9K
- O **C.** R9D
- O **D.** R9G

Question 26

BL was modified further to generate a "staurosporine warhead," and the kinetics of the resulting agent were analyzed.

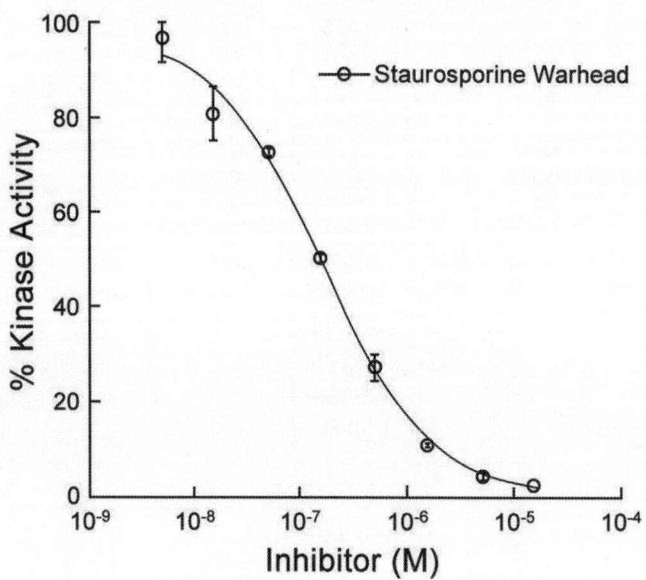

What is the approximate IC_{50} of the new compound?

- ○ **A.** 150 nM
- ○ **B.** 150 pM
- ○ **C.** 10 mM
- ○ **D.** 100 μM

The following questions are NOT based on a descriptive passage (Questions 27–30).

Question 27

When blood moves through arteries, the viscosity of blood produces a resistive force. The following equation is used to relate force and viscosity η:

$$F = -2\pi r l \frac{v}{R}\eta$$

where F is force, r is radius, *l* is length, v is speed, R is distance, and η is the viscosity. What are the dimensions of viscosity in the fundamental quantities of mass (M), length (L), and time (T)?

- ○ **A.** $M \cdot L^3 \cdot T^{-3}$
- ○ **B.** $M \cdot L^{-1} \cdot T^{-1}$
- ○ **C.** $M \cdot L^2 \cdot T^{-1}$
- ○ **D.** $M \cdot L^{-2} \cdot T^{-2}$

Question 28

Water has a specific heat of 4.18 J/g·°C, while glass (Pyrex) has a specific heat of 0.78 J/g·°C. If 40.0 J of heat is added to 1.00 g of each of these, which will experience the larger temperature increase?

- ○ **A.** They will both experience the same change in temperature, because only the mass of a substance relates to the increase in temperature.
- ○ **B.** Neither would necessarily experience a temperature increase.
- ○ **C.** Water
- ○ **D.** Glass

Question 29

At a given temperature, T in kelvin, the relationship between the three thermodynamic quantities including the change in Gibbs free energy (ΔG), the change in enthalpy (ΔH), and the change in entropy (ΔS) can be expressed as follows:

$$\Delta G = \Delta H - T\Delta S$$

The sublimation of carbon dioxide occurs quickly at room temperature. What might be predicted for the three thermodynamic quantities for the reverse reaction?

- ○ **A.** Only ΔS would be positive.
- ○ **B.** Only ΔS would be negative.
- ○ **C.** Only ΔH would be negative.
- ○ **D.** Only ΔG would be positive.

Question 30

Doppler ultrasound is a noninvasive test that can be used to estimate blood flow through vessels by bouncing high-frequency sound waves (ultrasound) off circulating red blood cells (RBCs). A probe can be positioned such that blood in a vessel under investigation may appear to be moving toward or away from the probe.

Consider a sound wave emanating from a stationary Doppler ultrasound probe that bounces off RBCs in blood approaching the probe with velocity, v. Assuming the Doppler ultrasound waves are only transmitted through fluid, the original wave relative to the reflected wave has:

- ○ **A.** a higher wavelength but a lower velocity.
- ○ **B.** a lower wavelength and the same velocity.
- ○ **C.** a higher wavelength and the same velocity.
- ○ **D.** a lower wavelength but a higher velocity.

Passage 6 (Questions 31–34)

Plasma pH is normally maintained at 7.4. A pH less than 7.35 is acidosis, whereas a pH of greater than 7.45 is alkalosis. Either condition can be a result of respiratory or metabolic changes.

Although buffers in the body fluids help resist changes in pH, the respiratory system and the kidneys regulate the pH of the body fluids. Malfunctions of either the respiratory system or renal system can result in acidosis or alkalosis, which may be beyond the capacity of the buffers to repair without the intervention of one of these organ systems.

Respiratory acidosis occurs with an increase in concentration (= partial pressure) of carbon dioxide (e.g., impaired breathing or ventilation as seen in chronic obstructive pulmonary disease, COPD, which includes chronic bronchitis and emphysema). The result is a lowered ratio of bicarbonate to pCO_2 resulting in a decrease in pH (acidosis). The acidosis is reversed gradually when kidneys increase the rate at which they secrete hydrogen ions into the filtrate and increase the absorption of bicarbonate.

Metabolic acidosis can result from the loss of bicarbonate ions (e.g., severe diarrhea) or the accumulation of metabolic acids (e.g., lactic acid, keto acids). This can lead to severe metabolic complications warranting intravenous bicarbonate therapy. The reduced pH stimulates the respiratory center, which causes hyperventilation. During hyperventilation, carbon dioxide is eliminated at a greater rate.

Respiratory alkalosis occurs during hyperventilation; when excessive carbon dioxide is eliminated from the system (which lowers pCO_2), the pH of the blood increases, resulting in alkalosis. This can be seen in conditions such as hysteria, stroke, and hepatic (liver) failure. The kidneys help to compensate for respiratory alkalosis by decreasing the rate of hydrogen ion secretion into the urine and the rate of bicarbonate ion reabsorption.

Metabolic alkalosis generally results when bicarbonate levels are higher in the blood. This can be observed, for example, after sustained vomiting of acidic gastric juices. Kidneys compensate for alkalosis by increasing the excretion of bicarbonate ions. The increased pH inhibits respiration. Reduced respiration allows carbon dioxide to accumulate in the body fluids.

Question 31

Diabetic ketoacidosis is an example of which of the following imbalances?

○ **A.** Respiratory acidosis
○ **B.** Respiratory alkalosis
○ **C.** Metabolic acidosis
○ **D.** Metabolic alkalosis

Question 32

Vomiting normally results in the expulsion of gastric contents, but prolonged vomiting may also include the expulsion of contents from the upper small intestine. Consider a person who begins vomiting and then the process becomes prolonged. That person would be expected to have experienced all of the following EXCEPT one. Which one is the EXCEPTION?

○ **A.** Metabolic alkalosis
○ **B.** Dehydration
○ **C.** Metabolic acidosis
○ **D.** Respiratory alkalosis

Question 33

Normal CO_2 is 40 mmHg with the normal range being 35–45 mmHg. If a patient's pH is 7.3 and pCO_2 is 50 mmHg, the patient must have:

- ○ **A.** respiratory acidosis.
- ○ **B.** respiratory alkalosis.
- ○ **C.** metabolic acidosis.
- ○ **D.** metabolic alkalosis.

Question 34

According to the passage, the active responses of the kidney to respiratory alkalosis are not directly associated with filtration. As such, the kidney's active responses in this case are LEAST likely to occur at the level of the:

- ○ **A.** glomerulus.
- ○ **B.** loop of Henle.
- ○ **C.** distal convoluted tubule.
- ○ **D.** proximal convoluted tubule.

Passage 7 (Questions 35–39)

The ninhydrin reaction is a useful analytical detection method for alpha-amino acids. The reaction is used in forensics for the detection of human contact to objects, such as fingerprints. The reagent ninhydrin produces a characteristic blue color with primary alpha-amino acids via the following series of reactions (*see* Figure 1):

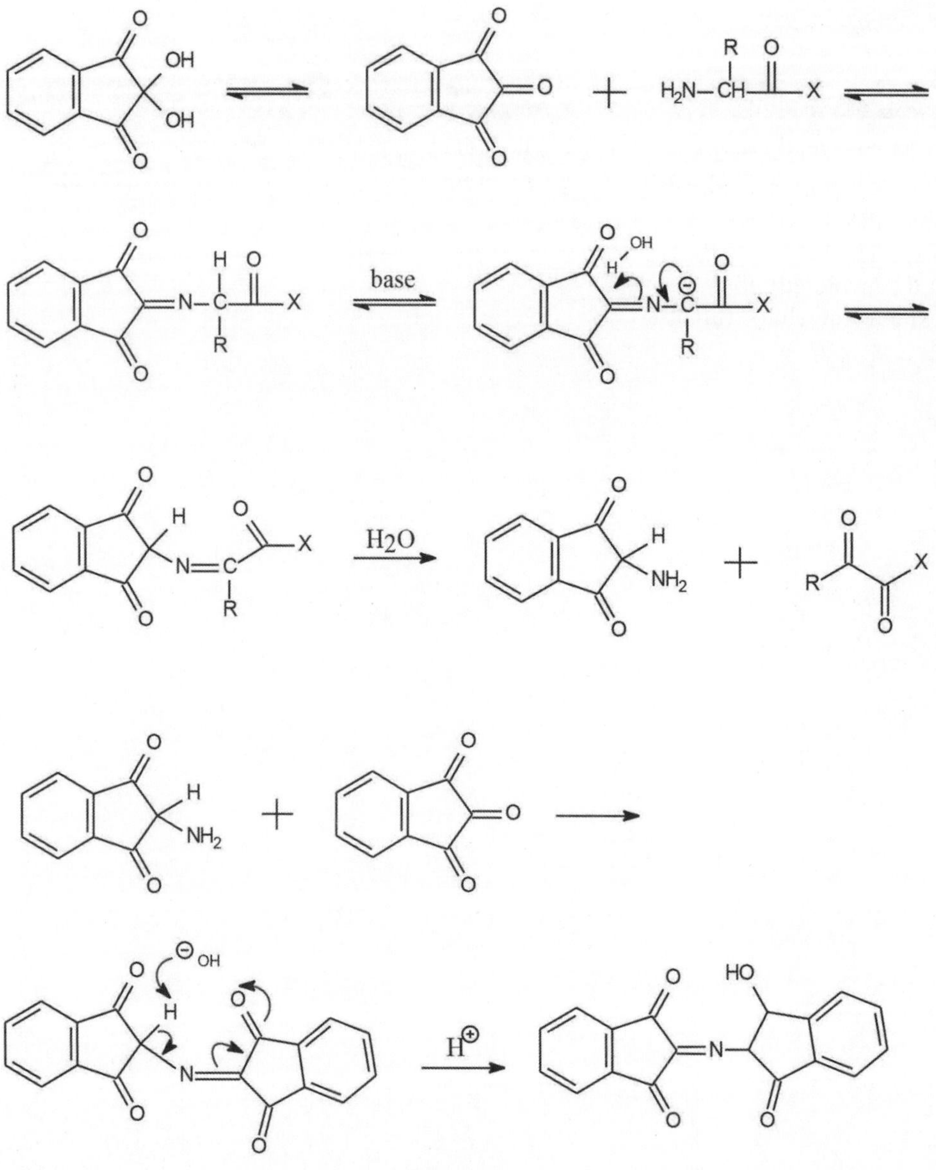

Figure 1

Question 35

In the first reaction of Fig. 1, the inorganic product, which is not written, is:

- A. CO_2
- B. H_2O
- C. HCl
- D. H_2O_2

Question 36

Which of the following compounds would be isotopically labeled if $H_2{}^{18}O$ were the only isotype source in the ninhydrin reaction?

- ○ A. 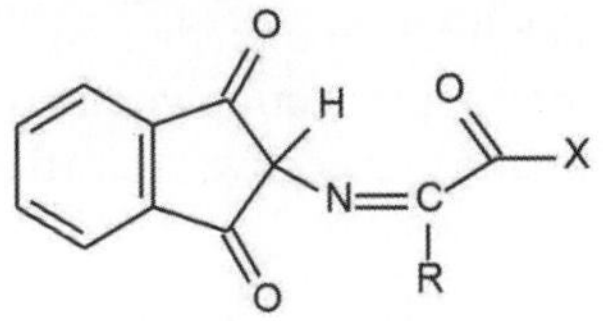
- ○ B. 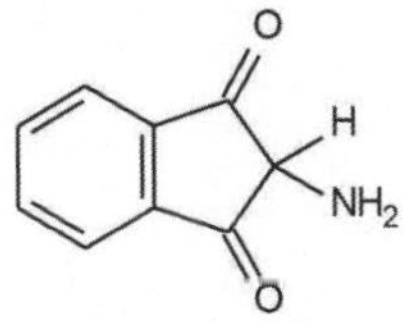
- ○ C. 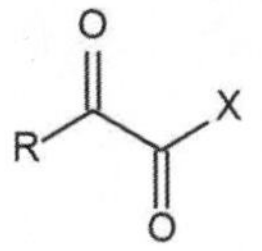
- ○ D.

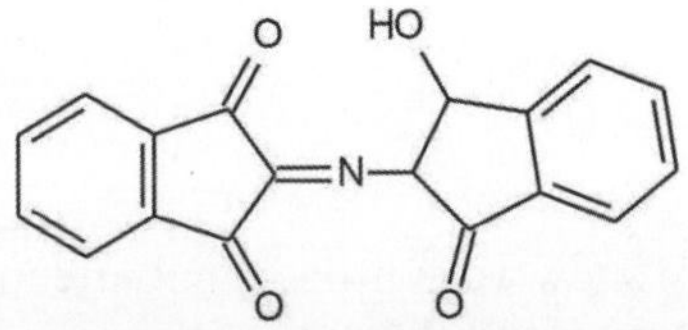

Question 37

Polypeptides sloughed off in fingerprints react with ninhydrin. Which of the following tetrapeptides would likely be most reactive with ninhydrin?

- ○ A. K-G-K-N
- ○ B. Y-V-V-T
- ○ C. H-D-E-E
- ○ D. C-C-G-C

Question 38

A mixture of alanine and benzoyl chloride is treated with dilute aqueous sodium hydroxide to yield compound Q. What functional group would be present in compound Q?

- ○ A. Ester
- ○ B. Aldehyde
- ○ C. Amide
- ○ D. Ether

Question 39

Base treatment of an amino acid usually results in the conversion of the acid to a derivative via the amino-carboxylate salt.

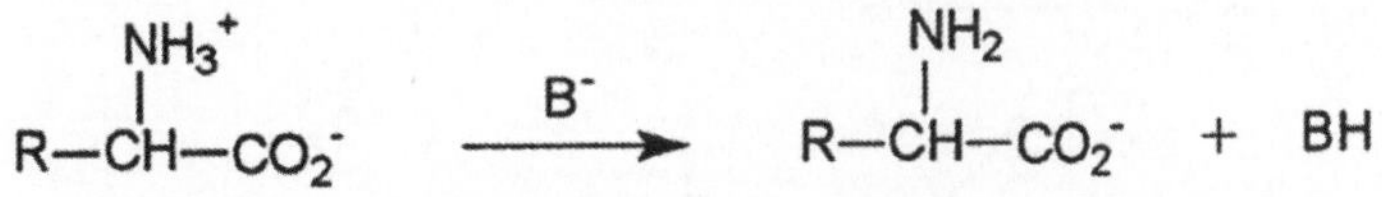

$$\text{R–CH(NH}_3^+\text{)–CO}_2^- \xrightarrow{B^-} \text{R–CH(NH}_2\text{)–CO}_2^- + \text{BH}$$

The above procedure:

- ○ A. decreases the rate of electrophilic reaction of the free amino group.
- ○ B. decreases the rate of nucleophilic reaction of the free amino group.
- ○ C. enhances the rate of nucleophilic reaction of the free amino group.
- ○ D. enhances the rate of electrophilic reaction of the free amino group.

Passage 8 (Questions 40–43)

The optical fiber is one type of optical waveguide or structure used to guide light waves to a designated location. The optical fiber is a long, thin, flexible rod made of silica, allowing waves to be guided along any path. The fiber consists of an inner *core* surrounded by an outer *cladding* layer, both of which are made of dielectric materials. Because of the difference in the index of refraction of the two layers, total internal reflection confines the waves within the core of the fiber. Sometimes the optical fiber is also coated with an opaque protective layer (the 'coating', *see* Figure 1).

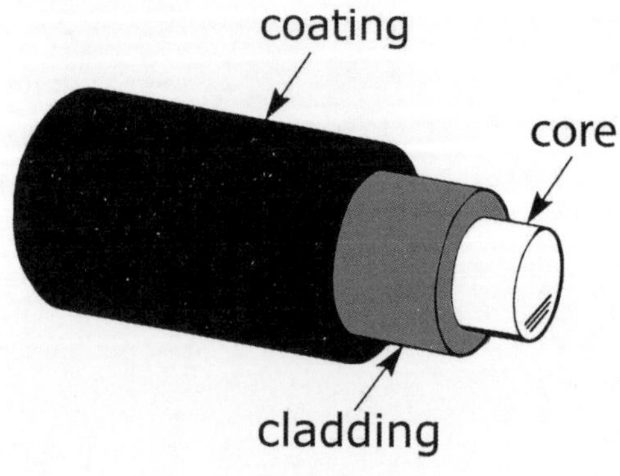

Figure 1

The main application for optical fibers is communication, because they show very little signal attenuation and very high bandwidth. However, the discovery of optical fibers also revolutionized the approach to diagnosis and treatment of certain gastrointestinal and pulmonary diseases through the use of endoscopy (physicians using optical fibers to relay images from internal organs).

A model for a segment of an optical fiber in longitudinal section is shown in Figure 2. A beam of light enters one end of the fiber at an angle of θ with the axis of the fiber. Assume that the interface between the air and the optical fiber is a flat plane. Figure 3 reflects the relationship between the index of refraction of silica and the wavelength of the light passing through it.

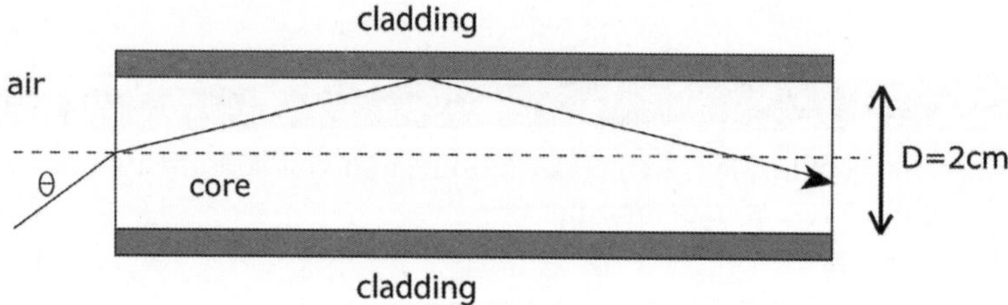

Figure 2

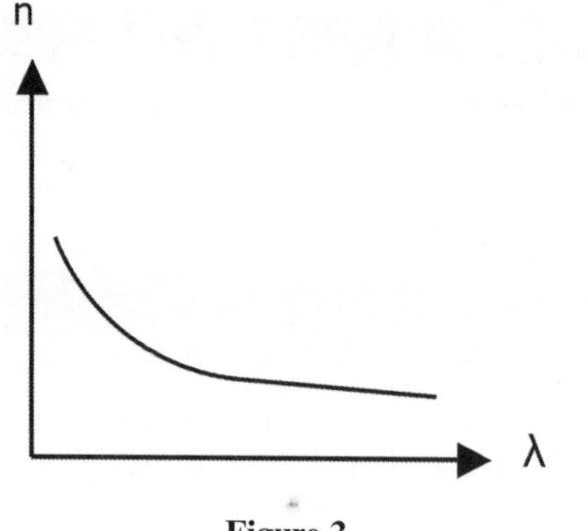

Figure 3

Question 40

What condition of the cladding will ensure that light signals are confined in the core?

- O **A.** The cladding must be conducting.
- O **B.** The dielectric nature of the cladding.
- O **C.** The cladding must have a higher index of refraction than the core.
- O **D.** The cladding must have a lower index of refraction than the core.

Question 41

If the critical angle in medium 1 is larger than that in medium 2, both measured with respect to an interface with air, which of the following statements is exact?

- O **A.** Medium 1 has a higher index of refraction than medium 2.
- O **B.** Medium 1 has a lower index of refraction than medium 2.
- O **C.** Medium 1 can never exhibit total internal reflection.
- O **D.** We do not have enough information to say which medium has a higher index of refraction.

Question 42

Consider that the critical angle at the interface between the core and the cladding is 60°. If the core has an index of refraction of 1.50, what is the index of refraction of the cladding?

- O **A.** 0.75
- O **B.** 1.06
- O **C.** 1.30
- O **D.** 1.76

Question 43

We know that for silica, the index of refraction varies nonlinearly with the wavelength of the light passing through it; this relation is illustrated in Figure 3. Suppose now that the incident light signal has a fixed angle of incidence. How does the angle of refraction in the optical fiber vary if the wavelength of the incoming signal increases steadily?

- O **A.** The angle of refraction in the optical fiber increases.
- O **B.** The angle of refraction in the optical fiber decreases.
- O **C.** The angle of refraction in the optical fiber does not vary.
- O **D.** We do not have enough information to decide.

The following questions are NOT based on a descriptive passage (Questions 44–47).

Question 44

Which of the following represents two structures that are equivalent?

○ A.

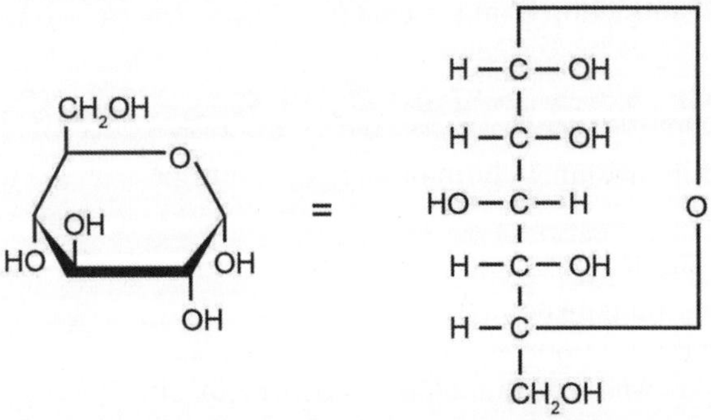

○ B.

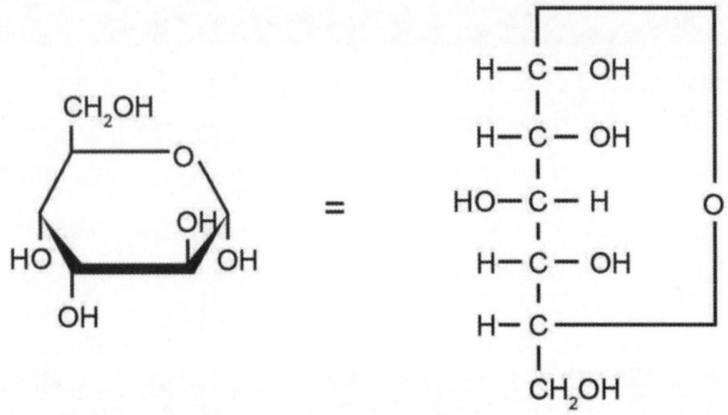

○ C.

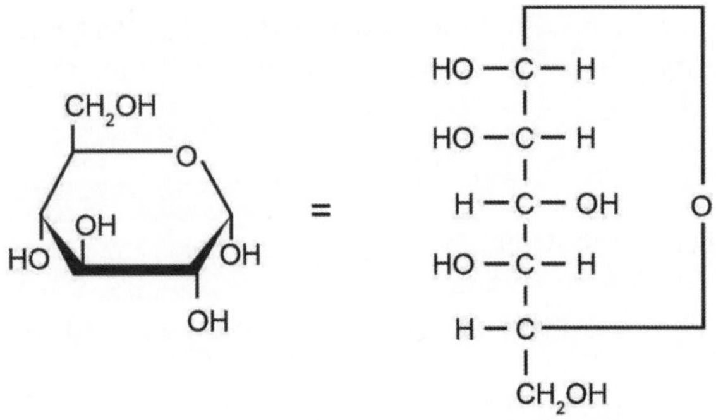

○ D.

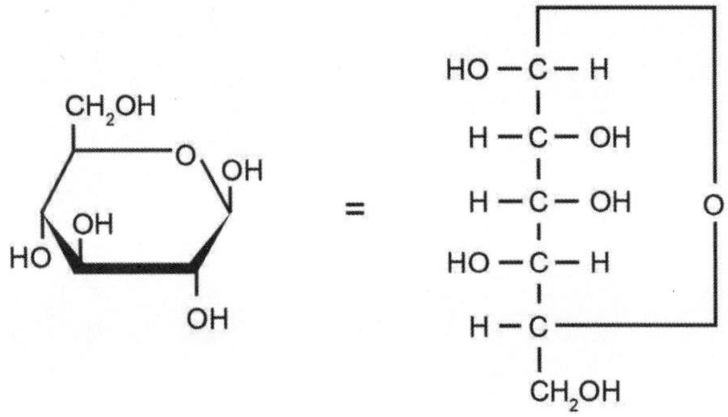

Question 45

Consider a solution containing a globular protein dissolved in water to produce a concentration of 120 g/L. If the osmotic pressure of the solution is 0.0224 atm at 27 °C, what would be the approximate molecular weight of the globular protein? (The universal gas constant can be approximated as 0.082 L atm K^{-1} mol^{-1}.)

- ○ **A.** 28,000
- ○ **B.** 48,000
- ○ **C.** 72,000
- ○ **D.** 144,000

Question 46

The standard changes in Gibbs free energy for the reactions below are given.

Phosphocreatine $\rightarrow$ creatine + P_i $\Delta G° = -43.0$ kJ/mol

ATP $\rightarrow$ ADP + P_i $\Delta G° = -30.5$ kJ/mol

Determine the overall $\Delta G°$ for the following reaction.

Phosphocreatine + ADP $\rightarrow$ creatine + ATP

- ○ **A.** –12.5 kJ/mol
- ○ **B.** +12.5 kJ/mol
- ○ **C.** –73.5 kJ/mol
- ○ **D.** +73.5 kJ/mol

Question 47

The intensity of sound X is 1000 times that of sound Y. What is the difference in the intensity levels of X and Y in terms of decibels?

- ○ **A.** 1000
- ○ **B.** 3
- ○ **C.** 100
- ○ **D.** 30

Passage 9 (Questions 48–52)

Catechol (benzene-1,2-diol) is a disubstituted organic compound with the molecular formula $C_6H_4(OH)_2$. Consider its structure below.

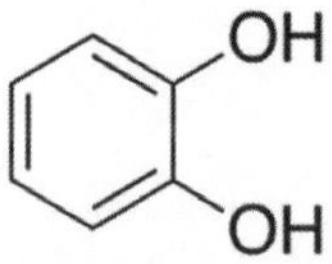

Catecholamines are composed of a catechol with an amine as the third substituent to the ring. The wide variety of catecholamines in humans are all derived from the amino acid tyrosine. Catecholamines are known to cause physiological responses to prepare the body for physical activity.

Consider the following catecholamines.

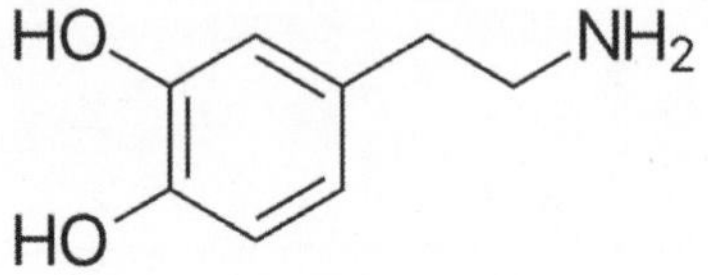

Dopamine 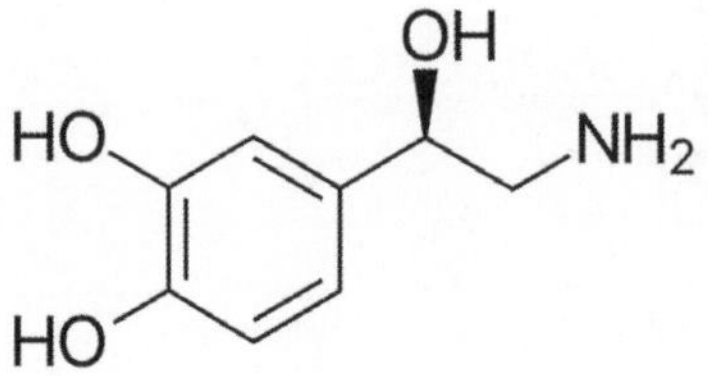 | Norepinephrine 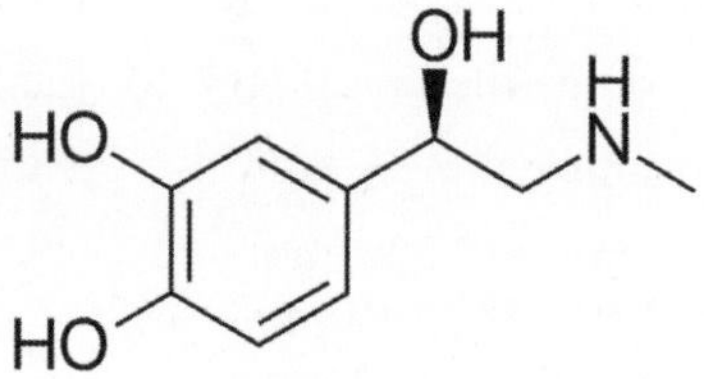 | Epinephrine

Question 48

Assuming that one equivalent of electrophile, X, reacts with catechol, how many trisubstituted isomers of catechol (i.e., with the molecular formula $C_6H_3(OH)_2X$) are possible?

- ○ **A.** Two
- ○ **B.** Three
- ○ **C.** Four
- ○ **D.** More than four

Question 49

Among the catecholamines, dopamine, norepinephrine, and epinephrine, how many possess a chiral center?

- ○ **A.** All three contain more than a single chiral center each.
- ○ **B.** All three contain a single chiral center each.
- ○ **C.** Only two contain a single chiral center each.
- ○ **D.** Only one contains a single chiral center.

Question 50

Adrenergic receptors are a class of G protein–coupled receptors that are targets of catecholamines. Binding of a catecholamine to the receptor will generally stimulate the sympathetic nervous system. A key component of the active site has two linked, identical amino acid residues that can donate an H-bond to the agonist. Which of the following would be most consistent with the described component of the active site of adrenergic receptors?

- ○ **A.** Glu-Glu
- ○ **B.** Ile-Ile
- ○ **C.** Ser-Ser
- ○ **D.** Met-Met

Question 51

Radiolabeled ligands represent a sensitive method for probing receptor binding. The interaction between norepinephrine and the adrenergic receptors is to be examined. Which of the following sites would be ideal for tritium (^3H) labeling?

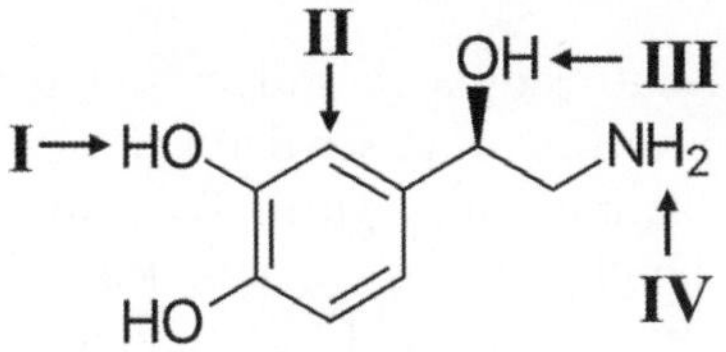

- ○ **A.** I
- ○ **B.** II
- ○ **C.** III
- ○ **D.** IV

Question 52

A derivative of dopamine with a less activated aromatic ring is reacted with *isatin* forming a thermodynamic mixture of 2 isomers: Product A and Product B.

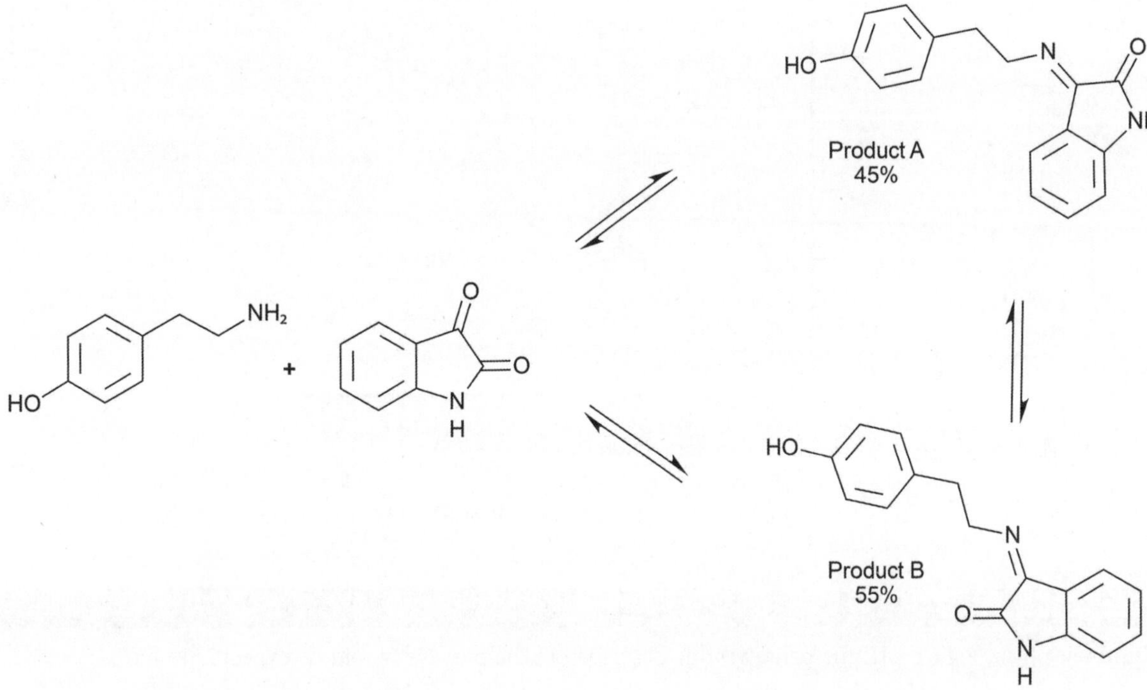

What is likely to be true regarding the relative thermodynamic stabilities of the two products?

I. Product A is less stable than Product B.
II. Product B is the thermodynamic product.
III. The kinetic product must be the more stable of the two products.

- ○ **A.** I only
- ○ **B.** II only
- ○ **C.** I and II only
- ○ **D.** I, II and III

Catecholamines/isomers: Ref. Vélez, Díaz-Oviedo, Quevedo; Journal of Molecular Structure Volume 1133, 5 April 2017, Pages 430-435.

Passage 10 (Questions 53–56)

Researchers working with a novel enzyme X-VUR identified several short peptide fragments that were hypothesized to bind with the enzyme's active site. Amongst them, a pentapeptide with amino acid sequence ANLEQ was of particular interest, due to its apparent interactions between it and the active site.

Generally speaking, 'docking' is carried out using a computer program in order to dock computer-generated depictions of small molecules to a receptor (or to a user-defined part thereof, for example: the active site of an enzyme), followed by evaluation of the molecules with respect to complementarity in terms of shape and properties, such as electrostatics. Good complementarity of a molecule indicates that the molecule is potentially good at binding to the structure under investigation. The outcome of a docking exercise normally includes some sort of affinity prediction for the molecules investigated, yielding a relative rank-ordering of the docked compounds with respect to affinity.

Computer docking experiments of the pentapeptide ANLEQ predicted that the carboxyl side group of the glutamate shared a hydrogen bond from a nearby serine, but the interaction appeared to be pH-dependent.

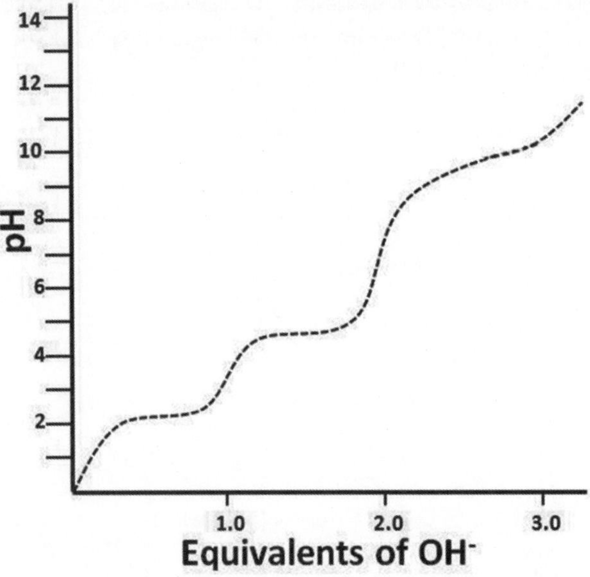

Figure 1 Titration curve for ANLEQ

Question 53

In solution at physiological pH, the pentapeptide described in the passage would be expected to have:

- O **A.** a net positive charge.
- O **B.** a net negative charge.
- O **C.** a net neutral charge.
- O **D.** a variable charge.

Question 54

Binding experiments with X-VUR were conducted at pH 8, where the enzyme shows optimal activity. The data is summarized in Table 1.

Table 1 Binding equilibria (dissociation, association; approximate values) at pH 8 with free energy for ANLEQ binding to the active site of X-VUR

Kd (M)	Ka (M^{-1})	ΔG° (kJ/mol)
10^{-7}	10^{7}	-43

At pH 8, X-VUR's active site would reasonably be expected to have which of the following?

I. A polar region
II. A non-polar region
III. A net positive charge

○ **A.** I only
○ **B.** I and III only
○ **C.** I and II only
○ **D.** I, II and III

Question 55

ANLEQ is overexpressed in cell cultures as part of a short peptide sequence VSPGSANLEQ that is cleaved into two fragments and purified using ion exchange chromatography. Using a buffer of pH 7, the best purification strategy would be to use:

○ **A.** anion exchange chromatography.
○ **B.** cation exchange chromatography.
○ **C.** size exclusion chromatography.
○ **D.** gel filtration.

Question 56

X-VUR has been shown to go through a multi-step activation cycle with multiple intermediate conformations. In one conformation, the glutamate in bound ANLEQ becomes protonated, even at physiological pH. What is a possible explanation for this occurrence?

○ **A.** The experiment is always conducted in a highly acidic buffer.
○ **B.** The microenvironment changes, such that the pKa of the glutamate side chain becomes significantly raised.
○ **C.** An adjacent residue forms a salt bridge with the glutamate side chain.
○ **D.** Conformation changes result in a highly hydrophilic environment.

The following questions are NOT based on a descriptive passage (Questions 57–59).

Question 57

The reaction P + 3Q $\rightarrow$ R was studied and the data in Table 1 collected.

Table 1

Exp.	[P] in M	[Q] in M	Initial rate of reaction
A	0.30	0.90	5.0×10^{-6}
B	0.30	1.80	1.0×10^{-5}
C	0.90	0.90	4.5×10^{-5}

The rate-determining step in this reaction probably involves:

- O **A.** two molecules of P and two molecules of Q.
- O **B.** three molecules of P and one molecule of Q.
- O **C.** one molecule of P and three molecules of Q.
- O **D.** two molecules of P and one molecule of Q.

Question 58

The freezing point of a solution of lactose was determined. Subsequently, lactase - an enzyme involved in the hydrolysis of lactose into its monomers - was added to the lactose solution. The enzyme was eventually removed from the solution. How would the freezing point of the post-lactase solution compare with that of the original solution?

- O **A.** It would be lower.
- O **B.** It would be higher.
- O **C.** It would be the same.
- O **D.** It cannot be determined from the information given.

Question 59

The following are among the imaging tools used to examine the interior of the human body: computed tomography (CT) scan, which uses X-rays; magnetic resonance imaging (MRI), which uses the same principle as nuclear magnetic resonance (NMR) in addition to radio waves; and positron emission tomography (PET) scan, which uses a radioactive tracer.

Ionizing radiation, in which there is enough energy to liberate electrons from atoms or molecules, can damage tissue and particularly DNA. Which of the following does NOT emit ionizing radiation?

- O **A.** CT scan
- O **B.** MRI
- O **C.** PET scan
- O **D.** All three emit ionizing radiation.

CANDIDATE'S NAME ____________________________________

RAW SCORE AND SCALED SCORE ____________________________

GS-1
Mock Exam 1 of 7
Solutions at MCAT-prep.com

GS-1 Section II: Critical Analysis and Reasoning Skills (CARS)

Questions: 1-53
Time: 90 minutes

INSTRUCTIONS: This test contains nine passages, each of which is followed by several questions. After reading the passage, select the best answer to each question. If you are unsure of the answer, eliminate the alternatives you know to be false then select an answer from the remaining alternatives. To indicate your selection, use a pencil to blacken the corresponding circle next to the answer choice and/or you can use the answer document at the back of this book. No marks are deducted for wrong answers.

The computer-based real MCAT has an on-screen highlighter function and ~~STRIKEOUT~~ function. These tools help to spotlight text or assist in the process of elimination. You may use a yellow highlighter for this paper-based exam and/or a pen (or preferably a pencil to make it easier should you change your mind) to mark text. At the time of publishing, both highlighting and strikeout functions can be used for passages, questions and answer choices. You can also flag a question to review later should time remain.

For the real exam, you will be provided with a dry erase board which is a white laminated noteboard booklet accompanied by a fine point marker. The noteboard includes 9 graph-lined pages for you to write though you cannot erase. You can simulate the experience with a fine point marker on a noteboard or with 8" x 14" plain graph paper.

Please note: For the real MCAT, a small number of field-tested questions will remain unscored.

This practice test has been designed exclusively to test knowledge and thinking skills. This exam may contain hypothetical statements and/or express controversial ideas. Statements contained herein do not necessarily reflect the policy, position, or view of RuveneCo Inc. or MCAT-prep.com.

START EXAM ONLY WHEN TIMER IS READY.

Passage 1 (Questions 1–5)

No one was less surprised by the news about St. John's wort than Stephen Barrett, 67, a retired psychiatrist who for nearly 30 years has made it his business to sniff out health-related frauds, fads, myths, and fallacies. Through newsletters, books, and now the World Wide Web, he has become one of America's premier debunkers of what he likes to call quackery. Barrett long ago wrote off St. John's wort as a treatment for severe depression, posting a dispassionate analysis of the evidence for and against it on his website, www.quackwatch.com, alongside similar dismissals of such nostrums as bee pollen, royal jelly, and "stabilized oxygen." His site - filled with useful links, cautionary notes and essays on treatments ranging from aromatherapy to wild-yam cream - is widely cited by doctors and medical writers and draws 100,000 hits a month. It has also made Barrett a lightning rod for herbalists, homeopaths, and assorted true believers, who regularly vilify him as dishonest, incompetent, a bully, and a Nazi.

None of these seems to daunt Barrett, who has been exposing bogus health claims since the late 1970s, when he first surveyed health-related mail-order ads in national magazines and discovered that none of them lived up to their claims. His findings spurred legislation that authorizes the federal government to levy penalties of $25,000 a day on repeat mail-order offenders. His big breakthrough - or, as he calls it, his "first Babe Ruth" - came in 1985, when he went after the hair analysis industry. He sent samples from the heads of two healthy girls to 13 laboratories that claimed they could measure nutritional needs based on a scientific analysis of an individual's hair. The reports were so off base and contradictory that his debunking report was published in the *Journal of the American Medical Association* and picked up by the national press. "It left the hair analysis industry with egg on its face," says Barrett. "Half the labs shut down."

Other Babe Ruth moments followed, none more satisfying to Barrett than the 1998 publication in *JAMA* of a report by Emily Rosa, an 11-year-old Colorado girl who for a school science project devised a simple test of therapeutic touch. It demonstrated that practitioners were unable to detect the "human energy field" on which their technique is based. Hearing of Emily's project, Barrett helped edit a report, got it published, and was rewarded with worldwide press coverage.

Barrett is underwhelmed by today's New Age celebrities. Dr. Andrew Weil, for example, is "very slick but makes glaring errors and hardly ever admits anything is quackery. I call him a 'rubber ducky.'" Deepak Chopra he dismisses as a purveyor of "Ayurvedic mumbo jumbo." (Chopra, for his part, calls Barrett "a self-appointed vigilante for the suppression of curiosity.")

Chiropractors too have felt Barrett's sting. While he sees benefits in chiropractic manipulation, he wonders about "a whole profession based on an idea - subluxations - that isn't true." He especially deplores the fact that some chiropractors claim that their manipulations can treat infectious diseases and prescribe homeopathic remedies, which he considers worthless. Barrett retired from his psychiatric practice in 1993 to devote himself full time to quackbusting. Along the way, he honed his communication skills and now considers himself an investigative journalist taking full advantage of the power of the internet. "Twenty years ago, I had trouble getting my ideas through to the media," he says. "Today, I am the media."

Source: Adapted from L. Jaroff, "The Man Who Loves to Bust Quacks." Copyright 2011 Time.

Question 1

According to the passage, the main result of Barrett's "quackbusting" has been to:

- O **A.** put many healthcare providers in danger of bankruptcy.
- O **B.** reveal many alternative healthcare claims to be fraudulent.
- O **C.** change the definition of medical quackery.
- O **D.** show alternative medicine practitioners are not knowledgeable about medicine.

Question 2

Many health advertisements contain testimonials. Stephen Barrett would probably want consumers to know that these testimonials:

- O **A.** are mostly reliable.
- O **B.** may claim "scientific proofs" that are false.
- O **C.** do not have the approval of the FDA.
- O **D.** can only be judged true if they are endorsed by real people.

Question 3

In regards to the therapeutic effects of some procedures, the author's main opinion is that:

- O **A.** mail order ads are mostly fallacious.
- O **B.** consumers should be skeptical of health care claims.
- O **C.** chiropractors lie about their abilities.
- O **D.** consumers should always believe Stephen Barrett.

Question 4

Which of the following hypothetical findings would most challenge Stephen Barrett's view of chiropractic practitioners?

- O **A.** Chiropractic practice is based on subluxations.
- O **B.** Chiropractors testify that their manipulations and homeopathic remedies have treated various infectious diseases.
- O **C.** A magazine cites chiropractic manipulation as a popular alternative treatment.
- O **D.** An experiment shows that chiropractic treatment reduces more the symptoms of tendinitis than nonsteroidal anti-inflammatory drugs.

Question 5

The passage argues that in evaluating the assertions of medical products or services claiming amazing benefits, one should consider which of the following?

- O **A.** The reliability of the claim
- O **B.** Worldwide media popularity
- O **C.** Endorsement from a medical society
- O **D.** Testimonials of consumers who have used a product or undergone a treatment

Passage 2 (Questions 6–12)

"The fox knows many things, but the hedgehog knows one big thing." So survives the epigrammatic aphorism of war poet, rhapsode, and paid mercenary Archilochus (seventh century BC). Only fragments of his wit and poetry survive, and what is known about the man himself is interspersed with conjecture. Revered as the finest poet in antiquity next to Homer, Archilochus is remembered mainly as the poet of abuse. Archilochus wrote direct and fierce innovative verses, fashioned as diatribes, which greatly influenced many poets and dramatists who followed him. He was also credited by the ancients with creating satire, elegiac couplets, and iambics. Horace speaks of the "rage" of Archilochus, and Hadrian describes his verses as "raging iambics." His iambics are the earliest known examples of satire, demonstrating his thorough mastery of the genre, though it is doubtful he actually created iambics. The bitter attacks of Archilochus, surviving only as fragments, helped his name endure through the centuries. What has endeared him to the modern world is his uncanny sense of self-expression and the interesting interpretations of his poetry and aphorisms.

For example, the fox and the hedgehog. As Arvan Harvat has written, "Basically, human beings are categorized as either 'hedgehogs' or 'foxes.' A hedgehog's life is an embodiment of a single, central vision of reality according to which they 'feel,' breathe, experience and think — 'system addicts,' in short. Foxes live centrifugal rather than centripetal lives, pursuing many divergent ends and, generally, possess a sense of reality that prevents them from formulating a definite grand system of 'everything,' simply because they 'know' that life is too complex to be squeezed into any Procrustean unitary scheme." This dichotomy of the two anthropomorphisms can be found in discussions of musicians, professors, students, and even Fortune 500 companies, or of general outlooks on life.

A renewal of enthusiasm in Archilochus' studies was caused by the discovery of a lengthy fragment, first published in 1974, rife with examples of Archilochus' "scorpion tongue." Sometimes his war poems, dispersed, scattered, and mangled, are ironic, often ambiguous, and sometimes full of disillusionment. Ambiguity in his verses and fragments has provided the impetus for a multitude of interpretations, in much the same way Nietzsche's aphorisms burst off the page, decentering and displacing univocal meaning into a Pentecostal polyphony of readings. His self-assessments and introspection in his city songs have provided comfort for a new host of readers who find themselves in the whirlwind of changing fortunes and circumstances, with cadences of hope in the midst of despair.

Fact and fiction, blurred together, have given Archilochus "legend" status. Not much is really known except for the scant accounts given by fellow Greek rhapsodes and philosophers and what is left of his writings. He left his birthplace to live on the remote island of Thasos, which was founded by his father. There he served as a noble soldier and wrote war poetry. Legend has it that he developed satires so bitter that usurpers and soldiers of the opposite army, deniers of his love, and the trifling family of that denier (Lycambes, Neobule, and her sisters) committed suicide. Supposedly killed by a man named Crow in battle, Archilochus was also important in instilling Bacchic worship at Paros, for which he composed lewd songs to Dionysus.

Although many historians have done so, critics point out that it is inadvisable to draw factual conclusions from fragments of Archilochus' poetry because lines that appear to be autobiographical may actually be instances of the poet adopting a mask or persona. As a cruel war poet and mercenary, he would suffer the fate of his karmic ill-begotten and debauched slanderous misfortunes, writing "Wretched I lie, dead with desire, pierced through my bones, with the bitter pains the Gods have given me."

Berlin, Sir Isaiah (1953). *The Hedgehog and the Fox*, New York, Simon & Schuster. Reproduced in part from: Archilocus. *New World Encyclopedia*. (2016, April 12). Retrieved from http://www.newworldencyclopedia.org/entry/Archilocus

Question 6

The author of the passage repeatedly refers to Archilochus' poetry as fragments in order to:

- ○ **A.** emphasize how little we know about Archilochus.
- ○ **B.** emphasize that Archilochus' existence cannot be established.
- ○ **C.** recognize Archilochus as the pioneer of satirical poems.
- ○ **D.** recognize Archilochus as an ancient poet.

Question 7

The passage asserts, "Fact and fiction, blurred and mixed together, have given Archilochus 'legend' status." Which of the following does the author most likely mean by describing Archilochus as a "legend"?

- o **A.** Archilochus' life is primarily known through the accounts of other writers.
- o **B.** Archilochus' recorded feats are similar to those of legendary war heroes.
- o **C.** Lines from Archilochus' poetry could be instances of the poet's adopting a mask or persona.
- o **D.** There are no records of his existence.

Question 8

Suppose that a new piece of evidence confirmed that Archilochus never existed at all. In response to this information, the author would probably suggest that scholars should:

- o **A.** abandon any study of the poetry attributed to Archilochus.
- o **B.** study the poetry formerly attributed to Archilochus only if the real author could be identified.
- o **C.** conclude that the ancient sources discussing Archilochus were forgeries.
- o **D.** continue to study the poetry even though its true author is unknown.

Question 9

It can be inferred from the passage that Archilochus wrote about satirical topics and crude violence because:

- o **A.** he wanted to dignify and glorify his occupation as a soldier.
- o **B.** he wanted to express his insights about the life to which he was constantly exposed.
- o **C.** he wanted to express his perceptions about warfare.
- o **D.** he wanted to leave a legacy for the next generation.

Question 10

In the final paragraph, the author of the passage quotes Archilochus a second time in order to:

- o **A.** prove Archilochus' excellence in writing war poetry.
- o **B.** highlight the characteristic bitterness found in Archilochus' writing.
- o **C.** re-focus the discussion on Archilochus' work.
- o **D.** criticize Archilochus' admirers.

Question 11

The passage suggests that Archilochus' poetry was outstanding at the time it was written because:

- o **A.** it contained violence and diatribe.
- o **B.** it was fraught with emotions and evoked varied interpretations among its readers.
- o **C.** his writing style was uniquely fierce in expressing bitter irony.
- o **D.** his verses strongly affected his audience.

Question 12

In reference to the discussion of Archilochus' aphorism in paragraph 2, the passage author interprets the fox and the hedgehog to represent personalities that are, respectively:

- o **A.** eclectic and systematizing.
- o **B.** carefree and focused.
- o **C.** skeptical and credulous.
- o **D.** liberal and conservative.

Passage 3 (Questions 13–18)

Humankind lingers unregenerately in Plato's cave, still reveling, its age-old habit, in mere images of the truth. But being educated by photographs is not like being educated by older, more artisanal images. For one thing, there are a great many more images around, claiming our attention. The inventory started in 1839 and since then just about everything has been photographed, or so it seems. This very insatiability of the photographing eye changes the terms of confinement in the cave, our world. In teaching us a new visual code, photographs alter and enlarge our notions of what is worth looking at and what we have a right to observe. They are a grammar and, even more importantly, an ethics of seeing. Finally, the most grandiose result of the photographic enterprise is to give us the sense that we can hold the whole world in our heads—as an anthology of images.

To collect photographs is to collect the world. Movies and television programs light up walls, flicker, and go out; but with still photographs the image is also an object, lightweight, cheap to produce, easy to carry about, accumulate, store. In Godard's *Les Carabiniers* (1963), two sluggish lumpen-peasants are lured into joining the King's Army by the promise that they will be able to loot, rape, kill, or do whatever else they please to the enemy, and get rich. But the suitcase of booty that Michel-Ange and Ulysse triumphantly bring home, years later, to their wives turns out to contain only picture postcards, hundreds of them, of Monuments, Department Stores, Mammals, Wonders of Nature, Methods of Transport, Works of Art, and other classified treasures from around the globe. Godard's gag vividly parodies the equivocal magic of the photographic image. Photographs are perhaps the most mysterious of all the objects that make up, and thicken, the environment we recognize as modern. Photographs really are experience captured, and the camera is the ideal arm of consciousness in its acquisitive mood.

To photograph is to appropriate the thing photographed. It means putting oneself into a certain relation to the world that feels like knowledge - and, therefore, like power. A now notorious first fall into alienation, habituating people to abstract the world into printed words, is supposed to have engendered that surplus of Faustian energy and psychic damage needed to build modern, inorganic societies. But print seems a less treacherous form of leaching out the world, of turning it into a mental object, than photographic images, which now provide most of the knowledge people have about the look of the past and the reach of the present. What is written about a person or an event is frankly an interpretation, as are handmade visual statements, like paintings and drawings. Photographed images do not seem to be statements about the world so much as pieces of it, miniatures of reality that anyone can make or acquire.

Photographs, which fiddle with the scale of the world, themselves get reduced, blown up, cropped, retouched, doctored, tricked out. They age, plagued by the usual ills of paper objects; they disappear; they become valuable, and get bought and sold; they are reproduced. Photographs, which package the world, seem to invite packaging. They are stuck in albums, framed and set on tables, tacked on walls, projected as slides. Newspapers and magazines feature them; cops alphabetize them; museums exhibit them; publishers compile them.

Sontag, S. (2010). *On Photography* (In Plato's Cave). New York: Picador.

Question 13

The author's main purpose in discussing the prevalence of photography is to demonstrate that:

- ○ **A.** photographic images capsulize and modify our perception of reality.
- ○ **B.** photographs describe reality more objectively than artisanal images.
- ○ **C.** photographs are handy objects that serve different purposes.
- ○ **D.** photography has lost its sense as an art because almost anyone can take pictures.

Question 14

In paragraph 2, the author states, "Godard's gag vividly parodies the equivocal magic of the photographic image." This insight by the author on Godard's *Les Carabiniers* rests on the assumption that:

- O **A.** photographs do not show the negative side of what they want to portray.
- O **B.** compared to films, photographs are practical tools in recording experience.
- O **C.** photographs are unbiased recordings of real life.
- O **D.** photographs are subjective representations of experiences.

Question 15

Which of the following lines in the passage best exemplifies the author's assertion that "being educated by photographs is not like being educated by older, more artisanal images"?

- O **A.** "They are a grammar and, even more importantly, an ethics of seeing."
- O **B.** "To photograph means putting oneself into a certain relation to the world that feels like knowledge — and, therefore, like power."
- O **C.** "Photographed images do not seem to be statements about the world so much as pieces of it."
- O **D.** "Photographs, which fiddle with the scale of the world, themselves get reduced, blown up, cropped, retouched, doctored, tricked out."

Question 16

One can infer that the author's statement, "To photograph is to appropriate the thing photographed," is intended to emphasize that photographs:

- O **A.** are almost exact reproductions of the world.
- O **B.** display the world as fragmented pieces selected by the artist.
- O **C.** are powerful tools in storing memories.
- O **D.** can help in identifying criminals and documenting factual information.

Question 17

Recent technological developments made photography easier and cheaper. Which claim from the passage is most strongly supported by this fact?

- O **A.** "The most grandiose result of the photographic enterprise is to give us the sense that we can hold the whole world in our heads — as an anthology of images."
- O **B.** "With still photographs, the image is also an object, lightweight, cheap to produce, easy to carry about, accumulate, store."
- O **C.** "Photographs, which package the world, seem to invite packaging."
- O **D.** "Photographs really are experience captured, and the camera is the ideal arm of consciousness in its acquisitive mood."

Question 18

The author would most likely agree with which idea about photography?

- O **A.** Photography is not merely a hobby or a science, but a visual art generically similar to sculpture.
- O **B.** Photography preserves well-loved memories, making it a popular art.
- O **C.** Photography makes people feel that they know about faraway places they have never seen.
- O **D.** Photography is merely a hobby, with little aesthetic value.

Passage 4 (Questions 19–23)

Much education in the postmodern and global era is online. Shifts in communication networks (for instance, between student and teacher) have taken place, becoming decentered, displaced. There is no real center to education in this exchange, and the process of communication is certainly not linear, but process-oriented. Simultaneous causes and effects take place which cannot really be separated in a simple stimulus response model or unidirectional arrow. Feedback loops are turned inside out like a Moebius strip or a fractal cascade - really no beginning and no end. Communication can be seen as a phenomenon which blossoms onto itself, delights itself in its own dance and ontological presence.

Leibniz invented a model of communication, albeit a tragic model, which formally proclaimed that no one really communicates with any one. Philosopher of science Michel Serres informs us that this can be mathematically formalized. While it is a bit out of my reach, I understand him to mean that misunderstanding received noise is the norm; meaning is never the same as a speaker's intent or meaning. This is somewhat like the common claim that students hardly ever remember the teachings, but we remember the teacher's personality. For Leibniz, the one-to-one model of generating meaning (interpersonal) was simply an act of God - a miracle. To this we can ascribe the same processual values and variables. The unidirectional model, traveling one way, was certainly a model of politics and religion. What about a model of one to the many? To some extent, this is how communication has historically been seen in academia. Of course, this model is still used, but it is starting to pale in comparison to a digital model of "many to many." Blogs. Forums. Facebook. We call it a network - but even that term still rings of the one-way arrow, except that there are simply more arrows, pointed towards a center. This seems facile and obviously simplistic, or analog, if you will.

With the emergence of digital technologies, we have witnessed a miraculous event - a model where the many communicate with the many, and at the same time. This, of course, would have profound implications for the educational process. How are we to know what we know when everyone is talking at the same time? What power shifts have occurred because of this displacement? How has this global medium radically changed our sense of self, other, meaning and knowledge?

How are we to understand communication? By focusing on misunderstanding? That would only enhance the negation of meaning. By trying to map out the plurality of voices on the internet? That would be quite a mess to sort out. Perhaps we could start with a flowchart which outlines this plurality of voices, not only online, but offline as well, within a specific context.

If we work or play online, we often say "keep me in the loop": that is, let me blossom with all the rest of the people in this fractal and digital blossom or dance. If we enter a chat room, everyone is continually transmitting and receiving messages, whether with a cloak of anonymity or five different webcams glaring across the LCD.

Professors have always been "out there." But also "in there." Subjective. Heads full of treatises and books, formulas and equations, the power slang of science and mathematics which keeps them apart from the student masses and hoi polloi. Out there. In there. In the digital and fractal dance blossoming onto itself, and out there with the procreation of meaning. Apart of and apart from, like a thumb in relation to the other fingers.

Source: Adapted from American Rhizomes & Rhapsodes (unpublished).

Question 19

Which of the following underlying assumptions about online communication is implied by the passage argument?

- O **A.** Perfect communication is impossible since the receiver of the information may interpret the message differently than the sender intended.
- O **B.** The World Wide Web has destroyed real communication, resulting in "received noise."
- O **C.** Communication has become underrated and taken for granted.
- O **D.** Modern technology has set new standards on what is real communication, rendering old standards obsolete.

Question 20

The tone of the author's discussion of teacher-learner communication can be described as:

- O **A.** bewildered.
- O **B.** thoughtful.
- O **C.** objective.
- O **D.** mocking.

Question 21

Which of the following schemes would the author most likely endorse to help us understand communication in the educational setting?

- O **A.** Giving each student a personality test to determine their communication style
- O **B.** Creating case studies of incidents where misunderstandings took place to determine what went wrong
- O **C.** Helping teachers and students express their ideas in the most objective possible way
- O **D.** Making a diagram that shows all communication sources and levels, both face-to-face and electronic

Question 22

What is the author's guiding metaphor for understanding communication in today's global era of digital technology?

- O **A.** Numerous arrows pointing toward a center
- O **B.** A fractal flower dance which blossoms
- O **C.** A miraculous act of God
- O **D.** A signal with a high proportion of noise

Question 23

The author's main concern about education in the online era relates to the fact that:

I. the interaction between students and teachers is hindered by the internet.
II. education has become dynamic, making any new information quickly obsolete.
III. there seems to be no established center for all communications in the classroom.

- O **A.** I only
- O **B.** II and III only
- O **C.** I and III only
- O **D.** III only

Passage 5 (Questions 24–28)

If Greek civilization seems more akin and "modern" to us now than that of any century before Voltaire, it is because the Hellene loved reason as much as form, and boldly sought to explain all nature in nature's terms.

The liberation of science from theology and the independent development of scientific research were parts of the heady adventure of the Greek mind. Greek mathematicians laid the foundations of trigonometry and calculus; they began and completed the study of conic sections, and they brought three-dimensional geometry to such relative perfection that it remained as they left it until Descartes and Pascal.

Democritus illuminated the whole area of physics and chemistry with his atomic theory. In a mere aside and holiday from abstract studies, Archimedes produced enough new mechanisms to place his name with the highest in the records of invention. Hippocrates freed medicine from mysticism and philosophical theory, and ennobled it with an ethical code; Herophilus and Erasistratus raised anatomy and physiology to a point which - except in Galen - Europe would not reach again till the Renaissance.

But the lover of philosophy will only reluctantly yield to science and art the supreme places in our Grecian heritage. Greek science itself was a child of Greek philosophy - of that reckless challenge to legend, that youthful love of inquiry, which for centuries united science and philosophy in one adventurous quest. Never had men examined nature so critically and yet so affectionately; the Greeks did no dishonor to the world in thinking that it was a cosmos of order and therefore amenable to understanding. They invented logic for the same reason that they made perfect statuary; harmony, unity, proportion, and form, in their view, provided both the art of logic and the logic of art.

Curious of every fact and every theory, they not only established philosophy as a distinct enterprise of the European mind, but they conceived nearly every system and every hypothesis and left little to be said on any major problem of life. Realism and nominalism; idealism and materialism; monotheism, pantheism, and atheism; feminism and communism; the Kantian critique and the Schopenhauerian despair; the primitivism of Rousseau and the immoralism of Nietzsche; the synthesis of Spencer and the psychoanalysis of Freud - all the dreams and wisdom of philosophy are here in the age and land of its birth.

Civilization does not die, it migrates; it changes its habitat and its dress, but it lives on. The decay of one civilization, as of one individual, makes room for the growth of another; life sheds the old skin and surprises death with fresh youth. Greek civilization is alive; it moves in every breath of mind that we breathe; so much of it remains that none of us in one lifetime could absorb it all.

We know its defects - its insane and pitiless wars, its stagnant slavery, its subjugation of women, its lack of moral restraint, its corrupt individualism, its tragic failure to unite liberty with order and peace. But those who cherish freedom, reason and beauty will not linger over these blemishes. They will hear behind the turmoil of political history the voices of Solon and Socrates, of Plato and Euripides, of Phidias and Praxiteles, of Epicurus and Archimedes; they will be grateful for the existence of such men and will seek their company across alien centuries.

They will think of Greece as the bright morning of that Western civilization which, with all its kindred faults, is our nourishment and our life.

Durant, W. Will Durant: The Glory of Greece. (2004). Retrieved from http://will-durant.com/greece.htm

Question 24

According to the passage, which of the following played a role in the development of science in ancient Greece?

I. The Greeks' curious minds
II. Greek philosophy
III. Greek logic

- ○ **A.** I only
- ○ **B.** I and II only
- ○ **C.** I, II, III
- ○ **D.** II only

Question 25

It may be inferred from the passage that the development of science and art reveals which of the following?

- ○ **A.** We live in an age that is almost identical to the classic Greek civilization.
- ○ **B.** Much of contemporary civilization is a reflection of Greek civilization.
- ○ **C.** The Western world would not have flourished if not for the Greek civilization.
- ○ **D.** All the scientific advances as well as the ills of society can be attributed to the Greek civilization.

Question 26

The age of Voltaire (18th century) is associated with the development of empirical science and with critique of Christianity and superstition. Based on this, which of the following statements in the passage most strongly supports the claim that "Greek civilization seems more akin and 'modern' to us now than that of any century before Voltaire"?

- ○ **A.** "The liberation of science from theology and the independent development of scientific research were parts of the heady adventure of the Greek mind."
- ○ **B.** "Greek mathematicians laid the foundations of trigonometry and calculus."
- ○ **C.** "Democritus illuminated the whole area of physics and chemistry with his atomic theory."
- ○ **D.** "Hippocrates freed medicine from mysticism and philosophical theory, and ennobled it with an ethical code."

Question 27

Which of the following statements most strongly supports the author's view that "civilization does not die, it migrates; it changes its habitat and its dress, but it lives on"?

- ○ **A.** All fields of science are the brainchildren of Greek philosophers and thinkers.
- ○ **B.** We are still living in the Hellenistic period.
- ○ **C.** The end of one civilization is the birth of another.
- ○ **D.** Western civilization still bears great similarity to Greek civilization.

Question 28

The author implies that the Greek civilization did not fully cease to exist. This claim could be supported by which of the following assumptions?

- ○ **A.** The legacy of Greek civilization is obsolete and not applicable to our modern time.
- ○ **B.** What the Greeks have done should be a reminder for all of us that nothing lasts forever.
- ○ **C.** A civilization only changes appearance; it lives on under a different name and ruler.
- ○ **D.** The legacy of Greek civilization is found in architecture, sculpture, mathematics, philosophy, and other modern human endeavors.

Passage 6 (Questions 29–34)

I can honestly say that I had no idea that the National Wildlife Federation came into being because of one cartoonist. Ding Darling used his cartoons to promote conservation ethics as far back as 1930 and was instrumental in creating the government agency that pioneered the practice of scientific management for fish and wildlife. As an interesting side note, Mr. Darling also led the development of the federal duck stamp that is still the primary source of revenue for waterfowl management and must be purchased by all waterfowl hunters to this day. Darling pointed out that while many people cared about wildlife conservation, there was no organized way to advocate or influence policy decisions. His work and input emphasized the importance of multiple stakeholder participation, accepting the attitudes, values, and beliefs of many groups. And his dream came true in 1936 when he "convinced President Franklin Roosevelt to invite over 2,000 hunters, anglers, and conservationists from across the country to the first North American Wildlife conference in Washington, D.C." (according to the National Wildlife Federation website). This is where the General Wildlife Federation, later changed to the National Wildlife Federation, was formed, with the idea of uniting all outdoor and wildlife enthusiasts behind a common goal of conservation, and where Ding Darling became the first president of the organization.

Darling's quest to unite all voices concerning conservation was the basis for many laws and policies that are present today at the national level. The National Wildlife Federation returns every year to Washington, D.C. to provide governance, vision, and grassroots efforts needed to achieve joint conservation goals.

The National Wildlife Federation is presently one of the nation's largest conservation organizations, with approximately 4,000,000 supporters that are committed to sustaining America's wilderness for the benefit of people and of wildlife. It covers 47 state affiliates along with their 4,000,000 supporters and partners in many communities across the country to help protect and restore wildlife habitat, confront global warming, and connect with nature. NWF works diligently to be (in their words) "the voice of conservation for diverse constituencies, which include hunters, anglers, gardeners, birdwatchers, scientists, and families raising the next generation of habitat stewards."

The National Wildlife Federation has the professional expertise and grassroots power to make a difference for wildlife and our children's future. None of this happened by chance - from climate change to mining reform, from the wilderness to energy development, from backyard habitats to connecting people to nature. What started out as a cartoonist's dream became one of the largest grassroots conservation organizations in the country.

The Natural Wildlife Federation demands strategic planning that can accommodate change. There must be acceptance of varying attitudes, values, and beliefs, and the group must encourage a collaborative approach to conservation, while at the same time, promoting lifelong learning and growth. With cooperation from state affiliates, the National Wildlife Federation today continues in its quest for change. One of the benefits of using an integrated stakeholder-based model is effective engagement of members over a broad constituent base.

Darling's original ideas are still a mainstay of conservation imperatives, goals, and objectives. So without a concerned citizen who happened to be a cartoonist, there would probably not be an organization like the National Wildlife Federation in today's society.

National Wildlife Federation. (n.d.). Retrieved from https://www.nwf.org/

Question 29

The author of the passage would most likely argue that to be successful, social movements should:

- O **A.** enlist artists to change public opinion.
- O **B.** work for the restoration of polluted rivers and waterways.
- O **C.** write petitions to the government urging them to make legislative changes.
- O **D.** enlist the participation of ordinary citizens in advancing social change.

Question 30

Based on passage information, which of the following would Ding Darling have been LEAST likely to do?

- O **A.** Publish cartoons that condemned the destruction of the waterfowl habitat
- O **B.** Organize a conference attended by environmental advocates from diverse backgrounds
- O **C.** Serve in a government agency involved in studies and management of wildlife and their habitats
- O **D.** Rally against the National Rifle Association's agenda on encouraging ownership of hunting rifles

Question 31

What is the author's most likely purpose for writing the passage?

- O **A.** To trace the history of the National Wildlife Federation and other related groups
- O **B.** To stress the importance of Ding Darling and his cartoons
- O **C.** To illustrate the influential role of Darling in helping establish the National Wildlife Federation
- O **D.** To encourage the average hunter to join the National Wildlife Association

Question 32

Based on passage information, which of the following would Ding Darling have most likely considered as a theme for one of his cartoons at the beginning of his career?

- O **A.** The pleasure of birdwatching
- O **B.** A condemnation of smuggling rare species of birds in the Amazon
- O **C.** A discussion between citizens, including Native Americans, about the importance of the buffalo
- O **D.** A call for organized civic action to combat global warming

Question 33

Which of the following is the National Wildlife Association involved in?

I. Organizing groups and communities to advance wildlife and habitat conservation goals
II. Spearheading government lobbying efforts that promote respect for diverse constituencies
III. Facilitating activities that bring people closer to nature

- O **A.** I
- O **B.** I and II
- O **C.** I and III
- O **D.** I, II, and III

Question 34

What is the main idea of the passage?

- O **A.** Ding Darling dedicated his craft to advancing his environmental cause.
- O **B.** Ding Darling was the seminal force behind the creation of the National Wildlife Federation.
- O **C.** The National Wildlife Federation became the most influential conservationist group in the United States.
- O **D.** The National Wildlife Federation sought to unite all outdoor enthusiasts and wildlife supporters for a common cause of saving the environment.

Passage 7 (Questions 35–41)

Just as the framers believed that the government needed to be protected from the people, they also believed that giving the government too much power would infringe on the God-given rights of the people. Therefore, the people needed to be protected from the government. It is upon the basis of this belief that the Bill of Rights was included into the Constitution. Because of this inclusion, however, conflict of freedom versus power became an ongoing and very active conflict in our society, lasting up to this day.

There is a difference between the government giving citizens the freedom of speech and the belief that humans are born with those freedoms. This is really what the Bill of Rights is about—not that the government grants its citizens certain rights, but instead that the government shall not take away these fundamental rights. It is along this line that the Bill of Rights has much in common with the Declaration of Independence, which states that God has given everyone certain rights and that chief among them are life, liberty, and the pursuit of happiness. The Bill of Rights was designed to protect those freedoms that were laid out in the Declaration of Independence.

The Constitution, however, gave the federal government more power than was originally planned during the American Revolution and under the Articles of Confederation. There became a need for a much stronger federal government due to rebellion and economic instability that could have torn the nation apart. Because of this need for a stronger government, built into the Constitution is an inherent conflict between the power that is given to the government and the freedom of the people.

This problem still exists in our society today, and probably always will, which can cause us problems internationally. More recent examples have shown that American citizens will take their freedom of speech to extreme measures, such as hate speech at military funerals by the Westboro Baptist Church or the burning of the Koran by Terry Jones. Because the Bill of Rights ensures these liberties, it can create large problems for the federal government, such as diplomatic difficulties and the endangerment of American lives. This also creates conflict between the federal government and its own citizens.

Such conflict between the government and its people causes the government to attempt to assume (and often succeed in assuming) more power unto itself, thus creating problems domestically. In fact, the government has grown so powerful that it believes it has the power to tell a person what kind of plant they can put in their body or grow in their garden. This is important to understand, because when a government becomes so repressive that it tries to control what a person can put in their own God-given body or grow on their own property, then it shows how far we are away from true liberty in this country and represents a radical departure from ideas of freedom set forth by many of our founding fathers, according to President Abraham Lincoln.

Due to overregulation, we have turned otherwise good people into hardened criminals through incarceration for such things as small as passing a bad check or putting something in one's body that the government does not like. Unless the power of the federal government is reduced, these problems in our society will only grow worse. The sad reality is that unless this conflict between liberty and power is resolved in our Constitution, then liberty will be suppressed as the government gains more power, and as Thomas Jefferson wrote, it will only be won back through blood.

Question 35

Which of the following BEST represents the passage's main topic?

- ○ **A.** The perennial expansion of governmental powers and the decrease of civil liberties
- ○ **B.** The increase of civil liberties and the decrease of federal powers due to underregulation
- ○ **C.** Apparent overregulation due to the increase of big business and government
- ○ **D.** The ongoing conflict between federal power and the people's freedom in American society

Question 36

When the author discusses legislation of the growth and consumption of plants, he/she manifests agreement with:

- O **A.** more government power.
- O **B.** less government power.
- O **C.** winning back lost rights through blood.
- O **D.** God's censorship of the use of cannabis.

Question 37

According to the passage, the Bill of Rights provides balance between:

- O **A.** government and business.
- O **B.** personal liberty and federal power.
- O **C.** freedom and self-control.
- O **D.** big governments and small governments.

Question 38

According to the passage, individual rights can be reduced over time by historical forces including:

I. civil unrest.
II. collective armed violence.
III. economic crises.

- O **A.** I and III
- O **B.** I and II
- O **C.** II and III
- O **D.** I, II, and III

Question 39

Which of the following historical incidents could most convincingly be used to contest the author's argument?

- O **A.** In some ancient civilizations, citizens rioted to overturn oppressive governments.
- O **B.** In the 1920s, rural southerners were jailed for brewing homemade liquor without paying the required tax.
- O **C.** In the 1950s, the federal government used its power to enforce laws defending black civil rights.
- O **D.** In 2014, police enforced a nightly curfew in response to the growing protests and outrage on the shooting of an African-American teenager by a white police officer.

Question 40

Which of the following hypothetical examples would BEST represent the idea that freedom of speech, when taken to its extreme, might have harmful effects on society?

- O **A.** A pro-Second Amendment rally supporting greater gun rights
- O **B.** A picket line protesting working conditions at a textile factory
- O **C.** A radio talk show host making insulting remarks about a recently murdered civil rights leader
- O **D.** A nonviolent sit-in in front of a bank accused of loan mortgage scalping

Question 41

What is the writer's main goal in writing the passage?

- O **A.** Encouraging readers to take up arms against the government
- O **B.** Educating readers about the founders' understanding of God-given rights
- O **C.** Redefining the meaning of "conflict" as it pertains to individual rights
- O **D.** Informing readers that the current amount of government power is excessive

Passage 8 (Questions 42–46)

Charles Ponzi, creator of the infamous Ponzi scheme, was really nothing more than a small-time operator who got lucky. Even while he was enjoying his doomed moment of fame, he was being outclassed in every respect by a Swede named Ivar Krueger. Instead of postal reply coupons, Krueger built his rainbow bridge to the sky on an even more modest item—the safety match.

Krueger was born in 1880 in the town of Kalmar, Sweden, where his family ran a number of match factories. When he was 20, he graduated from the Stockholm Royal Institute of Technology with degrees in both civil and mechanical engineering, and then worked in various countries, particularly the USA. He came back home in 1907 and set up a construction firm to exploit the latest advances in steel–concrete construction methods. After starting this venture, he then picked up the family match business, which was having financial problems, and gradually consolidated an international match conglomerate that controlled 75 percent of the world's match production.

Krueger's wealth was generated by the kind of imaginative financial engineering that in modern times would be associated with the Enron oil company scandal: false front companies, fake reports of profits, and acquiring businesses simply to loot their treasuries; he even forged large quantities of Italian government bonds. However, his core scheme was not all that different conceptually from Ponzi's.

Europe was financially strapped after World War I while the USA was wealthy, and Krueger signed up American investors in legions to support his International Match Company (IMCO), paying them handsome dividends on tax-exempt foreign investments. Despite Krueger's monopoly position in many national markets, IMCO didn't have the profitability to support such dividends, but his ingenious financial trickery kept outsiders from getting wise—though they should have become suspicious when he bluntly told the press that he would explain nothing about his finances, which didn't exactly suggest that he was operating on principles of scrupulous accounting transparency.

The stock market crash of 1929 basically gave the flimsy system the blow needed to knock it down, though given the size of Krueger's empire it took a couple of years for its unavoidable doom to become obvious to its master. He bought a 9-millimeter pistol, spent the night with a pretty Finnish girlfriend and then shot himself through the heart while lying on his bed in a trim pinstriped suit.

At his death, Krueger's businesses owed more than the Swedish national debt. Many investors were ruined by his downfall. In Sweden, where Krueger was regarded as an inspiring national hero, a government fell and there was a clear uptick in suicides. It took five years for investigators to trace through the wreckage, and they concluded that Krueger had robbed backers of the equivalent of hundreds of millions of dollars. In 1933, in the wake of the Krueger incident and other financial scandals, the U.S. government implemented the Securities Act to impose disclosures on companies selling stock. The relaxation of the rules in the 1990s led to the Enron scandal, which was the biggest financial fraud in the USA since Krueger's spectacular implosion.

Like Ponzi, Krueger was a crook whose games caught up with him, but he played in a much higher league than Ponzi. The American economist John Kenneth Galbraith once wrote of the Match King: "Boiler-room operators, peddlers of stocks in the imaginary Canadian mines, mutual fund managers whose genius and imagination are unconstrained by integrity, as well as less exotic larcenists, should read about Krueger. He was the Leonardo of his craft."

Partnoy, F. (2010). *Match King - Ivar Kreuger and the Financial Scandal of the Century*. Penguin books.

Question 42

What is the author's purpose in writing the passage?

- ○ **A.** To present Krueger as the finest of financial swindlers
- ○ **B.** To examine Krueger's methods of fraud
- ○ **C.** To provide a biography and historical overview of Krueger
- ○ **D.** To compare and contrast Krueger and Ponzi

Question 43

The passage suggests that:

I. not all swindlers are criminal masterminds.
II. Krueger's machinations left a huge impact on economic markets.
III. economics is always accompanied by forms of dishonesty.

- ○ **A.** I only
- ○ **B.** I and II
- ○ **C.** II and III
- ○ **D.** I, II, and III

Question 44

The author would probably warn investors to be wary of buying shares from companies that:

- ○ **A.** heavily rely on small-scale products.
- ○ **B.** do not comply with the required corporate disclosures.
- ○ **C.** do not pay taxable dividends.
- ○ **D.** trade government bonds.

Question 45

Which of the following would NOT count as an example of a change that would reduce the incidence of successful fraud?

- ○ **A.** Increased legislation on financial disclosure
- ○ **B.** Greater caution among investors
- ○ **C.** More integrity among financial operators
- ○ **D.** Prevention of crashes like the 1929 stock market crash

Question 46

Which of the following pieces of evidence, if true, would undermine the author's argument about Krueger's fraudulent financial scheme?

- ○ **A.** Krueger and his backers actually suffered the majority of their losses by investing in other fraudulent businesses.
- ○ **B.** Everyone in banking and finance was corrupt during that time.
- ○ **C.** Krueger was also heavily involved in legitimate businesses.
- ○ **D.** There was a genuine demand and huge payoff for the safety match in general.

Passage 9 (Questions 47–53)

The U.S. Marines wrote an interesting footnote to the history of codes and ciphers in World War II when they adopted one of the most unusual and impenetrable ciphers ever used in warfare: the language of the Navajo tribe, native to the American Southwest.

While the U.S. military made effective use of cipher machines, they were often too slow for combat use. Trying to encrypt and decrypt messages during a running battle was too difficult to be practical, and when things got hot enough, messages had to be shouted over the radio or field phone "in the clear," allowing the enemy to intercept them.

In early 1942, Philip Johnston, a World War I veteran then working as an engineer in Los Angeles, California, came to the Marine Corps with a proposal. Johnston was the son of a missionary who had grown up on the Navaho tribal reservation. He was one of the few outsiders who could speak the language, which bears no close relationship to any European or Asian tongue. Johnston suggested that Navaho would make a good "real-time" code.

The idea was not new. The U.S. Army had employed at least 14 Choctaw tribesmen as radio operators during the First World War and had been pleased with the results. There were worries that the Germans had acquired expertise in American native languages in the intervening years, but the Marines were intrigued and, after conducting a few simple trials, decided to set up a program to train and deploy Navaho tribesmen as radio operators for Marine units in the field. Navaho tribal leaders patriotically cooperated with the effort. The first Navaho "code talkers," as they were known, went ashore with the Marines at Guadalcanal in August 1942.

One of the issues with code talking was that the tribal languages didn't have their own words for modern concepts such as "tanks," "machine guns," "battleships," "radar," and so on. Instead of using the English terms, which would have rendered the "code" almost useless, the code talkers invented their own terms for such things, for example, using the Navaho words for "iron fish" for a submarine, "hummingbird" for a fighter plane, "eggs" for bombs, and so on. The Choctaw code talkers had come up with a similar scheme during WWI. At first the list of Navaho code words had 274 entries, though this was later expanded to 508. For terms with no Navaho equivalent that weren't covered in the list, a "phonetic alphabet" was devised, using the Navaho equivalents of English words whose first letters spelled out the phrase: "ant" for "A," "bear" for "B," "cat" for "C," and so forth.

After the war, the chief of Imperial Japanese Army intelligence, Lieutenant General Seizo Arisue, told American interrogators, "We couldn't break your codes at all." That was something of an exaggeration, since they did penetrate some low-level codes, but the code talkers were certainly far beyond their abilities. A total of 420 Navaho code talkers served with the Marines in World War II. The Army also used 50 Choctaw and about 17 Comanche code talkers in the invasion of Europe, and a number of other tribes contributed small numbers of code talkers to the war effort as well. In each case, the code talkers used their own tribal language.

The code talkers remained unpublicized and unknown for decades, partly because the military wanted to keep the idea secret so it could be used again in the future; but with the increased emphasis on diversity in the U.S. in the late 20th century, the story of the code talkers became widely known, and now it is one of the most famous episodes in the history of cryptology.

Dahl, Amanda (2016). The Navajo Code Talkers of World War II: The Long Journey Towards Recognition. *Historical Perspectives: Santa Clara University Undergraduate Journal of History*, Series II: Vol. 21, Article 11.

Question 47

The author's main suggestion in the passage is that:

○ **A.** Native Americans were enlisted extensively during the war.
○ **B.** code breaking by Native Americans was an essential step in winning the War.
○ **C.** the Navaho code talkers served an important function in World War II.
○ **D.** code breaking during the war was marked by diversity and complexity.

Question 48

What is the author's purpose for writing the passage?

- O **A.** To highlight the effectiveness of codes in wartime situations
- O **B.** To highlight the importance of Navaho code talkers during the war
- O **C.** To compare and contrast the codes used by America and Germany during the war
- O **D.** To explain why the Navaho language is so difficult for non-native speakers to learn

Question 49

Based on the information in the passage, what is NOT a possible reason for Germany's failing to crack the US military code?

- O **A.** They had no native Navaho speakers to help them break the code.
- O **B.** They did not know that the US radio codes were based on Navaho.
- O **C.** They lacked access to skilled code breakers.
- O **D.** They lacked access to Navaho dictionaries and language books.

Question 50

The author likely mentions the need to find Navaho terms for modern military concepts in order to:

- O **A.** illustrate the rudimentary nature of the Navaho language.
- O **B.** demonstrate that Navaho was an imperfect choice for the task.
- O **C.** emphasize that warfare presents a unique challenge to cryptologists because of its specialized vocabulary.
- O **D.** emphasize the challenge of adapting a tribal language for modern warfare.

Question 51

Based on the information in the passage, the U.S. Army would likely not have needed the Navaho code-talkers if which of the following had been available?

- O **A.** Fluent speakers of more well-known languages
- O **B.** Faster cipher machines
- O **C.** Better training in the use of cipher machines
- O **D.** Clearer radio and field phone reception

Question 52

According to passage information, the Navaho did not have words for many of the military weapons which were being used, such as tanks and submarines. Instead, they used:

- O **A.** abstract mythic notions.
- O **B.** euphemisms.
- O **C.** metaphors.
- O **D.** the words of the most similar Navaho weapons.

Question 53

Based on passage information, which of the following was NOT a problem with cipher machines?

- O **A.** They were more difficult to use than just shouting messages over the radio.
- O **B.** They were impractical to use during the chaos of battle.
- O **C.** They were too slow for combat use.
- O **D.** The encrypted messages could be easily intercepted by the enemy.

CANDIDATE'S NAME ______________________

RAW SCORE AND SCALED SCORE ______________________

GS-1
Mock Exam 1 of 7
Solutions at MCAT-prep.com

GS-1 Section III: Biological and Biochemical Foundations of Living Systems

Questions: 1-59
Time: 95 minutes

INSTRUCTIONS: Of all the questions on this test, most are organized into groups preceded by a passage. After evaluating the passage, select the best answer to each question in the group. Fifteen questions are independent of any descriptive passage or each other. Similarly, select the best answer to these questions. If you are unsure of an answer, eliminate the alternatives that you know to be incorrect and select an answer from the remaining alternatives. To indicate your selection, use a pencil to blacken the corresponding circle next to the answer choice and/or you can use the answer document at the back of this book. No marks are deducted for wrong answers.

The computer-based real MCAT has an on-screen highlighter function and ~~STRIKEOUT~~ function. These tools help to spotlight text or assist in the process of elimination. You may use a yellow highlighter for this paper-based exam and/or a pen (or preferably a pencil to make it easier should you change your mind) to mark text. At the time of publishing, both highlighting and strikeout functions can be used for passages, questions and answer choices. You can also flag a question to review later should time remain.

For the real exam, you will be provided with a dry erase board which is a white laminated noteboard booklet accompanied by a fine point marker. The noteboard includes 9 graph-lined pages for you to write though you cannot erase. You can simulate the experience with a fine point marker on a noteboard or with 8” x 14” plain graph paper.

You may consult the periodic table at any point during the science subtests.

Please note: For the real MCAT, a small number of field-tested questions will remain unscored.

This practice test has been designed exclusively to test knowledge and thinking skills. This exam may contain hypothetical statements and/or express controversial ideas. Statements contained herein do not necessarily reflect the policy, position, or view of RuveneCo Inc. or MCAT-prep.com.

START EXAM ONLY WHEN TIMER IS READY.

Passage 1 (Questions 1–4)

Preliminary attempts to characterize a new human protein, XBR, have suggested that it may influence the expression of specific genes, including the gene *pyx*. However, it was initially unclear whether this regulation was mediated via downstream transcription factors or direct interaction.

Experiment 1

An electrophoretic mobility shift assay was used to determine whether XBR directly interacts with *pyx* (Figure 1). Different amounts of XBR were incubated with the DNA promoter region of *pyx* and a middle section of the ampicillin resistance gene as a control. Each DNA fragment was labeled with a radioisotope, was identical in length (250 bp), and contained one promoter, as well as a transcriptional and translational start site.

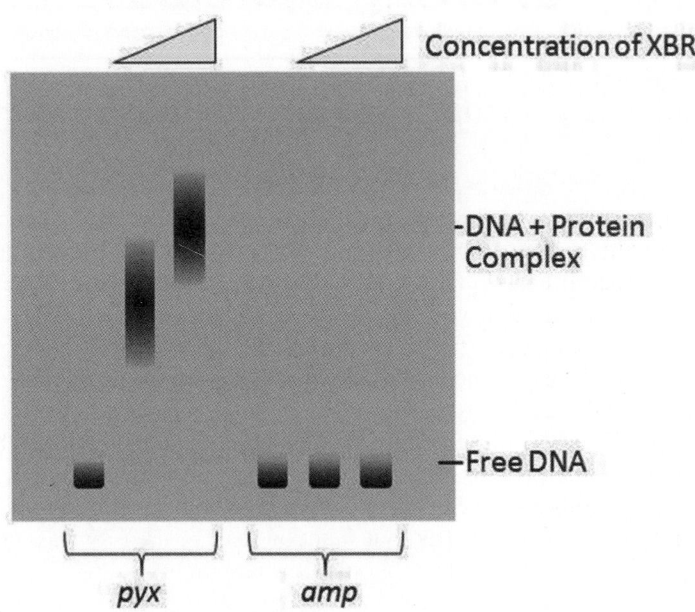

Figure 1 Interaction of XBR with *pyx* promoter and a fragment of the ampicillin resistance gene (*amp*) in an electrophoretic mobility shift assay

Experiment 2

Interaction of XBR with the *pyx* promoter region was studied *in vitro* using a β-galactosidase assay (Figure 2). Two plasmids were created, one that carried the β-galactosidase gene controlled by the *pyx* promoter, and one with the XBR operon connected with a *lacUV5* promoter. The *pyx* promoter plasmid was transformed into *E. coli* cells, both with and without the additional co-transformation of the XBR operon plasmid. Expression of the *lacUV5* promoter is regulated by the *lacI* repressor and can be induced with IPTG. Adding IPTG to the *E. coli* cultures containing the XBR plasmid induced the expression of XBR. To measure β-galactosidase expression, the *E. coli* cultures were given a solution that disrupted the cell membranes, but left the β-galactosidase intact. Samples were then treated with a synthetic color-reporting compound called ONPG, which was cleaved by β-galactosidase to yield a yellow compound. Activity of specific β-galactosidase is given in Miller units, a standardized measurement that quantifies β-galactosidase using ONPG.

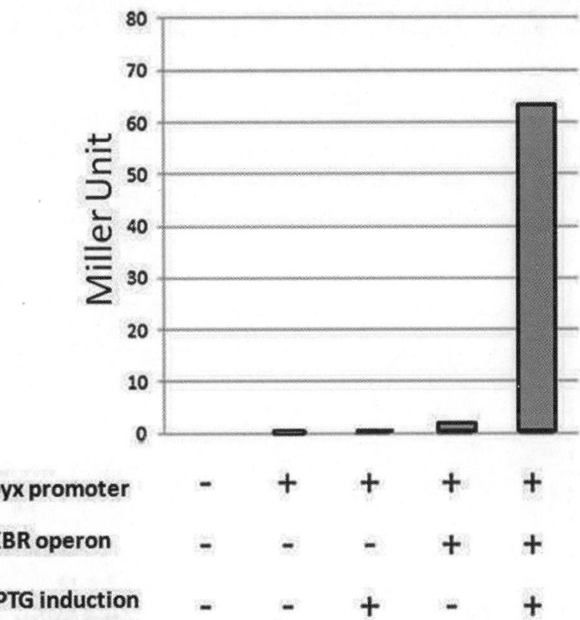

Figure 2 *In vitro* interaction between XBR and the *pyx* promoter region as detected with a β-galactosidase assay (Note: Since $k_2 << k_{-1}$, K_m is equal to the dissociation constant.)

Question 1

The results from Experiment 1 indicate that XBR:

- ○ **A.** binds directly to the promoter region of *pyx*.
- ○ **B.** induces the expression of *pyx*.
- ○ **C.** binds nonspecifically to DNA.
- ○ **D.** is more negatively charged than *pyx*.

Question 2

Expression of XBR in mammalian cells leads to all of the following EXCEPT:

- ○ **A.** upregulation of *pyx*.
- ○ **B.** direct interaction with the *pyx* promoter region.
- ○ **C.** translocation of XBR to the nucleus.
- ○ **D.** transcriptional regulation of *lacUV5*.

Question 3

Based on the results of both experiments, four regions of XBR were selected for mutagenesis studies. The goal was to eradicate the relationship between XBR and *pyx* by creating mutation(s) such that the XBR mutant would no longer be able to regulate *pyx* expression. Which of the following XBR amino acid sequences, if altered by mutation, presents the most promise for such a study?

- ○ **A.** Ala-Val-Phe-Leu-Ala-Val-Ile
- ○ **B.** Ala-Val-Asn-Leu-Gln-Val-Leu
- ○ **C.** Ala-Ile-Arg-Gly-Lys-Leu-Pro
- ○ **D.** Ala-Asp-Asn-Leu-Pro-Gly-Glu

Question 4

The rate of *pyx* expression in vitro can be modeled by the equation:

$$v = V_m A K_d + A$$

where V_m is the maximum rate of gene expression and A is the concentration of free transcription factor. The preceding is represented in graphic form as follows:

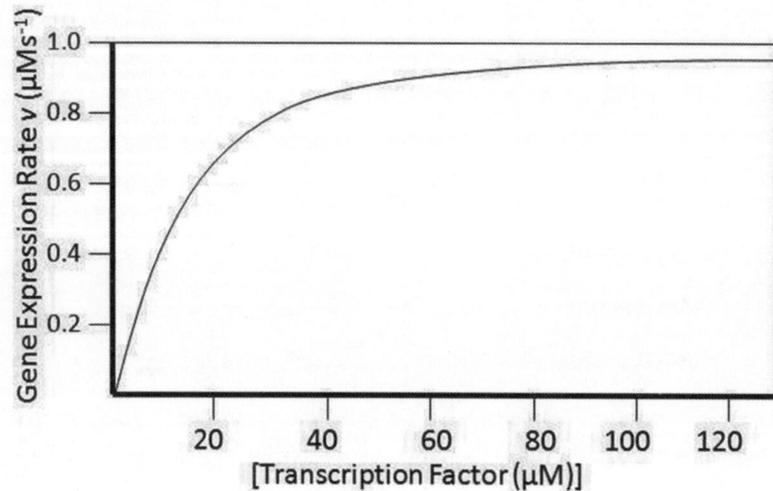

The dissociation constant K_d (M) is:

- A. 50
- B. 0.5
- C. 15
- D. 1.5×10^{-5}

Note: This page is left blank so that the passage would be visible without turning pages while assessing the passage-based questions.

Passage 2 (Questions 5–9)

The method of DNA replication proposed by James Watson and Francis Crick is known as semi-conservative replication since each new double helix retains one strand of the original DNA double helix. The evidence for this mechanism was provided by a series of classic experiments carried out by Meselson and Stahl in 1958 that proceeded as follows:

1. Cultures of the bacterium *E. coli*, which has a single circular chromosome, were grown for many generations in a medium containing the heavy isotope of nitrogen ^{15}N.
2. The cells containing the DNA labeled with ^{15}N were transferred to a culture medium containing the normal isotope of nitrogen (^{14}N).
3. After periods of time corresponding to the generation time for *E. coli* (50 min at 3 °C), samples were removed and the DNA extracted.
4. The DNA was then centrifuged at 40,000 times gravity for 20 h in a solution of cesium chloride (CsCl).

During centrifugation the heavy CsCl molecules began to sediment at the bottom of the centrifuge tubes, producing an increasing density gradient from the top of the tube to the bottom. The DNA settled out where its density equaled that of the CsCl solution. When examined under ultraviolet light, the DNA appeared in the centrifuge tube as a narrow band.

Two other hypotheses were advanced to explain the process of DNA replication. One is known as conservative replication and the other as dispersive replication. These hypotheses are summarized in Figure 1.

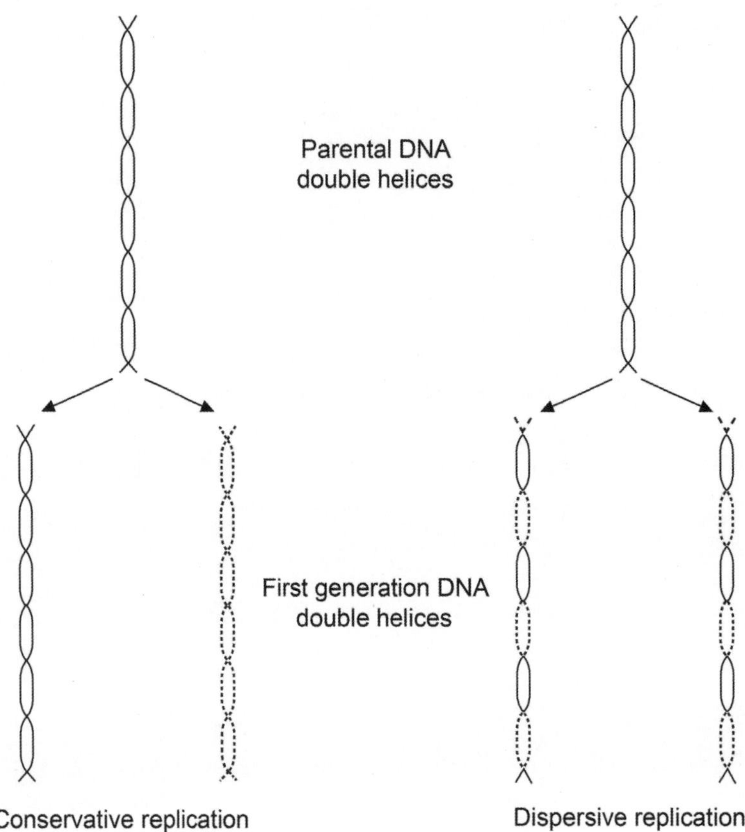

Figure 1

Question 5

Based on the passage, which of the following represents the appearance of the tubes after the cells had been allowed to grow in the ^{14}N for two generations?

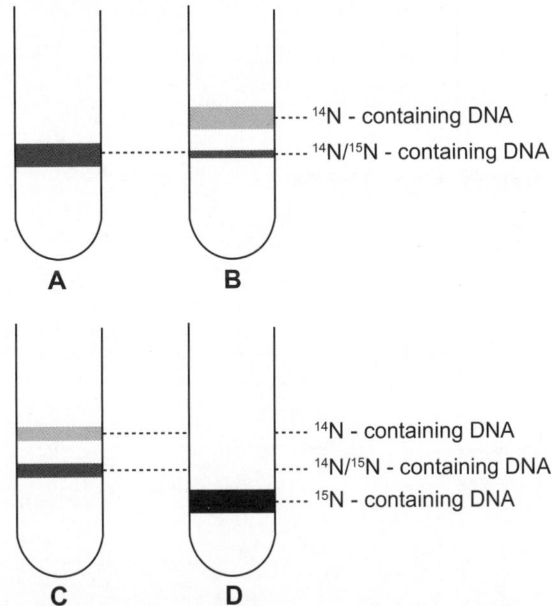

- O A.
- O B.
- O C.
- O D.

Question 6

Had conservative replication been the correct hypothesis, which of the following would represent the appearance of the tubes after the cells had been allowed to grow in the ^{14}N for one generation?

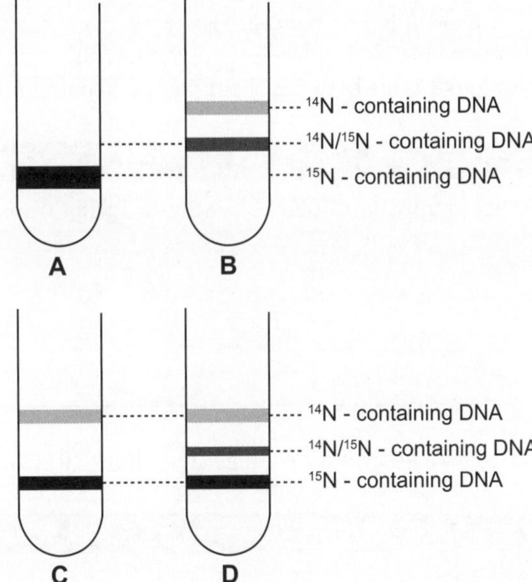

- O A.
- O B.
- O C.
- O D.

Question 7

Had dispersive replication been the correct hypothesis, which of the following would represent the appearance of the tubes after the cells had been allowed to grow in the ^{14}N for one generation?

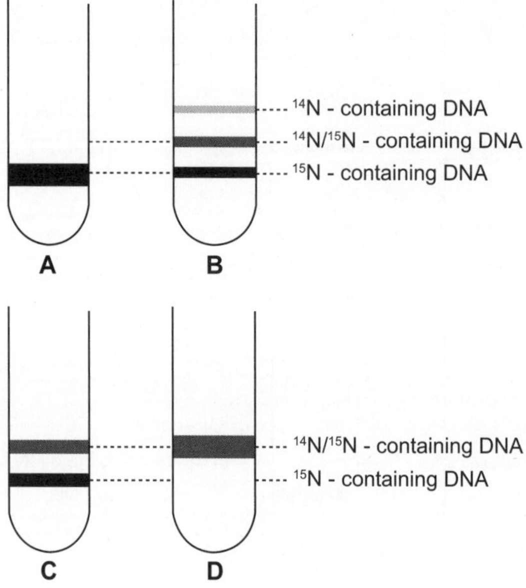

○ **A.**
○ **B.**
○ **C.**
○ **D.**

Question 8

Which of the following statements could be held LEAST accountable for DNA maintaining its helical structure?

○ **A.** Unwinding the helix would separate the base pairs enough for water molecules to enter between the bases, making the structure unstable.
○ **B.** The helix is stabilized by hydrogen bonds between bases.
○ **C.** The sugar phosphate backbone is held in place by hydrophilic interactions with the solvent.
○ **D.** C–G pairs have three hydrogen bonds between them, but A–T pairs only have two.

Question 9

Which of the following enzymes is most important in RNA synthesis during transcription?

○ **A.** DNA polymerase
○ **B.** RNA replicase
○ **C.** RNA polymerase
○ **D.** Reverse transcriptase

The following questions are NOT based on a descriptive passage (Questions 10–13).

Question 10

Glucose-1-phosphate is converted to glucose-6-phosphate during which of the following processes?

○ **A.** Glycogenolysis
○ **B.** Gluconeogenesis
○ **C.** Glycolysis
○ **D.** Glycogenesis

Question 11

A collection of nerve cell bodies in the central nervous system is generally referred to as a:

- O **A.** nerve.
- O **B.** Schwann node.
- O **C.** ganglion.
- O **D.** nucleus.

Question 12

Which of the following is true about muscle contraction?

- O **A.** Troponin and tropomyosin slide past each another, allowing the muscle to shorten.
- O **B.** Decreased intracellular [Ca^{++}] enhances the degree of muscular contraction.
- O **C.** Cardiac muscle fibers contain centrally located nuclei.
- O **D.** Neither actin nor myosin changes length during muscle contraction.

Question 13

Consider the following diagram that begins with a typical gene. The figure illustrates how such a gene leads to the synthesis of a protein identified as "p."

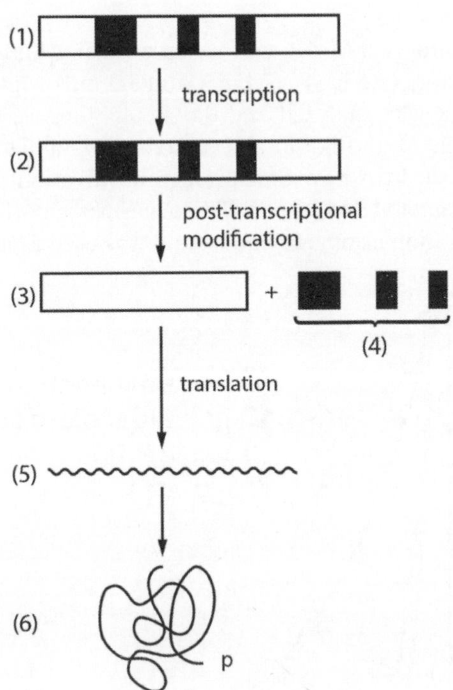

Regarding the diagram above, which of the following statements is true?

- O **A.** The thymine content of (1) and (2) is equal.
- O **B.** The number of nucleotide residues in (2) is twice the number of amino acid residues in (5).
- O **C.** The process occurring between (1) and (2) takes place in association with a ribosome.
- O **D.** The molecule (3) represents functional mRNA.

Passage 3 (Questions 14–17)

R-cembranoid (4R) is a natural compound that exerts neuroprotective effects by binding to nicotinic acetylcholine receptors (nAChRs). An important part of the preclinical development of all drugs is assessing their metabolism and pharmacokinetics. The structure of 4R is shown in Figure 1; it is a cembranoid that is metabolized into hydroxylated metabolites by cytochrome P450 enzymes.

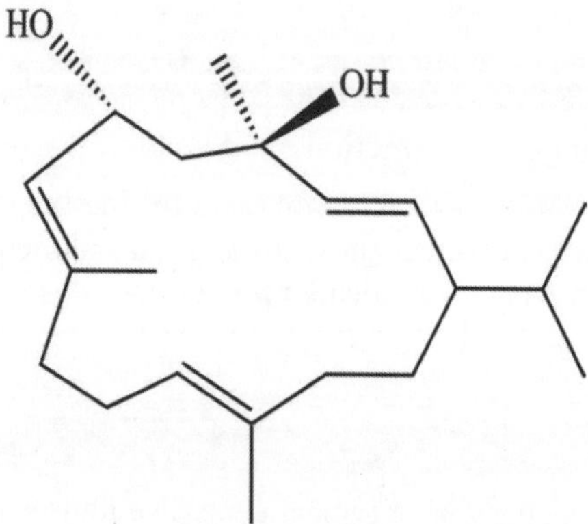

Figure 1 The structure of 4R

The metabolic stability of 1 μM and 10 μM 4R was assessed using male and female human and rat liver microsomes in the presence of cofactors (2.5 mM NADPH and 3.3 mM MgCl) at pH 7.4 for 0, 5, 15, 30, and 60 min at 37 °C. The metabolism of 4R was analyzed and the metabolites were identified using high-performance liquid chromatography (HPLC; Table 1) and liquid chromatography–tandem mass spectrometry (LC-MS/MS). The MS analysis was performed in electrospray ionization in positive ion mode (ESI+), and 4R was detected using the multiple reaction–monitoring (MRM) mode. The mean percent 4R at each incubation time point was compared with the baseline concentration at time 0; midazolam was used as a positive control.

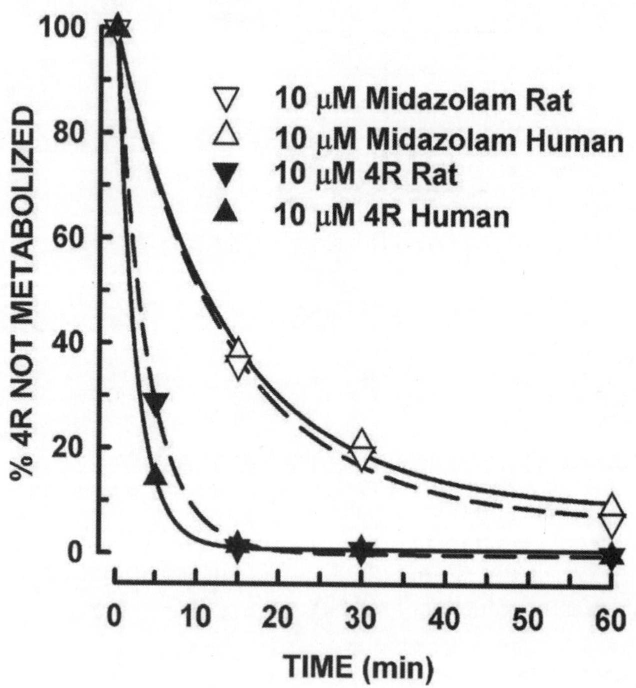

Figure 2 The metabolic stability of 4R was assessed in vitro using human and rat microsomes

The resulting metabolites identified are shown in Table 1, and their relative abundance is shown in Figure 3.

Table 1 The 4R Metabolites Detected with HPLC after Incubation in Human and Rat Liver Microsomes (a: retention time; b: the metabolites were identified using LC-MS/MS in MRM mode using a range of precursor masses with a common product ion mass of 95 m/z and a collision energy of 38 eV.

ID	RT[a] (min)	Major Precursor Mass[b] (m/z)	Precursor Form	Biotransformation
M1	6.29	303	$[M-2H_2O+H]^+$	di-hydroxylation
M2	7.02	303	$[M-2H_2O+H]^+$	di-hydroxylation
M3	7.93	321	$[M-H_2O+H]^+$	di-hydroxylation
M4	8.00	303	$[M-2H_2O+H]^+$	di-hydroxylation
M5	8.20	303	$[M-2H_2O+H]^+$	di-hydroxylation
M6	8.48	305	$[M-H_2O+H]^+$	hydroxylation
M7	8.76	287	$[M-2H_2O+H]^+$	hydroxylation
M8	9.11	321	$[M-H_2O+H]^+$	di-hydroxylation
M9	9.68	305	$[M-H_2O+H]^+$	hydroxylation
M10	9.92	305	$[M-H_2O+H]^+$	hydroxylation
4R	13.57	289	$[M-H_2O+H]^+$	(4R)

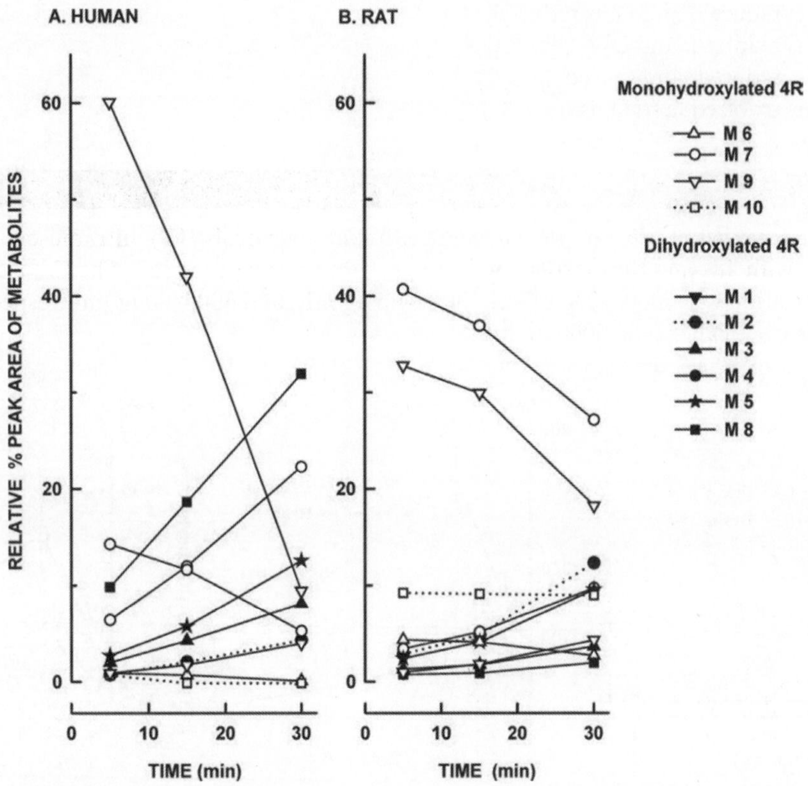

Figure 3 The relative abundance of 4R metabolites in human (A) and rat (B) microsomes, as determined using LC-MS/MS. The symbols represent the relative percent peak area of each metabolite, which was determined using the following equation:

(peak area of each metabolite per sample / total peak area of the 10 metabolites per sample) × 100

Source: Adapted from nih.gov, PMC4374761.

Question 14

According to the data presented in Figure 2, which of the following statements is NOT correct?

- ○ **A.** 4R is metabolized faster in human as opposed to rat microsomes.
- ○ **B.** 4R is metabolized faster than midazolam.
- ○ **C.** Midazolam is metabolized faster in human as opposed to rat microsomes.
- ○ **D.** 4R is metabolized completely within 20 minutes.

Question 15

HPLC with a polar stationary phase and a nonpolar mobile phase was used to separate 4R and its metabolites. Based on the data in Figure 3 and Table 1, which of the following statements describes the metabolites most accurately?

- ○ **A.** M1 is the most polar metabolite, and M10 is the least polar.
- ○ **B.** M10 is the most polar metabolite, and M1 is the least polar.
- ○ **C.** The dihydroxylated metabolites are more polar than the monohydroxylated metabolites.
- ○ **D.** There is no interconversion between di- and mono-hydroxylated metabolites.

Question 16

During the metabolism of 4R, cytochrome P450 enzymes metabolize 4R via the following reaction:

$$RH + O_2 + NADPH + H^+ \rightarrow ROH + H_2O + NADP^+$$

Which of the following chemical conversions occurs in the preceding reaction?

- ○ **A.** NADPH is reduced, and O_2 is reduced.
- ○ **B.** NADPH is oxidized, and O_2 is reduced.
- ○ **C.** NADPH is reduced, and O_2 is oxidized.
- ○ **D.** NADPH is oxidized, and O_2 is oxidized.

Question 17

To assess the clinical potential of 4R, rats were injected either intravenously (IV), intramuscularly (IM), or subcutaneously (SC) with 4R, and the plasma and brain distribution was assessed. The C_{max} achieved using IV, IM, and SC administration was 6000–8000 ng/mL, 300–400 ng/mL, and 300–400 ng/mL respectively. Tremors were observed with a C_{max} higher than 5000 ng/mL.

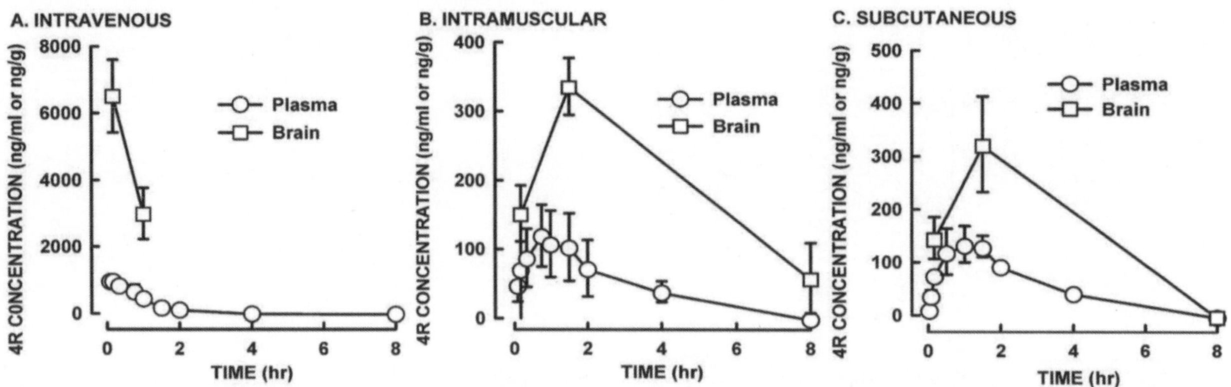

Which should be the first-choice and second-choice delivery routes in patients?

- ○ **A.** IV followed by IM
- ○ **B.** IV followed by SC
- ○ **C.** SC followed by IM
- ○ **D.** IM followed by SC

Note: This page is left blank so that the passage would be visible without turning pages while assessing the passage-based questions.

Passage 4 (Questions 18–22)

Initially, when there is no product, the addition of a small amount of substrate to an enzyme produces a rapid reaction. However, at a certain point, the addition of more substrate will not increase the rate any further. The K_m is the substrate concentration at which an enzyme-catalyzed reaction occurs at half its maximal velocity, $V_{max}/2$. K_m is called the Michaelis constant. Each enzyme has a unique K_m value.

A variety of molecules exist that can slow the rate of an enzyme-catalyzed reaction. They are called enzyme inhibitors. Inhibition may be reversible or irreversible. During competitive reversible inhibition, a compound structurally similar to the substrate associates with the enzyme's active site but is unable to react with it. While it remains there it prevents any molecules of true substrate from gaining access to the active site of the enzyme. However, if substrate concentration is increased, the rate of substrate-enzyme reaction also increases.

During noncompetitive reversible inhibition, the inhibitor forms an enzyme-inhibitor complex at a point on the enzyme other than its active site, preventing catalysis. When inhibitor saturation is reached, the rate of the reaction will be almost nil. Irreversible inhibitors completely inhibit enzymes, sometimes by causing the protein of the enzyme molecule to precipitate. Thus, a sufficiently high concentration of substrate negates the effect of the inhibitor.

Consider the data in the following table.

Table 1 Experimental Data Presenting the Rates of Protein Degradation (Rxn Rate) with Varying Concentrations of Trypsin and the Enzyme Inhibitor Inhibitin

Trial #	[trypsin] mmol/L	Rxn rate mmol $(Ls)^{-1}$	[inhibitin] mmol/L
1	5.6×10^{-4}	5.40	0
2	7.4×10^{-3}	5.45	3.6×10^{-6}
3	5.6×10^{-4}	1.98	7.2×10^{-6}
4	7.4×10^{-3}	2.02	1.1×10^{-5}
5	8.3×10^{-5}	0.04	1.4×10^{-5}

Question 18

What effect would a competitive reversible inhibitor be expected to have on V_{max} and K_m?

- O **A.** V_{max} would stay the same, but K_m would decrease.
- O **B.** V_{max} would stay the same, but K_m would increase.
- O **C.** K_m would stay the same, but V_{max} would decrease.
- O **D.** Both V_{max} and K_m would decrease.

Question 19

Extracts of the intestinal parasite *Ascaris* were found to contain irreversible noncompetitive inhibitors of human enzymes. The enzymes were likely:

- O **A.** HMG CoA synthetase and lyase.
- O **B.** NADH dehydrogenase and carboxypeptisomerase.
- O **C.** trypsin and pepsin.
- O **D.** hexokinase and vitamin D.

Question 20

Which of the following best accounts for the shape of the enzyme–substrate graph in the figure below?

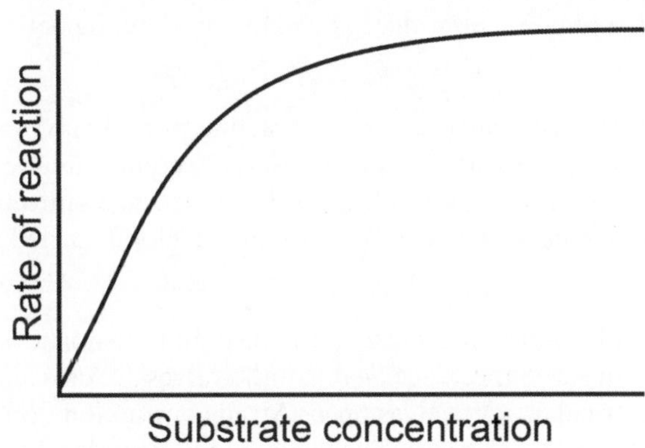

- O **A.** Enzyme–substrate specificity
- O **B.** Enzyme saturation
- O **C.** The formation of the enzyme–substrate complex
- O **D.** The K_m value unique to each enzyme

Question 21

Diisopropylfluorophosphate (DFP) acts as an irreversible inhibitor at the active site of acetylcholinesterase. This enzyme deactivates the chemical transmitter, acetylcholine. The main effect of DFP would be to:

- O **A.** prevent the passage of nerve impulses along the postsynaptic neuron.
- O **B.** prevent the entry of Ca^{2+} into the synaptic knob.
- O **C.** initiate muscular tetany.
- O **D.** generate a very large action potential.

Question 22

Given the data in Table 1, if researchers want to determine the effect that inhibitin has on the rate of product formation, Trial #3 should be compared with which of the following?

- O **A.** Trial #1
- O **B.** Trial #2
- O **C.** Trial #4
- O **D.** Trial #5

Passage 5 (Questions 23–27)

The process of depolarization triggers the cardiac cycle. The electronics of the cycle can be monitored by an electrocardiogram (EKG). The cycle is divided into two major phases, both named for events in the ventricle: the period of ventricular contraction and blood ejection, *systole*, followed by the period of ventricular relaxation and blood filling, *diastole*.

During the very first part of systole, the ventricles are contracting but all valves in the heart are closed thus no blood can be ejected. Once the rising pressure in the ventricles becomes great enough to open the aortic and pulmonary valves, the ventricular ejection or systole occurs. Blood is forced into the aorta and pulmonary trunk as the contracting ventricular muscle fibers shorten. The volume of blood ejected from a ventricle during systole is termed *stroke volume*.

During the very first part of diastole, the ventricles begin to relax, and the aortic and pulmonary valves close. No blood is entering or leaving the ventricles since once again all the valves are closed. Once ventricular pressure falls below atrial pressure, the atrioventricular (AV) valves open. Atrial contraction occurs towards the end of diastole, after most of the ventricular filling has taken place. The ventricle receives blood throughout most of diastole, not just when the atrium contracts. Figure 1 demonstrates the main events during the cardiac cycle.

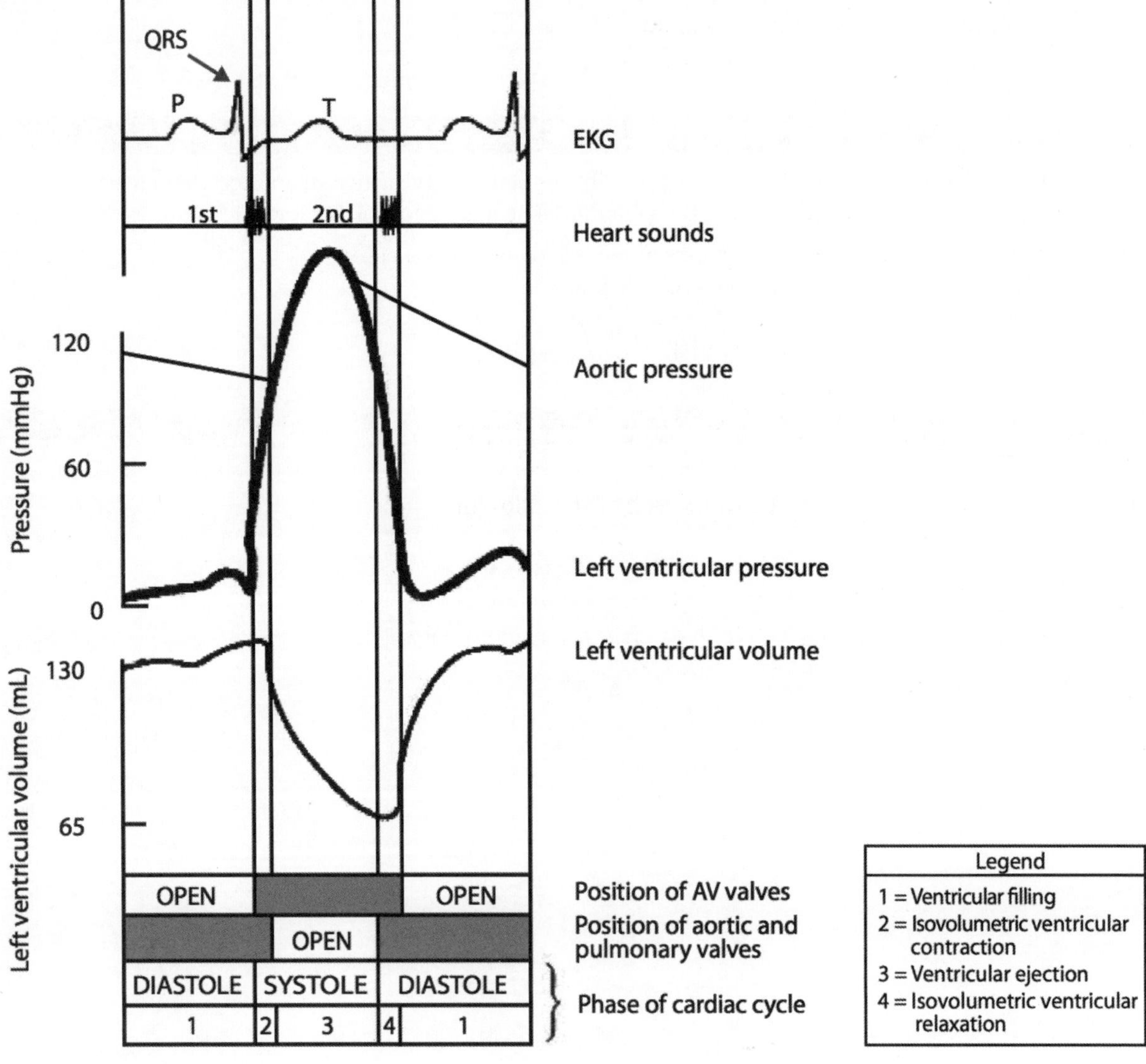

Figure 1 Electronic and pressure changes in the heart and aorta during the cardiac cycle.

Question 23

Position P on the EKG of Fig. 1 probably correspond to:

- O **A.** atrial contraction.
- O **B.** ventricular contraction.
- O **C.** the beginning of ventricular systole.
- O **D.** the beginning of ventricular diastole.

Question 24

The first heart sound represented in Fig. 1 is probably made when:

- O **A.** During ventricular systole, blood in the ventricle is forced against the closed atrioventricular valve.
- O **B.** During ventricular diastole, blood in the ventricles is forced through the aortic and pulmonary artery valves.
- O **C.** During ventricular diastole, blood in the ventricle is forced against the closed atrioventricular valve.
- O **D.** During ventricular systole, blood in the arteries is forced through the aortic and pulmonary artery valves.

Question 25

Would the walls of the atria or ventricles expected to be thicker?

- O **A.** Atria, because blood ejection due to atrial contraction is high.
- O **B.** Atria, because blood ejection due to atrial contraction is low.
- O **C.** Ventricles, because ventricular stroke volume is high.
- O **D.** Ventricles, because ventricular stroke volume is low.

Question 26

According to Fig. 1, the opening of the aortic and pulmonary valves is NOT associated with:

- O **A.** ventricular systole.
- O **B.** a rise and fall in aortic pressure.
- O **C.** a drop and rise in left ventricular volume.
- O **D.** the third phase of the cardiac cycle.

Question 27

The ejection fraction (EF) is defined as the ratio of the stroke volume to the volume of blood in the heart at the end of diastole (EDV), which is expressed as a percentage.

$$EF = (\text{Stroke Volume})/(EDV) \times 100\%$$

What is the best estimate of the ejection fraction indicated by Figure 1?

- O **A.** 40%
- O **B.** 50%
- O **C.** 60%
- O **D.** 100%

The following questions are NOT based on a descriptive passage (Questions 28–31).

Question 28

The developing fetus has a blood vessel, 'the ductus arteriosus', which connects the pulmonary artery to the aorta. When a baby is born, the ductus arteriosus closes permanently. Which of the following is the dominant feature found in a newborn baby whose ductus arteriosus did NOT obliterate?

- O **A.** Increased O_2 partial pressure in systemic arteries
- O **B.** Decreased CO_2 partial pressure in pulmonary arteries
- O **C.** Increased O_2 partial pressure in pulmonary arteries
- O **D.** Decreased O_2 partial pressure in systemic arteries

Question 29

Hemoglobin found in humans is composed of four chains that can each bind one oxygen molecule. Given a fully saturated hemoglobin molecule, the sigmoidal shape of the oxygen saturation curve in humans is an indication of which of the following?

- O **A.** The first oxygen molecule dissociates from the heme component, while the next three dissociate from the globin component.
- O **B.** It becomes easier to lose the second and third oxygen molecules.
- O **C.** It becomes more difficult to lose the second and third oxygen molecules.
- O **D.** The fourth oxygen molecule dissociates from the heme component, while the previous three dissociate from the globin component.

Question 30

When glucose monomers are joined together by glycosidic linkages to form a glycogen polymer, the changes in free energy, total energy, and entropy would be consistent with which of the following?

- O **A.** $+\Delta G$, $-\Delta H$, $-\Delta S$
- O **B.** $-\Delta G$, $+\Delta H$, $+\Delta S$
- O **C.** $+\Delta G$, $+\Delta H$, $-\Delta S$
- O **D.** $+\Delta G$, $+\Delta H$, $+\Delta S$

Question 31

Which of the following hormones found in the human menstrual cycle are produced in the ovary?

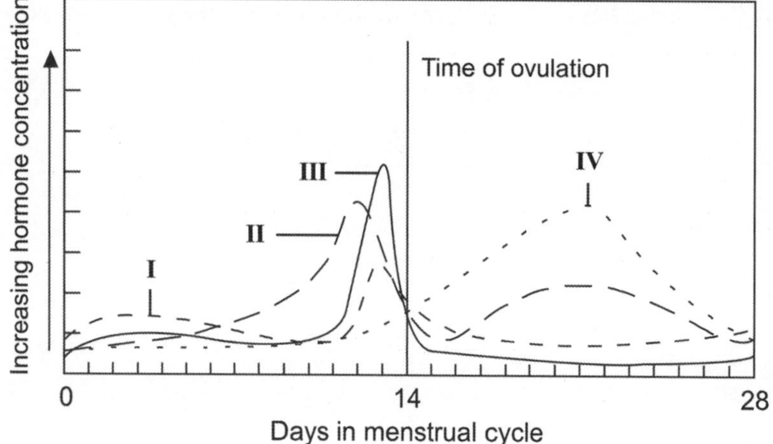

- O **A.** I and II
- O **B.** II and III
- O **C.** III and IV
- O **D.** II and IV

Note: This page is left blank so that the passage would be visible without turning pages while assessing the passage-based questions.

Passage 6 (Questions 32–35)

Mutations in the tumor suppressor protein p53 account for over 50% of all cases of human tumors. These mutations severely compromise the natural tumor suppression activity of the protein, often by causing instability followed by the unfolding of the protein or impeding the ability of the protein to bind to its target DNA sequences. Recent advances have turned to techniques such as thermal shift assays to find novel small-molecule compounds that can stabilize the protein by binding to structural cavities that are inadvertently caused by mutation.

Thermal shift assays measure the thermal stability of a protein, as well as any changes in the protein's melting temperature upon binding of a ligand. Protein samples are incubated in a buffer containing a fluorescent dye, such as Sypro Orange, which binds nonspecifically to hydrophobic surfaces. The fluorescence of the dye is typically quenched by water, but increases upon binding to the residues. The temperature is raised incrementally during the assay, and the fluorescence is read at each step. As the temperature approaches the protein's melting point, the protein unfolds, exposing the hydrophobic surfaces within the protein, leading to an increase in fluorescence. The midpoint value of the stability curve (Figure 1) marks the melting temperature, T_m.

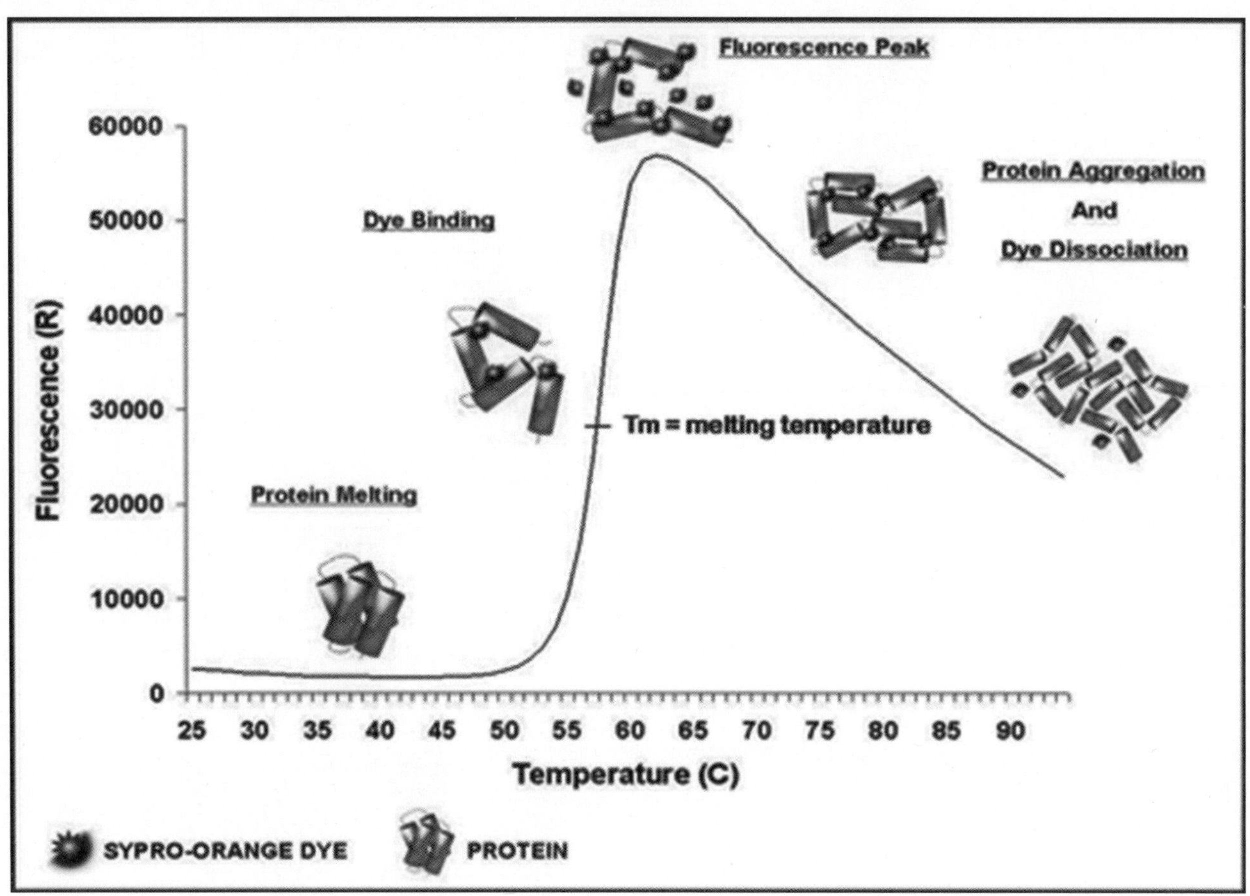

Figure 1 An example of a typical stability curve for a soluble protein

Experiment 1

Researchers identified one particular p53 mutant, p53A, which has a melting temperature lower than that of wild-type p53. Into four vials, 1 μM of p53A and Sypro Orange was aliquoted and stored at 4 °C. An hour before the assay, the vials were treated with either DMSO or a test drug, Stablivin, solubilized in DMSO in concentrations of 100 μM, 1 mM, or 10 mM. A fifth vial contained wild-type (WT) p53 as a positive control. The temperature was raised 0.5 °C per minute, and the fluorescence was read at each step (Figure 2).

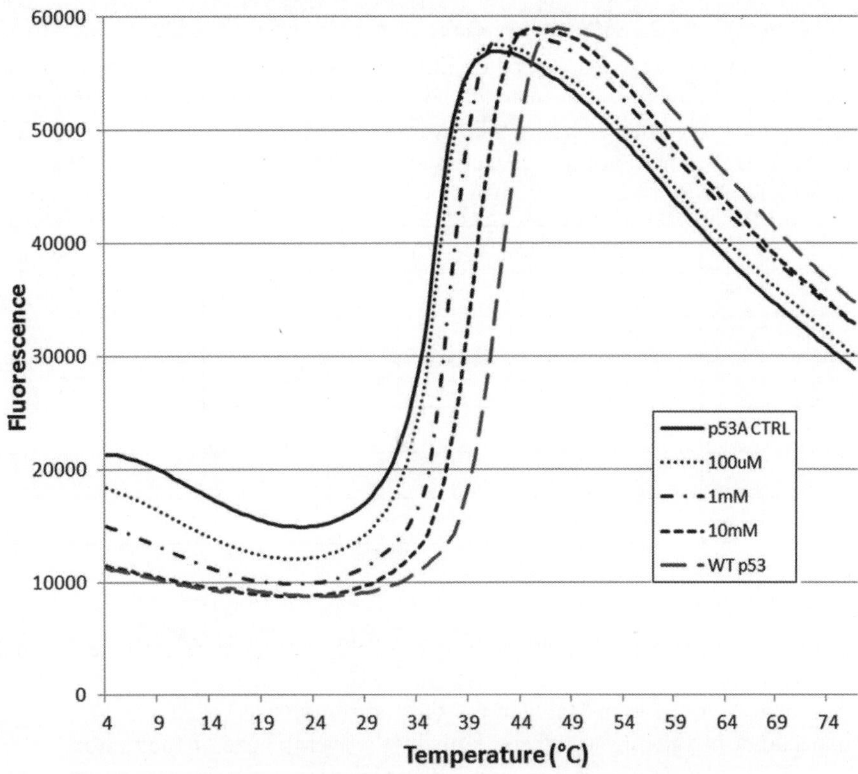

Figure 2 Thermal shift assay results for WT p53 and mutant p53A with or without increasing concentrations of Stablivin

The experiment was repeated multiple times, with results mirroring those shown in Figure 2. Subsequent assays showed that the addition of Stablivin did not affect p53A's ability to bind DNA.

Question 32

What effect does the addition of 10 mM Stablivin have on p53A?

- ○ **A.** It increases the T_m by 3 °C.
- ○ **B.** It increases the T_m by 9 °C.
- ○ **C.** It increases the T_m by 15 °C.
- ○ **D.** It restores wild-type functionality to p53A.

Question 33

Structural characterization of p53A shows that unlike some other p53 mutants, the DNA-binding region of p53A is unaffected. Given the experimental data and the information given in the passage, one might conclude that:

- ○ **A.** patients with the p53A mutation will not see adverse effects.
- ○ **B.** patients with the p53A mutation will be at a higher risk for tumor formation than those with no p53 mutations.
- ○ **C.** Stablivin binds to p53A's DNA-binding region.
- ○ **D.** the data in Figure 2 is irrelevant.

Question 34

Five groups of 10 mice each with already-developed p53A tumors were injected daily with Stablivin, and the results were recorded in a table. Stablivin was injected daily, as previous studies showed that the drug is removed from the bloodstream by the body after 24 hours. The average life expectancy was calculated with the first day of the experiment counted as Day 0; remaining mice were sacrificed after 60 days.

	Average tumor size (mm) after X days				Avg. life expectancy
Daily dose (mM)	0	10	20	30	
0.01	10	15	19	25	34
0.1	10	14	19	25	35
1	10	11	13	16	45
5	10	9	7	5	60
10	10	8	6	4	33

The researchers likely concluded that:

- ○ **A.** patients should receive dosages of Stablivin that would most likely restore the thermal stability of wild-type p53.
- ○ **B.** there is no correlation between Stablivin dosage and tumor size.
- ○ **C.** the life expectancy of the mice is affected only by the average size of the tumors.
- ○ **D.** Stablivin is toxic at daily dosages of around 10 mM.

Question 35

Thermal shift assays can be performed using a number of different fluorescent dyes. Some, such as Sypro Orange, are not suitable for usage with membrane proteins. Which of the following might be a suitable explanation?

- ○ **A.** Dyes cannot permeate through the lipid bilayer.
- ○ **B.** Membrane proteins have hydrophobic surfaces.
- ○ **C.** Sypro Orange does not bind to membrane proteins.
- ○ **D.** Membrane proteins are unstable at high temperatures.

Note: This page is left blank so that the passage would be visible without turning pages while assessing the passage-based questions.

Passage 7 (Questions 36–40)

The sequence of events during synaptic transmission at the neuromuscular junction can be summarized as follows.

The depolarization produced by an action potential in the synaptic terminal opens voltage-dependent calcium channels in the terminal membrane. Calcium ions enter the terminal down their concentration and electrical gradients, inducing synaptic vesicles filled with acetylcholine (ACh) to fuse with the plasma membrane facing the muscle cell. The ACh is thereby dumped into the synaptic cleft, and some of it diffuses across the cleft to combine with specific receptors on ACh-activated channels. When ACh is bound, the channel opens and allows sodium and potassium ions to cross the membrane. This depolarizes the muscle membrane and triggers an all-or-none action potential in the muscle cell. The action of ACh is terminated by the enzyme acetylcholinesterase, which splits ACh into acetate and choline.

In order to determine how and under what conditions ACh works, the following experiments were done.

Experiment 1

Determining the Effect of the Timing of Calcium Action on Transmitter Release

Calcium ions were removed from the bathing solution of a muscle cell so that release of ACh in response to nerve stimulation was virtually abolished. Calcium ions were then applied to the nerve terminal by ionophoresis from a micropipette close to the terminal just before the nerve was stimulated (N), without nerve stimulation, and just after the nerve was stimulated. The results obtained are shown in Figure 1.

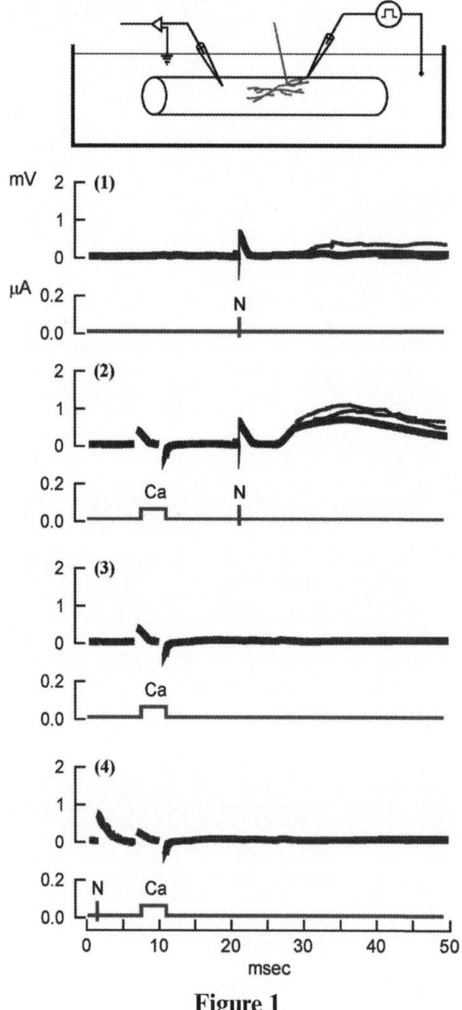

Figure 1

Experiment 2

Determining the Effect of ACh on Neuromuscular Transmission and Its Subsequent Action on the Postsynaptic Membrane

Stimulating electrodes were placed on the nerve, and a pair of recording electrodes was placed on the muscle. One of the electrodes was placed very close to the end plate region. First curare and then eserine were added to the solution bathing the muscle. The action potentials produced on stimulating the nerve were recorded. The results obtained are shown in Figure 2.

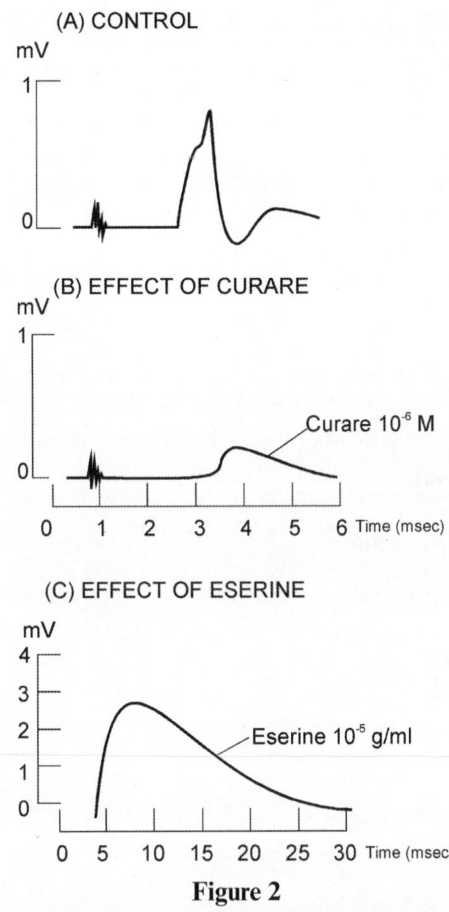

Figure 2

Question 36

At the neuromuscular junction, the receptors on the ACh-activated channels are likely located:

- o **A.** on the tubule of the T system.
- o **B.** in the sarcolemma.
- o **C.** on the muscle surface.
- o **D.** in the synaptic cleft.

Question 37

The depolarization across the muscle membrane triggers an all-or-none action potential in the muscle cell. This suggests that an increase in the amount of transmitter released at the neuromuscular junction would change:

- o **A.** the amplitude of the action potential.
- o **B.** the frequency of the nerve impulses.
- o **C.** the direction of the action potential.
- o **D.** the speed at which nerve impulses travel along the muscle cell.

Question 38

A mutation in the gene that codes for acetylcholinesterase would likely inhibit all, but which of the following processes?

- ○ **A.** A hyperpolarization in the postsynaptic membrane
- ○ **B.** A depolarization in the postsynaptic membrane
- ○ **C.** The passage of a series of nerve impulses along the axon of the postsynaptic neuron
- ○ **D.** The development of an inhibitory postsynaptic potential

Question 39

According to Figure 1, which of the following conclusions was confirmed by the experiment?

- ○ **A.** For transmitter release to occur, calcium ions need only be present after the depolarization of the presynaptic membrane.
- ○ **B.** The presence of calcium ions is the only variable that affects transmitter release at the synapse.
- ○ **C.** For transmitter release to occur, calcium ions must be present before and after depolarization of the presynaptic membrane.
- ○ **D.** For transmitter release to occur, calcium ions must be present before depolarization of the presynaptic membrane.

Question 40

In the control of Figure 2, the part of the curve between 4 and 5 msec is most consistent with:

- ○ **A.** the absolute refractory period.
- ○ **B.** the relative refractory period.
- ○ **C.** the depolarization of the membrane.
- ○ **D.** saltatory conduction.

Note: This page is left blank so that the passage would be visible without turning pages while assessing the passage-based questions.

Passage 8 (Questions 41–44)

Rhodopsin, also called visual purple because of its purple hue, is the main pigment found in mammalian rod photoreceptors in the retina. The membrane protein belongs to the G protein–coupled receptor family and is extremely sensitive to light. Exposure to light causes the isomerization of a bound retinal molecule in the center of the protein, which triggers a rapid conformational change that triggers an intracellular signaling cascade.

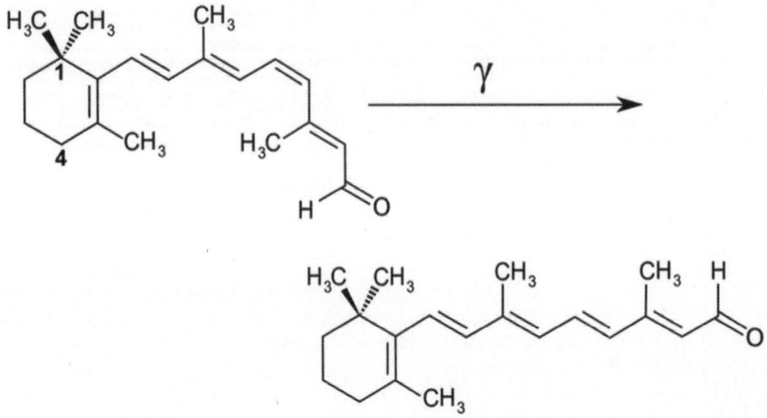

Figure 1 The photoisomerization of retinal with annotation of C-1 and C-4 (note that the numbering of carbons in retinoids begins in the ring and then continues in sequence)

Changes to rhodopsin's shape cause retinal to be ejected, photobleaching the rhodopsin. Eventually, the protein plus retinal complex is regenerated to its original state, a cycle that can take up to 45 minutes.

Researchers are able to determine the kinetics of this photobleaching reaction by measuring the amount of regenerated rhodopsin as a function of time after a flash of bright light.

The recovery of rhodopsin is given by the following equation, where p is the amount of pigment still present and the time, t, is in seconds:

$$1 - p = e^{-(t/400)}$$

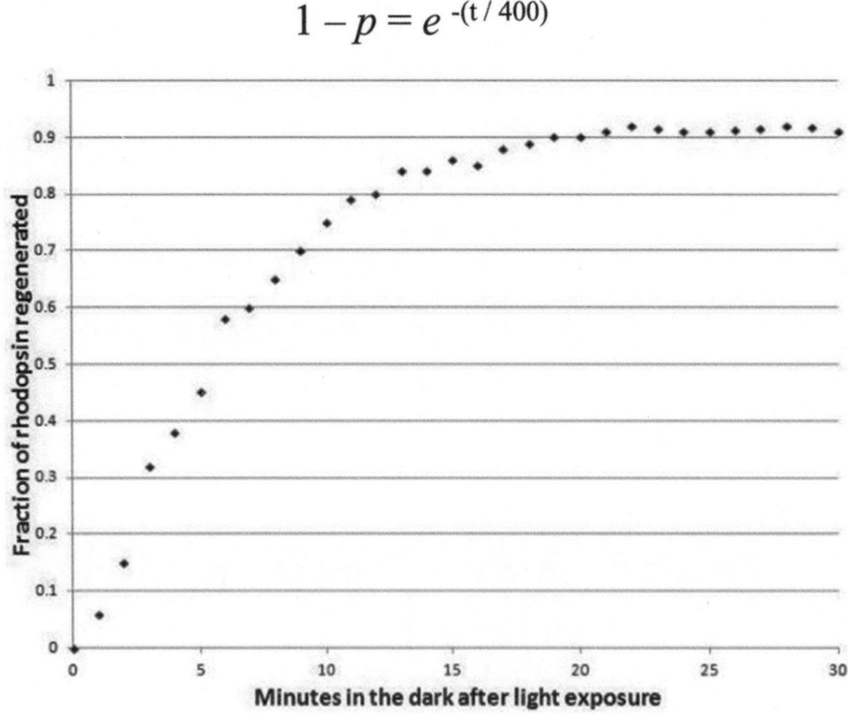

Figure 2 Regeneration of rhodopsin in the dark after initial light exposure as a measure of time

Question 41

When light falls on rod cells:

○ **A.** all-*cis*-retinal is converted to 11-*trans*-retinal.
○ **B.** 11-*cis*-retinal is converted to 11-*trans*-retinol.
○ **C.** 11-*trans*-retinal is converted to all-*trans*-retinal.
○ **D.** 11-*cis*-retinal is converted to all-*trans*-retinal.

Question 42

After 10 minutes in the dark, what fraction of rhodopsin is photobleached?

○ **A.** 0.10
○ **B.** 0.50
○ **C.** 0.25
○ **D.** 0.75

Question 43

The equation for the recovery of rhodopsin gives a time constant of 350 seconds. This represents:

○ **A.** the average amount of time required for half of the rhodopsin to be regenerated.
○ **B.** the time required for all of the rhodopsin to reach full regeneration.
○ **C.** the rate at which rhodopsin generates after light exposure.
○ **D.** the maximum velocity of rhodopsin regeneration.

Question 44

Retinitis pigmentosa is a group of inherited progressive disorders of rod cells that can lead to complete blindness. Which of the following is LEAST likely to be associated with retinitis pigmentosa?

○ **A.** A mutation in the gene coding for rhodopsin
○ **B.** Increase in the minimum time for regeneration after light exposure
○ **C.** Color blindness in the early stages of disease presentation
○ **D.** A mutation in rhodopsin pre-mRNA splicing factors

The following questions are NOT based on a descriptive passage (Questions 45–48).

Question 45

Consider Figure 1, where the black dots represent the active form of enzyme M and the white dots represent the active form of enzyme N at varying pH values and temperatures.

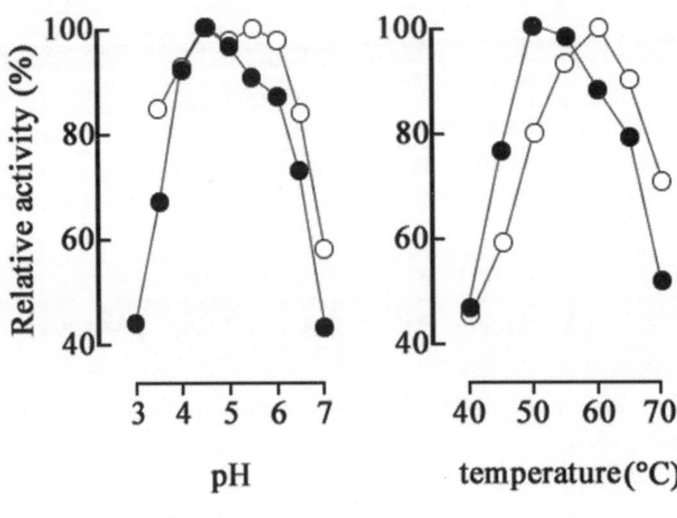

Figure 1

Which of the following can be correctly determined from Figure 1?

- O **A.** In reaching its peak, enzyme N exhibits the greater increase in activity per degree Celsius.
- O **B.** Enzyme M can sustain a percentage activity of more than 80% over a wider pH range.
- O **C.** Based on the data below 50 °C, extrapolating a linear regression line predicts that enzyme M would have less than 20% activity at 30 °C.
- O **D.** Given either a particular pH or temperature, there are instances of more than 30% difference in activity between the two enzymes under study.

Question 46

Which of the following is MOST consistent with the process of inhalation?

- O **A.** The thoracic cage moves inward as the diaphragm moves downward.
- O **B.** The internal pressure is positive with respect to atmospheric pressure.
- O **C.** The phrenic nerve is stimulated.
- O **D.** The diaphragm relaxes.

Question 47

The genetic basis of human blood types includes recessive (Z^O) and codominant alleles (Z^A and Z^B). Determine which of the following genotypes produce blood that agglutinates when combined with type O serum.

I. Z^AZ^A
II. Z^AZ^B
III. Z^AZ^O

- O **A.** I only
- O **B.** III only
- O **C.** I and II only
- O **D.** I, II, and III

Question 48

Both bacteria and eukaryotic cells may share all of the following features EXCEPT:

- ○ **A.** phospholipid bilayer.
- ○ **B.** cell wall.
- ○ **C.** ribosomes.
- ○ **D.** nuclear membrane.

Passage 9 (Questions 49–52)

The investigation of the mechanism and regulation of DNA replication in bacteria helps in the understanding and treatment of many infectious disorders. Models are sometimes produced to project possible drug actions or interactions.

Experimental Drug Model

The normal rate of DNA replication in *E. coli* approximates 750 nucleotides per second, which can be upregulated by protein Q (Prot Q), which can be blocked by P10-22, a drug under investigation. Enzyme C-rel downregulates gene expression of DNA Pol II and III through the inducing activity of Ruvase-2. Protein Q can bind C-rel, though the exact effect is not known. P10-22 leads to an increased activation of C-rel by upregulating Ruvase-2. The gene that produces C-rel is upregulated by the fourth-generation quinolone, Drovan (an antibiotic).

The following diagram summarizes the results of the main trials.

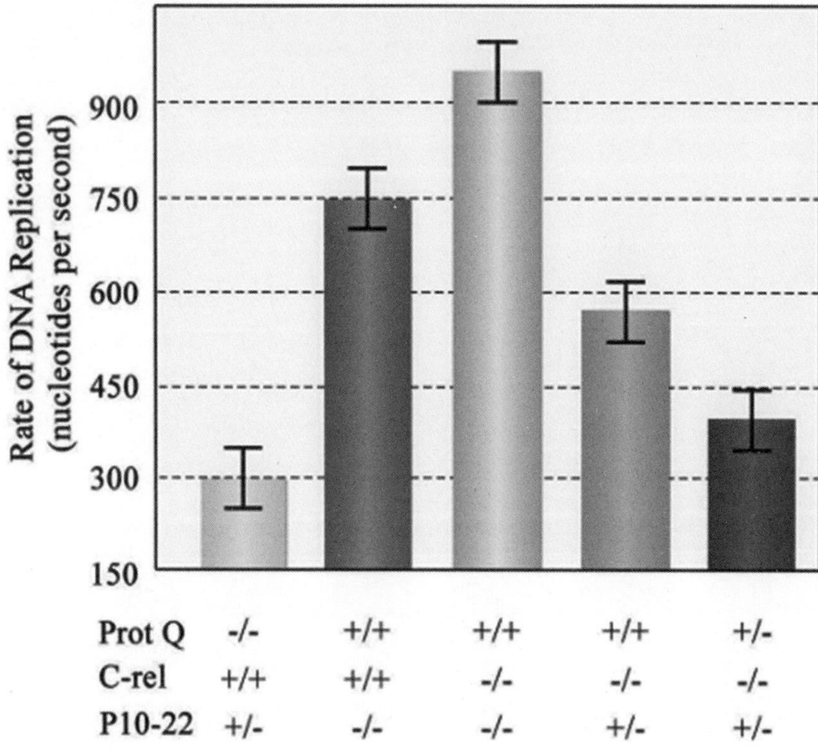

Figure 1 Summary of the effect of protein Q, C-rel and P10-22 on DNA replication in *E. coli*

Question 49

Which of the following pairs of compounds, when increased in concentration, can act independently of each other to reduce *E. coli* DNA replication?

- O **A.** C-rel, Drovan
- O **B.** Drovan, P10-22
- O **C.** P10-22, Prot Q
- O **D.** Prot Q, Ruvase-2

Question 50

Which of the following is most strongly suggested by Figure 1?

○ **A.** The first of the five bar diagrams is likely the control.
○ **B.** In the presence of a full concentration of Prot Q and absence of C-rel, giving P10-22 reduces the replication rate by 60%.
○ **C.** C-rel has more of an effect on DNA replication than P10-22.
○ **D.** C-rel is likely quite active in wild-type *E. coli.*

Question 51

Which of the following is most consistent with the information presented?

○ **A.** High concentrations of Prot Q in the presence of Drovan would be expected to have a greater effect than in the presence of P10-22.
○ **B.** Drovan's antibiotic resistance occurs with repeated trials.
○ **C.** If it were determined that Prot Q downregulated C-rel, then this would not be consistent with the overall effect of Prot Q.
○ **D.** If P10-22 does not have the substrate C-rel to activate, it has no observable effect on DNA replication.

Question 52

When the base composition of *E. coli* DNA was determined, 16% of the bases were found to be adenine. What is the G + C content?

○ **A.** 16%
○ **B.** 32%
○ **C.** 34%
○ **D.** 68%

Passage 10 (Questions 53–56)

The main regulatory molecules for acid secretion in the human stomach include three that stimulate acid secretion (acetylcholine, histamine, gastrin) and one that inhibits acid secretion (somatostatin). Acetylcholine is a neurotransmitter that can be released by enteric neurons via vagal stimulation. Histamine is a paracrine that is released from ECL (enterochromaffin-like) cells. Gastrin is a hormone that is released by G cells located in the gastric epithelium. Somatostatin, which can act as a paracrine or a hormone, is secreted by D cells of the gastric epithelium. The main interactions are summarized in Figure 1.

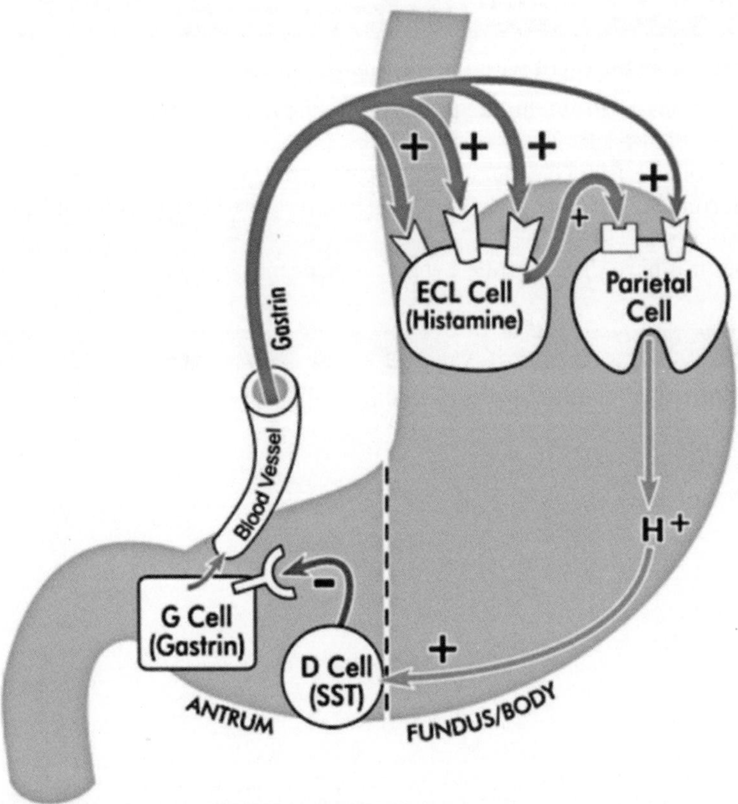

Figure 1 Regulation of gastric acid secretion by gastrin, histamine, somatostatin (SST), and acid in the gastric lumen

Cimetidine (Tagamet) was among the first of the rational drug-design structures, and the process began by assessing the structure of histamine. Cimetidine is now a popular, inexpensive antacid that can reduce the incidence of gastritis, reflux, and peptic ulcer disease. Major steps in the design of cimetidine include (1) using a histamine receptor model (H2) that led to the development of burimamide; (2) improving on the efficacy and safety of burimamide (see image below) by replacing sulfur with nitrogen with an additional functional group to reduce the protonated form of this antacid, which eventually resulted in the production of cimetidine. As one of the first rational drug designs, one of its main designers, who also discovered the heart medication, propanolol, won the 1988 Nobel Prize in Physiology/Medicine.

HN S N N N H H

Burimamide

Table 1 The pKa of Various Functional Groups

Functional group	Equilibrium	pKa
nitro	$C_6H_5N^{+}(=O)OH \rightleftharpoons C_6H_5N^{+}(=O)O^{-} + H^+$	-11.3
nitrile	$H_3C{-}C{\equiv}N^{+}{-}H \rightleftharpoons H_3C{-}C{\equiv}N{:} + H^+$	-10.1
ketone	$(H_3C)_2C{=}O^{+}{-}H \rightleftharpoons (H_3C)_2C{=}O + H^+$	-7.2
thiol	$H_3C{-}S^{+}H_2 \rightleftharpoons H_3C{-}S{-}H + H^+$	-6.8
phosphoric acid	$^{-}O{-}P(=O)(OH){-}OH \rightleftharpoons {}^{-}O{-}P(=O)(O^{-}){-}OH + H^+$	7.2
β-keto thioester	$H_3CH_2C{-}S{-}C(=O){-}CH_2{-}C(=O){-}CH_3 \rightleftharpoons H_3CH_2C{-}S{-}C(=O){-}C^{-}H{-}C(=O){-}CH_3 + H^+$	8.5
amide	$H_3C{-}C(=O){-}NH_2 \rightleftharpoons H_3C{-}C(=O){-}N^{-}H + H^+$	15.0
alcohol	$H_3CH_2C{-}O{-}H \rightleftharpoons H_3CH_2C{-}O^{-} + H^+$	15.9

Source: Image of the regulation of gastric acid secretion from the collection of Professor Mitchell L. Schubert, with the acknowledgement of Mary Beatty-Brooks (medical illustrator).

Question 53

In addition to stimulating gastric chief cells, cholinergic activity from the vagus nerve increases acid production by stimulating parietal cells. Yet another action of the cholinergic activity from the vagus, consistent with the information provided, would likely be which of the following?

- O **A.** Sensitizing ECL cells to gastrin
- O **B.** Sensitizing parietal cells to somatostatin
- O **C.** Desensitizing ECL cells to gastrin
- O **D.** Desensitizing parietal cells to histamine

Question 54

Given the information about burimamide and Table 1, which of the following functional groups added to the nitrogen replacing the sulfur atom in burimamide would be the most rational in the production of cimetidine?

- A. Nitrile
- B. Thiol
- C. Phosphoric acid
- D. Amide

Question 55

Cimetidine likely functions by:

- A. not binding to the histamine receptor and acting as an agonist.
- B. not binding to the histamine receptor and acting as an antagonist.
- C. binding to the histamine receptor and acting as an agonist.
- D. binding to the histamine receptor and acting as an antagonist.

Question 56

Various cimetidine–copper complexes have been evaluated for a superoxide dismutase (SOD)–like activity. SODs are important antioxidants that catalyze the dismutation (or partitioning) of the potentially damaging superoxide (O_2^-) radical into either ordinary molecular oxygen (O_2) or hydrogen peroxide (H_2O_2), which is less damaging than superoxide.

Consider the following kinetic parameters obtained with cimetidine complex–catalyzed dismutation in the presence of fluoride anions.

Cimetidine Complex 1		Cimetidine Complex 2	
$[F^-]$, μM	k_{cat}, s^{-1}	$[F^-]$, μM	k_{cat}, s^{-1}
0	8.4 +/- 0.5	0	8.3 +/- 0.5
10	8.6 +/- 0.5	10	2.7 +/- 0.3
20	8.5 +/- 0.5	20	~ 0

Based on these data, which of the following best describes the effect of fluoride on cimetidine complexes in the presence of superoxide?

I. Fluoride acts as an agonist of one of the two complexes.
II. Fluoride acts as an inhibitor of one of the two complexes.
III. Fluoride likely displaces the copper component of at least one of the cimetidine complexes.

- A. I only
- B. II only
- C. II and III only
- D. I, II, and III

The following questions are NOT based on a descriptive passage (Questions 57–59).

Question 57

Which of the following is NOT associated with a large negative free energy of hydrolysis?

- O **A.** Phosphoenolpyruvate
- O **B.** 3-Phosphoglycerate
- O **C.** 1,3-Diphosphoglycerate
- O **D.** ADP

Question 58

Huntington's disease is an autosomal dominant disorder. If the frequency of the dominant allele for Huntington's disease is 0.6 in a particular isolated population, what proportion of the population is free of the disease?

- O **A.** 0.06
- O **B.** 0.16
- O **C.** 0.36
- O **D.** 0.40

Question 59

The structure of D-glucose is shown below:

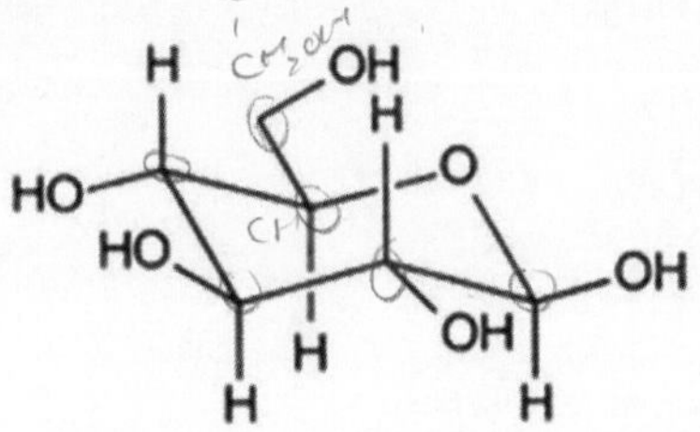

An alternative projection system often used in carbohydrate chemistry is the Fischer system. Fischer projections are particularly useful devices for depicting the absolute configuration at the various stereocenters of a compound. Which of the following most accurately represents the modified Fischer projection of D-glucose?

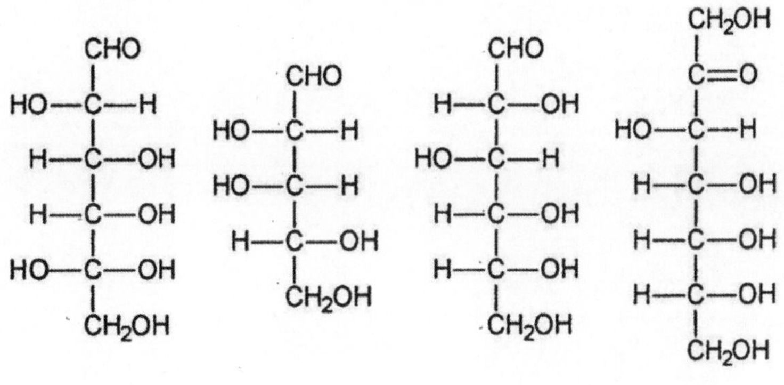

A. B. C. D.

- O **A.**
- O **B.**
- O **C.**
- O **D.**

CANDIDATE'S NAME ______________________________

RAW SCORE AND SCALED SCORE ______________________

GS-1
Mock Exam 1 of 7
Solutions at MCAT-prep.com

GS-1 Section IV: Psychological, Social, and Biological Foundations of Behavior

Questions: 1-59
Time: 95 minutes

INSTRUCTIONS: Of all the questions on this test, most are organized into groups preceded by a passage. After evaluating the passage, select the best answer to each question in the group. Fifteen questions are independent of any descriptive passage or each other. Similarly, select the best answer to these questions. If you are unsure of an answer, eliminate the alternatives that you know to be incorrect and select an answer from the remaining alternatives. To indicate your selection, use a pencil to blacken the corresponding circle next to the answer choice and/or you can use the answer document at the back of this book. No marks are deducted for wrong answers.

The computer-based real MCAT has an on-screen highlighter function and ~~STRIKEOUT~~ function. These tools help to spotlight text or assist in the process of elimination. You may use a yellow highlighter for this paper-based exam and/or a pen (or preferably a pencil to make it easier should you change your mind) to mark text. At the time of publishing, both highlighting and strikeout functions can be used for passages, questions and answer choices. You can also flag a question to review later should time remain.

For the real exam, you will be provided with a dry erase board which is a white laminated noteboard booklet accompanied by a fine point marker. The noteboard includes 9 graph-lined pages for you to write though you cannot erase. You can simulate the experience with a fine point marker on a noteboard or with 8" x 14" plain graph paper.

Please note: For the real MCAT, a small number of field-tested questions will remain unscored.

This practice test has been designed exclusively to test knowledge and thinking skills. This exam may contain hypothetical statements and/or express controversial ideas. Statements contained herein do not necessarily reflect the policy, position, or view of RuveneCo Inc. or MCAT-prep.com.

START EXAM ONLY WHEN TIMER IS READY.

Passage 1 (Questions 1–4)

Schizophrenia is one of the most severe and disabling psychiatric diagnoses, affecting about 1% of the American population. It is usually characterized by its cognitive symptomatology (e.g., hallucinations and delusions). Yet deficits in social functioning can also help to diagnose this disorder. This social symptomatology is found in relatives of diagnosed schizophrenics and in people with other psychopathological conditions, namely diagnosed autists and suicide attempters.

Impaired social functioning in diagnosed schizophrenics helps to predict relapses, poor illness course, and unemployment. Assessed areas include deficits in personal hygiene, community functioning, and social cognition. For example, face processing, voice processing, and facial and vocal emotion recognition are aspects of social cognition that have been found to be impaired both in diagnosed schizophrenics and in individuals with schizoid personality traits.

An investigation of the consequences of facial and voice recognition deficits in 20 diagnosed schizophrenics with no comorbidity, and in matched healthy controls adopted the following measures: facial recognition; facial affect recognition; neutral face recognition; vocal affect recognition; pitch perception; and a social functioning scale, assessing the domain of public self (behavior, appearance, and social presentation), independent living, occupational functioning, family relationships, important relationships other than family, community/leisure/recreation, acceptance and adherence to health regimens, communication, and locus of control. Results confirmed the previous findings associating face-related and voice-related deficits with the disorder. Table 1 shows correlations between some of this study's measures.

A study of the neural correlates of social cognition compared data from 146 autism spectrum disorder participants (autism group), 336 schizophrenic participants (schizophrenia group), and 492 healthy control subjects (control group). During functional magnetic resonance imaging (fMRI), participants performed two tasks: facial emotion recognition (FER) and theory of mind (ToM) paradigms. The autism group showed more pronounced medial prefrontal hypoactivation. The hypoactivation of the amygdala was found in both the schizophrenia and autism groups, specifically during FER for the schizophrenia group and during more complex ToM tasks for the autism group. Both groups also showed hypoactivation within the superior temporal sulcus during ToM tasks, though its hypoactivation was higher during FER in the autism group. Finally, somatosensory engagement was higher in the schizophrenia group and lower in the autism group.

Table 1 The Correlation Matrix for the Cognitive Tasks and Specific Domains of Social Functioning

	Face Affect	Vocal Affect	Test of Facial Recognition
Face Affect Recognition			
Vocal Affect Recognition	0.35		
Test of Facial Recognition	0.43*	0.47*	
Communication Dysfunction	−0.59**	−0.1	0.1
Occupational Dysfunction	−0.56**	−0.58**	−0.2
Public Self	−0.46*	−0.1	−0.04

* $p \leq 0.1$ (2-tailed, unadjusted)
** $p \leq 0.05$ (2-tailed, unadjusted)

Sources: Adapted from S.M. Couture, D.L. Penn, and D.L. Roberts, "The Functional Significance of Social Cognition in Schizophrenia: A Review." Copyright 2006 Schizophrenia Bulletin; G. Sugranyes, M. Kyriakopoulos, R. Corrigallet et al., "Autism Spectrum Disorders and Schizophrenia: Meta-analysis of the Neural Correlates of Social Cognition." Copyright 2011 PloS one; C. Hooker and S. Park, "Emotion Processing and Its Relationship to Social Functioning in Schizophrenia Patients." Copyright 2002 Psychiatry Research; K. Szanto, A.Y. Dombrovski, B.J. Sahakian et al. "Social Emotion Recognition, Social Functioning, and Attempted Suicide in Late-life Depression." Copyright 2012 American Journal of Geriatric Psychiatry.

Question 1

The *Diagnostic and Statistical Manual of Mental Disorders, Fifth Edition* (*DSM-5*), specifies which symptoms help to diagnose people with "Schizophrenia Spectrum and Other Psychotic Disorders." Which of the following would be a negative symptom for this category?

- ○ **A.** Avolition
- ○ **B.** Hallucinations
- ○ **C.** Disorganized speech
- ○ **D.** Catatonic behavior

Question 2

The findings in Figure 1 describe the neural fMRI correlates of social cognition, for two groups (autism, and schizophrenia), in two conditions (Facial emotion recognition, and Theory of mind). Yet, the names of the groups were omitted, and replaced with the letters A and B. Using the passage information, and the neural hypoactivation comparison results in Figure 1 which identify the least active areas per task for each group, it could be said that the letter A most likely corresponds to:

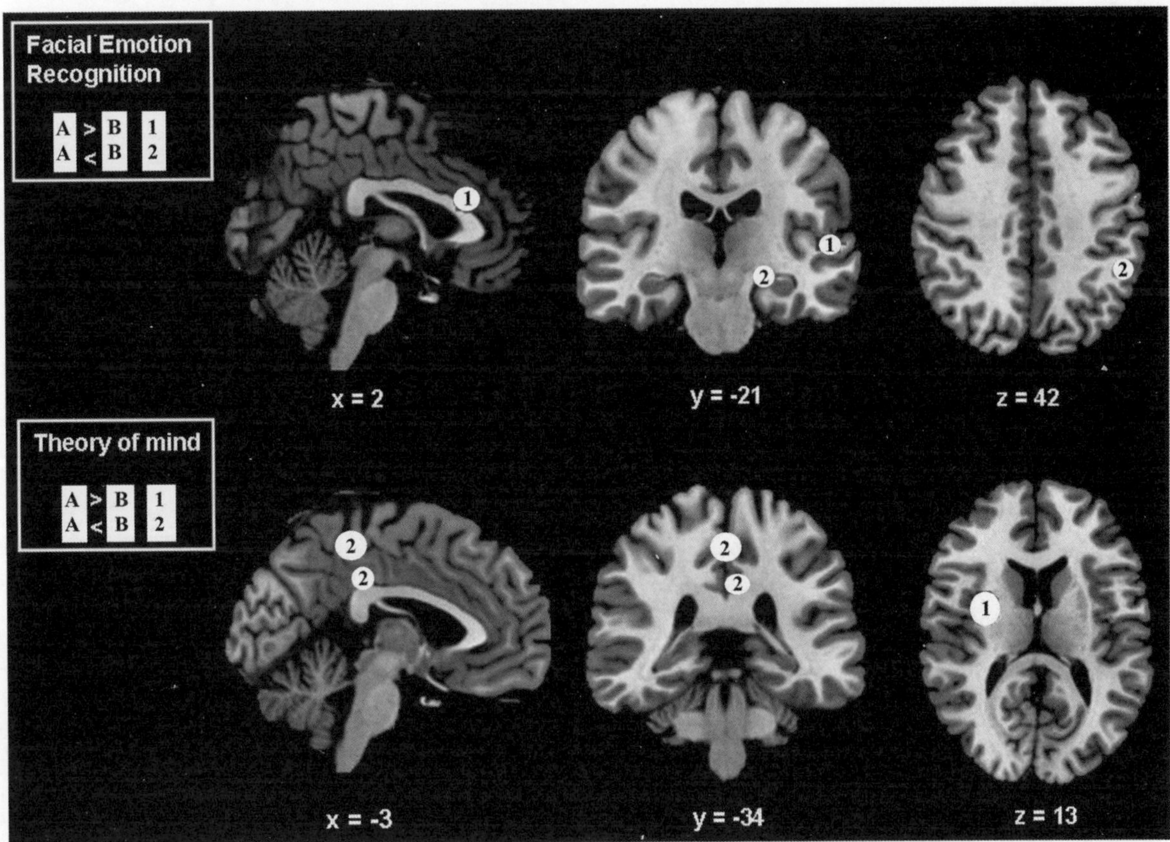

Figure 1 Neural hypoactivation for two groups (Schizophrenia, and Autism) while performing social cognition tasks

Source: *Adapted from G. Sugranyes, M. Kyriakopoulos, R. Corrigall, E. Taylor, & S. Frangou "Autism Spectrum Disorders and Schizophrenia: Meta-Analysis of the Neural Correlates of Social Cognition." Copyright 2011 PLOS one*

- ○ **A.** schizophrenia group.
- ○ **B.** control group.
- ○ **C.** autism group.
- ○ **D.** either the schizophrenia or the autism group, depending on the specific social cognition task.

Question 3

According to the findings in Table 1, which social cognition skill most affects social daily functioning?

- O **A.** Occupational dysfunction
- O **B.** Face affect recognition
- O **C.** Vocal affect recognition
- O **D.** Communication dysfunction

Question 4

In the context of a perspective-taking and theory of mind experiment, a child in Jean Piaget's pre-operational stage is told that someone swapped the location of a toy while the other person was not looking, moving it from a white to a black box. That child would likely think that the person behind whose back the toy had been swapped would firstly look for the toy:

- O **A.** in the white box.
- O **B.** in his or hers own pockets.
- O **C.** in the black box.
- O **D.** in the pockets of the person who had swapped the ball.

Note: This page is left blank so that the passage would be visible without turning pages while assessing the passage-based questions.

Passage 2 (Questions 5–8)

People with disabilities have always had to face a range of violations of their human rights. Over the course of history, several different cultures invented eugenics programs to get rid of criminals and mentally ill and disabled people. Although now disabled people in most developed cultures are guaranteed human rights, their ability to participate in society is still challenged by social distance, stigma, and prejudice.

A study was carried out to find out how authoritarianism (the belief that people with mental illness cannot care for themselves) and benevolence (the belief that people with mental illness are innocent and childlike) influence social distance from people with mental illnesses. Authoritarianism and benevolence were measured with a questionnaire that used different statements about the presentation and treatment of mental illness. Participants rated those statements on a six-point agreement scale. The higher the score on the final scale, the greater the disagreement with the prejudicial attitude was. Furthermore, the study conducted a path analysis to understand the influence of familiarity with mental illness and ethnicity on social distance. The results are displayed in Figure 1.

Some disability studies try to shed light on the underlying assumptions that surround disability. They are closely related to the disability movement and challenge perceptions about the normal body and the normal brain. These studies recognize the disabled body as a cultural construct. An example is the changes in the deaf community that took place between 1860 and the beginning of the 20th century. Historical research points out that the flourishing sign language communities of the earlier 19th century experienced a rapid decline when the political idea of assimilation became prominent. It describes how an "oralism" imperative led to a ban on teaching sign language in the classroom, an imperative to only use lip reading and speech. Eventually this led to a decline in people's ability to communicate in sign language. Their modes of expression were significantly reduced.

Although the situation has improved over the years, people with disabilities and mental illnesses tend to be defined socially in a way that overshadows all other aspects of their personality. They further still tend to suffer discrimination and prejudice on a daily basis.

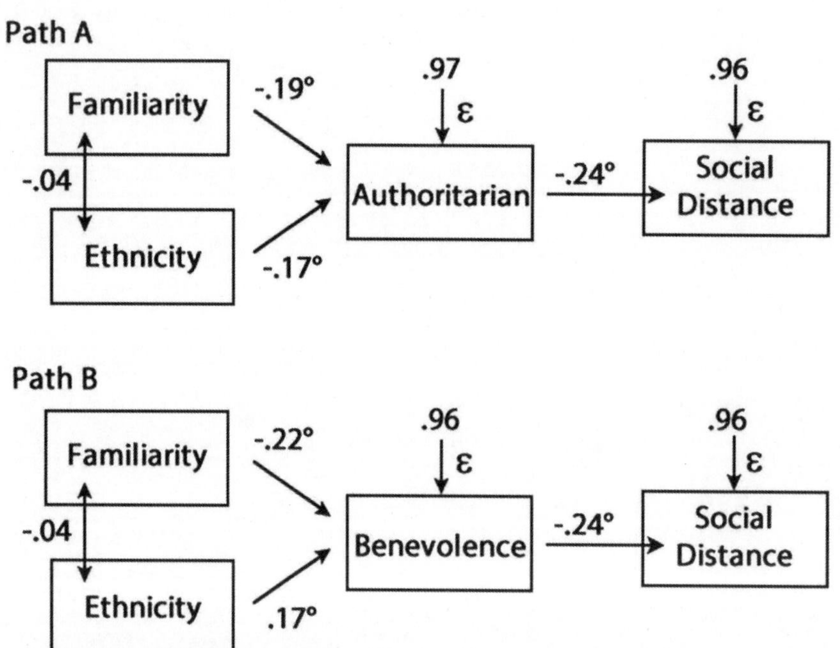

Figure 1 Causality paths relating familiarity and ethnicity with authoritarian (Path A) and benevolent (Path B) attitudes and social distance

Source: Adapted from D. Baynton, "A Silent Exile on This Earth: The Metaphorical Construction of Deafness in the Nineteenth Century." Copyright 2006 The Disability Studies Reader. Figures adapted from P. Corrigan, A. Edwards, A. Green et al., "Prejudice, Social Distance, and Familiarity with Mental Illness." Copyright 2001 Schizophrenia Bulletin.

Question 5

What was probably the reason for including benevolence as a variable in the study design, and what are the results, as described in the passage and in Figure 1?

- ○ **A.** They used benevolence as a control variable to better understand the effects of ethnicity and familiarity. In this sample ethnicity has a stronger effect.
- ○ **B.** They wanted to investigate the impact of benevolent prejudicial attitudes. They found that they can lead to greater social distance.
- ○ **C.** They used benevolence as a control variable to better understand the effects of ethnicity and familiarity. In this sample familiarity has a stronger effect.
- ○ **D.** They wanted to investigate the impact of benevolent prejudicial attitudes. They found that they can lead to lower social distance.

Question 6

According to Table 1, which of the conclusions below about validity is most pertinent?

Table 1 Demographics and Measures

Variable	Mean/frequency	SD
Gender		
Female	81.9%	
Male	18.1%	
Age (yrs)	37.9	11.7
Education		
HS	16.2%	
SC	39.5%	
AA	10.5%	
BA	18.0%	
> BA	15.6%	
Ethnicity		
White	77.9%	
Nonwhite	22.1%	
Familiarity	8.1	2.5
Authoritarianism	110.2	12.9
Benevolence	17.2	5.3
Social Distance	9.3	3.7

Note.—AA = associate's degree; BA = bachelor's degree; > BA = some graduate school education; HS = high school; OMI = Opinions of Mental Illness; SC = some college; SD = standard deviation.
[1] Familiarity is the score from the Level of Contact Report. Authoritarianism and benevolence are the factors from the OMI Questionnaire. Higher OMI scores represent greater disagreement with the prejudicial attitude. Social distance is the total score from the Social Distance Scale.

- ○ **A.** The study lacks internal validity.
- ○ **B.** The study is highly likely to be subjected to confounding bias.
- ○ **C.** The study is highly likely to be subjected to social desirability bias.
- ○ **D.** The study lacks external validity.

Question 7

In the passage, it is mentioned that "people with disabilities and mental illnesses tend to be defined socially in a way that overshadows all other aspects of their personality." This kind of ascription is most consistent with which of the following?

- O **A.** Sick status
- O **B.** Master status
- O **C.** Master role
- O **D.** Sick role

Question 8

As discussed in the passage, many disability studies perceive the disabled body as a cultural construct. This means that those studies believe that:

- O **A.** disability is something that bodies display.
- O **B.** society and culture can be major facilitators or barriers for people affected by disabilities.
- O **C.** even someone with a severe disability could cope better if the culture was adjusted to their needs.
- O **D.** disability is not an inevitable result of biology but highly contingent on social and historical processes.

The following questions are NOT based on a descriptive passage (Questions 9–12).

Question 9

A couple went to Africa, met a young boy, and decided to pay for his schooling. Helping the boy gave the couple a sense of meaning and purpose, made them feel happy, and decreased their inflammation levels. What type of happiness is being described?

- O **A.** Positive happiness
- O **B.** Agape happiness
- O **C.** Eudaimonic happiness
- O **D.** Hedonic happiness

Question 10

If someone holds anti-alcohol attitudes, in which of the following situations might they experience cognitive dissonance?

- O **A.** When discussing with peers their alcohol consumption habits
- O **B.** When considering the pros and cons of drinking alcohol
- O **C.** When partying with friends
- O **D.** When celebrating by drinking a glass of champagne

Question 11

Some cultural groups and societies are matrifocal, which means that:

- O **A.** a woman can have multiple husbands.
- O **B.** a married pregnant mother will move into her mother's home.
- O **C.** the authority and power structure are run by women.
- O **D.** women are forbidden to marry partners who do not belong to their clan.

Question 12

A correlational survey study found that the greater the depressive symptomatology, the worse affective communication and problem-solving skills were. Which of the following observations about these findings can be made?

- O **A.** Depression causes dysfunctional communication and problem solving.
- O **B.** Affective communication and depression both tap into affective states, and therefore there is high collinearity. The findings are tentative.
- O **C.** Greater impairment in affective communication leads to higher levels of depression.
- O **D.** It is not clear whether poor communication and problem solving lead to depressive symptoms or depression leads to poor communication and problem solving.

Passage 3 (Questions 13–17)

Commitment as a value is inherent in romantic relationships such as long-term dating and marriage. Infidelity is defined as a violation of the commitment that binds together the partners, both emotionally and sexually. This violation then threatens the trust, stability, and security of the relationship. Infidelity can sever relationships, and among 160 cultures in the world, the most commonly cited reason for divorce is infidelity. The partner who is betrayed experiences great emotional pain, distress, and confusion.

National surveys using representative samples estimate that 20–25% of males and 10–15% of females have been sexually unfaithful during their marriage. Other studies forecast that anywhere from 30% to 60% of all married couples will be unfaithful at some time during the course of their marriage.

Motivations as to why people cheat are complex. Some posit that infidelity is inevitable, while others assert that infidelity and hookups are due to individual factors such as a lack of self-control. In one interesting experiment, researchers manipulated research subjects' level of ego depletion. All the research subjects were in mutually exclusive relationships. In the experimental condition, subjects were told to eat radishes but not chocolate while doing some tasks. Within a few minutes after the completion of those tasks, a confederate texted the subjects asking whether they would like to meet up for coffee and if they would give out their phone number. Figure 1 shows that those in the experimental condition who succumbed to eating chocolate, thereby demonstrating ego depletion, were more likely to accept the coffee date and give out their phone number.

Because of the feelings of anger, pain, and betrayal, some therapists recommend the concept of forgiveness be woven into interventions for couples who have experienced infidelity. Forgiveness refers to the victim's willingness to move toward prosocial feelings and behaviors, forfeiting feelings of resentment and negative judgment toward the offender.

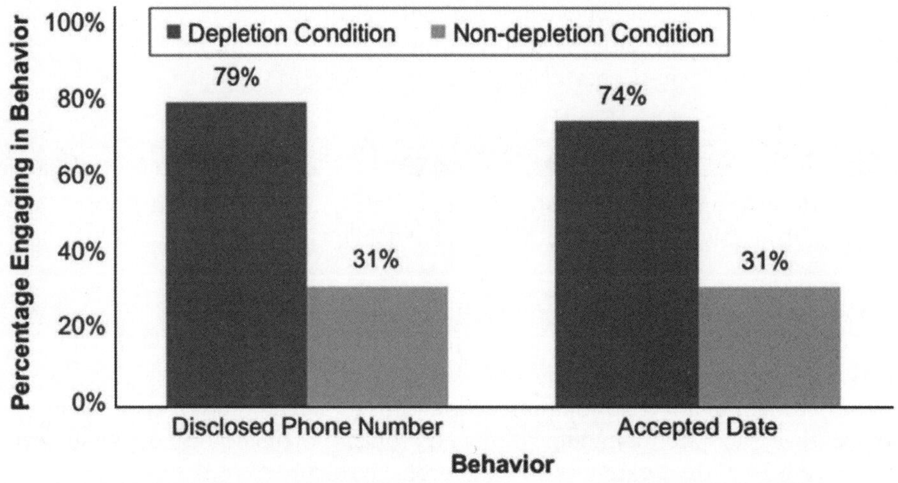

Figure 1 Percentage of participants engaging in behavior by condition

Source: Adapted from N.J. Ciarocco and J. Echevarria, "Hungry for Love: The Influence of Self-regulation on Infidelity." Copyright 2012 Journal of Social Psychology.

Question 13

"Time heals all wounds." The pain of the extramarital affair fades over time because the harm done has faded in the victim's memory. The memory of this event is stored in the victim's:

- O **A.** episodic memory.
- O **B.** semantic memory.
- O **C.** multi-store memory.
- O **D.** procedural memory.

Question 14

From the perspective of ego depletion theory, what conclusion can be drawn from Figure 1?

- ○ **A.** The subjects who were asked to eat the radishes and not the chocolate exerted selective avoidance energy. Thus, their energies were distracted and made them more likely to accept the date.
- ○ **B.** The subjects who were informed that they could eat the chocolate did not experience any cognitive dissonance; they did not have to alter their behavior. This made them more likely to reject the date.
- ○ **C.** The subjects who were told to eat the radishes but not the chocolate experienced greater psychological fatigue. Thus, they had less self-control to refrain from accepting the date.
- ○ **D.** The subjects who were told that they could eat the chocolate experienced greater levels of conscientiousness. Thus, they had greater self-control to refrain from accepting the date.

Question 15

It has been speculated that men would be more likely to engage in extramarital affairs because of the higher potential reproductive rate with lower costs of reproduction. This type of speculation has been advanced by:

- ○ **A.** social cognitive psychologists.
- ○ **B.** attachment-oriented psychologists.
- ○ **C.** behavioral psychologists.
- ○ **D.** evolutionary psychologists.

Question 16

Consider a study that has, as a last step, the task of imagining in writing, in a videotaped room, how one would feel when betraying one's partner. Which prior procedures below would best test the facial feedback hypothesis for the emotions of guilt and grief?

- ○ **A.** Subjects are randomly assigned to a control condition, where nothing happens, or to an experimental condition, where they are exposed to videos of diseased people.
- ○ **B.** During pre-screening, research participants are photographed both smiling and frowning. They are then randomized to the condition described in the question stem or to the control condition of describing the room they are in.
- ○ **C.** Research subjects are randomized to a condition in which they are injected with a drug that temporarily paralyzes the muscles involved in facial expressions, and a condition in which they are injected with a placebo drug that does not paralyze any facial expressions.
- ○ **D.** Research subjects are randomized to a condition in which they smell shirts worn by ovulating women, and a condition in which they smell freshly laundered shirts.

Question 17

In the ego depletion study, research subjects were further randomly exposed to nature scenes. The study found that nature exposure moderated the effect of ego depletion on the frequency of research subjects agreeing to a coffee date with the confederate. How could the researchers interpret this finding?

- ○ **A.** Agreeing to a coffee date can now be fully explained by another variable.
- ○ **B.** The strength of the effect of the level of ego depletion on acceptance of a coffee date is altered.
- ○ **C.** There is no longer a relationship between level of ego depletion and agreeing to a coffee date.
- ○ **D.** The dependent variable—agreeing to a coffee date—is no longer the dependent variable, as the dependent variable is now exposure to nature scenes.

Passage 4 (Questions 18–21)

Macroeconomic, company-level, and/or individual factors can be behind involuntary unemployment, job loss, job insecurity, and job displacement. These phenomena usually accompany macroeconomic recessive trends. During expansion periods, layoffs tend to be associated with the workers' lack of competence and poor character. The below-average productivity stigma is milder during economic recessions.

The impact of the Great Recession (from the end of 2007 to mid-2009) is under intense scrutiny. Major individual, social, economic, cultural, worldwide, short- and long-term repercussions have been identified. Unemployment doubled in the U.S. from 2001 (around 5%) to 2010 (around 10%). Currently, the unemployment rate is once more slowly declining.

The consequences of unemployment are generally negative. Few positive outcomes have been named, specifically increased self-employment and start-up activity. Economic and non-economic negative outcomes include lower quality of life, economic distress, strained relations with colleagues, friends, family, and/or community members, and relatives' lower attainments, and workers' lower self-esteem, anxiety, depressive symptoms, suicide, physical illnesses, and social withdrawal. Thus unemployment leads to marked decay in psychological and physical health for workers and those around them. This is illustrated in Figures 1 and 2.

Figure 1, compiled by Oesch and Lipps, illustrates how well-being tends to decrease with unemployment duration in two European countries. Participants, aged between 20 and 60 years, were in paid employment at the date of the first single-item measurement of subjective well-being. Oesch and Lipps' study further showed how "becoming unemployed hurts as much when regional unemployment is high as when it is low." That is, unemployment's negative consequences do not seem to be minimized during recessions by its being a shared phenomenon. Figure 2 reinforces these observations, by showing how happiness varies significantly in accordance with one's work arrangements.

These negative consequences do nothing but hinder reemployment. Moreover, re-employment is found to merely minimize some of these consequences; it does not eliminate them. For example, economic distress was found to last for around 20 years after the job loss event. It is of the utmost importance that unemployment is subjected to primary, secondary, and tertiary preventive measures that not only attempt to prevent job losses from occurring but also provide the tools required to deal with such events and minimize their generalized negative consequences.

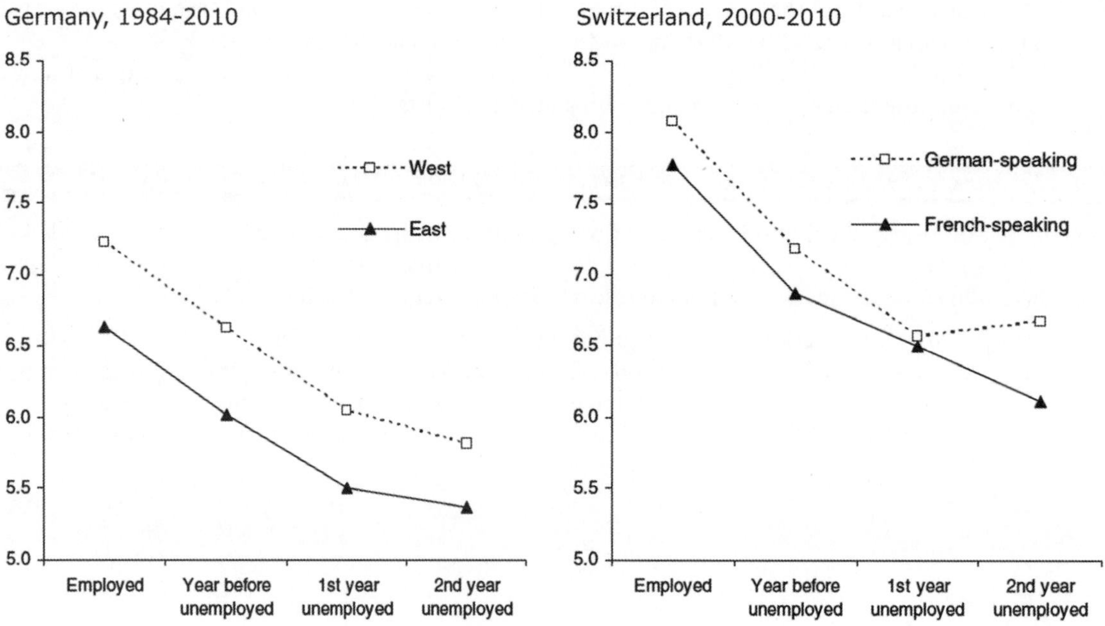

Figure 1 Subjective well-being (measured on a scale from 0 to 10) and employment status—results from a pooled cross-sectional analysis

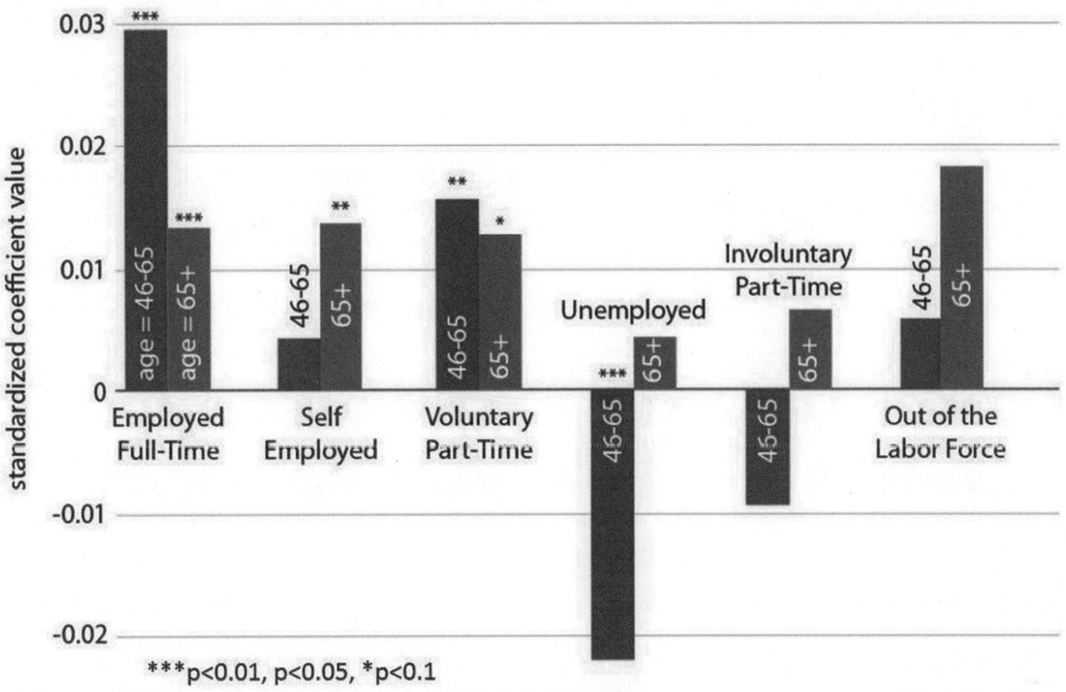

Figure 2 BPL (happiness) of 15- to 46-year-olds (reference group) per late-life work and employment arrangements

Notes: The numbers are based on the fully standardized coefficient estimates from an OLS regression from 2009-2012 using country and year dummies. The dependent variable measures the respondents' assessment of their current life relative to their best possible life on a scale of 0 (worst possible life) to 10 (best possible life). *References/sources au verso.*

Question 18

Which of the following topics would be the most interesting from a macrosociological perspective?

- O **A.** The psychological distress caused by the Great Recession to unemployed parents
- O **B.** The cross-cultural worldwide impact of the Great Recession on family structures
- O **C.** The social impact of the Great Recession on American men's practices
- O **D.** The worldwide impact of the Great Recession on the functioning of the banking industry

Question 19

A longitudinal study followed the workers of a plant until it closed. The study began as soon as the news of the impending closure was announced and finished one year after the closure. Which of the following would affect the least the validity and reliability of the study?

- O **A.** Generalizability
- O **B.** Selection bias
- O **C.** Endowment effect
- O **D.** Attrition bias

Question 20

Figure 1 and Figure 2 put together illustrate how:

- O **A.** the fact that we are "one of a million" unemployed people does not make the situation any better. However, being employed is associated with higher levels of happiness and well-being.
- O **B.** the majority of unemployed people are discontented with their lives. Most do not start to feel better about unemployment in the long run or show great signs of improvement in well-being.
- O **C.** everyone reacts badly to unemployment. However, there are great and statistically significant national disparities in the way people react to unemployment.
- O **D.** people are generally happy when employed. There is only a decline in well-being after they lose their jobs.

Question 21

The passage mentioned an unemployed "stigma," principally when times are prosperous. Stigma is:

- ○ **A.** the social rejection of people who are thought to possess some negative attribute due to a held social group membership.
- ○ **B.** the belief that someone who belongs to some specific social group possesses an attribute or characteristic that is generally assigned to the whole group.
- ○ **C.** the process of labeling someone as a deviant "outsider" simply because they do not act like the dominant, more powerful group.
- ○ **D.** the strict set of moral and ethical norms about mandatory behaviors people should exhibit.

Sources: Adapted from J.E. Brand, "The Far-Reaching Impact of Job Loss and Unemployment." Copyright 2014 California Center for Population Research; D. Oesch and O. Lipps, "Does Unemployment Hurt Less If There Is More of It Around? A Panel Analysis of Life Satisfaction in Germany and Switzerland." Copyright 2012 European Sociological Review; C. Graham and M. Nikolova, "Employment Arrangements, Late-Life Work, and Happiness." Copyright 2010–2013 Gallup World Poll.

Passage 5 (Questions 22–26)

Social media, social network engagement, and their relationship with identity have raised considerable research interest. It is argued that people's identities trigger certain publications in social media. However, social media can also influence what people remember and how narratives are told. It can thus shape both collective and individual identities.

Table 1 Hierarchical Regression on Social Media Use with (Model 1) and without (Model 2) Personality Variables

	Model 1				Model 2			
	Beta	Standard error	Degrees of freedom	*p* value	Beta	Standard error	Degrees of freedom	*p* value
Gender	−.01	0.38	6	0.88	0.02	0.38	9	0.63
Race	−.08	0.49	6	0.007	−.10	0.49	9	0.001
Education	−.03	0.13	6	0.47	−.03	0.14	9	0.35
Income	−.01	0.05	6	0.87	−.01	0.05	9	0.87
Age	−.32	0.02	6	0	−.29	0.02	9	0.00
Life satisfaction	−.06	0.03	6	0.05	−.06	0.03	9	0.11
R^2	12.50%							
Extraversion					0.13	0.04	9	0.00
Emotional stability					−.08	0.05	9	0.02
Openness					0.08	0.05	9	0.01
R^2					15.70%			

Sources: *Adapted from B. Hogan, "The Presentation of Self in the Age of Social Media: Distinguishing Performances and Exhibitions Online." Copyright 2010 Computers in Human Behavior; table adapted from T. Correa, A.W. Hinsley, and H.G. Zúñiga, "Who Interacts on the Web?: The Intersection of Users' Personality and Social Media Use." Copyright 2010 Computers in Human Behavior.*

On a collective level, social movements can display information that shapes the group identity. For example, they can show who publicly supports or likes the movement, they can use particular linguistic styles, and display logotypes and other visuals that will become associated in memory with the movement. They can materialize their identity more easily via social media. A similar effect is observed on an individual level. Social media networks provide the possibility of displaying curated identities through functions such as photo albums, tagging, and timelines. Identities shape and are shaped while enacting these functions.

A recent study investigated whether different personality traits could explain how and to what extent people engage in social media networks. The study found that factors such as extraversion, emotional stability, and openness to experience can predict how people engage online. Furthermore, it has been found that gender and age work as intermediating factors. Table 1 shows the regression analysis that was carried out on a sample of 959 participants. The study tested three different hypotheses: (1) people who are more extraverted will use social media more frequently; (2) people who are more emotionally stable will use social media less frequently; and (3) people who are more open to new experiences will use social media more frequently.

Question 22

According to Table 1, what are the outcomes for the three hypotheses tested in the study that was carried out to investigate whether personality traits can predict social network use?

- ○ **A.** Hypothesis 3 was supported; hypothesis 1 and hypothesis 2 were not supported. Openness explained 15.70% of the variance in social media use.
- ○ **B.** Hypothesis 1, hypothesis 2, and hypothesis 3 were not supported; life satisfaction was the strongest predictor of social media use.
- ○ **C.** Hypothesis 1 was supported; hypothesis 2 and hypothesis 3 were not supported; 12.5% of the variance was explained by demographic factors and life satisfaction.
- ○ **D.** Hypothesis 1, hypothesis 2, and hypothesis 3 were supported; extraversion is the strongest personality predictor of social media use.

Question 23

The study referred to in Table 1 uses extraversion, openness, and emotional stability as descriptors of personality. Which personality model was utilized for this study?

- ○ **A.** Big Five personality traits
- ○ **B.** Myers–Briggs Type Indicator
- ○ **C.** Minnesota Multiphasic Personality Inventory
- ○ **D.** Hans Eysenck's personality theory

Question 24

It was argued in the passage that social media networks have a curating function in creating narrative identities. Posts such as pictures reinforce memories about a particular situation. Memories that are not captured in a timeline tend to fade away more quickly. What is the most likely explanation for these observations?

- ○ **A.** The retrieval of information is highly dependent on the person's psychological or physical state. When there is a mismatch between the emotional or physical states at the moments of memorization and retrieval, recall might fail.
- ○ **B.** The brain can only store a limited amount of information. The memory that has been stored the longest is displaced by new memories when the storage is full. Social media timelines provide the possibility of restoring the event as a fresh memory at the beginning of the chain.
- ○ **C.** Recall is highly dependent on the availability of contextual cues. Social media works as a contextual cue, and as such enhances recall.
- ○ **D.** When the brain is recording information, neurons form patterns of excitatory stimulation and inhibition. Social media posts available in the timeline lead to the formation of inhibition patterns.

Question 25

In accordance with the mere exposure effect, frequent interaction on social media networks would most likely lead to:

- O **A.** a weaker bond with people who are not members of that particular social media network.
- O **B.** a greater affinity for connections who frequently post content.
- O **C.** a more positive social connection between members who do not like each other's posts.
- O **D.** a change in attitude when confronted with posts that strongly oppose someone's original position.

Question 26

Social movements profit from collective memory because it enables them to act as a cohesive community. The collective awareness of shared traits and circumstances is called:

- O **A.** herd behavior.
- O **B.** groupthink.
- O **C.** collective unconscious.
- O **D.** collective identity.

The following questions are NOT based on a descriptive passage (Questions 27–30).

Question 27

Which of the following sensory receptors is involved in pain perception, and which lobe is thought to be responsible for processing that information (sensory receptor, lobe, respectively)?

- O **A.** Rods, temporal lobe
- O **B.** Dendrites, temporal lobe
- O **C.** Nociceptors, parietal lobe
- O **D.** Meissner corpuscles, parietal lobe

Question 28

Which of the following problem-solving techniques is most likely adopting a manager with a "thinking" Jungian personality type, who, when faced with a decision, analyzes similar past situations and their outcomes?

- O **A.** Incubation
- O **B.** Insight
- O **C.** Analogies
- O **D.** Means–end analysis

Question 29

One of Robert Merton's self-fulfilling prophecies examples was about how a false rumor about the insolvency of a bank led investors to retract their money from the bank, and the formerly financially solid bank was left in financial difficulties. Which of the following statements is an INCORRECT observation about such a phenomenon?

- O **A.** Self-fulfilling prophecies involve the shaping of individual and social realities via held beliefs.
- O **B.** Self-fulfilling prophecies involve a possibly false definition of a situation that triggers new behavior, one that ultimately makes the belief come true.
- O **C.** Self-fulfilling prophecies involve a false assumption by a perceiver about a target, one that ultimately causes the target to exhibit expectancy-consistent behaviors.
- O **D.** Confronting the false assumption with the truth (e.g., a social campaign) is the most effective way of breaking the vicious self-fulfilling circle.

Question 30

Ants are eusocial animals that form superorganisms; they live in groups, do not survive when alone over extended periods of time, show division of labor, and have highly specialized skills. How did the sociologist Herbert Spencer understand superorganisms like the ants within human society?

- O **A.** He explained that superorganisms, because of their division of labor, would form an evolutionary disadvantage for human societies.
- O **B.** He criticized the concept of superorganisms, as it does not apply to the extremely individualistic human society.
- O **C.** He used the term to explain how nature influences social structures.
- O **D.** He used it to explain how human societies form structures that are not organic but social.

Passage 6 (Questions 31–35)

Religion and spirituality are social phenomena found in different forms across cultures. Both are an expression of one's connection, beliefs, practices, and rituals related to the transcendent. Science has often been regarded as being at odds with religion, principally for nonbelievers. Nonbelievers sometimes discard believers' stances as unworthy of scientific attention.

For example, two decades ago, the idea that religion might influence psychological and/or physical health outcomes "was greeted with skepticism and even hostility by many medical researchers." Religion also sometimes had a social taboo status. Moreover, religious practices were linked to psychiatric disorders and thereafter taken as a sign of mental illness.

Whatever the reason, religion undoubtedly was a controversial, understudied topic. This state of affairs has changed. There is a clear rising tendency worldwide to study the impact of religion on mental and physical health (Figure 1). Generally, positive associations have been found. Few studies report negative relationships. Nowadays, religion and spirituality are recognized as psychosocial factors in health, and are recommended in patient care.

For example, a recent study used priming to show that believing that body and mind are separate entities (body–mind dualism) led people more often to adopt unhealthy behaviors and attitudes. Further, when participants were primed with healthy behaviors, they more often adopted metaphysical views.

Religion was formerly often measured via the use of simple, often single-item questions such as "Are you a religious person?" Currently, multidimensional scales are beginning to be used. Findings are still unclear. For example, a study showed how religious feeling, but not attendance, favored the remission of major depressive disorder symptoms among hospital inpatients. Another study found that attendance and church support protected African Americans from depressive disorders.

Some explanative mechanisms for the effects of religion/spirituality on health have been proposed. These involve aspects such as coping resources and behaviors, self-esteem and self-efficacy, positive emotions, personal lifestyles, self-control, and social support. Some findings are more difficult to explain via such mechanisms. For example, a double-blind randomized control trial showed that distant prayer for hospitalized cardiac care patients, in comparison with non-prayed-for patients, was associated with statistically significantly better health conditions in several measures (e.g., use of antibiotics, cardiopulmonary arrest, and pneumonia).

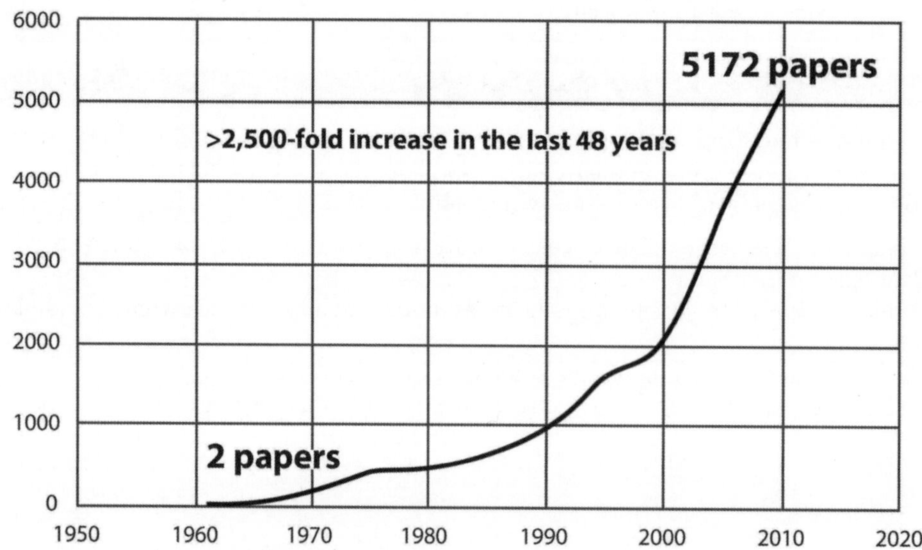

Figure 1 PubMed publications on the relationship between religion and health

For full references for this passage, see over (after Question 35).

Question 31

The passage described how religion was sometimes regarded as a taboo. Which of the following is NOT the aim or purpose of a social taboo?

- ○ **A.** To prevent the sacred from being defiled
- ○ **B.** To increase self-awareness and social facilitation
- ○ **C.** To enact systems of social control
- ○ **D.** To prevent ordinary people from performing dangerous actions

Question 32

Making use of the information provided in the passage, which would be the most valid, reliable, and ethical research design for studying the effects of primed religious beliefs on surveyed attitudes toward healthy lifestyles, as described, when alone in a room where chips were at easy reach, by randomly selected, informed, and consenting participants?

- ○ **A.** Group A and group B read a text about the importance of religion. Afterward every participant fills out the survey. They are then debriefed, thanked, and sent home.
- ○ **B.** Group A is asked to perform a free-recall task associated with the target word "atheism" and group B with the target word "theism." Afterward the participants fill out the survey. Each participant is then thanked and sent home.
- ○ **C.** Participants fill out the survey. Afterward group A is subliminally presented with the sentence "Art is beautiful" and group B is subliminally presented with the sentence "God exists", both while watching a video clip about a music band. They are then debriefed, thanked, and sent home.
- ○ **D.** Group A is subliminally presented with the sentence "Art is beautiful" and group B is subliminally presented with the sentence "God exists", both while watching a video clip about a music band. Afterward, participants fill out the surveys. They are then debriefed, thanked, and sent home.

Question 33

According to the information provided in the passage, which of the following statements about the use of multidimensional scales is the LEAST correct?

- ○ **A.** Such scales highlight how religion and spirituality have many dimensions, each possibly responsible for different effects on health.
- ○ **B.** The use of such scales has yielded conflicting results, and additional research is required for understanding which dimension is responsible for which health effects.
- ○ **C.** The use of such scales shows how the single-item assessment of religiousness led to confounding results and disconfirms past findings.
- ○ **D.** Such scales involve the development of several items for assessing people's religiousness and spirituality, adding to the complexity of the research field.

Question 34

As noted in the passage, the effects of religion/spirituality on health have been explained by several mechanisms or mediators. How could the variable "positive emotions" be used to explain such effects?

- ○ **A.** Believing in the transcendent gives people the psychological means, attitudes, and behaviors to enable them to better deal with adverse life circumstances.
- ○ **B.** Believing in the transcendent makes people feel more integrated and assisted by the wider group of believers to which they belong.
- ○ **C.** Believing in the transcendent helps people choose healthy and pacific over unhealthy and distressful attitudes and behaviors.
- ○ **D.** Believing in the transcendent gives people hope for the resolution of their problems and instills optimistic attitudes.

Question 35

The passage described a double-blind randomized control trial about the health effects of praying for hospitalized patients. What biasing phenomenon/-a did the double-blind procedure most likely try to prevent?

- ○ **A.** Conformity and deindividuation
- ○ **B.** Social desirability biases
- ○ **C.** Confirmatory expectations
- ○ **D.** Social loafing

Sources: Adapted from M. Forstmann, P. Burgmer, and T. Mussweiler, "The Mind Is Willing, but the Flesh Is Weak: The Effects of Mind-Body Dualism on Health Behavior." Copyright 2012 Psychological Science; S.A. Kharitonov, "Religious and Spiritual Biomarkers in Both Health and Disease." Copyright 2012 Creative Commons; E.L. Idler, M.A. Musick, C.G. Ellison et al., "Measuring Multiple Dimensions of Religion and Spirituality for Health Research: Conceptual Background and Findings from the 1998 General Social Survey." Copyright 2003 Sage Publications; C.G. Ellison and J.S. Levin, "The Religion-Health Connection: Evidence, Theory, and Future Directions." Copyright 1998 Health Education & Behavior; H.G. Koenig, "Religion, Spirituality, and Health: The Research and Clinical Implications." Copyright 2012 ISRN Psychiatry.

Passage 7 (Questions 36–40)

A common way to measure income inequality within a country or between countries is the Gini index (also called the Gini coefficient). This is a measure of statistical dispersion that was developed by the Italian sociologist Corrado Gini to quantitatively assess the lack of purity of categories (i.e., how many incorrectly classified individuals are included within a certain category). As applied to social inequality, this lack of purity is concerned with how many individuals are not in an equality situation. It varies on a scale of 0 (everyone receives the same income) to 1 (one person receives all the income). Greater Gini indices indicate greater inequality, and the value itself represents the amount of deviation or distance from an equality situation.

A Lorenz curve is used to determine the cumulative percentages of total income received against the cumulative number of earners, beginning with the poorest and ending in the richest or greatest earner. The area between the Lorenz curve and a hypothetical line of absolute equality illustrates the Gini index, expressed as a percentage of the maximum area under the line. Tables 1a, 1b, 1c, and 1d display the proportions of the total income earned by different quantiles of the population in four different fictional countries. The line at 45 degrees is the line of equality.

Global or worldwide income is distributed very unevenly, with the richest 20% of the population earning 80% of the total global income. The global Gini coefficient is around 0.6 (i.e., 60%). Inequalities in social status, illustrated by the Gini index, have been shown to lead, on an individual, national, or global level, to inequalities in health status. The social gradient in health tries to quantify these health status-related differences. It is composed of socioeconomic and demographic indicators.

Table 1a, 1b, 1c, 1d Lorenz Curve for Four Fictitious Countries (A, B, C, and D)

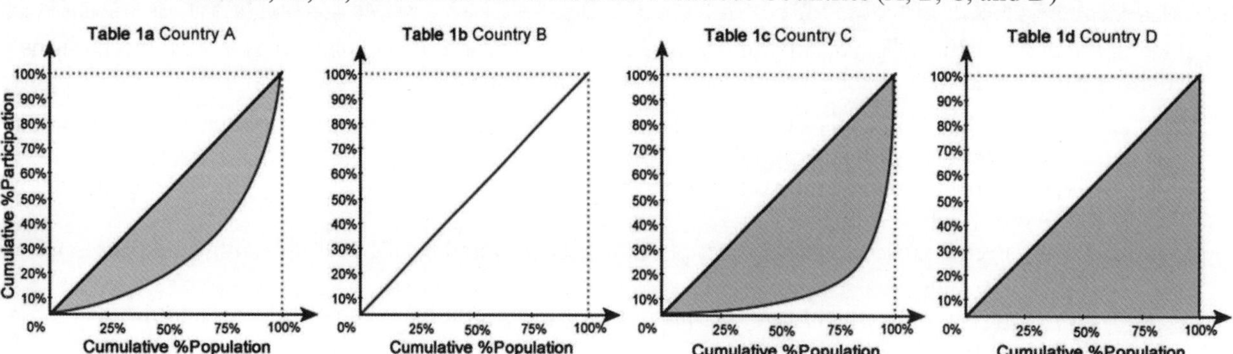

Source: Adapted from J. Kosteniuk and H. Dickinson, "Tracing the Social Gradient in the Health of Canadians: Primary and Secondary Determinants." Copyright 2003 Social Science & Medicine.

Question 36

How should the countries shown in Table 1a, 1b, 1c, and 1d be ordered, according to their degree of income inequality, descending from the country with the greatest equality?

- ○ **A.** Country B, country A, country C, country D
- ○ **B.** Country A, country C, country D, country B
- ○ **C.** Country A, country B, country C, country D
- ○ **D.** Country D, country A, country C, country B

Question 37

The Gini coefficient can provide information about:

- ○ **A.** how the informal economy of a country affects equality.
- ○ **B.** how the earnings of people in different countries increase or decrease over time.
- ○ **C.** whether the number of people living in absolute poverty increases or decreases.
- ○ **D.** whether there are more or less inequalities in health in a population.

Question 38

The passage mentions socioeconomic and demographic indicators are used for determining the social gradient in health. Which of the following indicators would not fall under this definition?

- ○ **A.** Education
- ○ **B.** Self-esteem
- ○ **C.** Housing
- ○ **D.** Unemployment

Question 39

What would be the primary proposal put forth by conflict theory to reduce the social gradient in health?

- ○ **A.** Give more power to the patients
- ○ **B.** Redefine malnutrition in order to fight obesity
- ○ **C.** Give health providers more freedom to adjust to the needs of patients
- ○ **D.** Put hospitals under state control rather than market control

Question 40

Which one of the following is NOT a factor that modernization theory would point to in order to explain poverty and inequalities?

- ○ **A.** Population growth
- ○ **B.** Global power relationships
- ○ **C.** Technology
- ○ **D.** Cultural patterns

Passage 8 (Questions 41–44)

Today the concept of wellness is very popular. Consumers' health care marketplace is estimated at $502 billion, led by disease preventing and wellness products such as organic foods, vitamins, fortified beverages, nutritional supplements, and weight management products. Wellness has even been introduced into the tourism industry, targeting customers who want to focus on and maintain wellness and health during their travels. Many hotels, for example, have stand-up desks or feature rooms with eucalyptus-scented towels to calm their guests.

An increasing number of workplaces have also implemented wellness programs, with categories that include (1) screenings to identify health risks, (2) disease management programs to prevent the onset of chronic conditions or assist in controlling or managing existing conditions, and (3) 'promotion of health' activities such as time for exercise, vouchers for the gym, and the installation of bike racks. People also hire wellness coaches who are experts trained in working alongside clients to facilitate lifestyle changes and thereby promote personal growth and wellness.

In the discussion of wellness and prevention, the topics of brain health and sleep health also emerge. What are brain and sleep health? Though defining these terms would seem easy and one might assume that textbooks abound with definitions, the reality is that grasping the general concept of health is quite complicated. What is known is that promoting brain health involves a holistic approach that facilitates emotional, cognitive, spiritual growth, and the maximization learning and self-fulfillment. The concept of brain health stresses that the brain is resilient and that it requires multi-stimulus environmental stimulation.

Defining and measuring sleep health is also a challenge. For example, does its definition for health care professionals rely on the absence of a sleep disorder? Or perhaps it involves duration of sleep time or, conversely, the duration in which one feels alert during nonsleeping periods? One thing that is known is that poor sleep has health consequences, including cardiovascular problems. Table 1 shows the studies used to assess the effects of short sleep duration on the risk of developing or dying of coronary heart disease, as illustrated by Figure 1. The same investigation compared the results associated with the effects of short and long sleep duration. Long sleep duration was associated with a mean risk of 1.38, with the confidence interval also set at 95%. The associated heterogeneity coefficient was p = 49% (p=0.028), and the Egger's test results were p=0.92.

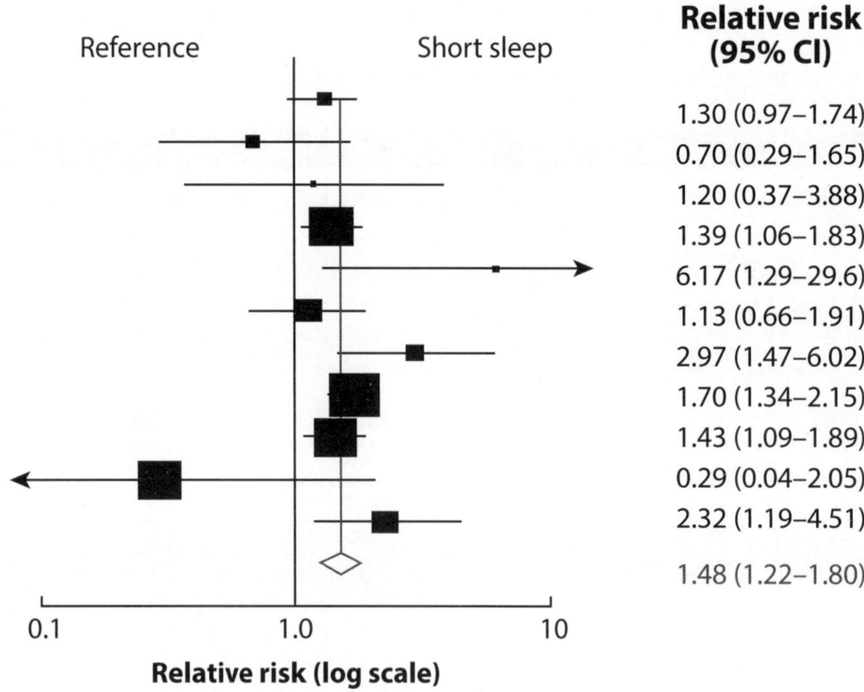

Figure 1 Forest plots of the risk of developing or dying of coronary heart disease associated with short duration of sleep compared with the reference group

Table 1 Description of Selected Studies about the Risk of Developing or Dying of Coronary Heart Disease Associated with Short Duration of Sleep

First author	Year	Country	Sample size	Total CHD events	Follow-up (years)
Qureshi	1997	USA	7,844	413	10.0
Mallon (men)	2002	Sweden	906	71	12.0
Mallon (women)	2002	Sweden	964	20	12.0
Ayas	2003	USA	71,617	934	10.0
Amagai (men)	2004	Japan	4,419	26	8.2
Meisinger (men)	2007	Germany	3,508	295	10.1
Meisinger (women)	2007	Germany	3,388	85	10.1
Shankar (men)	2008	Singapore	25,552	846	7–13
Shankar (women)	2008	Singapore	32,492	570	7–13
Ikehara (men)	2009	Japan	41,489	508	14.3
Ikehara (women)	2009	Japan	57,145	373	14.3
Combined effect: $P < 0.0001$			249,324	4,141	
Heterogeneity: $I^2 = 44\%$; $P = 0.059$ Egger's test: $P = 0.95$					

Source: Adapted from C.L. Jackson, S. Redline, and K.M. Emmons, "Sleep as a Potential Fundamental Contributor to Disparities in Cardiovascular Health." Copyright 2015 Annual Review of Public Health.

Question 41

What type of research methodology was used for the study depicted in Figure 1?

- ○ **A.** Solomon four-group design
- ○ **B.** Longitudinal cohort design
- ○ **C.** Ethnography
- ○ **D.** Meta-analysis

Question 42

Which of the following approaches to health is more commonly equated with traditional, unorthodox medicine?

- ○ **A.** Holistic approach
- ○ **B.** Treating diseases
- ○ **C.** Biopsychosocial approach
- ○ **D.** Boosting wellness

Question 43

According to information from Figure 1 and the passage, what conclusion can be drawn from the sleep study?

- ○ **A.** There are no risks associated with the duration of sleep for coronary heart disease.
- ○ **B.** Short sleep duration is associated with greater risk of coronary heart disease. Long sleep duration is not.
- ○ **C.** Both longer and shorter durations of sleep are associated with a greater risk of coronary heart disease.
- ○ **D.** Gender is a statistically significant predictor of developing or dying from coronary heart disease.

Question 44

A wellness coach instructed her trainee to keep a daily diary of food items consumed, item-by-item caloric intake, and of the circumstances and thoughts experienced during food cravings. Which of the following schools of thought in Psychology is likely guiding the coach's work?

- O **A.** Existential
- O **B.** Psychodynamic
- O **C.** Cognitive behavioral
- O **D.** Mindfulness

The following questions are NOT based on a descriptive passage (Questions 45–48).

Question 45

In looking at the Figure, which Gestalt grouping principle for perceptual organization is used?

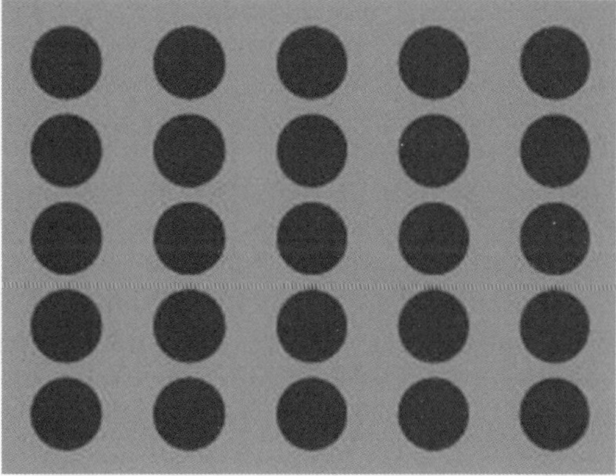

- ○ **A.** Proximity
- ○ **B.** Symmetry
- ○ **C.** Common region
- ○ **D.** Similarity

Question 46

Timothy Leary coined the term "reality tunnel." It describes how every individual's perception of the world is filtered through his or her own experiences and beliefs. Which psychological concept or theory is most closely related to this idea?

- ○ **A.** Talcott Parson's gloss
- ○ **B.** Benjamin Bloom's taxonomy
- ○ **C.** Donald Broadbent's attention model
- ○ **D.** Metacognition

Question 47

Rods are responsible for which type of vision?

- ○ **A.** Day vision
- ○ **B.** Color vision
- ○ **C.** Scotopic vision
- ○ **D.** Accurate vision

Question 48

In a study that used a voxel-based morphometry of 160 adults, all of whom had no history of psychiatric illnesses, half of them did have a history of childhood maltreatment. What were the findings that were most probably uncovered?

- ○ **A.** There is a correlation between childhood maltreatment and sleep disorders.
- ○ **B.** There is a statistically significant correlation between proprioceptors' sensitivity and childhood maltreatment.
- ○ **C.** There is a relationship between childhood maltreatment and reduced hippocampal volumes.
- ○ **D.** There is a relationship between childhood maltreatment and medulla oblongata decay.

Passage 9 (Questions 49–52)

Today there are at least 48 states in the U.S. that have some form of legal gambling. Five types of gaming are legal in the United States. The first is charitable gaming. Regardless of who runs it, it must ultimately benefit nonprofit organizations. Bingo is an example of charitable gaming. The second type is casino gambling. Atlantic City and Las Vegas probably come to mind; Nevada was the first state in the United States to legalize casino gambling. The third type is lotteries, which date back to colonial times. The fourth category encompasses Native American gaming, which is often operated by tribes. The last type is pari-mutuel wagering; examples of this include horse racing and dog racing.

Slot machines are a growing industry: the share of slot machines in the "gaming pie" has grown from approximately 40% to 70% during a 35-year time period. Most gamblers report that slot machines are their favorite form of gambling, so much so that innovative ways of countering the negative financial repercussions that gamblers might experience have been put into place. Pop-up messages, for example, have been employed, which come up when gamblers are approaching their predetermined limit. In one laboratory experiment with 59 individuals randomized to one of two conditions (a monetary limit pop-up reminder and no pop-up reminder), the experimental group subjects were more likely to stick to their predetermined monetary limit than the control group.

Bingo is often the first type of gambling to which a child might be introduced. It is also largely dominated by women. The stereotypical image of a bingo player is that of an elderly woman with a lot of time on her hands who plays to pass the time—a fun and innocuous form of entertainment. One study found that the predictors of more money spent on bingo were being female, being older, living in a rented apartment/house, receiving government income, and reporting more health problems.

Internet sweepstakes cafes are also surfacing rapidly. These are storefront operations that advertise long-distance phone minutes or Internet to customers, but in reality, gamblers play on computers that mimic slot machines and video poker game experiences. On entering, the sounds of slot machines ring out, giving customers the feel of being in a casino. In some Internet sweepstakes cafes, customers have to sign a waiver stating that they are not gambling before signing on to a computer.

Question 49

In the study about the pop-up messages in the slot machines, the researchers hypothesize that the pop-up messages will be effective in disrupting gamblers':

- O **A.** dissociative state.
- O **B.** repressive state.
- O **C.** depressive state.
- O **D.** anxiety state.

Question 50

A couple, being informed of overspending trends in Las Vegas, and having thus set, a priori, a budget limit, ended up overspending because they kept believing that their chances would soon change. Which of the following phenomena might have the opposite cognitive and behavioral effects to those of the gambler's fallacy just described?

- O **A.** Automatic processing
- O **B.** Foot-in-the door
- O **C.** Personalization
- O **D.** Representativeness heuristic

Question 51

In the laboratory experiment examining the effectiveness of pop-up messages in slot machines, some have raised the concern that, in a casino, gamblers' attention may be diverted from the pop-up messages because of the vast amount of external stimuli (e.g., noise, and bright lights). These critics are raising questions about the study's:

- O **A.** construct validity; that is, whether the experimental procedures measure ways of overcoming distractions such as the bright lights and noise.
- O **B.** internal validity; that is, whether the bright lights and noise can cause attrition.
- O **C.** ecological validity; that is, whether in the real world the pop-up messages would be effective, because in a casino the bright lights and noise can be distracting.
- O **D.** predictive validity; that is, the extent to which the bright lights and noise in a casino can predict whether gamblers continue to play.

Question 52

In a study about the third-person effect and its role in gambling advertising, which is a plausible hypothesis to test?

- O **A.** After watching a gambling commercial, research subjects are likely to indicate that other women will be less vulnerable to the persuasive message than their male counterparts.
- O **B.** After watching a gambling commercial, research subjects are more likely to rate that the commercial has little influence on them but that others will be more influenced by the message.
- O **C.** After research subjects watch a gambling commercial, perceptions of influence of the commercial on problem gamblers will be found to be consistently greater than perceptions of influence on non-problem gamblers.
- O **D.** After watching a gambling commercial, research subjects will perceive that influence is predicted by controversial-content and brand-name advertisements.

Passage 10 (Questions 53–56)

Every individual in a society belongs to various groups. Rites of passage may be performed to mark the passing from one group to another, as in the passing from childhood to adolescence. Some rites of passage are more universal, while others only exist in specific communities. Common rites of passage are connected to adulthood, pregnancy, childbirth, college graduation, engagement, marriage, and death.

Rites of passage play an important part in socialization. They are shaped by social institutions and different symbols are used to express the meaning of the transition for the individual and the community. While rites of passage further serve the purpose of stabilizing a person's identity in a new role, some of them can be dangerous for health and psychological well-being. One example is female genital mutilation, which in some countries forms part of the rituals that surround the transition from childhood to adolescence. This rite of passage assigns higher social status to young women in their culture but can simultaneously pose a serious risk to their health.

In the modern globalized world, it has been observed that certain rites of passage get adopted by cultures other than those where these were originally performed. Sometimes, they get slightly modified, and are found in very unexpected contexts.

Question 53

In accordance with Auguste Comte, what is the most important question to be asked in order to understand and interpret rites of passage?

- O **A.** How do rites of passage maintain stability in society?
- O **B.** How do rites of passage prompt and facilitate social inequalities within society?
- O **C.** How do rites of passage serve to oppress women in society?
- O **D.** How do rites of passage change in modern society?

Question 54

In many Western cultures, the bride wears a white dress on her wedding day and the female wedding guests neither wear white, black, nor red but are expected to wear bright colors. This dress code signifies (a):

- O **A.** rite of passage.
- O **B.** social institution.
- O **C.** social norm.
- O **D.** ethnocentrism.

Question 55

According to the passage, what is the relationship between rites of passage, social institutions, and culture?

- O **A.** Rites of passage can vary based on culture but are always defined by social institutions.
- O **B.** Rites of passage are often defined by social institutions rather than culture.
- O **C.** Rites of passage reinforce culture by spreading across social institutions.
- O **D.** The influence of rites of passage on culture is mediated by social institutions.

Question 56

Which of the following is an example of indirect cultural diffusion?

- O **A.** A 3-year-old child who attends church for the first time and learns the appropriate behavior in religious places through a mixture of advice from her parents and her own observations of the churchgoers
- O **B.** A mother telling her daughter about the rituals that were performed on her wedding day and the daughter deciding to set up her own wedding rituals in a similar way
- O **C.** The traditionally Western ritual of the bride and groom exchanging wedding rings becoming more and more popular as a part of Chinese wedding ceremonies
- O **D.** The popularity of playing both hockey and baseball in the border region between Canada and the United States

---

The following questions are NOT based on a descriptive passage (Questions 57–59).

Question 57

Some have argued that mandating school uniforms is a way to increase a sense of community and belonging among students in a school. Ultimately this could foster school safety and promote learning. Which theory or concept best supports such an argument?

- O **A.** Authoritarian personality
- O **B.** Contact hypothesis
- O **C.** Self-efficacy
- O **D.** Group membership

Question 58

Individuals with damage to the anterior cingulate cortex tend to demonstrate:

- O **A.** impulsivity and unchecked aggression.
- O **B.** inability to send messages to the adrenal gland to produce the hormone for "fight or flight."
- O **C.** difficulty expressing their beliefs or thoughts verbally.
- O **D.** challenges with vision and hearing.

Question 59

Longitudinal data on baby name choices has shown that names that are popular with higher-class parents are subsequently chosen by lower-class parents for their children. Usually when this happens the name goes out of fashion for parents from higher classes. Georg Simmel observed a similar tendency in the fashion industry and described this phenomenon as:

- O **A.** social transmission.
- O **B.** proletarian drift.
- O **C.** false consciousness.
- O **D.** trickle-down effect.

Full-length MCAT Practice Test GS-2

Periodic Table of the Elements

You may consult this page anytime you wish during the following exam sections:

- Section I: Chemical and Physical Foundations of Biological Systems
- Section III: Biological and Biochemical Foundations of Living Systems

On the real exam, the computer-based shortcut to see the periodic table is Alt + T.

1 **H** 1.0																	2 **He** 4.0
3 **Li** 6.9	4 **Be** 9.0											5 **B** 10.8	6 **C** 12.0	7 **N** 14.0	8 **O** 16.0	9 **F** 19.0	10 **Ne** 20.2
11 **Na** 23.0	12 **Mg** 24.3											13 **Al** 27.0	14 **Si** 28.1	15 **P** 31.0	16 **S** 32.1	17 **Cl** 35.5	18 **Ar** 39.9
19 **K** 39.1	20 **Ca** 40.1	21 **Sc** 45.0	22 **Ti** 47.9	23 **V** 50.9	24 **Cr** 52.0	25 **Mn** 54.9	26 **Fe** 55.8	27 **Co** 58.9	28 **Ni** 58.7	29 **Cu** 63.5	30 **Zn** 65.4	31 **Ga** 69.7	32 **Ge** 72.6	33 **As** 74.9	34 **Se** 79.0	35 **Br** 79.9	36 **Kr** 83.8
37 **Rb** 85.5	38 **Sr** 87.6	39 **Y** 88.9	40 **Zr** 91.2	41 **Nb** 92.9	42 **Mo** 95.9	43 **Tc** (98)	44 **Ru** 101.1	45 **Rh** 102.9	46 **Pd** 106.4	47 **Ag** 107.9	48 **Cd** 112.4	49 **In** 114.8	50 **Sn** 118.7	51 **Sb** 121.8	52 **Te** 127.6	53 **I** 126.9	54 **Xe** 131.3
55 **Cs** 132.9	56 **Ba** 137.3	57 **La*** 138.9	72 **Hf** 178.5	73 **Ta** 180.9	74 **W** 183.9	75 **Re** 186.2	76 **Os** 190.2	77 **Ir** 192.2	78 **Pt** 195.1	79 **Au** 197.0	80 **Hg** 200.6	81 **Tl** 204.4	82 **Pb** 207.2	83 **Bi** 209.0	84 **Po** (209)	85 **At** (210)	86 **Rn** (222)
87 **Fr** (223)	88 **Ra** (226)	89 **Ac**** (227)	104 **Unq**** (261)	105 **Unp** (262)	106 **Unh** (263)	107 **Uns** (262)	108 **Uno** (265)	109 **Une** (267)									
			*	58 **Ce** 140.1	59 **Pr** 140.9	60 **Nd** 144.2	61 **Pm** (145)	62 **Sm** 150.4	63 **Eu** 152.0	64 **Gd** 157.3	65 **Tb** 158.9	66 **Dy** 162.5	67 **Ho** 164.9	68 **Er** 167.3	69 **Tm** 168.9	70 **Yb** 173.0	71 **Lu** 175.0
			**	90 **Th** 232.0	91 **Pa** (231)	92 **U** 238.0	93 **Np** (237)	94 **Pu** (244)	95 **Am** (243)	96 **Cm** (247)	97 **Bk** (247)	98 **Cf** (251)	99 **Es** (252)	100 **Fm** (257)	101 **Md** (258)	102 **No** (259)	103 **Lr** (260)

CANDIDATE'S NAME ______________________________

RAW SCORE AND SCALED SCORE ______________________

GS-2
Mock Exam 2 of 7
Solutions at MCAT-prep.com

GS-2 Section I: Chemical and Physical Foundations of Biological Systems

Questions: 1-59
Time: 95 minutes

INSTRUCTIONS: Of all the questions on this test, most are organized into groups preceded by a passage. After evaluating the passage, select the best answer to each question in the group. Fifteen questions are independent of any descriptive passage or each other. Similarly, select the best answer to these questions. If you are unsure of an answer, eliminate the alternatives that you know to be incorrect and select an answer from the remaining alternatives. To indicate your selection, use a pencil to blacken the corresponding circle next to the answer choice and/or you can use the answer document at the back of this book. No marks are deducted for wrong answers.

The computer-based real MCAT has an on-screen highlighter function and ~~STRIKEOUT~~ function. These tools help to spotlight text or assist in the process of elimination. You may use a yellow highlighter for this paper-based exam and/or a pen (or preferably a pencil to make it easier should you change your mind) to mark text. At the time of publishing, both highlighting and strikeout functions can be used for passages, questions and answer choices. You can also flag a question to review later should time remain.

For the real exam, you will be provided with a dry erase board which is a white laminated noteboard booklet accompanied by a fine point marker. The noteboard includes 9 graph-lined pages for you to write though you cannot erase. You can simulate the experience with a fine point marker on a noteboard or with 8” x 14” plain graph paper.

You may consult the periodic table at any point during the science subtests.

Please note: For the real MCAT, a small number of field-tested questions will remain unscored.

This practice test has been designed exclusively to test knowledge and thinking skills. This exam may contain hypothetical statements and/or express controversial ideas. Statements contained herein do not necessarily reflect the policy, position, or view of RuveneCo Inc. or MCAT-prep.com.

START EXAM ONLY WHEN TIMER IS READY.

Passage 1 (Questions 1–4)

An elevated concentration of plasma LDL cholesterol is a major risk factor for the development of coronary heart disease. Cholesterol is biosynthesized in a series of 25 separate enzymatic reactions that initially involves 2 successive condensations of three acetyl-CoA units to form the compound HMG-CoA. This is reduced and then converted in a series of reactions to the isoprenes that are building-blocks of squalene (a terpene) - the immediate precursor to sterols - which cyclizes and is further metabolized to cholesterol.

Lovastatin is a cholesterol-lowering agent isolated from the fungus *Aspergillus terreus*. Its metabolite is an inhibitor of HMG-CoA reductase which catalyzes an early and rate limiting step in the biosynthesis of cholesterol.

Consider the structure of lovastatin.

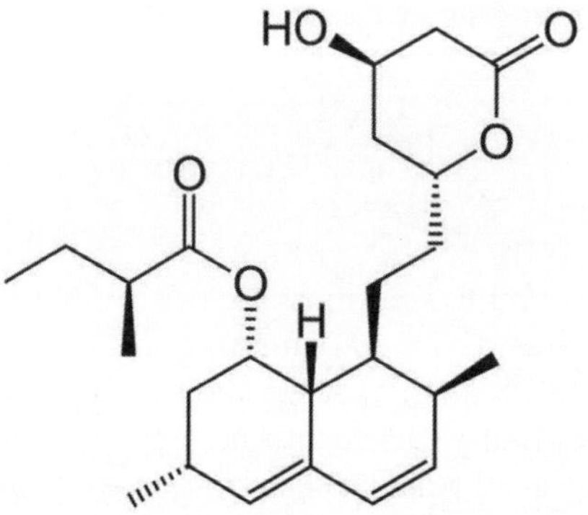

Figure 1 Structure of Lovastatin. Note that the bicyclic moiety of lovastatin is referred to as the hexahydro-naphthalene ring.

Question 1

The HMG moiety in the molecule HMG-CoA has how many carbons?

- ○ **A.** 4
- ○ **B.** 6
- ○ **C.** 9
- ○ **D.** 18

Question 2

How many chiral centers does lovastatin have?

- ○ **A.** Fewer than 8
- ○ **B.** 8
- ○ **C.** 9
- ○ **D.** More than 9

Question 3

Lovastatin has 2 double bonds in the hexahydro-naphthalene moeity. From left to right, which of the following is consistent with the configuration at the 2 double bonds?

- O **A.** *E, E*
- O **B.** *E, Z*
- O **C.** *Z, E*
- O **D.** *Z, Z*

Question 4

In the segments of lovastatin that are outside of the hexahydro-naphthalene moiety, as compared to *R* configuration chiral centers, lovastatin has:

- O **A.** one more *S* configuration chiral center.
- O **B.** one fewer *S* configuration chiral center.
- O **C.** the same number of *S* chiral centers.
- O **D.** None of the above since Lovastatin has no *S* chiral centers.

Passage 2 (Questions 5–8)

An electron transport chain (ETC) is a series of compounds that transfer electrons from electron donors to electron acceptors via redox reactions, and couples this electron transfer with the transfer of protons across a membrane. ATP synthase is an integral protein consisting of several different subunits, which as a group, is directly responsible for the production of ATP via chemiosmotic phosphorylation.

A student took notes outlining the basic elements of the ETC and illustrated the result as follows:

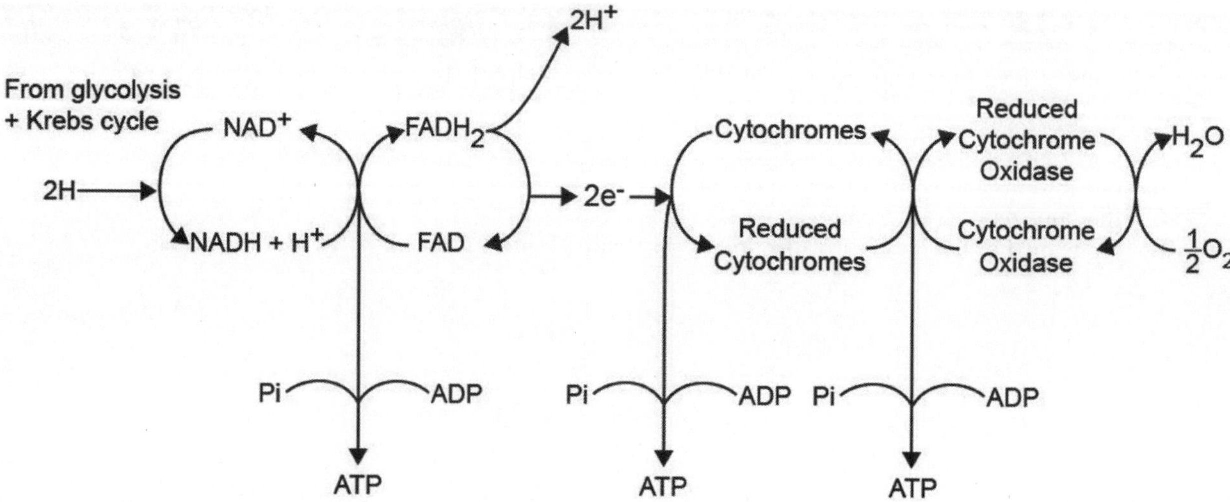

Next, the student tabulated some standard results of reduction potentials for several important metabolic reactions.

Table 1 Standard half-reaction reduction potentials.

Reduction: Half Reactions	$E^{o\prime}$ (V)
Acetyl CoA + CO_2 + H^+ + $2e^-$ → Pyruvate + CoA	-0.48
$2H^+ + 2e^- \rightarrow H_2$	-0.42
α-Ketoglutarate + CO_2 + $2H^+$ + $2e^-$ → Isocitrate	-0.38
NAD^+ + $2H^+$ + $2e^-$ → NADH + H^+	-0.32
FAD + $2H^+$ + $2e^-$ → $FADH_2$	-0.22
FMN + $2H^+$ + $2e^-$ → $FMNH_2$	-0.22
Acetaldehyde + $2H^+$ + $2e^-$ → Ethanol	-0.20
Pyruvate + $2H^+$ + $2e^-$ → Lactate	-0.18
Oxaloacetate + $2H^+$ + $2e^-$ → Malate	-0.17
Cytochrome b_5^{3+} + e^- → Cytochrome b_5^{2+}	0.02
Fumarate + $2H^+$ + $2e^-$ → Succinate	0.03
Ubiquinone (Q) + $2H^+$ + $2e^-$ → Ubiquinol (QH_2)	0.04
Cytochrome c^{3+} + e^- → Cytochrome c^{2+}	0.23
Cytochrome a^{3+} + e^- → Cytochrome a^{2+}	0.39
1/2 O_2 + $2H^+$ + $2e^-$ → H_2O	0.82

Question 5

Which of the following would best explain why the student's illustration shows 2 electrons funneled into the ETC but Table 1 shows only one electron per cytochrome b, c and a, respectively?

- O **A.** The student made an error.
- O **B.** The electron pair is shared between 2 different cytochromes: one electron from the electron pair goes to one cytochrome as the other electron goes to a different cytochrome.
- O **C.** The metal ion in cytochrome is a one-electron acceptor requiring 2 molecules of each cytochrome per electron pair entering the ETC.
- O **D.** The cytochromes have half of the molecular weight of the precursors in the ETC.

Question 6

Based on Table 1, in the absence of coenzyme A, which of the following is the strongest reducing agent?

- O **A.** Lactate
- O **B.** Pyruvate
- O **C.** Malate
- O **D.** Succinate

Question 7

How many voltaic cells with a voltage of at least 1200 mV can be made using the standard half-cell reactions listed in Table 1?

- O **A.** 0
- O **B.** 1
- O **C.** 2
- O **D.** 3

Question 8

Which of the following statements best describes why the ETC is effective in achieving an overall electron transfer?

- O **A.** Each step involves the pumping of protons across the inner mitochondrial membrane.
- O **B.** The E° value of each carrier becomes more positive than the previous carrier.
- O **C.** All reactions are based on the interconversion of the ferrous ion to the ferric ion.
- O **D.** NADH and oxygen come into contact only on the matrix side producing water.

The following questions are NOT based on a descriptive passage (Questions 9–12).

Question 9

20 mL of 0.05 M Mg^{2+} in solution is desired. It is attempted to achieve this by adding 5 mL of 0.005 M $MgCl_2$ and 15 mL of $Mg_3(PO_4)_2$. What is the concentration of $Mg_3(PO_4)_2$?

- O **A.** 0.065 M
- O **B.** 0.022 M
- O **C.** 0.150 M
- O **D.** 0.100 M

Question 10

Which of the following is the strongest reducing agent?

Electrochemical reaction	E° value (V)
$MnO_2 + 4H^+ + 2e^- \leftrightarrow Mn^{2+} + 2H_2O$	+1.23
$Fe^{3+} + e^- \leftrightarrow Fe^{2+}$	+0.771
$N_2 + 5H^+ + 4e^- \leftrightarrow N_2H_5^+$	-0.230
$Cr^{3+} + e^- \leftrightarrow Cr^{2+}$	-0.410

- O **A.** Cr^{3+}
- O **B.** Cr^{2+}
- O **C.** Mn^{2+}
- O **D.** MnO_2

Question 11

Given that the hydrolysis of ATP has a ΔG° of -32.5 kJ/mol, and the hydrolysis of glucose-6-phosphate has a ΔG° of -11.6 kJ/mol, what is the overall ΔG° for the phosphorylation of glucose by ATP?

- O **A.** +20.9 kJ/mol
- O **B.** -20.9 kJ/mol
- O **C.** +44.1 kJ/mol
- O **D.** -44.1 kJ/mol

Question 12

The biceps muscle holds the forearm and any load held by the hand, if present. There are forces at the elbow joint where the humerus meets the radius. The human forearm can be considered as a set of levers as illustrated below.

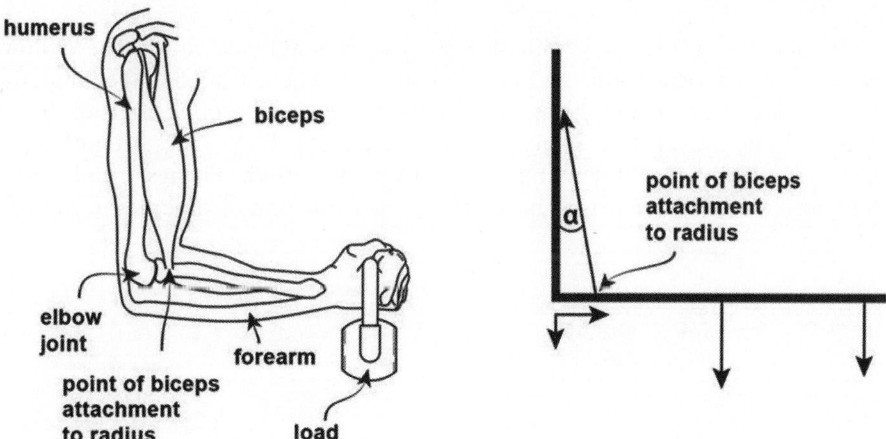

Consider that the arm is in rotational and translational equilibrium, as the load held in the hand increases, what would be the expected change in the vertical and horizontal components of the forces at the elbow, respectively?

- O **A.** Decreased, increased
- O **B.** Increased, does not change
- O **C.** Increased, increased
- O **D.** Decreased, does not change

Passage 3 (Questions 13–16)

Motor vehicle crashes account for nearly 1.3 million deaths every year and is the 9th leading cause of death. While the first mass-produced car was sold in 1903, it wasn't until the mid-1960s that vehicle safety standards were implemented, including the use of crash test dummies.

Crash test dummies, which are anthropomorphic devices used in simulated car crashes, allow companies to measure the forces a driver experiences during and after impact. These tests help car manufacturers design cars to keep passengers safe by minimizing the amount of force they feel during a collision. In a research study sponsored by the National Highway Traffic Safety Administration (NHTSA), a test dummy in a Dodge Grand Caravan SE was crashed into a barrier with an impact velocity of 56.3 km/h. The test dummy was prepared with a head accelerometer which recorded the driver's head velocity as a function of time as shown in Figure 1.

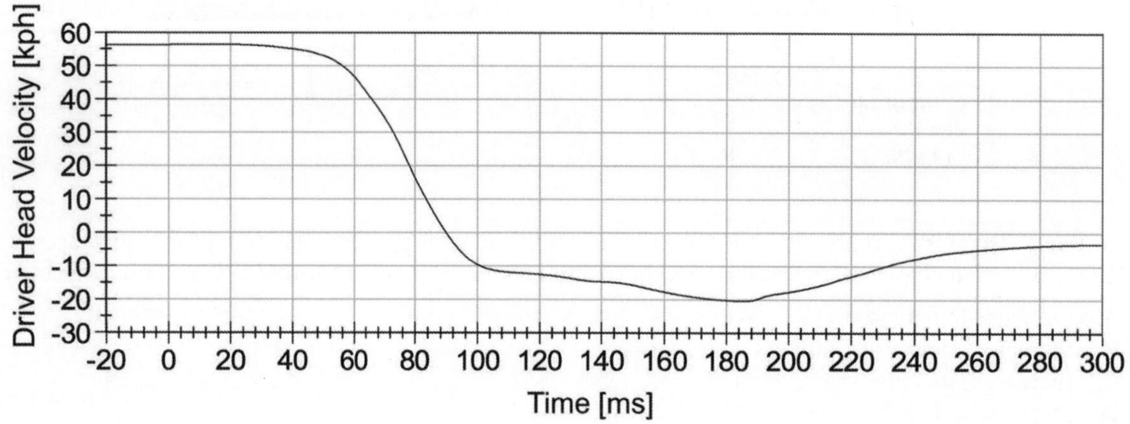

Figure 1 Velocity [kph] vs. time [ms] of the translational motion [along one axis] of the head of the test dummy.

Car manufacturers use measures such as the Head Injury Criterion (HIC) to determine the likelihood of a head injury in a collision. The HIC is proportional to the force the driver feels and the time duration of the acceleration. Crash test dummies provide a means for measuring the HIC of various cars and are used to determine the NHTSA star rating for automobile safety. Cars with larger HIC values are ranked less safe.

Question 13

What is the maximum deceleration felt by the driver?

- ○ **A.** 0.5 km/s^2
- ○ **B.** 1.5 km/s^2
- ○ **C.** 10 km/s^2
- ○ **D.** 1500 km/s^2

Question 14

During which time interval did the driver experience the highest risk of a head injury?

- ○ **A.** 10-20 ms
- ○ **B.** 70-80 ms
- ○ **C.** 100-110 ms
- ○ **D.** 180-190 ms

Question 15

If the speed of the car described in the passage increased by a factor of two, the energy in the crash will:

- ○ **A.** increase by 2.
- ○ **B.** increase by 4.
- ○ **C.** decrease by 2.
- ○ **D.** decrease by 4.

Question 16

Which of the following graphs best illustrates the driver's head deceleration after the impact?

○ **A.**

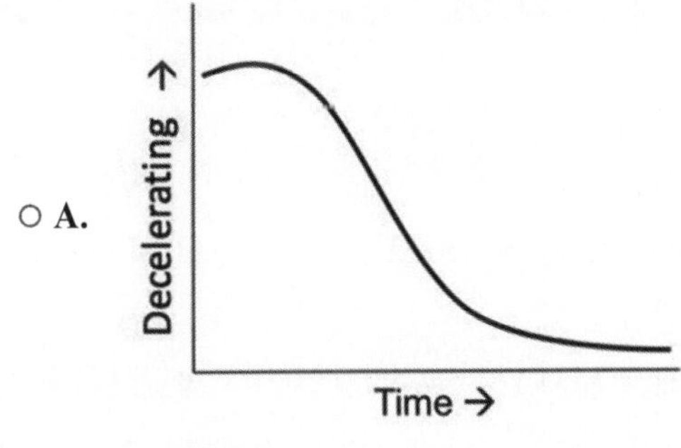

○ **B.**

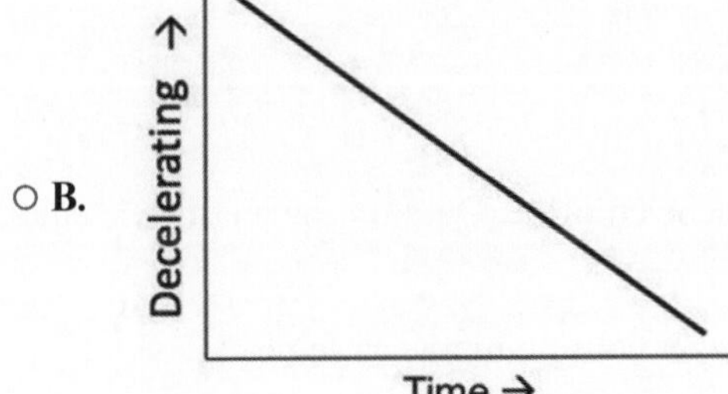

○ **C.**

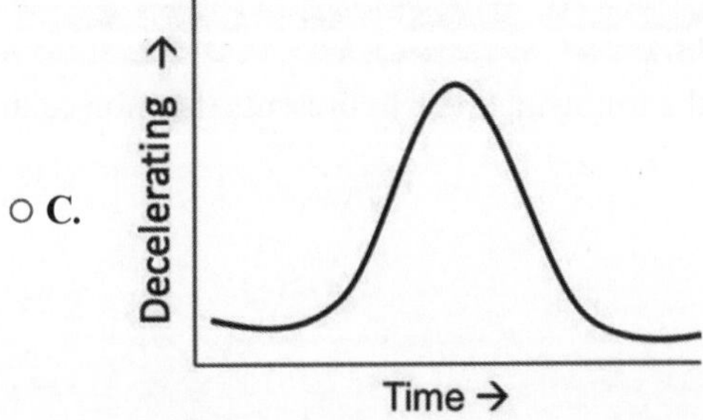

○ **D.**

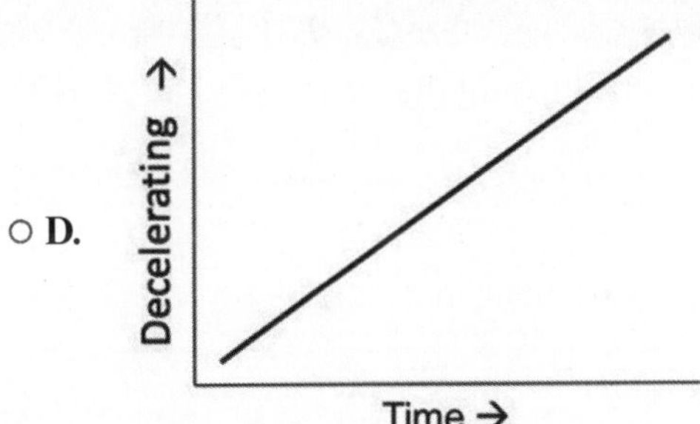

Passage 4 (Questions 17–22)

A stimulant found in tea leaves is caffeine ($C_8H_{10}N_4O_2$). Tea leaves contain 3% caffeine by weight and a trace amount of theophylline, a homolog lacking the methyl group at position 7. The structure for caffeine can be seen in Figure 1.

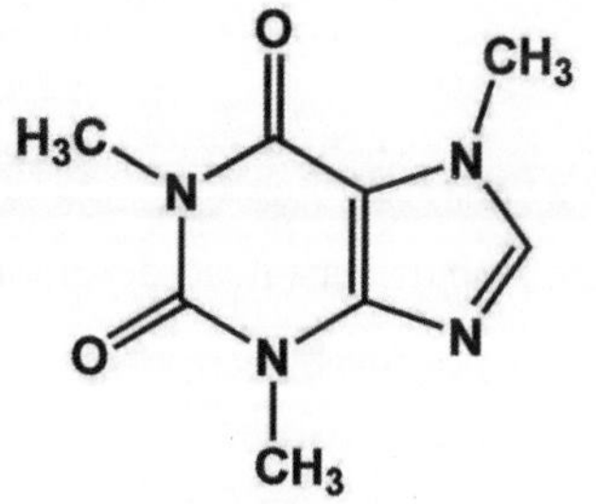

Figure 1

A student decided to investigate properties of caffeine. To begin, she attempted to extract caffeine from tea leaves by following the protocol below.

1. Add 50 g dry tea leaves, 15 g powered $CaCO_3$, and 300 ml of 80 °C H_2O to a 500 ml flask.
2. Boil the mixture for 20 minutes.
3. Filter the hot mixture with a Buckner funnel.
4. Cool the aqueous extract to 15 - 20 °C.
5. Transfer the extract to a separatory funnel containing methylene chloride. Data on the methylene chloride: molecular weight - 84.93; density - 1.33 g/ml; vapor density - 2.9.
6. Shake the funnel, let the layers separate, remove the desired layer containing the caffeine.

Question 17

Caffeine and theophylline are both neutral compounds. Which of the following likely represents the molecular formula for theophylline?

- O **A.** $C_9H_{13}N_4O_2$
- O **B.** $C_8H_{13}N_4O_2$
- O **C.** $C_7H_7N_4O_2$
- O **D.** $C_7H_8N_4O_2$

Question 18

Which of the following best explains why the protocol requires the student to add the tea leaves to 80 °C H_2O in Step 1?

- O **A.** H_2O at 80 °C serves to dampen the dry tea leaves.
- O **B.** Caffeine is relatively soluble in H_2O at 80 °C.
- O **C.** H_2O at 80 °C serves as a solvent for the reaction of calcium carbonate and caffeine.
- O **D.** H_2O at 80 °C is below the boiling point.

Question 19

Caffeine is best characterized as a:

- O **A.** steroid.
- O **B.** pyrimidine.
- O **C.** purine.
- O **D.** nitrogenous base.

Question 20

The solvent used to do the extraction should do all of the following EXCEPT:

- O **A.** be sparingly soluble in the liquid from which the solute is to be extracted.
- O **B.** readily dissolve the substance to be extracted.
- O **C.** react chemically with the solute to form a complex product.
- O **D.** be easily separated from the solute after extraction.

Question 21

Which of the following best states the relationship between methylene chloride and the aqueous extract?

- O **A.** Methylene chloride will make up the bottom layer of liquid and aqueous extract the top layer in the separatory funnel.
- O **B.** The aqueous extract will make up the bottom layer and methylene chloride the top layer in the separatory funnel.
- O **C.** The aqueous extract is soluble in the methylene chloride.
- O **D.** Impurities in the mixture are extracted from the methylene chloride to the aqueous extract.

Question 22

In the absence of caffeine and when a person is awake and alert, little is expressed by CNS neurons. However, during a continued wakeful state, over time, adenosine accumulates in the neuronal synapses resulting in the binding to and the activation of adenosine receptors found on certain CNS neurons; when activated, these receptors produce cellular responses that ultimately increase drowsiness. Thus it can be concluded that when caffeine is consumed, it acts as an adenosine:

- O **A.** chaperone.
- O **B.** promoter.
- O **C.** receptor agonist.
- O **D.** receptor antagonist.

Passage 5 (Questions 23–28)

Streptavidin is a bacterial protein that is routinely used in biological applications as a binding partner for biotin, a water-soluble B-vitamin. The structure of a biotin-binding site of streptavidin is complex and irregular. In the naturally occurring streptavidin, the biotin-binding site contains amino acids N23 and S27 (numbers represent the positions of the amino acids in the primary structure). Side chains of these amino acids participate in the formation of hydrogen bonds with ureic oxygen of biotin. In certain applications, it is necessary to alter the ligand binding specificity of streptavidin.

Experiment: Streptavidin Binding to Biotin and its Analogs

The biotin-binding site of streptavidin was redesigned to weaken its interactions with biotin while maintaining a strong affinity to the two other biotin analogs, 2-iminobiotin and diaminobiotin. To alter its biotin binding specificity, different mutations were introduced in the biotin-binding site of streptavidin. These mutations disrupted the hydrogen bonds formed between N23 and S27 side chains of streptavidin and biotin.

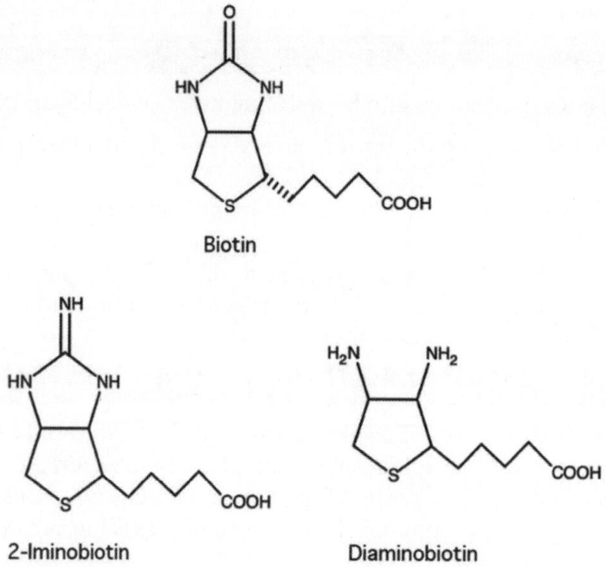

O
HN NH
S COOH
Biotin

NH
HN NH
S COOH
2-Iminobiotin

H_2N NH_2
S COOH
Diaminobiotin

Figure 1 Schematic chemical representation of biotin and its analogs: 2-iminobiotin and diaminobiotin

The streptavidin-biotin interaction was determined to be as follows in the cases identified as I, II, III and IV.

I. Natural streptavidin complexed with biotin

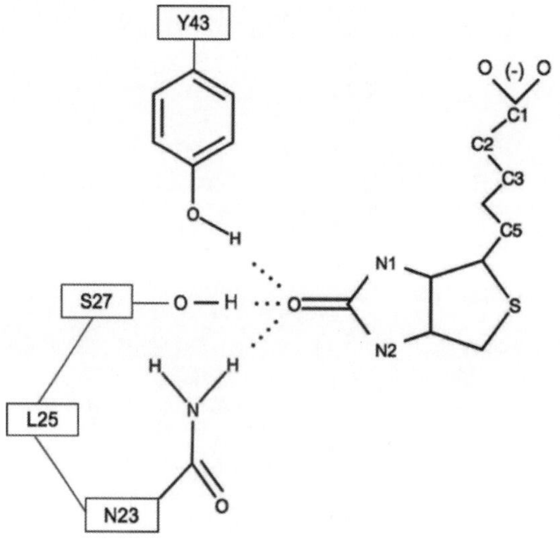

Y43
O (-) O
C1
C2
C3
C5
O H
N1
S27 O — H ··· O
S
N2
H H
N
L25
N23 O

II. Natural streptavidin complexed with 2-iminobiotin

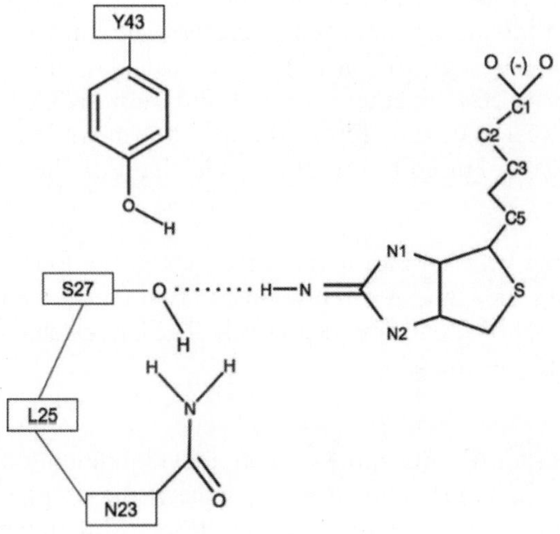

III. Streptavidin mutant complexed with biotin

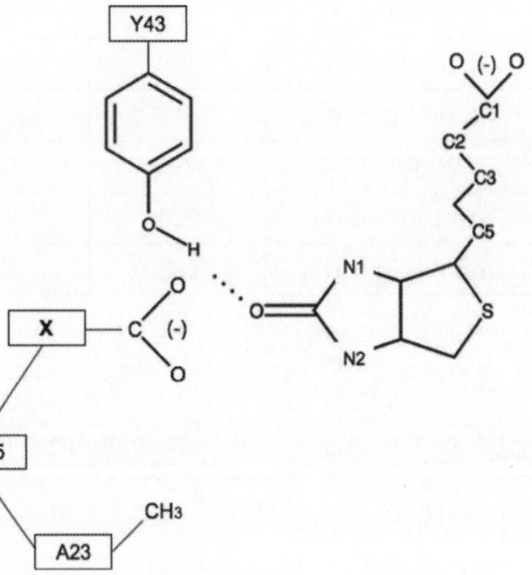

IV. Streptavidin mutant complexed with 2-iminobiotin

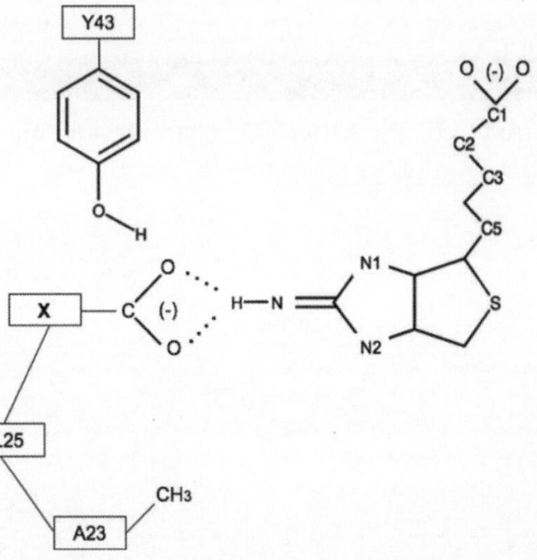

When designing streptavidin mutants, the difference in a local electrostatic charge distribution between biotin and the two different biotin analogs was used to predict the effect of changing amino acids on biotin-binding potential. S27 in the biotin-binding site is the amino acid residue known to have the largest electrostatic contribution to the binding free energy. Based on free energy calculations, it was predicted that introducing a negative charge at the position of S27 together with the mutation N23A (Mutant A23X27) would disrupt the hydrogen bonds formed between natural streptavidin and biotin while allowing a formation of a strong bond between the imino hydrogen of amino biotin and a side chain of the new amino acid at position 27 of streptavidin.

To evaluate the binding free energy between biotin and streptavidin, the following formula was used: $\Delta G = \Delta E + \Delta G_d + \Delta G_{const} - T\Delta S_c$, where ΔE, ΔG_d, and ΔS_c represent internal energy change, the desolvation free energy change, and the change in conformational entropy respectively. The energy change, ΔE is the sum of electrostatic, van der Waals, and the internal energy values.

Table 1 Measured values for ΔE, ΔG and K_a for streptavidin binding to biotin and its analogs are shown. Mutations refer to the amino acid sequence of the streptavidin with None for the natural streptavidin and Mutant for the streptavidin mutant A23X27.

Mutations	Ligand	ΔE	ΔG	K_a (M^{-1})
None	Biotin	-	-	2.5×10^{13}
	2-Iminobiotin	1.8	1.0	8×10^6
	Diaminobiotin	4.2	3.4	ND
Mutant	Biotin	10.3	-0.1	1.4×10^4
	2-Iminobiotin	6.4	1.1	1×10^6
	Diaminobiotin	6.2	3.5	2.7×10^4

Adapted from Reznik et al. A streptavidin mutant with altered ligand-binding specificity. 1998. PNAS, Vol. 95, pp. 13525-13530.

Question 23

How many stereocenters does biotin possess?

- O **A.** 0
- O **B.** 1
- O **C.** 2
- O **D.** 3

Question 24

What amino acid is likely to be introduced at position 27 in a streptavidin mutant (labeled as X in illustration III and IV)?

- O **A.** D or E
- O **B.** A or W
- O **C.** R or D
- O **D.** H or K

Question 25

The binding free energy, ΔG can be calculated using experimental approach and it depends on a number of factors including which of the following?

- ○ **A.** The internal energy change within a molecule
- ○ **B.** The electrostatic energy of the binding surface
- ○ **C.** The change in the conformational entropy
- ○ **D.** All of the above

Question 26

2-iminobiotin shows a drastically lower binding affinity to the natural streptavidin as compared to biotin. Also, the streptavidin mutant has a significantly lower binding affinity to biotin as compared to the 2-iminobiotin, which is reflected by K_a values in the table. The main reason for such difference could be due to which of the following?

- ○ **A.** The protonation change in the 2-iminobiotin affecting the formation of hydrogen bonds.
- ○ **B.** The difference in electrostatic properties as defined by the presence of the guanidino group in 2-iminobiotin and the absence of the ureic group in biotin.
- ○ **C.** The change in thermal energy in 2-iminobiotin as compared to biotin.
- ○ **D.** The structural differences between the biotin and its analogs.

Question 27

The high ΔE value measured for biotin complexed with the streptavidin mutant could be explained by:

- ○ **A.** the loss of van der Waals bonds formed between biotin analogs and streptavidin.
- ○ **B.** the introduction of structural strains in the complex.
- ○ **C.** the electrostatic attraction between biotin and the mutant being weak.
- ○ **D.** the electrostatic attraction between biotin and the mutant being strong.

Question 28

According to the information provided, the drastic reduction of the K_a measured for the streptavidin mutant complexed with biotin was likely due to which of the following?

I. The disruption of hydrogen bonds formed by the side chains between biotin and streptavidin
II. The conformational change within the molecule reducing the binding surface between biotin and streptavidin mutant
III. The change in the charge of the biotin-binding site of the streptavidin mutant

- ○ **A.** I only
- ○ **B.** II and III only
- ○ **C.** I and III only
- ○ **D.** I, II and III

The following questions are NOT based on a descriptive passage (Questions 29–32).

Question 29

Astatine is the last member of Group VII and is radioactive with a half-life of 8 hours. Astatine is an alternative to radioactive iodine for the diagnosis and treatment of thyroid conditions.

Consider the transport of an astatine sample which took 20 hours. What proportion of the sample had undergone radioactive decay?

- O **A.** 0.58
- O **B.** 0.18
- O **C.** 0.82
- O **D.** 0.42

Question 30

75 grams of glucose ($C_6H_{12}O_6$) and 75 grams of sucrose ($C_{12}H_{22}O_{11}$) were each added to beakers of water (beaker 1 and beaker 2, respectively). Which of the following would be true?

- O **A.** Boiling point elevation for beaker 1 would be greater than the boiling point elevation for beaker 2.
- O **B.** Boiling point elevation for beaker 1 would be less than the boiling point elevation for beaker 2.
- O **C.** The same degree of boiling point elevation will occur in both beakers.
- O **D.** No boiling point elevation would be observed in either of the beakers.

Question 31

What would the freezing point in kelvin of a solution which is 0.50 molal in sucrose and 0.50 molal in acetic acid be?

(K_f of water = 2.0 °C mol^{-1} and freezing point of water = 0 °C)

- O **A.** -1.0 K
- O **B.** -2.0 K
- O **C.** 272 K
- O **D.** 271 K

Question 32

Nitric oxide (NO) is a free radical which is well known as a powerful vasodilator with a short half-life of only a few seconds in blood. Consider the equilibrium shown below which was established within the confines of a closed system.

Reaction I

$4NH_3(g) + 5O_2(g) \leftrightarrow 4NO(g) + 6H_2O(g)$

$\Delta H_{rxn} = -1100 \text{ kJ mol}^{-1}$

What effect will increasing the pressure have on this system?

- O **A.** The equilibrium will shift to the left.
- O **B.** The equilibrium will shift to the right.
- O **C.** The equilibrium position will remain the same.
- O **D.** The equilibrium position will depend on whether a catalyst is present or not.

Note: This page is left blank so that the passage would be visible without turning pages while assessing the passage-based questions.

Passage 6 (Questions 33–36)

Local anaesthetics prevent or relieve pain by interrupting nerve conduction. All local anaesthetics are membrane stabilizing drugs; they reversibly decrease the rate of depolarization and repolarization of excitable membranes. They bind to specific receptor sites on the sodium channels in nerves and block the movement of ions through these pores. Structural features of local anaesthetics are shown in Figure 1.

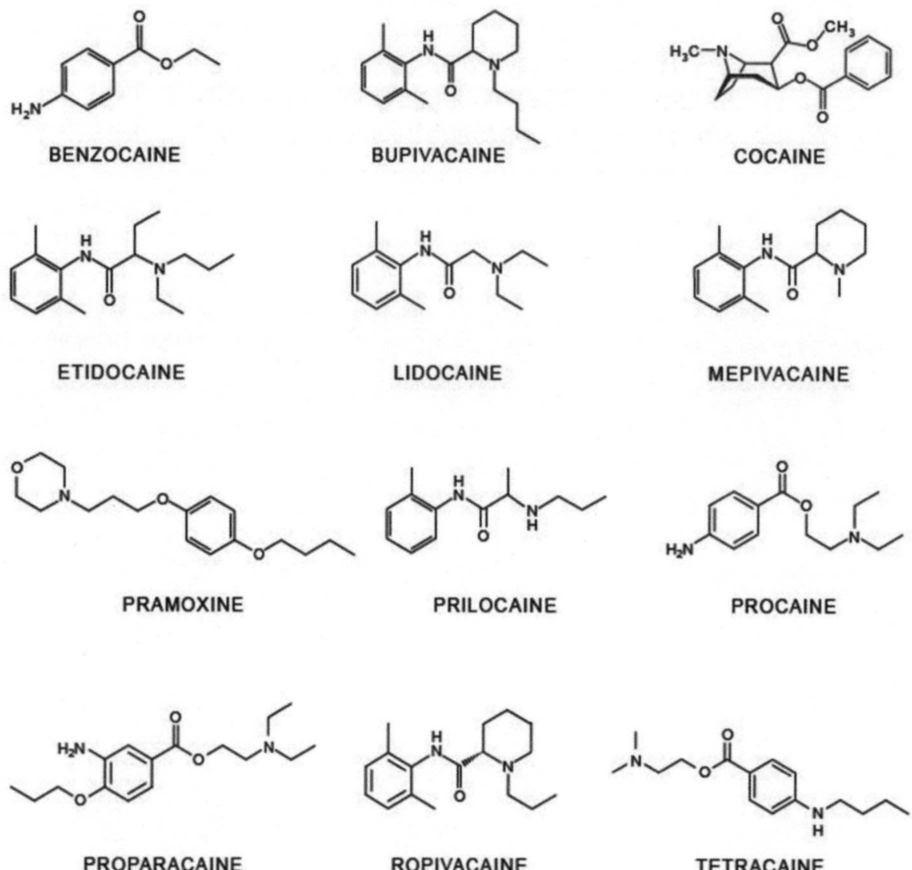

Figure 1 Structures of 12 of the most commonly used local anaesthetics

Both the chemical and pharmacologic properties of local anaesthetic drugs determine their clinical properties. Local anaesthetic agents are weak bases, and exist in ionized and unionized forms.

During manufacture they are precipitated as powdered solids which are relatively insoluble. For this reason, they are produced as water-soluble salts to allow them to be injected. These are usually hydrochloride salts which produce a mildly acidic solution that is stable and can be injected. Sodium bicarbonate ($NaHCO_3$) is often added to local anaesthetics as part of their manufacture.

Table 1 The pKa of several local anaesthetic agents

Anaesthetic	pKa
Mepivacaine	7.6
Etidocaine	7.7
Articaine	7.8
Lidocaine	7.9
Prilocaine	7.9
Bupivacaine	8.1
Procaine	9.1

Local anaesthetics must pass through the nerve membrane in a non-ionized lipid-soluble base form, and once they are within the nerve, they must equilibrate into an ionic form to be active (Figure 2). The fraction of the base form is inversely related to how long it takes these anaesthetics to act (onset time). The pH of normal body tissue is 7.4, but active infections can increase the acidity of surrounding tissues considerably.

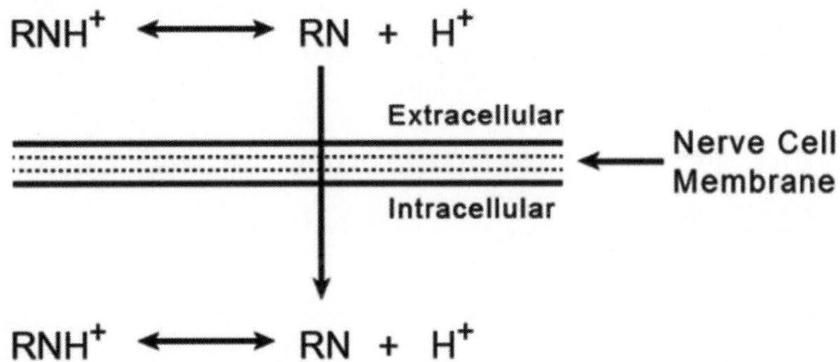

Figure 2 Movement of local anaesthetic ions through the cell membrane of a nerve cell which leads to local analgesia. The receptor site for activity is thought to be located at the cytoplasmic (inner) portion of the sodium channel.

Question 33

At normal tissue pH of 7.4, which of the anaesthetics in Table 1 would have the highest percentage of diffusible form available to penetrate the cell membrane?

- O **A.** Procaine
- O **B.** Mepivacaine
- O **C.** Bupivacaine
- O **D.** Either lidocaine or prilocaine

Question 34

Why would sodium bicarbonate be added to local anaesthetics?

- O **A.** To inhibit the formation of the base form so they take longer to work.
- O **B.** To increase the amount of the base form which shortens the time it takes to work.
- O **C.** To increase the amount of cationic form present and so it becomes less painful to inject.
- O **D.** To equilibrate the amounts of cationic and base form present.

Question 35

What effect would injecting lidocaine into an infected site have on the onset time of analgesia?

- O **A.** It would decrease it.
- O **B.** It would have no effect.
- O **C.** It would increase it.
- O **D.** It would have a result more like mepivacaine.

Question 36

Amide-linked local anaesthetics such as lidocaine are metabolized by amine dealkylation in the liver by the cytochrome P450 system. Which of the following is likely to be a metabolite of lidocaine?

○ A.

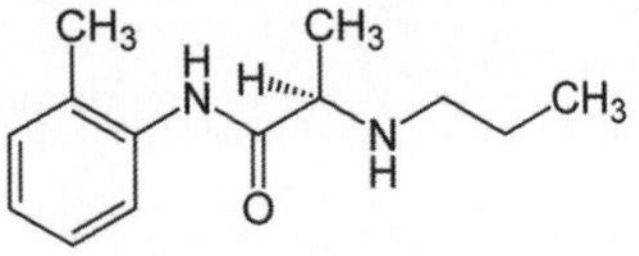

○ B.

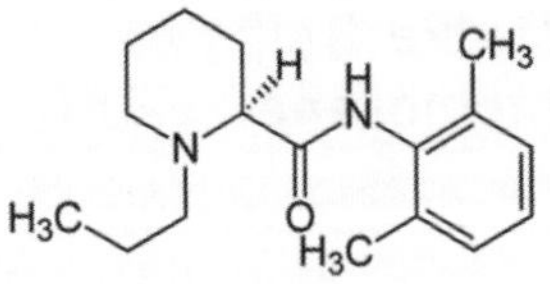

○ C.

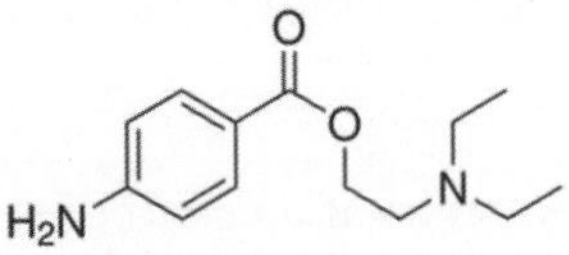

○ D.

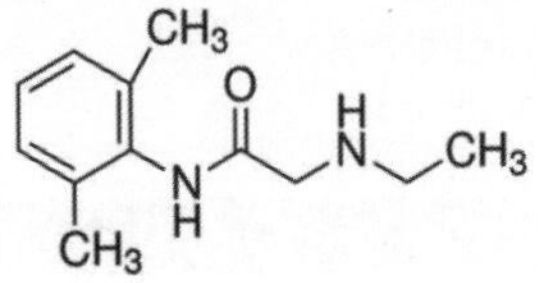

Passage 7 (Questions 37–40)

The invention of the compound microscope by Jansen in the late 1500's truly revolutionized the world of science, particularly the field of cellular and molecular biology. The discovery of the cell as the fundamental unit of living organisms and the insight into the bacterial world are two of the contributions of this instrument to science.

It is unseemly that such a relatively simplistic apparatus took generations to be developed. Its main components are two convex lenses: one acts as the main magnifying lens and is referred to as the objective, and another lens called the eyepiece. The two lenses act independently of each other when bending light rays. The actual lens set-up is depicted in Fig.1.

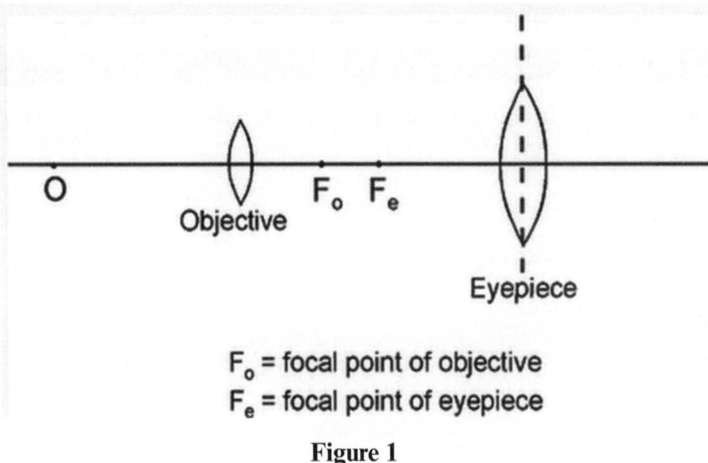

Figure 1

Light from the object (O) first passes through the objective and an enlarged, inverted first image is formed. The eyepiece then magnifies this image. Usually the magnification of the eyepiece is fixed (either x10 or x15) and three rotating objective lenses are used: x10, x40 and x60. The most recent development in microscope technology is the electron microscope which uses a beam of electrons instead of light. Photographic film must be used otherwise no image would be formed on the retina. This microscope has a resolution about a hundred times that of the light microscope.

Question 37

Based on the passage, what type of image would have to be produced by the objective magnification?

- **A.** Either virtual or real
- **B.** Virtual
- **C.** Real
- **D.** It depends on the focal length of the lens

Question 38

Two compound microscopes A and B were compared. Both had objectives and eyepieces with the same magnification but A gave an overall magnification that was greater than that of B. Which of the following is a plausible explanation?

- **A.** The distance between objective and eyepiece in A is greater than the corresponding distance in B.
- **B.** The distance between objective and eyepiece in A is less than the corresponding distance in B.
- **C.** The eyepiece and objective positions were reversed in A.
- **D.** The eyepiece and objective positions were reversed in B.

Question 39

The magnification of the eyepiece of a compound microscope is x15. The image height is 25 mm and the magnification of the objective is x40. What is the object height?

- **A.** 1.67 mm
- **B.** 0.60 mm
- **C.** 0.38 mm
- **D.** 0.04 mm

Question 40

What is the refractive power of an objective lens with a focal length of 0.50 cm?

- **A.** 0.2 diopters
- **B.** 2.0 diopters
- **C.** 20 diopters
- **D.** 200 diopters

Passage 8 (Questions 41–44)

The cortex of the adrenal gland is a source of corticosteroids. They are derived from cholesterol by oxidation, with cleavage of a portion of the alkyl substituent bonded to the carbon at the number 17 position.

Cholesterol

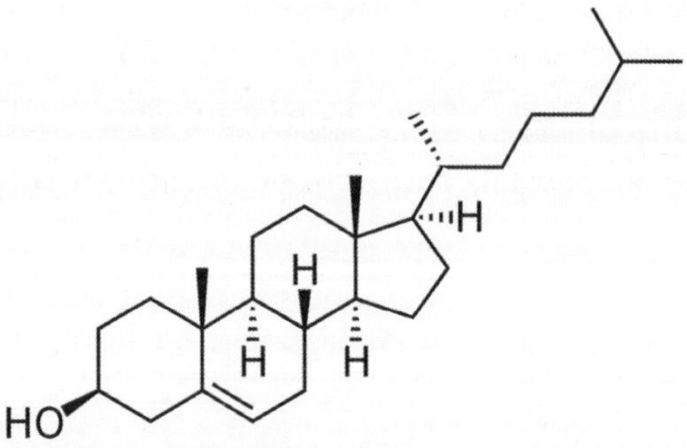

Two common corticosteroids are cortisol and cortisone.

Cortisol

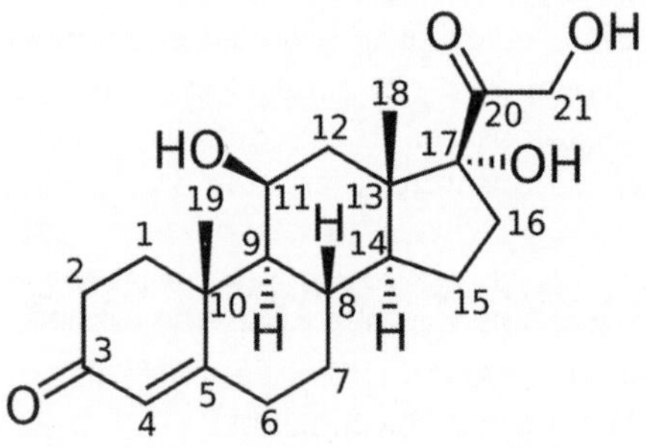

Cortisone

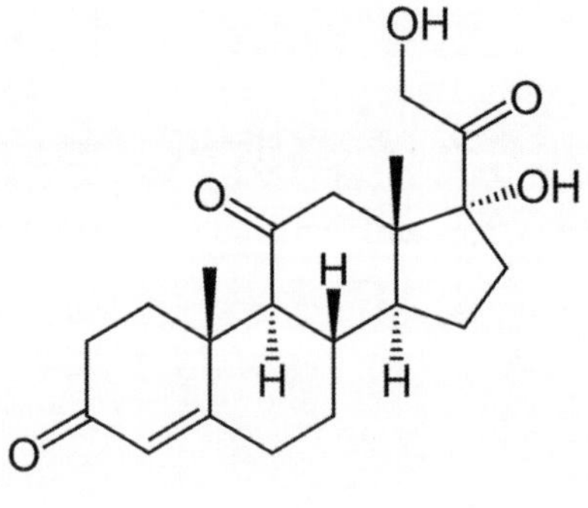

After attempting to separate the two corticosteroids by gas-liquid chromatography, the identity of each sample was determined by infrared spectroscopy.

Question 41

Cholesterol, cortisone and cortisol are best identified as:

- ○ **A.** cholesterols.
- ○ **B.** corticosteroids.
- ○ **C.** bile acids.
- ○ **D.** steroids.

Question 42

Which of the following would explain the non-separation of cortisol from cortisone by the method of gas-liquid chromatography (GLC)?

- ○ **A.** The solid material in the column of the GLC, through which substances pass in their mobile phase, absorbs cortisol and cortisone equally well.
- ○ **B.** Cortisol and cortisone have relatively high boiling points.
- ○ **C.** Cortisol and cortisone have very similar boiling points.
- ○ **D.** Cortisol moves through the column of the GLC, through which substances pass in their mobile phase, at a much quicker rate than cortisone.

Question 43

Which of the following absorption frequency ranges would be present in the IR spectrum of cortisone, but not cholesterol?

- ○ **A.** 1620 - 1680 cm^{-1}
- ○ **B.** 3200 - 3600 cm^{-1}
- ○ **C.** 2100 - 2200 cm^{-1}
- ○ **D.** 3350 - 3500 cm^{-1}

Question 44

In the body tissues, cortisol is likely converted to cortisone by which of the following enzymes?

- ○ **A.** 11-Hydroxysteroid dehydrogenase
- ○ **B.** 11-Oxysteroid isomerase
- ○ **C.** Steroid ligase
- ○ **D.** Transferases

The following questions are NOT based on a descriptive passage (Questions 45–48).

Question 45

In the reoxidation of QH_2 by the enzyme Complex III ubiquinone-cytochrome c reductase, the stoichiometry of the reaction requires 2 moles of cytochrome c per mole of QH_2 for which of the following reasons?

- O **A.** Cytochrome c is present in Complex III as 2 separate molecules.
- O **B.** Cytochrome c is a one-electron acceptor, whereas QH_2 is a two-electron donor.
- O **C.** Cytochrome c is a two-electron acceptor, whereas QH_2 is a one-electron donor.
- O **D.** As a result of the entropic penalty, twice as much cytochrome c as compared to QH_2 is required.

Question 46

Studies were carried out to determine the inhibition activities of the chemotherapeutic medications mocetinostat, belinostat, and entinostat for three types of histone deacetylases: HDAC1, HDAC2, and HDAC3.

Drug	IC_{50} HDAC1	IC_{50} HDAC2	IC_{50} HDAC3
Mocetinostat	0.15 μM	0.29 μM	1.66 μM
Belinostat	27 nM	27 nM	27 nM
Entinostat	0.51 μM	100 μM	1.7 μM

Which of the following is (are) the most potently inhibited by all three medications?

- O **A.** HDAC1
- O **B.** HDAC2
- O **C.** HDAC3
- O **D.** HDAC1 and HDAC2

Question 47

Four compounds - allyl alcohol, benzoic acid, 2-butanone and butyraldehyde - were identified and stored in separate bottles. By accident, the labels were lost from the sample bottles. The following information was obtained via infrared spectroscopy and was used to identify and relabel the sample bottles.

Infrared absorption peaks (cm^{-1})

Bottle I	Bottle II	Bottle III	Bottle IV
1700 (sharp)	1710	1730 (sharp)	3333 (broad)
-	3500-3333 (broad)	2730	1030 (small)

Which of the following most accurately represents the contents of bottles I, II, III, and IV, respectively?

- O **A.** Butyraldehyde, 2-butanone, benzoic acid, allyl alcohol
- O **B.** Benzoic acid, butyraldehyde, allyl alcohol, 2-butanone
- O **C.** 2-Butanone, butyraldehyde, allyl alcohol, benzoic acid
- O **D.** 2-Butanone, benzoic acid, butyraldehyde, allyl alcohol

Question 48

The ^{1}HNMR of compound X is shown in Fig. 1.

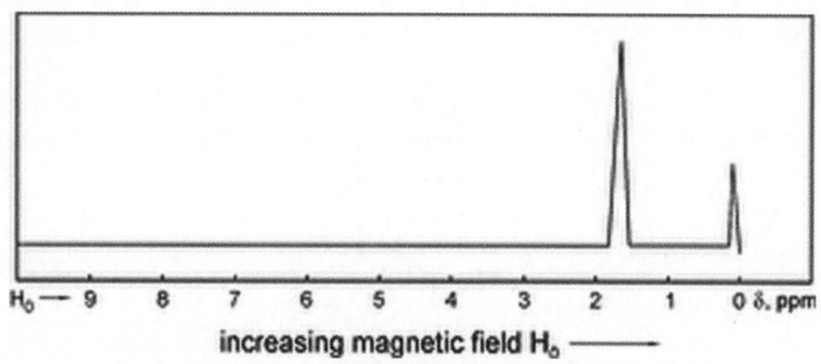

Figure 1

Compound X has the molecular formula C_6H_{12} and chemical tests revealed that the compound was an alkene. Which of the following best represents the structure of compound X?

- A. $CH_3—CH{=}CH—CH_2–CH_2–CH_3$
- B. $CH_3—C(CH_3){=}C(CH_3)—CH_3$
- C. $(CH_3)_2C{=}C(H)CH_2CH_3$
- D. (cyclohexene)

Passage 9 (Questions 49–52)

Figure 1 illustrates chemical methods often used by organic chemists for qualitative analysis of water soluble unknowns. Table 1 lists characteristic chemical tests of organic compounds. For instance, Fehling's tests that are positive are indicative of an aldehyde.

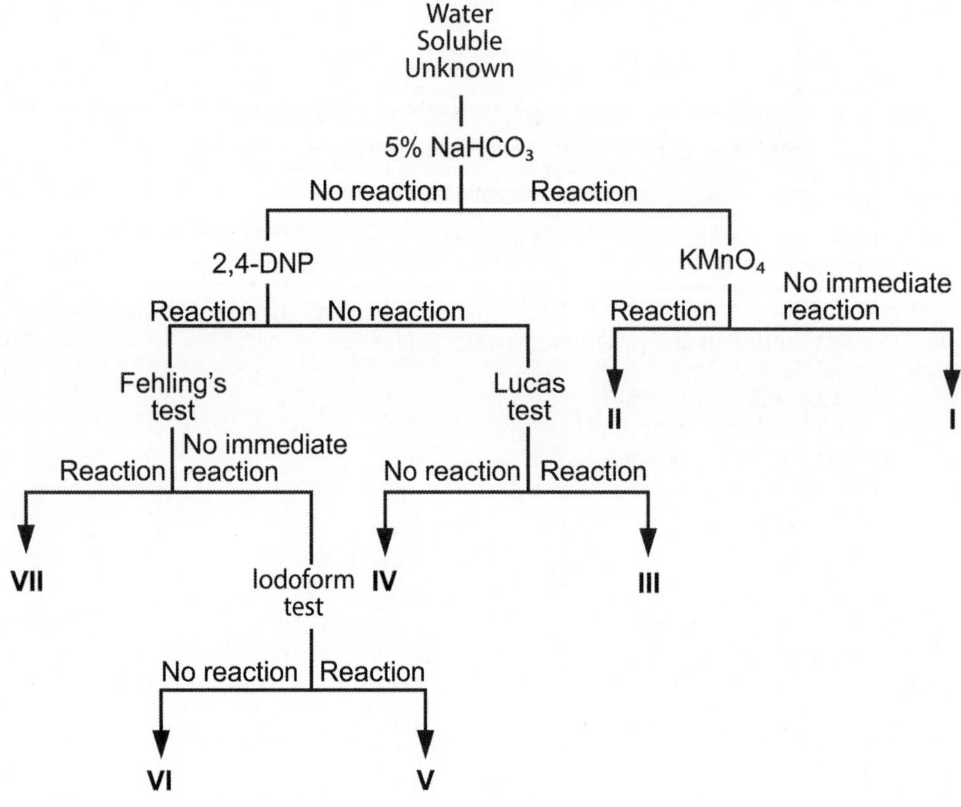

Figure 1

Chemical Test	Compounds
Sodium hydroxide	Organic acids: carboxylic acids and phenols
Lucas	Alcohols with 5 or less carbon atoms
Sodium bicarbonate	Carboxylic acids
2,4-Dinitro-phenylhydrazine (DNP)	Aldehydes and ketones
Fehling's solution	Aldehydes
Iodine in sodium hydroxide (Iodoform)	Acetaldehydes and ketones with the CH_3-CO- group Alcohols with the $CH_3CH(OH)$- as a structural feature
Sulfuric acid	Alcohols, ethers, alkenes Soluble Lewis bases

Table 1

Question 49

Cyclohexanol should fall into which of the following groups?

- O **A.** I
- O **B.** II
- O **C.** III
- O **D.** IV

Question 50

A water soluble unknown is unreactive in the presence of sodium bicarbonate, gives a positive 2,4-DNP test and negative Fehling's and Iodoform tests. In which of the following classes should this compound be classified?

- O **A.** Aldehyde
- O **B.** Ketone
- O **C.** Carboxylic acid
- O **D.** Alcohol

Question 51

When an ether solution of an aldehyde is added to an ether solution of lithium aluminum hydride ($LiAlH_4$), the carbonyl group of the aldehyde will be:

- O **A.** reduced to the corresponding primary alcohol.
- O **B.** hydrated to the corresponding diol.
- O **C.** reduced to the corresponding secondary alcohol.
- O **D.** deoxygenated to the corresponding alkane.

Question 52

Acetone should give positive test results for which of the following chemical tests?

- O **A.** Lucas and sodium bicarbonate
- O **B.** 2,4-DNP and Fehling's
- O **C.** Iodoform and 2,4-DNP
- O **D.** Iodoform and potassium permanganate

Passage 10 (Questions 53–56)

Various rules of thumb have been proposed by the scientific community to explain the mode of radioactive decay by various radioisotopes. One of the major rules is called the n/p ratio. If all the known isotopes of the elements are plotted on a graph of number of neutrons (n) versus number of protons (p), it is observed that all isotopes lying outside of a "stable" n/p ratio region are radioactive as shown in Figure 1.

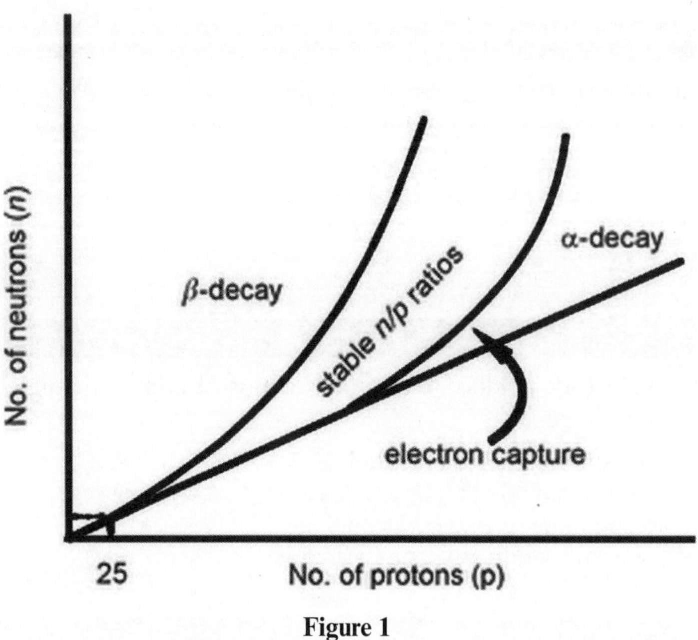

Figure 1

The graph exhibits straight line behavior with unit slope up to p = 25. Above p = 25, those isotopes with an n/p ratio lying below the stable region usually undergo electron capture while those with n/p ratios lying above the stable region usually undergo beta decay. Very heavy isotopes (p > 83) are unstable because of their relatively large nuclei and they undergo alpha decay. Gamma ray emission does not involve the release of a particle. It represents a change in an atom from a higher energy level to a lower energy level.

Question 53

How do gamma rays behave in an electric field?

- ○ **A.** They are not deflected in any direction.
- ○ **B.** They are deflected toward the positive plate.
- ○ **C.** They are deflected toward the negative plate.
- ○ **D.** They oscillate between plates, that is, they are attracted to one plate and then the other.

Question 54

How would the radioisotope of magnesium with mass number 27 undergo radioactive decay?

- ○ **A.** Electron capture
- ○ **B.** Alpha decay
- ○ **C.** Beta decay
- ○ **D.** Gamma ray emission

Question 55

The half-life of cobalt-60 is 5.2 years. If a sample's activity is 250 millicuries after 15.6 years, what must its original activity have been?

- O **A.** 500 millicuries
- O **B.** 1000 millicuries
- O **C.** 2000 millicuries
- O **D.** 5000 millicuries

Question 56

In a hypothetical radioactive series, Tl-210 undergoes 3 beta decay processes, 1 alpha decay process and 1 gamma ray emission to yield a stable product. What is the product?

- O **A.** $^{214}_{76}Os$
- O **B.** $^{214}_{84}Po$
- O **C.** $^{206}_{86}Rn$
- O **D.** $^{206}_{82}Pb$

The following questions are NOT based on a descriptive passage (Questions 57–59).

Question 57

All of the following contribute to the large, negative, Gibbs free energy change upon hydrolysis of "high energy" compounds EXCEPT one. Which one is the exception?

- O **A.** Stabilization of products by solvation
- O **B.** Stabilization of products by extra resonance forms
- O **C.** Low activation energy of the forward reaction
- O **D.** Electrostatic repulsion within the reactant

Question 58

Capillaries tend to be more permeable than most semipermeable membranes. The only significant plasma constituents that capillaries do not allow to pass are proteins. Given that the concentration of protein in plasma is approximately 1.5 mmol/L and the concentration of all solutes in plasma approximates 300 mmol/L, what is the oncotic pressure of plasma at the approximate body temperature of 37 °C with respect to capillaries? [The universal gas constant can be approximated as 60 L Torr $K^{-1}mol^{-1}$.]

- O **A.** 28 mmHg
- O **B.** 37 mmHg
- O **C.** 47 mmHg
- O **D.** 5.6×10^3 mmHg

Question 59

A novel enzyme DFL87G-1 catalyzes a reaction with k_{cat} equal to 500 s^{-1} and a specificity constant, k_{cat}/K_m, equal to 10^6 $M^{-1}s^{-1}$. At what concentration of the substrate would DFL87G-1 achieve half of the maximum velocity?

- O **A.** 5×10^{-4} μM
- O **B.** 2.5×10^{-4} μM
- O **C.** 500 μM
- O **D.** 250 μM

CANDIDATE'S NAME ______________________________

RAW SCORE AND SCALED SCORE ______________________

GS-2
Mock Exam 2 of 7
Solutions at MCAT-prep.com

GS-2 Section II:
Critical Analysis and Reasoning Skills (CARS)

Questions: 1-53
Time: 90 minutes

INSTRUCTIONS: This test contains nine passages, each of which is followed by several questions. After reading the passage, select the best answer to each question. If you are unsure of the answer, eliminate the alternatives you know to be false then select an answer from the remaining alternatives. To indicate your selection, use a pencil to blacken the corresponding circle next to the answer choice and/or you can use the answer document at the back of this book. No marks are deducted for wrong answers.

The computer-based real MCAT has an on-screen highlighter function and ~~STRIKEOUT~~ function. These tools help to spotlight text or assist in the process of elimination. You may use a yellow highlighter for this paper-based exam and/or a pen (or preferably a pencil to make it easier should you change your mind) to mark text. At the time of publishing, both highlighting and strikeout functions can be used for passages, questions and answer choices. You can also flag a question to review later should time remain.

For the real exam, you will be provided with a dry erase board which is a white laminated noteboard booklet accompanied by a fine point marker. The noteboard includes 9 graph-lined pages for you to write though you cannot erase. You can simulate the experience with a fine point marker on a noteboard or with 8" x 14" plain graph paper.

Please note: For the real MCAT, a small number of field-tested questions will remain unscored.

This practice test has been designed exclusively to test knowledge and thinking skills. This exam may contain hypothetical statements and/or express controversial ideas. Statements contained herein do not necessarily reflect the policy, position, or view of RuveneCo Inc. or MCAT-prep.com.

START EXAM ONLY WHEN TIMER IS READY.

Passage 1 (Questions 1–7)

Unlike some other classical figures (e.g. Auguste Comte, Émile Durkheim), Max Weber did not attempt, consciously, to create any specific set of rules governing social sciences in general, or sociology in particular. Compared to Durkheim and Marx, Weber was more focused on individuals and culture, and this is clear in his methodology. Whereas Durkheim focused on the society, Weber concentrated on the individuals and their actions, whereas Marx argued for the primacy of the material world over the world of ideas, Weber valued ideas as motivating actions of individuals, at least in the big picture.

Weber was concerned with the question of objectivity and subjectivity. Weber distinguished social action from social behavior, noting that social action must be understood through how individuals subjectively relate to one another. Study of social action through interpretive means must be based upon understanding the subjective meaning and purpose that the individual attaches to their actions. Social actions may have easily identifiable and objective means, but much more subjective ends, and the understanding of those ends by a scientist is subject to yet another layer of subjective understanding (that of the scientist). Weber noted that the importance of subjectivity in social sciences makes creation of full-proof, universal laws much more difficult than in natural sciences, and that the amount of objective knowledge that social sciences may achieve is precariously limited. Overall, Weber supported the goal of objective science, but he noted that it is an unreachable goal—although one definitely worth striving for.

> There is no absolutely "objective" scientific analysis of culture.... All knowledge of cultural reality... is always knowledge from particular points of view.... An "objective" analysis of cultural events, which proceeds according to the thesis that the ideal of science is the reduction of empirical reality to "laws," is meaningless... [because]... the knowledge of social laws is not knowledge of social reality but is rather one of the various aids used by our minds for attaining this end. (Max Weber, "Objectivity in Social Science," 1897)

The principle of "methodological individualism," which holds that social scientists should seek to understand collectivities (such as nations, cultures, governments, churches, corporations, etc.) solely as the result and the context of the actions of individual persons, can be traced to Weber, particularly to the first chapter of Economy and Society, in which he argues that only individuals "can be treated as agents in a course of subjectively understandable action." In other words, Weber argued that social phenomena can be understood scientifically only to the extent that they are captured by models of the behavior of purposeful individuals, models which Weber called "ideal types," from which actual historical events will necessarily deviate due to accidental and irrational factors. The analytical constructs of an ideal type never exist in reality, but provide objective benchmarks against which real-life constructs can be measured.

> We know of no scientifically ascertainable ideals. To be sure, that makes our efforts more arduous than in the past, since we are expected to create our ideals from within our breast in the very age of subjectivist culture.
>
> - Max Weber, 1909

Weber's methodology was developed in the context of a wider argument within sociology, the Methodenstreit (debate over methods). Weber's position was close to historicism, as he understood social actions as being heavily tied to particular historical contexts and believed their analysis required the understanding of subjective motivations of individuals (social actors). Thus Weber's methodology emphasizes the use of comparative historical analysis. Therefore Weber was more interested in explaining how a certain outcome was the result of various historical processes, rather than predicting an outcome of those processes in the future.

Weber, M. (1949). Objectivity in Social Science and Social Policy. *The Methodology of the Social Sciences*. Glencoe, IL: Free Press.
Reproduced in part from Political Economist Karl Emil Maximilian "Max" Weber, 1864. (2014, April 21). Retrieved from http://voutsadakis.com/GALLERY/ALMANAC/Year2014/Apr2014/04212014/2014apr21.html

Question 1

Which of the following sociological studies would be expected to most interest Weber?

- ○ **A.** A report on repercussions of President Bush's "War on Terror" policy
- ○ **B.** An objective study of social behavior among victims of domestic violence
- ○ **C.** An analysis of the Napoleon's reasons for waging the Napoleonic Wars
- ○ **D.** A predictive analysis forecasting how President Obama's foreign policy will affect diplomacy

Question 2

Weber's attitude toward objectivity in the social sciences is that:

- O **A.** it is almost completely non-existent.
- O **B.** it is nothing more than an ideal.
- O **C.** it can be achieved through study of social laws.
- O **D.** there is no clear dividing line between objective and subjective.

Question 3

According to Weber, the analysis of culture:

- O **A.** assumes institutions as agents.
- O **B.** is based on a set of rules.
- O **C.** is always marked by subjective perspective.
- O **D.** makes accurate predictions about future events.

Question 4

According to passage information, which of the following concepts DOES NOT point toward a difference between Weber and other classical figures in the social sciences?

I. Weber was interested in individual social actions.
II. Weber valued the ideas that drive individual actions.
III. Weber created subjective standards for understanding society.

- O **A.** I and II
- O **B.** I only
- O **C.** III only
- O **D.** II and III

Question 5

It can be inferred from the passage that Methodenstreit (debate over methods) was:

- O **A.** a debate about how to define concepts like "social action."
- O **B.** a debate about how to make sense of social actions in history.
- O **C.** a debate over whether to be primarily objective or subjective.
- O **D.** a debate over what caused certain individuals to behave the way they did.

Question 6

Weber would most likely agree with which of the following types of text?

- O **A.** An analysis that strives to make sense of historical events by discussing the forces that act on nation-states and empires
- O **B.** An analysis that makes sense of historical events through human universals like the death drive and will to power
- O **C.** An analysis that makes sense of historical events based on laws of supply and demand and the circulation of resources
- O **D.** An analysis that explains how the culture of a given historical moment influences ordinary people's beliefs and priorities

Question 7

According to passage information, Weber's concept of methodological individualism is best exemplified by the way he:

- O **A.** conceives large-scale institutions as the product of many small acts by individuals.
- O **B.** focuses on how social action can be understood through subjective interpretation.
- O **C.** interprets "ideal types" on the basis of debate over methods.
- O **D.** rejects Marx and Durkheim's interpretation of social action.

Passage 2 (Questions 8–12)

The dissection of humans has always been an object of controversy among the stakeholders of religious and civilized society. There are many who consider dissection to be the ultimate insult to the dead and the most extreme breach of privacy of a person. Some philosophers label dissection as a "blasphemous" violation of humanity itself and the "last act of torment" ever possible. Still, cadaver dissection has continued in the medical curriculum because of the obvious benefits of delivering firsthand, unabridged and original morphological information of the human body. The diverging schools of thought have not deterred practical and clinically oriented medical/surgical institutions in continuing their cadaver-oriented studies.

Presently, the medical education community has polarized into two belief systems: the "pro-dissection traditionalists" who consider dissection as an integral part of anatomy education and the "anti-dissection modernists" who regard dissection as obsolete and dispensable.

The enormous advances of computer-based learning cannot be undermined. However, despite all their technology, computers can never simulate the "real" in terms of establishing structural concepts. They cannot achieve the variations, pathology and biodynamics of man's body, and, with all their advancements, will still remain an artificial synthetic medium. Hence they cannot instill core anatomy knowledge among up-and-coming health personnel in the same way a cadaver can. The student who is deprived of cadaver-based learning will only see the appearance or location of a body structure, but he or she will never be able to feel the texture, friability, toughness or elasticity of that structure.

Such learning will be superficial, protocol-oriented learning, and hence cannot be regarded as a deep approach to learning. The replacement of active dissection time by digital labs might produce a generation of confused, ill-informed physicians and surgeons who have been spoon-fed on "intangible, abridged concepts," and who are unfamiliar with the complete reality of human body and life. This gamble on technology may be too risky in terms of patients' safety and wellbeing, which will lie solely in the hands of these future caretakers of health. Hence modern technological amenities should be reassessed in terms of their functional, cognitive utility rather than their convenience.

The cadaver has survived the most important test of pedagogical fitness—the test of time. Dissection is unparalleled as an educational tool for instilling gross anatomy concepts. There are long-term cognitive benefits to the students of an active learning process involved in cutting through various layers to expose morphologic details in a stepwise manner. It provides an ideal training ground for future biomedical applications, clinical endeavors and invasive procedures. The psycho-visual-tactile multi-sensory stimuli that are part of a dissection ritual leave an indelible mark on the minds of learners. This hypothesis has been statistically proved by improved exam scores of cadaver dissection groups as compared to intervention groups using other learning alternatives.

Computers provide intricate multidimensional spatial configurations, while cadavers instill psychomotor dexterity, lexical enhancement and bioethical values. They reflect two different approaches to learning, and combined together, they produce doctors who can work more effectively towards an ideal fulfillment of the Hippocratic oath.

Hassan, T. (2011). Is Dissection Humane? *Journal of Medical Ethics and History of Medicine, 4*(4).

Question 8

Based on passage information, which of the following statements would anti-dissection modernists be UNLIKELY to agree with?

- ○ **A.** Digital labs produce a learning experience roughly comparable to cadaver dissections
- ○ **B.** The dignity of the dead outweighs the needs of the living
- ○ **C.** Dissection was necessary in the past only because people lacked other ways to learn anatomy
- ○ **D.** Medical schools can adapt to new technologies while still obeying the Hippocratic Oath

Question 9

What is the main purpose of this passage?

- ○ **A.** To inform readers about the debate over cadaver dissection
- ○ **B.** To create outrage over the disappearance of cadaver dissection in medical schools
- ○ **C.** To persuade readers that dissection is a key part of medical education
- ○ **D.** To evaluate both sides of the cadaver dissection debate

Question 10

Suppose a study demonstrated that dissecting cadavers as a medical student improved performance in surgeons, but not family physicians. What effect would this have on the author's argument?

- ○ **A.** It would suggest the author should refine her argument to distinguish between different kinds of medical practitioners.
- ○ **B.** It would disprove the author's argument by showing that dissecting cadavers does not guarantee excellence in medical practice.
- ○ **C.** It would be irrelevant to the author's argument because it does not address the claim that dissection is an assault on human dignity.
- ○ **D.** It would strengthen the author's argument by showing that virtual labs promote shallow, protocol-based learning.

Question 11

In context, the phrase "protocol-oriented learning" (paragraph 4) most closely means which of the following?

- ○ **A.** Learning to obey an authority figure, rather than trust one's own intuition
- ○ **B.** Learning according to a series of predetermined steps, rather than the learner's interests and talents
- ○ **C.** Learning to follow a procedure, rather than internalizing the deep-seated knowledge of a true expert
- ○ **D.** Learning that instills technical skills but does not inspire deep feelings

Question 12

Which of the following claims, if true, would most strongly undermine the author's argument?

- ○ **A.** Most people would never consent to being dissected by medical students after their death.
- ○ **B.** For some trainee physicians, cadaver dissection takes up lab time that could be used on training that will better help them serve their patients.
- ○ **C.** Computer simulations have been used to greatly improve education in many branches of science, including structural and chemical engineering.
- ○ **D.** Among patients surveyed, a large majority did not express a preference for doctors who had studied using cadavers as opposed to virtual labs.

Passage 3 (Questions 13–17)

"The Death of the Ball Turret Gunner" is a five-line poem by Randall Jarrell. It was about a gunner in a Sperry ball turret on a World War II American bomber aircraft, who was killed and whose remains were unceremoniously hosed out of the turret.

> From my mother's sleep I fell into the State,
> And I hunched in its belly till my wet fur froze.
> Six miles from earth, loosed from its dream of life,
> I woke to black flak and the nightmare fighters.
> When I died they washed me out of the turret with a hose.

Jarrell, who served in the Army Air Force, provided the following explanatory note:

> A ball turret was an acrylic glass sphere set into the belly of a B-17 or B-24, and inhabited by two .50 caliber machine-guns and one man, a short small man. When this gunner tracked with his machine-guns a fighter attacking the bomber from below, he revolved with the turret; hunched upside-down in his little sphere, he looked like the foetus in the womb. The fighters which attacked him were armed with cannon firing explosive shells. The hose was a steam hose.

Reviewer Leven M. Dawson says, "The theme of Randall Jarrell's 'The Death of the Ball Turret Gunner' is that institutionalized violence, or war, creates moral paradox, a condition in which acts repugnant to human nature become appropriate." Most commentators agree, calling the poem a condemnation of the dehumanizing powers of "the State," which are most graphically exhibited by the violence of war. Due partly to its short length, "The Death of the Ball Turret Gunner" poem has been widely anthologized. In fact, Jarrell came to fear that his reputation would eventually rest on it alone.

The basic figurative pattern of the poem is a paradoxical one of death being represented in terms of birth. The "belly" of the "State"—which is the name of the B-17 or B-24, but also represents the persona's "state" (condition or country)—has replaced the secure womb of the "mother's sleep" (the full sleep of complete battle fatigue dreaming of home, or the general security of peacetime existence), and the Gunner undergoes the birth trauma; he falls from [his] mother's sleep (the womb) and is awakened to the "nightmare" unnaturalness of institutionalized "life." (This birth may be seen as the rebirth of initiation into a mature vision of reality and evil.) But the birth of the Ball Turret Gunner is reversed in purpose, for "Six miles from earth" he is "loosed from its dream of life"; the birth in his "'state" is death.

The paradoxical structure as well as the imagery of "The Death of the Ball Turret Gunner" originates in Shelley's elegy for John Keats, "Adonais," stanza XXXIX:

> Peace, peace! he is not dead, he doth not sleep—
> He hath awakened from the dream of life—
> 'Tis we, who lost in stormy visions, keep
> With phantoms an unprofitable strife. . . .

The Ball Turret Gunner also awakens from the "'dream of life." As, paradoxically for Shelley, the death of Keats was birth, birth in the Gunner's new "state" is death; in his condition, life is an unnatural, insecure "dream" from which one awakens to "stormy visions" of "strife" with "phantoms" ("black flak and the nightmare fighters") and then dies. Ascension into the heavens is to find death, not apotheosis; and the "Six miles from earth," the ascent of the Gunner where he finds death, must suggest the reverse direction, a conventional burial six feet under the earth. Water, which is conventionally associated with rebirth and the womb, in the Gunner's condition is either cold or is used to eject, rather than secure, the individual in his protective container. The umbilical "hose" is reversed in function also, being used indifferently to eject the dead body of the gunner.

Dawson, L. M. (1972). 29. Jarrell's the Death of the Ball Turret Gunner. *The Explicator, 31*(4), 62-65. doi:10.1080/00144940.1972.11483141

Question 13

Among the following options, which is most accurate? The author of the passage refers to Shelley in the final paragraph in order to:

- O **A.** juxtapose the structure of both poems.
- O **B.** make a comparison of Keats and Jarrell's imagery.
- O **C.** contrast the meanings of death for Keats and Jarrell.
- O **D.** show how poetry progresses over time through the example of Keats and Jarrell.

Question 14

The author explains that "state" refers to the B-17 or B-24. It can be inferred that he includes this fact in order to:

- O **A.** point out the Army's use of abstruse jargon, which makes it seem like a different world from civilian life.
- O **B.** call attention to the multiple meanings and careful word choice in Jarrell's poem.
- O **C.** clarify that readers should not misinterpret "state" in this poem as meaning "nation."
- O **D.** show that this is an ambiguous poem in which nothing is as it seems.

Question 15

The author suggests that Jarrell's controlling metaphor in his poem is:

- O **A.** sleep.
- O **B.** death.
- O **C.** the "State."
- O **D.** the womb.

Question 16

A comparison of Jarrell's poem is made with Shelley's "Adonais" through:

- O **A.** meter and rhyme.
- O **B.** meaning and rhetoric.
- O **C.** metaphor and imagery.
- O **D.** genre and era.

Question 17

The passage suggests that the poem's main theme is:

- O **A.** man's inhumanity to man.
- O **B.** the dehumanizing nature of war from "the State."
- O **C.** the paradox of war's dilemmas.
- O **D.** the "State's" business of war.

Passage 4 (Questions 18–24)

The tulip—so named, it is said, from a Turkish word, signifying a turban—was responsible for a craze in Holland that is still apparent to this day. It was introduced into Western Europe sometime in the middle of the 16th century. Conrad Gesner, who claims the merit of having brought it into repute—little dreaming of the commotion it was shortly afterwards to make in the world—says that he first saw it in the year 1559, in a garden at Augsburg, belonging to the learned Counsellor Herwart, a man very famous in his day for his collection of rare exotics. The bulbs were sent to this gentleman by a friend at Constantinople, where the flower had long been a favourite. Ten or eleven years later, tulips were much sought after by the wealthy, especially in Holland and Germany. Rich people at Amsterdam sent for the bulbs direct to Constantinople, and paid the most extravagant prices for them.

The first roots planted in England were brought from Vienna in 1600. Until the year 1634 the tulip annually increased in reputation, until it was deemed a proof of bad taste in any man of fortune to be without a collection of them. Many learned men, including Pompeius de Angelis and the celebrated Lipsius of Leyden, the author of the treatise "De Constantia," were passionately fond of tulips. The rage for possessing them soon caught the middle classes of society, and merchants and shopkeepers, even of moderate means, began to vie for the rare flowers, no matter the preposterous price. A trader at Harlaem was known to pay one-half of his fortune for a single root, not with the design of selling it again at a profit, but to keep in his own conservatory for the admiration of his acquaintance.

One would suppose that there must have been some great virtue in this flower to have made it so valuable in the eyes of so prudent a people as the Dutch; but it has neither the beauty nor the perfume of the rose—hardly the beauty of the "sweet, sweet-pea;" neither is it as enduring as either. Beckmann, in his *History of Inventions*, says, "When it has been weakened by cultivation, it becomes more agreeable in the eyes of the florist. The petals are then paler, smaller, and more diversified in hue; and the leaves acquire a softer green colour. Thus this masterpiece of culture, the more beautiful it turns, grows so much the weaker, so that, with the greatest skill and most careful attention, it can scarcely be transplanted, or even kept alive."

Many persons grow insensibly attached to that which gives them a great deal of trouble, as a mother often loves her sick and ever-ailing child better than her more healthy offspring. Upon the same principle we must account for the unmerited encomia lavished upon these fragile blossoms. In 1634, the rage among the Dutch to possess them was so great that the ordinary industry of the country was neglected, and the population, even to its lowest dregs, dove into the tulip trade. As the mania increased, prices augmented, until, in the year 1635, many persons were known to invest a fortune of 100,000 florins in the purchase of forty roots. It then became necessary to sell them by their weight in *perits*, a small weight less than a grain. A tulip of the species called *Admiral Liefken*, weighing 400 *perits*, was worth 4400 florins; an *Admiral Van der Eyck*, weighing 446 *perits*, was worth 1260 florins; a *Childer* of 106 *perits* was worth 1615 florins; a *Viceroy* of 400 *perits*, 3000 florins, and, most precious of all, a *Semper Augustus*, weighing 200 *perits*, was thought to be very cheap at 5500 florins.

People who had been absent from Holland, and whose chance it was to return when this folly was at its maximum, were sometimes led into awkward dilemmas by their ignorance. There is an amusing instance of the kind related in Blainville's *Travels*. A wealthy merchant, who prided himself not a little on his rare tulips, received upon one occasion a very valuable consignment of merchandise from the Levant. Intelligence of its arrival was brought him by a sailor, who presented himself for that purpose at the couting-house, with bales of goods of every description. The merchant, to reward him for his news, munificently made him a present of a fine red herring for his breakfast. The sailor had, it appeared, a great partiality for onions, and seeing a bulb very like an onion lying upon the counter of this liberal trader, and thinking it, no doubt, very much out of its place among silks and velvets, he slyly seized an opportunity and slipped it into his pocket, as a relish for his herring. He got clear off with his prize, and proceeded to the quay to eat his breakfast. Hardly was his back turned when the merchant noticed his missing his valuable *Semper Augustus*, worth three thousand florins, or about 280 sterling. The whole establishment was instantly in an uproar; search was everywhere made for the precious root, but it was not to be found. Great was the merchant's distress of mind. The search was renewed, but again without success. At last, someone thought of the sailor.

The unhappy merchant sprang into the street at the bare suggestion. His alarmed household followed him. The sailor, simple soul! had not thought of concealment. He was found quietly sitting on a coil of ropes, masticating the last morsel of his "*onion.*" Little did he dream that he had been eating a breakfast whose cost might have regaled a whole ship's crew for a twelvemonth; or, as the plundered merchant himself expressed it, "might have sumptuously feasted the Prince of Orange and the whole court of the Stadtholder." The most unfortunate part of the business for him was that he remained in prison for some months on a charge of felony preferred against him by the merchant.

Mackay, C. (1852). *Memoirs of Extraordinary Delusions and the Madness of Crowds*. London: Richard Bentley.

Question 18

The main purpose of the passage is to:

- ○ **A.** trace the history of the tulip from its first discovery.
- ○ **B.** explain why it was surprising that Holland was the center of the tulip craze.
- ○ **C.** contrast the varying attitudes of the Dutch regarding the tulip craze.
- ○ **D.** tell about the reasons for and effects of the tulip craze in Holland.

Question 19

In context, what does the author most closely mean by the line "Many persons grow insensibly attached to that which gives them a great deal of trouble"?

- ○ **A.** People loved tulips because of the high prices they paid for them.
- ○ **B.** People loved tulips because they were more fragile and sickly than other flowers.
- ○ **C.** People loved tulips because of their rarity.
- ○ **D.** People loved tulips because they caused the country's economy to fall into chaos.

Question 20

We can infer from the passage that some items acquire a runaway popularity because:

- ○ **A.** they are finer and more luxurious than other items in their category.
- ○ **B.** they come from far away and remind people of exotic destinations.
- ○ **C.** they have an innate appeal for everyone from the aristocrats to the lowest dregs.
- ○ **D.** they initially catch on with a few elite tastemakers.

Question 21

What is the likely main point of the anecdote in the final two paragraphs?

- ○ **A.** To show the difference in cultural sophistication that existed at the time between wealthy merchants and uneducated workers
- ○ **B.** To illustrate the ironic difference in attitude between people who knew of tulips' value and those who did not
- ○ **C.** To demonstrate the cruelty and injustice of the seventeenth century legal system
- ○ **D.** To show that ignorance can lead to funny and awkward results

Question 22

The author's overall attitude to the tulip craze can be inferred to be:

- ○ **A.** nostalgia for a time when trends were set by learned men and intellectuals.
- ○ **B.** contempt for the idiocy of people who waste money on pointless items.
- ○ **C.** outrage at the extravagance of the wealthy who could afford to pay staggering prices for useless luxuries.
- ○ **D.** bemusement at an irrational overvaluation of what is now an ordinary item.

Question 23

According to the passage, which of the following did NOT play a role in the mania for tulips?

- O **A.** Popularity among wealthy and learned men
- O **B.** A belief that tulips were more beautiful than any other flower
- O **C.** A trickle-down cffcct from wealthy to middle-class to working class
- O **D.** A belief that not liking tulips betrayed bad taste

Question 24

The author would likely agree with which of the following claims?

- O **A.** The tulip craze was absurd because people did not actually like tulips, but only bought them to sell at a profit.
- O **B.** Popular crazes come to a natural endpoint based on the rational economic laws of supply and demand.
- O **C.** If wealthy people had not vouched for the tulips, they might never have been the object of a craze.
- O **D.** Early adapters intentionally start crazes in order to make a profit from an item that eventually becomes sought-after.

Passage 5 (Questions 25–29)

"I believe strictly in the Monroe Doctrine, in our Constitution, and in the laws of God," said Mary Baker Eddy in 1923, a century after Monroe proposed his doctrine. It's an interesting list, in an interesting order.

One of the virtues of Jay Sexton's *The Monroe Doctrine: Empire and Nation in Nineteenth-Century America*, a lucid and illuminating history of "Monroe's Doctrine," is the way he explains Eddy's passion for what was originally a narrow, prosaic compromise meant to address a specific set of demands in foreign and domestic policy. The Monroe Doctrine essentially states that the US is neutral on existing European colonies in the Americas, but opposed to the creation of any new ones. Sexton shows with clarity that Monroe's statement about the Americas is not a "Doctrine" or a "Declaration" but a site of controversy. It has been used to support pro- and anti-slavery causes, pro- and anti-imperialism ideologies, pro- and anti-interventionist policies. As every American leader has to coopt the Declaration and Constitution to their political ends, so too everyone has to genuflect before the Doctrine.

Another of Sexton's achievements is to demonstrate that Monroe did not actually accomplish his aim. His aim was accomplished, but not by him. Monroe warned off European powers from setting up new colonies in the Americas, but included no specifics about how the US would respond. As it turned out, it wasn't up to them anyway. Britain had already been making overtures to the US to cooperate against the freshly aggressive monarchist powers of the Continent, bound together in the Holy Alliance, and by siding with the US, Britain effectively ensured that no European power would even attempt to set up a beachhead in America's backyard. British leaders saw the commercial advantages of an American alliance; Americans saw that they could benefit from cooperation with Britain, both economically and in security terms. Not that anyone in Europe really wanted to colonize the Americas anyway, though the absence of threat did not keep politicians from milking rumors for their own purposes. "Plus choses changent, et plus elles restent le memes" [the more things change, the more they stay the same].

Sexton is also very good on noting the interactions between British policy and the US more generally. The British abolition of slavery, for example, sent tremors through Southern politicians: "Once the engine behind the slave trade and its entrenchment in North America, the world's most powerful nation now committed itself to ending slavery. It is hard to overstate the significance to the United State of the United Kingdom's Slavery Abolition Act of 1833, which began the process of emancipation in British possessions in the Caribbean. British abolition further radicalized both sides of the slavery debate in the United States," both encouraging radical abolitionists to demand an immediate end to slavery and making Southern politicians dig in their heels.

He also has these important observations about American exceptionalism: America thought itself unique, "yet it emerged and evolved in relation to the foreign policies of other expansionist powers. The British empire most often provided a model... both positive and negative... for nineteenth-century Americans. Its diverse forms allowed Americans to find in it what they wanted. Anticolonialists scored political points at home by condemning British practices in Ireland and India; proponents of nonintervention pointed to the state papers of Lord Castlereagh, which articulated this principle before the 1823 [Monroe] message; naval theorists such as Alfred Thayer Mahan marveled at the triumphs of the Royal Navy; businessmen and exporters mimicked the strategies employed by their British counterparts; American statesmen found inspiration in the tactics of 'informal imperialism' employed by the British in Latin America and East Asia. Though the Monroe Doctrine aimed to supplant British power in the Western Hemisphere, it drew deeply from the practices of the British Empire in Latin America."

Sexton, J. (2012). *The Monroe Doctrine: Empire and Nation in Nineteenth-Century America*. New York: Hill & Wang.

Question 25

The French phrase "plus choses changent, et plus elles restent le memes [the more things change, the more they stay the same]" is used in the third paragraph. What is the best inference of what this means within the context of the passage?

- O **A.** People change sides
- O **B.** Politicians have changed greatly since the nineteenth century
- O **C.** Politicians today still stir up fear for opportunistic reasons
- O **D.** Politicians are always willing to change sides to fit their purposes

Question 26

The relationship between the U.S. and Britain, according to the final paragraph, was largely marked by:

- O **A.** antagonism.
- O **B.** exploitation.
- O **C.** mutual influence.
- O **D.** one-way influence.

Question 27

The Monroe Doctrine in its original form, according to the passage, can be inferred to have been:

- O **A.** unrealistic wishful thinking.
- O **B.** pragmatic policy-setting.
- O **C.** a politically calculated statement of US power.
- O **D.** an unjust exploitation of US power.

Question 28

The author's overall attitude to politics within the passage can be described as:

- O **A.** patriotic.
- O **B.** skeptical.
- O **C.** vacillating.
- O **D.** emotional.

Question 29

According to passage information, Sexton's main argument would be most effectively refuted by a book proving that:

- O **A.** other countries such as Britain believe in their own "exceptionalism" just as strongly as the US does.
- O **B.** Monroe was actually instrumental in persuading Britain to ally with the US.
- O **C.** some British citizens supported American slaveowners and were against the abolition of slavery in Britain.
- O **D.** setting up colonies in South America would have been unprofitable for European powers.

Passage 6 (Questions 30–34)

In Jungian psychology, the shadow or "shadow aspect" is one of the many archetypes of the unconscious mind (or collective unconscious). It consists of patterns of behavior or modes of functioning related to repressed weaknesses, disliked personality traits, shortcomings, and instincts. It is one of the most recognizable archetypes, and the most accessible to the conscious mind. "Everyone carries a shadow," Jung wrote, "and the less it is embodied in the individual's conscious life, the blacker and denser it is." It may be (in part) one's link to more primitive animal instincts, which are superseded during early childhood by the conscious mind.

According to Jung, the shadow, in being instinctive and irrational, is prone to projection: turning a personal inferiority into a perceived moral deficiency in someone else. Jung writes that if these projections are unrecognized "the projection-making factor (the Shadow archetype) then has a free hand and can realize its object—if it has one—or bring about some other situation characteristic of its power." These projections insulate and cripple individuals by forming an ever thicker fog of illusion between the ego and the real world.

From one perspective, "the shadow... is roughly equivalent to the whole of the Freudian unconscious", and Jung himself considered that "the result of the Freudian method of elucidation is a minute elaboration of man's shadow-side unexampled in any previous age."

Jung also believed that "in spite of its function as a reservoir for human darkness—or perhaps because of this—the shadow is the seat of creativity"; so that for some, it may be, "the dark side of [a person's] being, his sinister shadow... represents the true spirit of life as against the arid scholar."

The shadow may appear in dreams and visions in various forms, and typically "appears as a person of the same sex as that of the dreamer." It is possible that it might appear with dark features to a person of any race, since it represents a distant, primitive and indiscriminate aspect of the mind. The shadow's appearance and role depend greatly on the living experience of the individual, because much of the shadow develops in the individual's mind rather than simply being inherited in the collective unconscious. Nevertheless, some Jungians maintain that "the shadow... contains, besides the personal shadow, the shadow of society... fed by the neglected and repressed collective values."

Interactions with the shadow in dreams may shed light on one's state of mind. A conversation with the shadow may indicate that one is concerned with conflicting desires or intentions. Identification with a despised figure may mean that one has an unacknowledged difference from the character; a difference which could point to a rejection of the illuminating qualities of ego-consciousness. These examples refer to just two of many possible roles that the shadow may adopt, and are not general guides to interpretation. Also, it can be difficult to identify characters in dreams—"all the contents are blurred and merge into one another [resulting in] 'contamination' of unconscious contents"—so that a character who seems at first to be a shadow might represent some other complex instead.

Jung also made the suggestion of there being more than one layer making up the shadow. Top layers contain the meaningful flow and manifestations of direct personal experiences. These are made unconscious in the individual by such mechanisms as the change of attention from one thing to another, simple forgetfulness, or repression. These more superficial layers are those that are more easily accessible to the conscious mind. Underneath these more superficial layers, however, are the psychic shadow contents of all human experiences. Jung described these deeper layers as "a psychic activity which goes on independently of the conscious mind and is not dependent even on the upper layers of the unconscious—untouched, and perhaps untouchable by personal experience" (Campbell, 1971).

Jung, C. G., & Campbell, J. (1988). *The Portable Jung*. New York: Penguin Books.

Question 30

Which of the following CANNOT be inferred from the final paragraph?

- ○ **A.** The bottom layers of the Shadow are deeper because they relate to more deeply rooted elements of being.
- ○ **B.** Every shadow layer contains elements of thought that the mind is not fully conscious of.
- ○ **C.** The top layers of the Shadow reflect universal attributes of human experience.
- ○ **D.** The top layers of the Shadow contain important experiences that may have been repressed.

Question 31

The author suggests that the shadow side is overall:

- ○ **A.** the embodiment of everything bad about humans.
- ○ **B.** a metaphor for the parts of ourselves we fear or want to keep hidden.
- ○ **C.** a negative and frightening aspect of the mind that is not tameable or passible of being analysed.
- ○ **D.** an unfamiliar and frightening aspect of the mind.

Question 32

Based on passage information, what was Jung's attitude towards Freud?

- ○ **A.** Jung knew of Freud but was dismissive of his work.
- ○ **B.** Jung completed his major work before Freud and was an influence on him.
- ○ **C.** Jung and Freud collaborated and held the same psychological theories.
- ○ **D.** Jung knew of and was influenced by Freud, but their theories were not identical.

Question 33

In paragraph 5 the author states that "Nevertheless, some Jungians maintain that 'The shadow... contains, besides the personal shadow, the shadow of society... fed by the neglected and repressed collective values.'" What does this suggest about the relationship between Jung and his followers?

- ○ **A.** Jung and his followers disagreed about how people should cope with the demands of society.
- ○ **B.** Jungians are continually reinterpreting Jung's ideas for modern times.
- ○ **C.** Jung and his followers sometimes disagreed about the respective importance of the individual and society.
- ○ **D.** Jung did not want his theories to be applied to societies, but some Jungians insist that he was wrong.

Question 34

Jung's theories on the shadow would probably be rejected by all of the following EXCEPT:

- ○ **A.** a cognitive behavioral therapist who believes negative patterns of thought are the result of conditioning and can be changed through mental training.
- ○ **B.** a Rousseauian thinker who believes humans are basically "noble savages" corrupted by civilization.
- ○ **C.** a primitivist who believes that modern life is superficial and people must get in touch with their instincts and dark thoughts.
- ○ **D.** a technological Utopian who believes that global communication is doing away with ancient prejudices and producing a more humane society.

Passage 7 (Questions 35–41)

Telling the history of opera analysis, naming its most famous practitioners, constitutes a background to a more complicated issue: understanding the ideological and aesthetic problems that underpin analytical writing on opera. The central problem remains the necessity to cope with an art that mixes various languages (visual, verbal, musical); this problem has affected every writer on opera, and can be said to twist their own interpretative languages. While opera combines three basic systems, an analytical methodology has yet to be developed that is capable of discussing these as they exist in experiential reality, as aspects of a single and simultaneously perceived entity. Virtually all operatic interpretation has been forced to dissect the operatic experience, focusing separately upon the music, the text and the visual form of any operatic passage (i.e. "while the text spoken is this, we see that on stage, and the music does this").

Opera analysis deals monophonically with what in performance is a visual-textual-musical polyphony. To be sure, analysis often seeks for a relationship between these systems, yet such a search is itself born of interpretation's inability directly to reflect or translate the complex simultaneities of opera. Analysing opera thus inevitably creates a fundamental schism, and its quest for relationships is perhaps driven by longing for a whole object that the act of analysis has itself unfused.

Analysis of the music of opera tends to display similar methodological ironies. The 19th-century formalists' view of operatic music as musical structure allowed our casual understanding of opera analysis as music analysis. While librettos have been seen as partial or incomplete texts, music has more often been regarded as a full text in its own right, needing no prosthetic aura (lent by the verbal or visual) to command our attention. The autonomy of operatic music is less secure than it might seem, and analysis of operatic music, like that of librettos, is often characterized by nervous sensitivity to the absent discursive systems, verbal and visual.

Adopting the two strategies established in the 19th century, the analysis of operatic music either assumes that music has the capacity to retrace meanings that originate in the visual or verbal systems and that analysis should seek these transpositions, or prefers to neutralize the question of representation, regarding operatic music as self-sufficient or exemplifying procedures found in instrumental music. In thus establishing the autonomy of music, theorists grant it prestige.

By invoking methodologies familiar in analysis of instrumental music, such readings plead (in the case of Lorenz, overtly) that operatic music fundamentally operates in ways identical with those of music uninflected by verbal or visual systems. This move strives to reinforce the notion that, in opera, music alone attains the status of a full text.

This repression of the non-musical is itself as complex a phenomenon as arguments about the musical consequences of symbolization. Operatic music has, over the course of its history, attracted to itself a rich fund of negative judgments: as formally uncontrolled, illogical, excessive, subjective, vulgar, immoral, feminine. Associating operatic music with instrumental music may seem straightforwardly to reflect an historical-stylistic reality (e.g. that da capo aria rhetoric resembles Baroque concerto forms). Yet whether accomplished through analytical demonstration or an act of naming (for example, by referring to Wagner's operas as 'symphonies'), it inevitably bespeaks a desire to purify operatic music through a purgative association with genres uncorrupted by non-musical systems; significantly, it reflects as well a recuperation of operatic music to a masculine objectivity.

This purifying gesture seems doomed to fail. Opera analysis will inevitably face the necessity of acknowledging the polyphony between visual, verbal and musical, in an object it seems compelled to unlayer.

Abel, S., & Abbate, C. (1992). Unsung Voices: Opera and Musical Narrative in the Nineteenth Century. *Theatre Journal*, 44(3), 422. doi:10.2307/3208572

Question 35

This passage does all of the following EXCEPT:

- ○ **A.** identify common threads within the complex history of opera analysis.
- ○ **B.** describe the unique difficulties inherent in analyzing opera.
- ○ **C.** offer an actual analytical approach to opera analysis.
- ○ **D.** identify weaknesses in existing opera analysis.

Question 36

The line "it reflects as well a recuperation of operatic music to a masculine objectivity" (paragraph 6) suggests that:

- O **A.** operatic music is primarily composed by men, whereas librettos and stage design are done by both men and women.
- O **B.** instrumental music has typically been seen as a more pure and logical genre than theater and narrative.
- O **C.** instrumental music appeals to male critics because it is inherently objective.
- O **D.** while it is true that opera music is the same as instrumental music, it is incorrect to see this quality as "masculine."

Question 37

Based on the passage, we can infer that the relationship between opera and instrumental music is that:

- O **A.** they are formally very different.
- O **B.** they are formally similar, but different in context.
- O **C.** opera music is formally the same as instrumental music, but with words and visuals.
- O **D.** instrumental music is formally controlled, but opera music is not.

Question 38

The author would probably respond as follows to a critic who considered opera a form of theater in which the music exists primarily to support the verbal text?

- O **A.** Positively, because this would counter criticism's tendency to disregard text
- O **B.** Negatively, because text is the least important aspect of opera production
- O **C.** Positively, because this approach views text and music as working together
- O **D.** Negatively, because this reinforces the criticized tendency to privilege one aspect of opera

Question 39

What is the main topic of the passage?

- O **A.** A heightened understanding of the operatic experience
- O **B.** A need for a holistic approach to the analysis of opera
- O **C.** An historical overview of operatic analysis and its limitations
- O **D.** Operatic analysis and art for art's sake

Question 40

Which of the following would the author be most likely to endorse?

- O **A.** A work of opera criticism that separated the parts of the opera that are permanent, including score and libretto, from those that change with performance, like costume and acting choices.
- O **B.** A work of opera criticism that analyzed a single scene, trying to show how music, story and visuals create a unified experience from the spectator's point of view
- O **C.** A work of criticism that aimed to tease apart which aspects of an opera were musically pure, and which were formally uncontrolled.
- O **D.** A work of opera criticism that focused on narrative and viewed music as an accessory to telling a story.

Question 41

According to passage information, what does the author see as problematic about opera criticism's failure to discuss all elements of a text?

- O **A.** By separating opera into different spheres, it makes the genre seem more complicated than it really is.
- O **B.** It analyzes form instead of content.
- O **C.** It fails to grasp the medium's artistic complexity and reproduces harmful ideological ideas.
- O **D.** It fails to grasp the aesthetic and ideological limitations of opera.

Passage 8 (Questions 42–46)

Speech is so familiar a feature of daily life that we rarely pause to define it. It seems as natural to man as walking, and only less so than breathing. Yet it needs but a moment's reflection to convince us that this naturalness of speech is but an illusory feeling. The process of acquiring speech is, in sober fact, an utterly different sort of thing from the process of learning to walk. In the case of the latter function, culture, in other words, the traditional body of social usage is not seriously brought into play. The child is individually equipped, by the complex set of factors that we term biological heredity, to make all the needed muscular and nervous adjustments that result in walking.

Indeed, the very conformation of these muscles and of the appropriate parts of the nervous system may be said to be primarily adapted to the movements made in walking and in similar activities. In a very real sense the normal human being is predestined to walk, not because his elders will assist him to learn the art, but because his organism is prepared from birth, or even from the moment of conception, to take on all those expenditures of nervous energy and all those muscular adaptations that result in walking. To put it concisely, walking is an inherent, biological function of man.

It is not so with language. It is of course true that in a certain sense the individual is predestined to talk, but that is due entirely to the circumstance that he is born not merely in nature, but in the lap of a society that is certain, reasonably certain, to lead him to its traditions. Eliminate society and there is every reason to believe that he will learn to walk, if, indeed, he survives at all. But it is just as certain that he will never learn to talk, that is, to communicate ideas according to the traditional system of a particular society. Or, again, remove the newborn individual from the social environment into which he has come and transplant him to an utterly alien one. He will develop the art of walking in his new environment very much as he would have developed it in the old. But his speech will be completely at variance with the speech of his native environment.

Walking, then, is a general human activity that varies only within circumscribed limits as we pass from individual to individual. Its variability is involuntary and purposeless. Speech is a human activity that varies without assignable limit as we pass from social group to social group, because it is a purely historical heritage of the group, the product of long-continued social usage. It varies as all creative effort varies — not as consciously, perhaps, but nonetheless as truly as do the religions, the beliefs, the customs, and the arts of different peoples. Walking is an organic, an instinctive function (not, of course, itself an instinct); speech is a non-instinctive, acquired, "cultural" function.

Sapir, E. (2014). *Language: An Introduction to the Study of Speech.* Bensenville, IL.: Lushena Books.

Question 42

Which of the following does NOT follow from Sapir's line of reasoning when he states that "speech is a human activity which varies without assignable limit"?

- ○ **A.** Speech varies as we pass from social group to other social groups.
- ○ **B.** Speech varies because of the social usages and history of cultural groups.
- ○ **C.** Speech varies more than the instinctive sounds and cries made by animals.
- ○ **D.** Speech varies based on a person's genetically determined capacity for complex grammar.

Question 43

What duality does the author NOT suggest is important to understanding speech?

- O **A.** Nature vs. society
- O **B.** Instinctual vs. learned
- O **C.** Biology vs. culture
- O **D.** Tradition vs. innovation

Question 44

In context, what does the author most likely mean by the line "his speech will be completely at variance with the speech of his native environment" (paragraph 3)?

- O **A.** The child will speak a language that is not understood in his adoptive country.
- O **B.** The child will grow up speaking the language of his adoptive tribe or country.
- O **C.** The child's way of speaking will anger and antagonize people in his native country.
- O **D.** The child's way of speaking will shift between two sets of customs.

Question 45

The linguist Noam Chomsky has argued that young children learn language surprisingly quickly from a relatively small amount of input, and that "A consideration of [the] narrowly limited extent of the available data [that children are exposed to] leave[s] little hope that much of the structure of the language can be learned by an organism initially uninformed as to its general character."

If true, what effect would this claim have on the argument in the passage?

- O **A.** Support it, because individual concepts are learned from a culture, but a language's "structure" is innate
- O **B.** Contradict it, because people do not learn language as thoroughly as Sapir argues they do
- O **C.** Contradict it, because people would have to be born with some innate knowledge of language's "natural character"
- O **D.** Contradict it, because babies are already born with innate concepts for all the words they will eventually learn in a language

Question 46

Which of the following pieces of information would NOT contradict the author's main claims in the passage?

- O **A.** A discovery that languages across the world share some features in common, such as nouns, verbs and similar grammatical structures
- O **B.** A deaf child raised without language input, who created her own gesture system that she used to form sentences
- O **C.** Two neighboring tribes who could not communicate with each other because each of their languages contained untranslatable concepts
- O **D.** The existence of an extended family who had average overall intelligence and normal upbringings, but were congenitally unable to learn language

Passage 9 (Questions 47–53)

Blake's beginnings as a poet are as normal as the beginnings of Shakespeare. His method of composition, in his mature work, is exactly like that of other poets. He has an idea (a feeling, an image), he develops it by accretion or expansion, alters his verse often, and hesitates often over the final choice. The idea, of course, simply comes, but upon arrival it is subjected to prolonged manipulation. In the first phase Blake is concerned with verbal beauty; in the second he becomes the apparent naïf, really the mature intelligence. It is only when the ideas become more automatic, come more freely and are less manipulated, that we begin to suspect their origin, to suspect that they spring from a shallower source.

The Songs of Innocence and of Experience, and the poems from the Rossetti manuscript, are the poems of a man with a profound interest in human emotions, and a profound knowledge of them. The emotions are presented in an extremely simplified, abstract form. This form is one illustration of the eternal struggle of art against education, of the literary artist against the continuous deterioration of language.

It is important that the artist should be highly educated in his own art; but his education is one that is hindered rather than helped by the ordinary processes of society which constitute education for the ordinary man. For these processes consist largely in the acquisition of impersonal ideas which obscure what we really are and feel, what we really want, and what really excites our interest. It is of course not the actual information acquired, but the conformity which the accumulation of knowledge is apt to impose, that is harmful. Tennyson is a very fair example of a poet almost wholly encrusted with parasitic opinion, almost wholly merged into his environment.

Blake, on the other hand, knew what interested him, and he therefore presents only the essential, only, in fact, what can be presented, and need not be explained. And because he was not distracted, or frightened, or occupied in anything but exact statement, he understood. He was naked, and saw man naked, and from the center of his own crystal. To him there was no more reason why Swedenborg should be absurd than Locke. He accepted Swedenborg, and eventually rejected him, for reasons of his own. He approached everything with a mind unclouded by current opinions. There was nothing of the superior person about him. This makes him terrifying.

But if there was nothing to distract him from sincerity there were, on the other hand, the dangers to which the naked man is exposed. His philosophy, like his visions, like his insight, like his technique, was his own. And accordingly he was inclined to attach more importance to it than an artist should; this is what makes him eccentric, and makes him inclined to formlessness.

> But most through midnight streets I hear
> How the youthful harlot's curse
> Blasts the new-born infant's tear,
> And blights with plagues the marriage hearse,

is the naked vision;

> Love seeketh only self to please,
> To bind another to its delight,
> Joys in another's loss of ease,
> And builds a Hell in Heaven's despite,

is the naked observation; and The Marriage of Heaven and Hell is naked philosophy, presented. But Blake's occasional marriages of poetry and philosophy are not so felicitous.

> He who would do good to another must do it in Minute Particulars.
> General Good is the plea of the scoundrel, hypocrite, and flatterer;
> For Art and Science cannot exist but in minutely organized particulars. . .

One feels that the form is not well chosen. The borrowed philosophy of Dante and Lucretius is perhaps not so interesting, but it injures their form less. Blake did not have that more Mediterranean gift of form which knows how to borrow as Dante borrowed his theory of the soul; he must need to create a philosophy as well as a poetry. A similar formlessness attacks his draughtsmanship.

Eliot, Thomas Stearns. *The Sacred Wood*. New York: Alfred A. Knopf, 1921; Bartleby.com, 1996.

Question 47

The author of the passage uses the word "naked" several times in reference to Blake, how he saw mankind, his poetry and his philosophy. Which of the following is NOT a meaning which can be inferred from passage information?

- ○ **A.** In all honesty
- ○ **B.** Stripped of pretension and illusion
- ○ **C.** Unmarked by artistry
- ○ **D.** Without the trappings of society and popular opinion

Question 48

According to information in the passage, Blake could have produced more first-rate poetry if he had:

- ○ **A.** written philosophical poems only about other philosophers' ideas.
- ○ **B.** used more poetic devices and philosophical concepts rather than presenting "naked concepts."
- ○ **C.** acquired fewer impersonal ideas.
- ○ **D.** believed less fervently in his self-created philosophy.

Question 49

If this author wrote an evaluation of Tennyson, we might expect him to argue that:

- ○ **A.** Tennyson was unable to choose the correct forms for his thoughts.
- ○ **B.** Tennyson was an average poet whose work does not stand out in any way.
- ○ **C.** Tennyson always expressed himself eloquently and in well-chosen forms, but he believed too many absurd ideas.
- ○ **D.** Tennyson always expressed himself eloquently, but included few interesting ideas because his beliefs were too conventional.

Question 50

The author writes that "There was nothing of the superior person about him. This makes him terrifying." In context, why does the author likely consider Blake terrifying?

- ○ **A.** Blake's ideas were brutally honest because he was uninterested in expressing himself in a way that made him look good.
- ○ **B.** Blake's rough manners and poor opinion of human nature made him unfit to socialize with "superior people."
- ○ **C.** Blake's sacrilegious ideas about the "marriage of heaven and hell" shocked the religious sensibilities of his day.
- ○ **D.** Blake aimed to scandalize and alarm people by showing how different his ideas were from those of "superior people."

Question 51

Based on the passage, what can we infer about Locke and Swedenborg?

- ○ **A.** Locke's theories were reasonable, but Swedenborg's became more absurd over time.
- ○ **B.** Other thinkers at the time regarded Locke as reasonable, and Swedenborg as eccentric.
- ○ **C.** Locke was popular, while Swedenborg was little-known.
- ○ **D.** Locke's work was based on science, while Swedenborg's was based on personal experience.

Question 52

Which of the following lines in the passage most strongly supports the author's claim that "the Songs of Innocence and of Experience, and the poems from the Rossetti manuscript, are the poems of a man with a profound interest in human emotions, and a profound knowledge of them"?

- ○ **A.** 'He accepted Swedenborg, and eventually rejected him, for reasons of his own."
- ○ **B.** "'Love seeketh only self to please,/ To bind another to its delight,/ Joys in another's loss of ease,/ And builds a Hell in Heaven's despite,' is the naked observation."
- ○ **C.** "His education is one that is hindered rather than helped by the ordinary processes of society which constitute education for the ordinary man."
- ○ **D.** "One feels that the form is not well chosen. The borrowed philosophy of Dante and Lucretius is perhaps not so interesting, but it injures their form less."

Question 53

Which of the following is NOT described as being part of the creative process?

- ○ **A.** An idea appears in the author's mind.
- ○ **B.** The poet tries different ways of expressing the original idea.
- ○ **C.** The poet has a divine flash of inspiration.
- ○ **D.** Over time, the poet learns about his chosen art form.

 END OF EXAM SECTION.

CANDIDATE'S NAME ______________________________

RAW SCORE AND SCALED SCORE ______________________

GS-2 Section III: Biological and Biochemical Foundations of Living Systems

Questions: 1-59
Time: 95 minutes

INSTRUCTIONS: Of all the questions on this test, most are organized into groups preceded by a passage. After evaluating the passage, select the best answer to each question in the group. Fifteen questions are independent of any descriptive passage or each other. Similarly, select the best answer to these questions. If you are unsure of an answer, eliminate the alternatives that you know to be incorrect and select an answer from the remaining alternatives. To indicate your selection, use a pencil to blacken the corresponding circle next to the answer choice and/or you can use the answer document at the back of this book. No marks are deducted for wrong answers.

The computer-based real MCAT has an on-screen highlighter function and ~~STRIKEOUT~~ function. These tools help to spotlight text or assist in the process of elimination. You may use a yellow highlighter for this paper-based exam and/or a pen (or preferably a pencil to make it easier should you change your mind) to mark text. At the time of publishing, both highlighting and strikeout functions can be used for passages, questions and answer choices. You can also flag a question to review later should time remain.

For the real exam, you will be provided with a dry erase board which is a white laminated noteboard booklet accompanied by a fine point marker. The noteboard includes 9 graph-lined pages for you to write though you cannot erase. You can simulate the experience with a fine point marker on a noteboard or with 8" x 14" plain graph paper.

You may consult the periodic table at any point during the science subtests.

Please note: For the real MCAT, a small number of field-tested questions will remain unscored.

This practice test has been designed exclusively to test knowledge and thinking skills. This exam may contain hypothetical statements and/or express controversial ideas. Statements contained herein do not necessarily reflect the policy, position, or view of RuveneCo Inc. or MCAT-prep.com.

START EXAM ONLY WHEN TIMER IS READY.

Passage 1 (Questions 1–4)

Arginine is one of the 20 most common natural amino acids. Most healthy people do not need to supplement with arginine because the body usually produces sufficient quantities. The pathway for arginine synthesis was studied using cells from a red bread mold. This natural form of arginine is illustrated below.

The red bread mold *Neurospora crassa* grows well on a cultural plate with "minimal" medium which is a fluid containing only a few simple sugars, inorganic salts, and vitamin. *Neurospora* that grows normally in nature (wild type) has enzymes that convert these simple substances into the amino acids necessary for growth. Mutating any one of the genes that makes an enzyme can produce a *Neurospora* strain that cannot grow on minimal medium. The mutant would only grow if the enzyme product were to be added as a supplement. On the other hand, if a "complete" medium is provided, containing all required amino acids, then *Neurospora* would grow, with or without mutation.

Figure 1 A synthesis pathway for the amino acid arginine. Each gene in italics in the diagram produces one enzyme necessary for the synthesis of this essential amino acid required for growth.

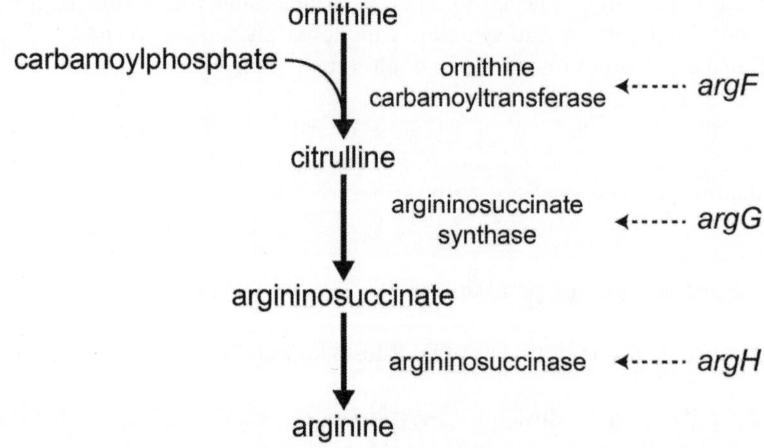

Table 1 Growth response of mutant strains in "minimal" media with supplements (ornithine, citrulline, argininosuccinate, and arginine) as indicated. Strain growth is indicated by (+) and no strain growth is indicated by (-).

mutant strain	nothing	ornithine	citrulline	argininosuccinate	arginine
P	-	-	-	+	+
Q	-	-	-	+	+

Question 1

Which of the following is NOT an accurate description of naturally-occurring arginine?

- O **A.** Acidic amino acid
- O **B.** *L*-Configuration
- O **C.** α-Amino acid
- O **D.** *S*-Configuration

Question 2

Which of the following is most likely consistent with the overall synthetic pathway for arginine (accounting for coupled reactions)?

- O **A.** $\Delta H < 0$
- O **B.** $\Delta G = 0$
- O **C.** net ATP production
- O **D.** $\Delta G > 0$

Question 3

According to the information provided, a conclusion that can be made with certainty is that neither mutant strain P nor Q have the defective enzyme:

- O **A.** carbamoyltransferase.
- O **B.** argininosuccinate synthase.
- O **C.** argininosuccinase.
- O **D.** None of the above enzymes are defective in either mutant strain P nor Q.

Question 4

Experiments using the two mutant strains P and Q, reveal that strain P accumulates citrulline, but strain Q does not. Which of the following statements is most consistent with the data provided?

- O **A.** Strain Q has only one mutation.
- O **B.** Strain P has a mutation in *argF* only.
- O **C.** Strain P has mutations in *argF*, *argG* and *argH*.
- O **D.** Strain P has a mutation in *argG* only.

Passage 2 (Questions 5–9)

Human serum albumin (HSA) is the most abundant protein in human plasma, and it is produced in the liver at a rate of approximately 10–15 g per day. It has a variety of important roles in the circulation, some of which are exploited during drug development. For example, many metal-bound radiopharmaceuticals bind to SA from different species, and with differing affinities. These copper chelates include Cu-ETS (ethylglyoxal bis(thiosemicarbazonato)copper(II)), Cu-PTSM (pyruvaldehyde bis(N^4-methylthiosemicarbazonato)copper(II)), and Cu-ATSM (diacetyl bis(N^4-methylthiosemicarbazonato)copper(II)). When copper interacts with sulfur to form organosulfur compounds, like the chelates shown in Figure 1, they usually form water insoluble compounds due to the atomic structure of copper and sulfur and their d orbital interaction. These molecules are pretty flat and chemists usually have to dissolve them in organic solvents.

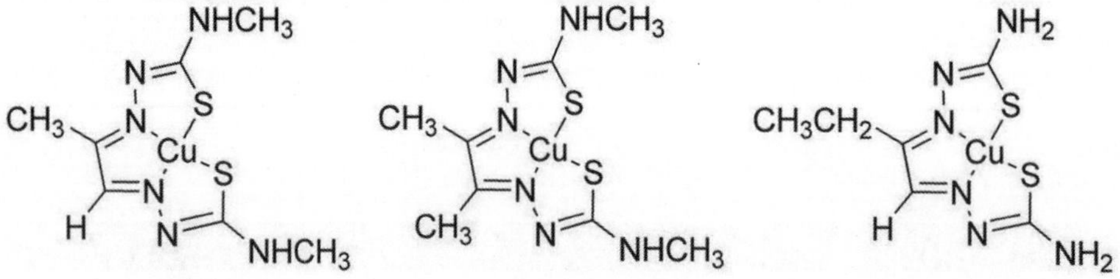

Cu-PTSM Cu-ATSM Cu-ETS

Figure 1 The structures of Cu-PTSM, Cu-ATSM, and Cu-ETS.

Drugs that bind to known sites in HSA can be evaluated to understand these differing affinities, including warfarin (which binds to site IIA of HSA via a hydrophobic interaction) and ibuprofen (which binds to site IIIA of HSA via an ionic interaction). Warfarin is an anticoagulant used in the prevention of thrombosis and thromboembolism, the formation of blood clots in the blood vessels and their migration elsewhere in the body, respectively. Ibuprofen is a pain reliever than can reduce inflammation.

Table 1 The percentage of free Cu-PTSM after displacement by warfarin and ibuprofen.

Molar ratio (drug:HSA)	Warfarin	Ibuprofen
0	4.0 ± 0.1	4.0 ± 0.1
0.5	4.6 ± 0.1	3.4 ± 0.1
1	5.8 ± 0.7	3.4 ± 0.3
2	7.7 ± 0.8	3.2 ± 0.5
4	14.8 ± 0.3	4.8 ± 0.2
8	20.1 ± 1.5	10.1 ± 0.6

Table 2 The displacement of Cu-ATSM and Cu-ETS from HSA by warfarin and ibuprofen.

Molar ratio (drug:HSA)	Cu-ATSM		Cu-ETS	
	Warfarin	Ibuprofen	Warfarin	Ibuprofen
0	5.9 ± 0.4	5.9 ± 0.4	40.6 ± 1.1	40.6 ± 1.1
0.5	7.3 ± 0.2	7.1 ± 0.6	42.8 ± 1.6	43.9 ± 2.2
1	9.4 ± 0.8	7.5 ± 0.8	44.2 ± 1.2	42.1 ± 2.7
2	12.4 ± 0.9	8.2 ± 1.1	45.2 ± 1.3	45.8 ± 2.6
4	14.5 ± 0.6	7.3 ± 0.8	42.8 ± 3.4	43.6 ± 3.1
8	19.0 ± 1.7	10.5 ± 1.1	44.7 ± 2.7	49.6 ± 1.2

Adapted from nih.gov: PMC2674521, PMC2388251 and PMC51166.

Question 5

The following represents the primary structure for an active subdomain of SA with all circles being amino acids, all connections being covalent bonds, and the highlighting of the connection between amino acids at various positions in the primary structure.

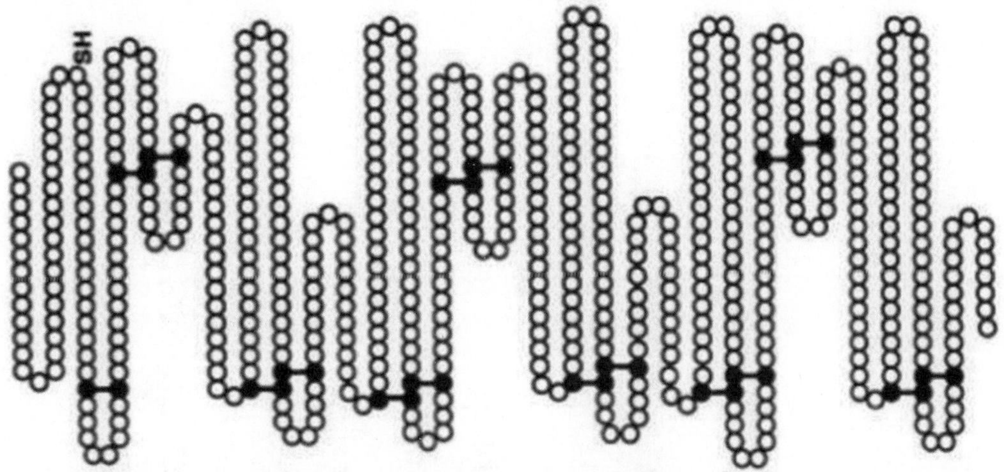

All of the following are true regarding the preceding diagram EXCEPT:

- O **A.** the diagram provides some information about the tertiary structure.
- O **B.** there are exactly 17 cystine residues.
- O **C.** there are at most 34 cysteine residues.
- O **D.** none of the black circles can represent methionine.

Question 6

As a group, the three copper chelates shown in Figure 1 can be best described as which of the following?

I. Basic
II. Neutral
III. Lipophilic

- O **A.** I only
- O **B.** I and III only
- O **C.** II and III only
- O **D.** I, II and III

Question 7

Changing the pH of binding reaction mixtures can have a dramatic effect on ligand-protein binding. Altering the pH of reactions between warfarin or ibuprofen and HSA is likely to:

- O **A.** affect both reactions equally.
- O **B.** affect warfarin-HSA binding but not ibuprofen-HSA binding.
- O **C.** affect ibuprofen-HSA binding but not warfarin-HSA binding.
- O **D.** not affect either interaction.

Question 8

The binding of Cu-PTSM, Cu-ATSM, and Cu-ETS to SA (40 mg/mL) from a variety of species was tested using radio thin layer chromatography (radio TLC) at 1 min, 30 min, and 24 hours.

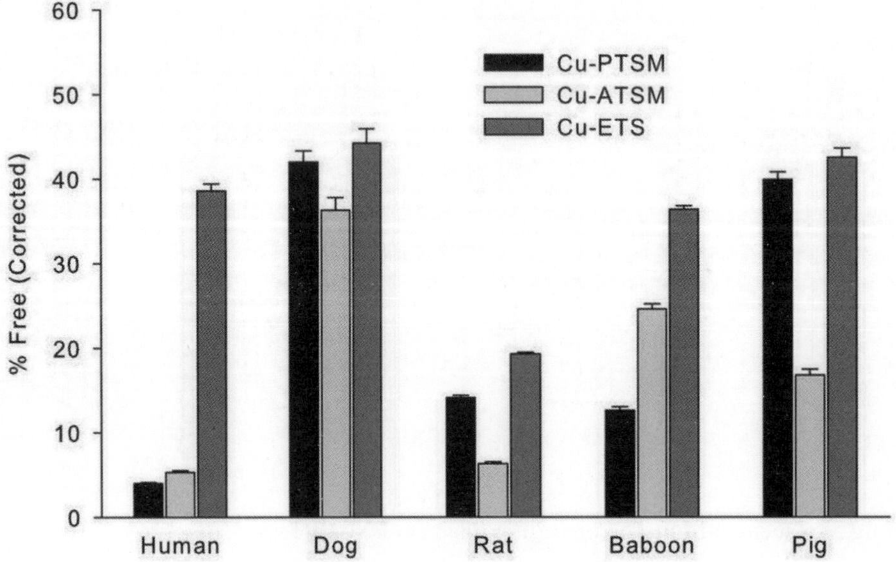

After 24-h of mixing the copper chelates with SA, radio TLC revealed only the presence of the intact radiopharmaceuticals. Based on this information, which of the following statements is most likely to be true?

- O **A.** The association between the radiopharmaceuticals and SA is reversible.
- O **B.** Radiocopper was lost to the protein by ligand exchange.
- O **C.** All serum albumin have identical binding sites, regardless of species.
- O **D.** The association between the radiopharmaceuticals and SA is irreversible.

Question 9

A patient is being treated for deep vein thrombosis using warfarin, but needs to undergo an imaging scan using a radiopharmaceutical tracer. Based on the data presented, which is likely to be the best tracer to use?

- O **A.** Cu-ETS
- O **B.** Cu-PTSM
- O **C.** Cu-ATSM
- O **D.** Either Cu-PTSM or Cu-ATSM

The following questions are NOT based on a descriptive passage (Questions 10–13).

Question 10

Which of the following statements is NOT true concerning a graph of reaction rate *v* vs. substrate concentration [S] for an enzyme that follows Michaelis-Menten kinetics?

○ **A.** K_m is the [S] at which $v = ½$ Vmax.
○ **B.** At very high [S], the velocity curve becomes a horizontal line that intersects the y-axis at K_m.
○ **C.** As [S] increases, the initial velocity of reaction, *v*, also increases.
○ **D.** The y-axis is a rate term with units such as μM/min.

Question 11

Apo-X is a drug which blocks prophase from occurring. When Apo-X is added to a tissue culture, in which phase of the cell cycle would most cells be arrested?

○ **A.** Mitosis
○ **B.** G_1
○ **C.** G_2
○ **D.** Synthesis

Question 12

All of the following are true about a blood pressure of 150/60 EXCEPT:

○ **A.** the value normally indicates the venous pressure in the arm.
○ **B.** 150 indicates the pressure as a consequence of ventricular contraction.
○ **C.** the pulse pressure is 90.
○ **D.** 60 indicates the diastolic pressure.

Question 13

Which complex in the electron transport chain does NOT contribute to the proton gradient?

○ **A.** Complex I
○ **B.** Complex II
○ **C.** Complex III
○ **D.** Complex IV

Passage 3 (Questions 14–17)

Sickle cell anemia in humans is an example of a mutation affecting a base in one of the genes involved in the production of hemoglobin. Hemoglobin, in adults, is made up of four polypeptide chains attached to the prosthetic group heme. The polypeptide chains influence the oxygen carrying capacity of the molecule. A change in the base sequence of the triplet coding for one amino acid out of the normal 146 amino acids in the beta chains gives rise to the production of sickle cell hemoglobin. The physiological effect of this is to lower the oxygen-carrying capacity of these red blood cells. In the heterozygous condition individuals show the sickle-cell trait. The red blood cells appear normal and only about 40% of the hemoglobin is abnormal.

A gene represented by two or more alleles within a population is said to be *polymorphic*. Allelic differences are caused by sequence differences, that is, the DNA itself is polymorphic and results in sequence differences between homologous regions of DNA in different individuals. These differences can be detected even when no other differences can be found and knowledge of this polymorphism could be used for the pre- or postnatal diagnosis for the sickle-cell gene.

Rather than directly sequencing a gene, differences called restriction fragment length polymorphisms (RFLPs) can be used to highlight the regions of sequence differences between individuals. The technique depends on a restriction enzyme making a cut at a site on the gene for normal hemoglobin, not present on sickle-cell hemoglobin, causing fragments cut by the given enzyme to be smaller than it is in individuals not possessing the site.

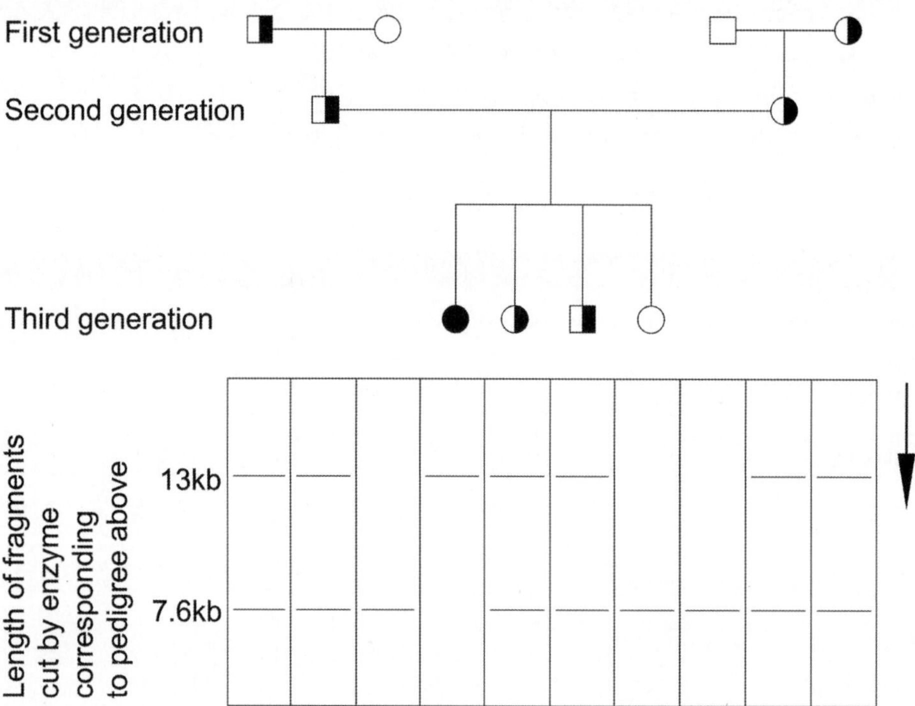

Figure 1 Inheritance pattern of an RFLP associated with sickle-cell disease. Males are represented by squares and females by circles. An open square or circle indicates an individual who is homozygous normal. A half-filled square or circle indicates an individual with sickle-cell trait. A filled square or circle indicates a homozygous individual with sickle-cell disease. The direction of electrophoresis is indicated by an arrow.

Question 14

In parts of the world where malaria is endemic, individuals with sickle-cell trait cannot contract the disease. Which of the following is the most likely explanation for this?

- O **A.** The protozoan which causes malaria needs the amino acid altered by the point mutation to survive.
- O **B.** A closely linked gene to the mutated gene in anemic patients confers resistance to malaria.
- O **C.** The protozoan which causes malaria cannot live in red blood cells containing the abnormal hemoglobin.
- O **D.** There is too little oxygen in sickle cell patients to support the protozoan which causes malaria.

Question 15

Figure 1 indicates that the fragment cut by the restriction enzyme in an individual who is homozygous for the sickle-cell condition is:

- O **A.** 7.6 kb long.
- O **B.** 13 kb long.
- O **C.** 20.6 kb long.
- O **D.** 5.4 kb long.

Question 16

If the heterozygous male in the first generation in Figure 1 was substituted with a homozygous male for the normal condition, the phenotypes of the third generation would be expected to be in the ratio of:

- O **A.** 1 normal : 2 sickle-cell trait : 1 sickle-cell disease.
- O **B.** 1 normal : 1 sickle-cell trait.
- O **C.** 2 normal : 1 sickle-cell trait : 1 sickle-cell disease.
- O **D.** 1 sickle-cell trait : 1 sickle-cell disease.

Question 17

Which of the following biological processes will be most affected by the presence of the mutant gene for sickle cell anemia in an individual?

- O **A.** Fermentation of pyruvate to lactate and ATP
- O **B.** Production of pyruvate and ATP in glycolysis
- O **C.** The production of carbon dioxide, water and ATP during the Krebs cycle and oxidative phosphorylation
- O **D.** The production of carbon dioxide and ATP from ADP in the electron transport chain

Passage 4 (Questions 18–21)

A large number of biological processes, both behavioral and physiological, follow a circadian rhythm, a 24-hour oscillation that displays an endogenous and entrainable pattern. Driven by a circadian clock, they have been observed in a wide range of life forms, including cyanobacteria as well as plants, fungi, and of course, animals.

Two genes in particular, Per1 and Per2, are responsible for encoding the proteins Period Circadian Protein Homolog 1 (PER1) and Period Circadian Protein Homolog 2 (PER2). Both are important for the maintenance of circadian rhythms in cells, and are themselves expressed in accordance with a daily oscillating rhythm. Mice with mutations in either Per1 or Per2 show an impaired circadian phenotype, though they maintain some regularity at least in the short term.

Researchers wanted to study the effect that mutations in both genes would cause, and created double-mutant mice with the genotype $Per1^{m/m}Per2^{m/m}$. Figure 1 shows the measured activities of two mice, one wild type and one $Per1^{m/m}Per2^{m/m}$, during a period of light-dark (shaded area responds to dark), followed by a prolonged period in continuous dim red light (shaded area after 6 days). Both mice were previously maintained in the dark.

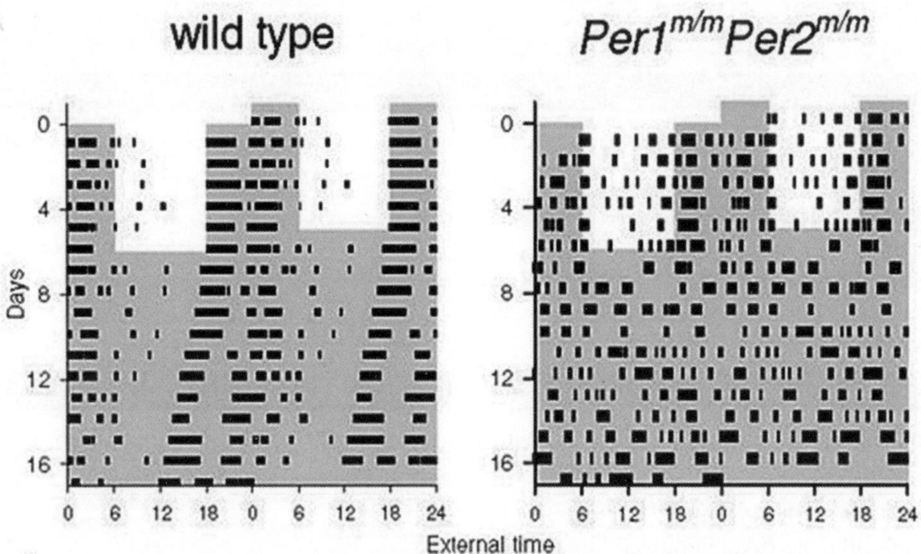

Figure 1 Measured activity of a wild type and $Per1^{m/m}Per2^{m/m}$ mouse during periods of light-dark, followed by continuous dim red light. Black bars correspond to periods of rest.

Adapted from D.R. van der Veen et al, "SCN-AVP release of mPer1/mPer2 double-mutant mice in vitro," *Journal of Circadian Rhythms* (2008).

Question 18

Activity patterns indicative of disrupted circadian rhythm appeared in $Per1^{m/m}Per2^{m/m}$ mice:

- O **A.** after 6 days after light-dark monitoring.
- O **B.** immediately upon light-dark monitoring.
- O **C.** after 16 days after light-dark monitoring.
- O **D.** after a full cycle of light-dark monitoring.

Question 19

If another wild-type mouse was measured alongside the experimental mouse, with the exception that it has never been exposed to any light-dark cycles, one might expect that the dark-adapted mouse would:

- O **A.** exhibit activity similar to the $Per1^{m/m}Per2^{m/m}$ mouse.
- O **B.** express neither Per1 nor Per2.
- O **C.** exhibit a similar circadian rhythm, varying only in pattern duration.
- O **D.** exhibit a circadian rhythm only after the activation of a dim red light.

Question 20

Researchers repeated the experiment with new mice, this time using a 30-hour schedule, with 15 hours each of period light and dark. They found that:

- O **A.** the wild type mouse adopted the 30 hour schedule, while the $Per1^{m/m}Per2^{m/m}$ mouse continued to be arrhythmic.
- O **B.** both the wild type and $Per1^{m/m}Per2^{m/m}$ mouse adopted the 30 hour schedule.
- O **C.** the wild type mouse remained on a 24 hour schedule, while the $Per1^{m/m}Per2^{m/m}$ mouse continued to be arrhythmic.
- O **D.** both the wild type and $Per1^{m/m}Per2^{m/m}$ mouse displayed arrhythmic behavior.

Question 21

Certain drugs are able to induce Per1 and Per2 gene expression, offering possible treatment options for those with circadian rhythm disorders. One would expect that periodic dosage of these drugs would:

- O **A.** restore regularly oscillating activity patterns to $Per1^{m/m}Per2^{m/m}$ mice.
- O **B.** have minimal effect on $Per1^{m/m}Per2^{m/m}$ mice.
- O **C.** restore the function of Per1 and Per2.
- O **D.** shorten the time of light-dark adaptation in $Per1^{m/m}Per2^{m/m}$ mice.

Passage 5 (Questions 22–26)

The combination of hemoglobin with oxygen can be affected not only by oxygen tension but also by pH, CO_2 and glycerate-2,3-biphosphate (GBP). GBP binds preferentially to the deoxygenated form of hemoglobin with a dissociation constant of about 10^{-5} M^{-1}. Its dissociation constant with HbO_2 is only about 10^{-3} M^{-1}. Since the concentrations of GBP and hemoglobin are both about 5 mM in the erythrocyte, we would expect most of the deoxy form to be complexed with GBP and most of the oxyhemoglobin to be free of GBP.

The net effect of the GBP is to shift the standard oxygen–hemoglobin dissociation curve to higher oxygen tensions. This shift is not sufficient to lower the binding of oxygen at the high oxygen tensions in the capillaries of the lungs, but it is sufficient to cause a substantially greater release of oxygen at the lower oxygen tensions that exist where it is needed, that is, in the rest of the body tissues.

The myoglobin molecule is widely distributed in animals. It displays a great affinity for oxygen and in fact only begins to release oxygen when the partial pressure of oxygen is below 20 mmHg. In this way it acts as a store of oxygen, only releasing it when supplies of oxyhemoglobin have been exhausted.

Question 22

Glycerate-2,3-biphosphate likely functions to shift the oxygen–hemoglobin dissociation curve by:

- ○ **A.** increasing the carbon dioxide concentration in the red blood cells.
- ○ **B.** altering the pH of the tissue fluid surrounding the red blood cells.
- ○ **C.** reducing the affinity between oxygen and hemoglobin at low oxygen concentrations.
- ○ **D.** forming a complex with oxygen at low oxygen concentrations.

Question 23

Which of the following graphs would you expect to represent the oxygen dissociation curve for myoglobin?

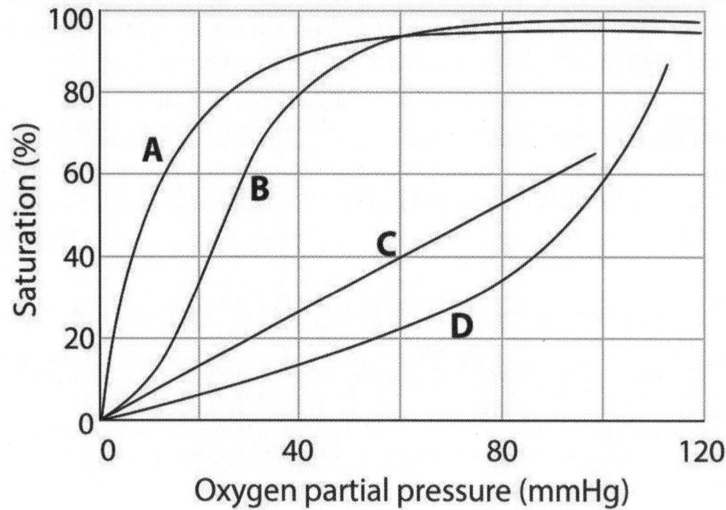

- ○ **A.**
- ○ **B.**
- ○ **C.**
- ○ **D.**

Question 24

Which of the following tissues most benefits from the shifts in the oxygen-dissociation curves caused by GBP and myoglobin?

- O **A.** Cardiac muscle tissue
- O **B.** Skeletal muscle tissue
- O **C.** Loose connective tissue
- O **D.** Intestinal wall tissue

Question 25

In regions with an increased partial pressure of carbon dioxide, the oxygen–hemoglobin dissociation curve is shifted to the right. This is known as the Bohr effect or shift. What is the physiological significance of this shift?

- O **A.** It counteracts the shift in the oxygen–hemoglobin dissociation curve caused by the presence of GBP.
- O **B.** It counteracts the shift in the oxygen–hemoglobin dissociation curve caused by the presence of myoglobin.
- O **C.** It increases the pH of actively respiring tissue.
- O **D.** It facilitates the delivery of increased quantities of oxygen from the blood to cells which produce energy.

Question 26

The Bohr shift can also occur in response to a low pH. Under such conditions, which of the following equations best describes the Bohr shift?

- O **A.** $CO_2 + H_2O \leftrightarrow H_2CO_3 \leftrightarrow H^+ + HCO_3^-$ (tissues)
- O **B.** $H^+ + HbO_2 \leftrightarrow HHb^+ + O_2$ (tissues)
- O **C.** $HCO_3^- + H^+ \leftrightarrow H_2CO_3 \leftrightarrow CO_2 + H_2O$ (lungs)
- O **D.** $HHB^+ + O_2 + HCO_3^- \leftrightarrow HBO_2 + CO_2 + H_2O$ (lungs)

The following questions are NOT based on a descriptive passage (Questions 27–30).

Question 27

Considering only the process described, which of the following cellular reactions would be consistent with a negative ΔS?

- O **A.** Dehydration
- O **B.** Respiration
- O **C.** Catabolism
- O **D.** Hydrolysis

Question 28

Which of the following does NOT follow the normal anatomical sequence?

I. gametogenesis → seminal vesicles → seminiferous tubules
II. seminiferous tubules → epididymis → vas deferens
III. vas deferens → ejaculatory duct → urethra

- O **A.** I only
- O **B.** II only
- O **C.** I and II only
- O **D.** II and III only

Question 29

A biologically active agent, which completely diffuses through capillary beds, is injected into the brachiocephalic vein of the left arm. Which of the following would be most affected by the agent?

- O **A.** Heart
- O **B.** Lung
- O **C.** Left arm
- O **D.** Left leg

Question 30

All of the following contain a phospholipid bilayer EXCEPT:

- O **A.** neurolemma.
- O **B.** sarcolemma.
- O **C.** basement membrane.
- O **D.** cell membrane.

Passage 6 (Questions 31–36)

Active transport is the energy-consuming transport of molecules against a concentration gradient. Energy is required because the substance must be moved in the opposite direction of its natural tendency to diffuse. Movement is usually unidirectional, unlike diffusion which is reversible.

When movement of ions is considered, two factors will influence the direction in which they diffuse: one is concentration, the other is electrical charge. An ion will usually diffuse from a region of its high concentration to a region of its low concentration. It will also generally be attracted towards a region of opposite charge, and move away from a region of similar charge. Thus ions are said to move down electrochemical gradients, which are the combined effects of both electrical and concentration gradients. Strictly speaking, active transport of ions is their movement against an electrochemical gradient powered by an energy source.

Research has shown that the cell surface membranes of most cells possess sodium pumps. Usually, though not always, the sodium pump is coupled with a potassium pump. The combined pump is called the sodium-potassium pump. This pump is an excellent example of active transport.

Table 1 Concentration of Na^+, K^+, and Cl^- inside and outside mammalian motor neurons.

Ion	Concentration (mmol/L H_2O)		Equilibrium potential (mV)
	Inside cell	Outside cell	
Na^+	15.0	150.0	+60
K^+	150.0	5.5	-90
Cl^-	9.0	125.0	-75
Resting membrane potential (V_m) = -70 mV			

Question 31

All of the following explain the ionic concentrations in Table 1 EXCEPT:

- O **A.** Na^+ and Cl^- ions passively diffuse more quickly into the extracellular fluid than K^+ ions.
- O **B.** Na^+ ions are actively pumped out of the intracellular fluid.
- O **C.** the negative charge of the cell contents repels Cl^- ions from the cell.
- O **D.** the cell membrane is more freely permeable to K^+ ions than to Na^+ and Cl^- ions.

Question 32

If cyanide was added to nerve cells, what would be expected to happen to the ionic composition of the cells?

- O **A.** Na^+ ions would be actively pumped into the cell and K^+ ions would be pumped out.
- O **B.** Intracellular Na^+ would increase since the sodium pump would be impaired.
- O **C.** The potential of the cell membrane would not be reversed so that Cl^- ions would freely enter the cell.
- O **D.** The cell membrane would become freely permeable to Na^+ and Cl^- ions.

Question 33

The temporary increase in the sarcolemma's permeability to Na^+ and K^+ ions that occurs at the motor end plate of a neuromuscular junction is immediately preceded by:

- O **A.** the release of acetylcholine from the motor neuron into the synaptic gap.
- O **B.** the release of adrenaline from the motor neuron into the synaptic gap.
- O **C.** the passage of a nerve impulse along the axon of a motor neuron.
- O **D.** the release of noradrenaline from a sensory neuron into the synaptic gap.

Question 34

The overall reaction which takes place at the sodium pump is given by the equation:

$$3Na^+_{(inside)} + 2K^+_{(outside)} + ATP^{4-} + H_2O \rightarrow 3Na^+_{(outside)} + 2K^+_{(inside)} + ADP^{3-} + P_i + H^+$$

When a muscle is very active, at the end of glycolysis, pyruvate is converted to lactate by the addition of H^+ ions. During vigorous exercise, how many ions of K^+ could be pumped into a cell per molecule of glucose?

- O **A.** 2
- O **B.** 4
- O **C.** 8
- O **D.** 12

Question 35

Active transport assumes particular importance in all but which of the following structures?

- O **A.** Cells of the large intestine
- O **B.** Alveoli
- O **C.** Nerve and muscle cells
- O **D.** Loop of Henle

Question 36

At inhibitory synapses, a hyperpolarization of the membrane known as an inhibitory postsynaptic potential is produced rendering V_m more negative. This occurs as a result of:

- O **A.** an increase in the postsynaptic membrane's permeability to Na^+ and K^+ ions.
- O **B.** an increase in the permeability of the presynaptic membrane to Ca^{2+} ions.
- O **C.** the entry of Cl^- ions into the synaptic knob.
- O **D.** an increase in the permeability of the postsynaptic membrane to Cl^- ions.

Passage 7 (Questions 37–40)

The Sanger method for sequencing DNA uses newly synthesized DNA that is randomly terminated. The method employs chain-terminating dideoxynucleotide triphosphates (ddXTPs) to produce a continuous series of fragments during catalyzed reactions. The ddXTPs act as terminators because while they can add to a growing chain during polymerization, they cannot be added onto.

When DNA is being sequenced, the appropriate enzymes are added to make a complementary copy of a primed single-stranded DNA fragment. By choosing an appropriate primer, the region of the nucleic acid that is copied can be predetermined. Synthetic reaction mixtures are then set up, each containing one or more radioactive deoxyribonucleoside triphosphates to label the fragments for detection by autoradiography. Each mixture contains a single, limiting amount of dideoxytrinucleoside triphosphate to randomly terminate the synthesized fragments at one of the four nucleotides. The products of four separate reaction mixtures, each containing a different dideoxynucleoside triphosphate, are analyzed.

Following synthesis, the reaction products are separated from the template by denaturation and fractionated by electrophoresis on polyacrylamide gels. After electrophoresis the positions of the fragments on the gel are detected by autoradiography. The sequence is read directly from the autoradiogram, starting with the fastest moving (*smallest*) fragment at the bottom, and then moving up the gel to larger fragments. In order to read the DNA sequence, the individual bands must be followed beginning at the bottom of the gel.

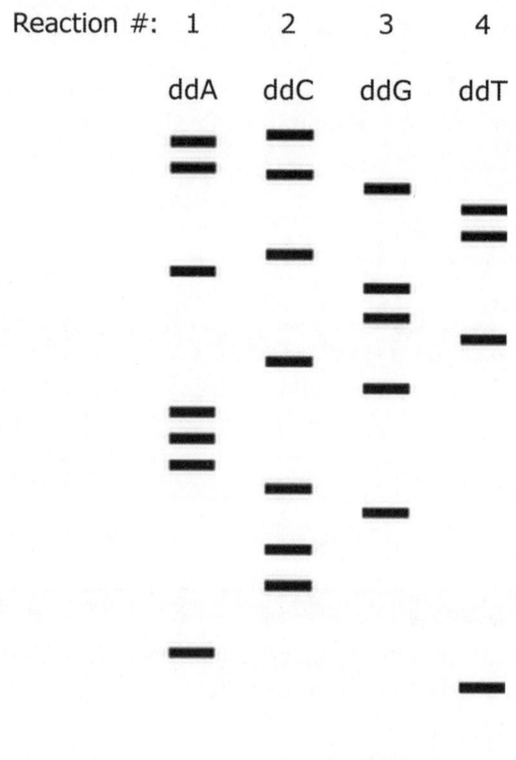

Figure 1 Autoradiogram of a fragmented DNA strand post-synthesis.

Question 37

The passage suggests that dideoxynucleoside triphosphates are able to be used in the Sanger method because they lack a:

- O **A.** hydroxyl group on their phosphoric acid component.
- O **B.** hydroxyl group on C1 of their ribose component.
- O **C.** hydroxyl group on C3 of their ribose component.
- O **D.** hydroxyl group on C5 of their ribose component.

Question 38

According to Figure 1, the newly synthesized DNA strand began and ended with:

- O **A.** an adenine and guanine residue, respectively
- O **B.** a cytosine and guanine residue, respectively
- O **C.** a guanine and cytosine residue, respectively.
- O **D.** a cytosine and adenine residue, respectively.

Question 39

Using data from Figure 1, the first 8 residues of the DNA template sequence were:

- O **A.** GTACCGCA.
- O **B.** GAAACGCC.
- O **C.** CATGGCGT.
- O **D.** CTTTGCGG.

Question 40

One of the latest adaptations of the Sanger method uses four different colored fluorescent derivatives attached to the four different ddXTP terminators. The most likely main advantage of this new approach is that:

- O **A.** electrophoresis treatment to the denatured DNA would no longer be necessary.
- O **B.** ddUTP can be used as a chain-terminating dideoxynucleotide triphosphate.
- O **C.** the technique would be faster and more economical.
- O **D.** all four reactions could be carried out simultaneously prior to electrophoresis and then can run on one gel.

Passage 8 (Questions 41–44)

The hepatitis C virus (HCV) contains a single-stranded positive-sense RNA genome that is translated into a single protein. The resulting protein is then cleaved into multiple additional proteins that are critical for the viral life cycle. The NS3 serine protease plays a key role in processing the viral pre-protein, as well as inactivating host adaptor proteins that are important for immune sensing.

Compound 1 is a serine protease inhibitor with the structure shown in Figure 1.

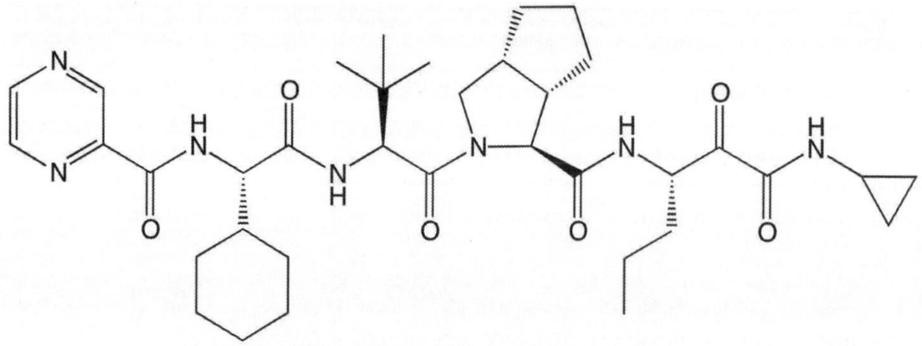

Figure 1 The structure of Compound 1

The effectiveness of anti-viral agents in infected patients can be measured using a variety of methods, including measuring the viral load in each cell. For HCV, specific single nucleotide polymorphism (SNPs) in the DNA sequence of the NS3 protease can directly affect the effectiveness of these drugs. The ability of Compound 1 to inhibit the viral load of infected patients with different mutations is shown in Figure 2.

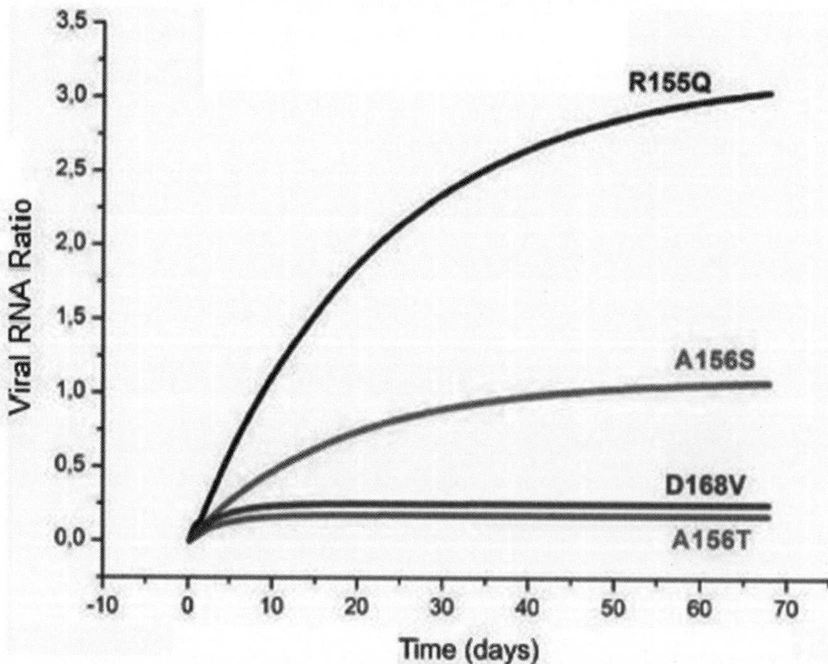

Figure 2 The ability of Compound 1 to inhibit the viral load, measured by RNA(+), of HCV patients with different genetic mutations. In wildtype, Compound 1 binds effectively to NS3 protease, reducing the viral load to negligible levels. Note: the designations associated with each curve indicates the wildtype amino acid first, the number is its location in the primary structure, and the second letter in each sequence is the amino acid present in the mutant.

To obtain effective therapeutic agents in patients who are resistant to Compound 1, two analogs were developed (Compound 1a and Compound 1b). The steady-state kinetics of both agents were then assessed in Patient Y (*see* Figure 3).

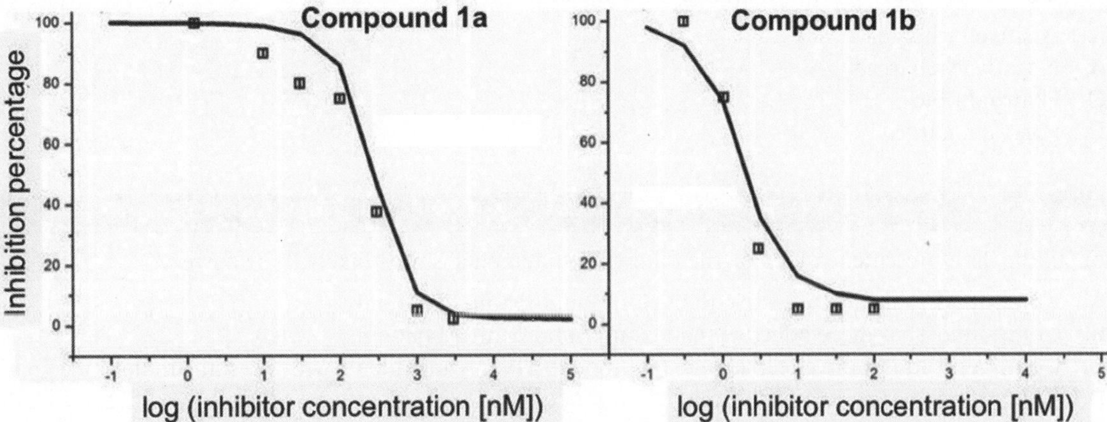

Figure 3 The kinetics of HCV replication inhibition in a patient who was unresponsive to Compound 1

Note that the effect of an inhibitor is measured as the percentage decrease in the reaction rate. Thus the inhibition percentage is determined by:

$$\text{Percent Inhibition} = \frac{\text{Rate without inhibitor} - \text{rate with inhibitor}}{\text{rate without inhibitor}} \times 100$$

Adapted from ema.europa.eu WC500115532 , and nih.gov PMC3958367.

Question 41

Viral inhibitors can be distinguished according to the mechanism by which they function. Based on the information provided, Compound 1 treats hepatitis C virus by functioning as:

- ○ **A.** an antagonist.
- ○ **B.** an agonist.
- ○ **C.** a catalyst.
- ○ **D.** a placebo.

Question 42

Final analysis of the kinetics of interaction between Compound 1 and NS3 revealed a K_i of 7 nM. Although this suggests effective inhibition, the development team undertook a project to identify more potent analogs of Compound 1 to reduce the dosing frequency in patients with hepatitis C. This resulted in the development of an additional four related compounds (Compounds 2–5). Which of the following compounds would be a more potent inhibitor?

- ○ **A.** Compound 2 (K_i = 7 μM)
- ○ **B.** Compound 3 (K_i = 10 nM)
- ○ **C.** Compound 4 (K_i = 8 nM)
- ○ **D.** Compound 5 (K_i = 100 pM)

Question 43

Patients with different mutations in NS3 protease exhibit different responsiveness to Compound 1. Based on the information presented, if the difference in binding was strictly due to the amino acid mutations outlined in Figure 2, what type of amino acids are most important for the inhibitory action?

- O **A.** Positively charged
- O **B.** Negatively charged
- O **C.** Hydrophobic
- O **D.** Polar uncharged

Question 44

Based on all the data presented, which of the following statements is most likely to be correct?

- O **A.** Compound 1a is more effective than Compound 1b in all patients.
- O **B.** Compound 1b is more effective than Compound 1a in all patients.
- O **C.** Compound 1a is more effective than Compound 1b only in patients with the same mutation as patient Y.
- O **D.** Compound 1b is more effective than Compound 1a only in patients with the same mutation as patient Y.

The following questions are NOT based on a descriptive passage (Questions 45–48).

Question 45

Cholecystokinin (CCK) is a family of peptide hormones, with varying numbers of amino acids, that stimulate the digestion of fat and protein in the GI system. A sulfated form of CCK, illustrated below, can activate the CCK receptor.

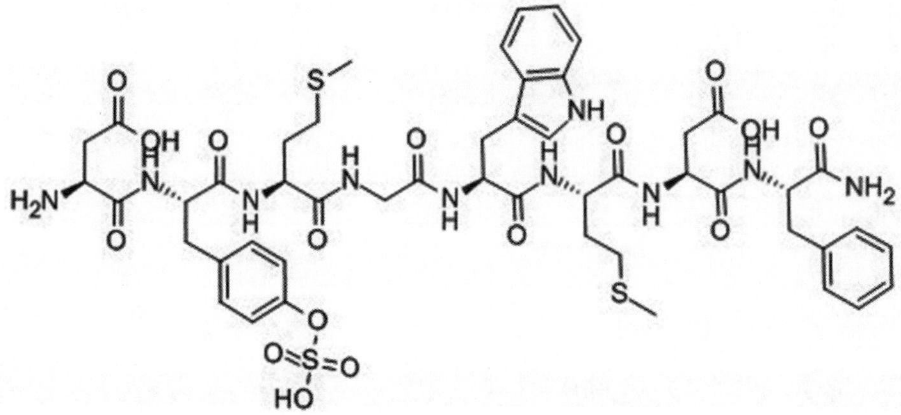

Given the structure of the sulfated form of CCK above, which of the following is the most accurate descriptor?

- O **A.** Pentapeptide
- O **B.** Hexapeptide
- O **C.** Heptapeptide
- O **D.** Octapeptide

Question 46

It has been found that proinsulin, the precursor molecule to insulin, contains a portion that is stabilized by disulfide bonds after folding. Such disulfide bonds pertain to what level of protein structure?

- O **A.** Primary structure
- O **B.** Secondary structure
- O **C.** Tertiary structure
- O **D.** Quaternary structure

Question 47

Almost all mammals, and certainly humans, are endotherms ("warm-blooded"). Consider radiant heat passing between an endotherm and its cooler environment. Heat would be expected to be radiated and absorbed in which of the following ways?

- O **A.** Only the endotherm radiates heat, which is then absorbed by the environment.
- O **B.** Only the environment radiates heat, which is then absorbed by the endotherm.
- O **C.** Heat exchange occurs in both directions: the endotherm radiates more and absorbs less heat per unit area than the environment.
- O **D.** Heat exchange occurs in both directions: the environment radiates more and absorbs less heat per unit area than the endotherm.

Question 48

One of the the possible injuries during a high speed motor vehicle accident includes a *traumatic hemothorax* in which blood accumulates in the pleural cavity. With regards to a traumatic hemothorax, which of the following would be of greatest concern?

- O **A.** High oxygenation due to an elevated diaphragm
- O **B.** Low oxygenation due to blood in the main bronchi
- O **C.** High oxygenation due to excess blood inside of the alveoli
- O **D.** Low oxygenation due to compression of the lung

Passage 9 (Questions 49–52)

Activin A, a cytokine synthesized by many cell types in the body, is known to be essential to developmental and repair processes. It plays a role in the inflammatory response, and is synthesized by monocytes upon stimulation with macrophage-activating inducers like GM-CSF and the cytokine IFNγ. Some cases of severe asthma show elevated levels of activin A in the serum, leading researchers to seek a relationship between alveolar macrophages (AM), macrophage stimulating factors like GM-CSF and IFNγ, and activin A.

Experiment 1

Wild-type AMs were cultured for 24 hours with 100 U/mL IFNγ. mRNA was extracted from the cells, and activin A expression was analyzed using quantitative-PCR. Figure 1 shows the relative fold change in the expression of activin A.

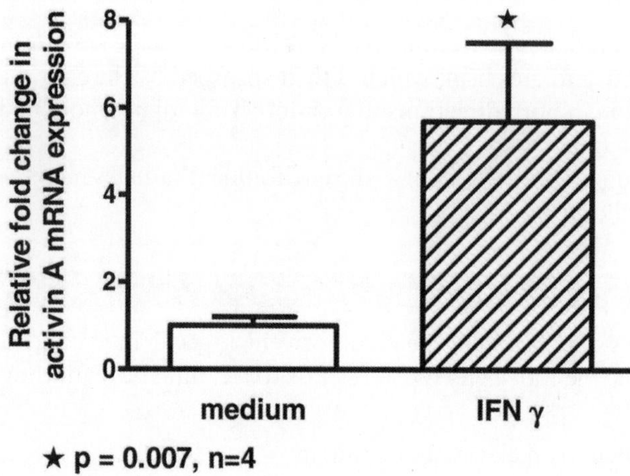

Figure 1 Expression of Activin A mRNA with and without IFNγ.

Experiment 2

To determine whether blocking IFNγ using a specific anti-IFNγ antibody would affect intrinsic activin A expression, AMs genetically unable to express GM-CSF were cultured for 24 hours with a control immunoglobulin (Ig) or anti-IFNγ.

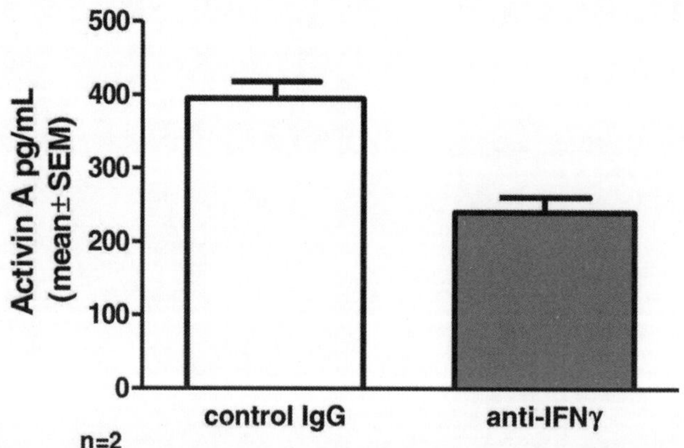

Figure 2 Expression of GM-CSF knockout alveolar macrophages incubated with anti-IFNγ antibody.

Adapted from H. Dalrymple, "Alveolar macrophages of GM-CSF knockout mice exhibit mixed M1 and M2 phenotypes," *BMC Immunology* (2013).

Question 49

A localized increase in IFNγ in lung tissue would lead to:

- ○ **A.** a decrease in activin A expression.
- ○ **B.** a disruption in T cell differentiation.
- ○ **C.** an inflammatory response.
- ○ **D.** negative regulation of activin A function.

Question 50

Before mounting an IFNγ-mediated response, alveolar macrophages may employ what process to protect the body against foreign bodies?

- ○ **A.** Phagocytosis
- ○ **B.** Apoptosis
- ○ **C.** Antigen presentation
- ○ **D.** Plasmolysis

Question 51

GM-CSF knockout mice with permanently disrupted GM-CSF have been found to exhibit an over-expression of IFNγ. Thus, IFNγ's relationship to activin A is that of a(n):

- ○ **A.** inhibitor.
- ○ **B.** positive regulator.
- ○ **C.** anti-inflammatory regulator.
- ○ **D.** transcription factor.

Question 52

IFNγ is 143 amino acids long and within its sequence is 11 amino acids divided into two clusters termed D1 and D2. These 2 clusters have an affinity for heparan sulfate (HS). HS occurs as two or three chains associated with cell surface proteins involved in regulating a wide variety of biological activities. Consider the HS subunit below.

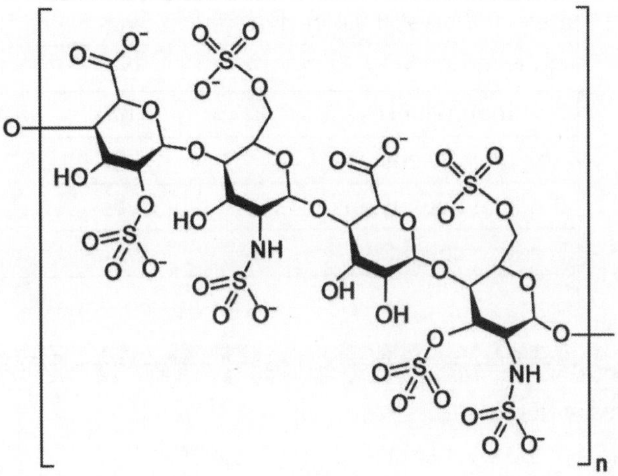

Which of the following is most consistent with the primary structures of D1 and D2, respectively?

- ○ **A.** KTGKRKR and RGRR
- ○ **B.** ATGAFAF and FGFF
- ○ **C.** YTGYWYW and WGWW
- ○ **D.** DTGEGEG and EGDD

Passage 10 (Questions 53–56)

Two antibiotics were tested for their effectiveness at killing a particular strain of bacteria that had been grown in media on culture plates. Antibiotic A was administered to 3 plates (P1, P2, and P3); antibiotic B was administered to 3 different plates (P4, P5, and P6); while an equivalent volume of water was added to another three plates (P7, P8, and P9).

The plates were incubated at 37 °C for five days in an incubator, after which the average number of bacteria still present on the plates was determined. The percentage of bacteria per plate relative to the original administration per plate is listed in Table 1.

Table 1

	0-10%	11-50 %	51-75 %	76-100 %	101 % or more
P1		X			
P2		X			
P3			X		
P4				X	
P5			X		
P6				X	
P7					X
P8					X
P9				X	

A series of tests were done on the bacteria prior to their being plated in the media. The results of the tests are listed in Table 2.

Table 2

Retained crystal violet dye	yes
Grew in presence of O_2	yes
Common pili present	no
Sex pili present	no
Produce hemolysins	yes
Produce coagulase	no

Question 53

Three of the plates were treated with water to:

- ○ **A.** account for bacteria that grow better in an aqueous medium.
- ○ **B.** account for bacteria that grow worse in an aqueous medium.
- ○ **C.** insure that any change in the number of bacteria were the result of the addition of antibiotics.
- ○ **D.** insure that all extraneous factors that could cause a change in bacteria number were eliminated.

Question 54

What is the likely feature of certain bacteria which allow them to retain dye upon being stained?

- ○ **A.** The presence of a bilayer nuclear membrane
- ○ **B.** Peptidoglycan in the cell wall
- ○ **C.** Pili on the surface of the cell wall
- ○ **D.** The presence of active Golgi bodies

Question 55

Which of the following could be inferred from the information given in the passage?

- ○ **A.** All the bacteria used in this experiment have a resistance to antibiotic B.
- ○ **B.** All the bacteria in this experiment have a resistance to both antibiotic A and antibiotic B.
- ○ **C.** The combination of antibiotic A and B would result in maximal mitochondrial inhibition resulting in the greatest number of bacteria dying.
- ○ **D.** Some of the remaining bacteria on plates 4 - 6 would be susceptible to antibiotic A.

Question 56

If five bacterial cells were plated on a culture dish, in a medium without any antibiotics, and incubated under ideal conditions, how many cells would most likely be present on the plate after 3 generations?

- ○ **A.** 8
- ○ **B.** 40
- ○ **C.** 60
- ○ **D.** 80

The following questions are NOT based on a descriptive passage (Questions 57–59).

Question 57

Which of the following gives rise to the skeletal system?

- ○ **A.** Ectoderm
- ○ **B.** Endoderm
- ○ **C.** Mesoderm
- ○ **D.** Pharyngeal gill slits

Question 58

Which of the following refers to a continuous partial contraction of a muscle?

- ○ **A.** Tetany
- ○ **B.** Tonus
- ○ **C.** Twitch
- ○ **D.** Tremor

Question 59

The difference between the bacterium *E. coli* and the fungus *Aspergillus* is:

- ○ **A.** *Aspergillus* contains ribosomes.
- ○ **B.** *E. coli* has a cell wall.
- ○ **C.** *Aspergillus* can undergo anaerobic metabolism.
- ○ **D.** *E. coli* does not have a nucleus.

CANDIDATE'S NAME ______________________________

RAW SCORE AND SCALED SCORE ______________________

GS-2
Mock Exam 2 of 7
Solutions at MCAT-prep.com

GS-2 Section IV: Psychological, Social, and Biological Foundations of Behavior

Questions: 1-59
Time: 95 minutes

INSTRUCTIONS: Of all the questions on this test, most are organized into groups preceded by a passage. After evaluating the passage, select the best answer to each question in the group. Fifteen questions are independent of any descriptive passage or each other. Similarly, select the best answer to these questions. If you are unsure of an answer, eliminate the alternatives that you know to be incorrect and select an answer from the remaining alternatives. To indicate your selection, use a pencil to blacken the corresponding circle next to the answer choice and/or you can use the answer document at the back of this book. No marks are deducted for wrong answers.

The computer-based real MCAT has an on-screen highlighter function and ~~STRIKEOUT~~ function. These tools help to spotlight text or assist in the process of elimination. You may use a yellow highlighter for this paper-based exam and/or a pen (or preferably a pencil to make it easier should you change your mind) to mark text. At the time of publishing, both highlighting and strikeout functions can be used for passages, questions and answer choices. You can also flag a question to review later should time remain.

For the real exam, you will be provided with a dry erase board which is a white laminated noteboard booklet accompanied by a fine point marker. The noteboard includes 9 graph-lined pages for you to write though you cannot erase. You can simulate the experience with a fine point marker on a noteboard or with 8" x 14" plain graph paper.

Please note: For the real MCAT, a small number of field-tested questions will remain unscored.

This practice test has been designed exclusively to test knowledge and thinking skills. This exam may contain hypothetical statements and/or express controversial ideas. Statements contained herein do not necessarily reflect the policy, position, or view of RuveneCo Inc. or MCAT-prep.com.

START EXAM ONLY WHEN TIMER IS READY.

Passage 1 (Questions 1–4)

The value of the arts in society has been under debate for the last several decades. Some researchers consider there to be two main classes of value: instrumental and intrinsic. Instrumental values of the arts include, at an individual level, aspects such as skills training, self-efficacy, and physical and/or mental health. From a broader social and economic level, they include aspects such as economic growth and academic performance. Intrinsic values of the arts include captivation, empathy, and aesthetic pleasure. Socially, these translate into an ability to create social bonds, an increase in cultural and social capital, and the expression of communal cultural meaning.

Art is also scientifically valuable. The most obvious example comes from the Berlin school of Gestalt psychology, greatly affected by Max Wertheimer's 1912 paper on the phi phenomenon of motion perception. Wertheimer demonstrated that people perceive images as unitary percepts (i.e., a Gestalt). The whole image cannot, at least initially, be decomposed into its constitutive visual elements. That is, the perceptual experience of the whole enters consciousness before the parts. For Wertheimer, this wholeness or Gestalt results from the functional relations or dynamics that exist between the parts (i.e., reciprocal dependency).

The idea that the whole is more than the sum of its parts was disseminated and sometimes applied to other fields, like psychotherapy. Yet many Gestalt psychologists and artists kept investigating and demonstrating varied principles of perceptual organization, often under the form of optical illusions, like Wertheimer's, or works of art, like Maurits Escher's impossible figures. These demonstrations are still currently used to illustrate interesting universal perceptual phenomena and their underlying principles. For example, psychopathological disorders such as autism and schizophrenia seem to be associated with impaired mechanisms of perceptual organization. Specifically, the ability to perceive the Gestalt, possibly also due to perceptual principles of grouping (seeing a set of elements as "going together"), is not as effective in these populations as it is in the typical population.

Figure 1 depicts the performance of two groups (control and diagnosed schizophrenics) in a task that involved detecting a letter (T or F) among many letter-resembling symbols (specifically ˥-). The target could be embedded (grouped with the symbols) or isolated (spatially distant from the symbols). Accuracy and latency were measured. As this recent study illustrates, Gestalt research on the neuropsychological translation of such universal perceptual principles continues to evolve.

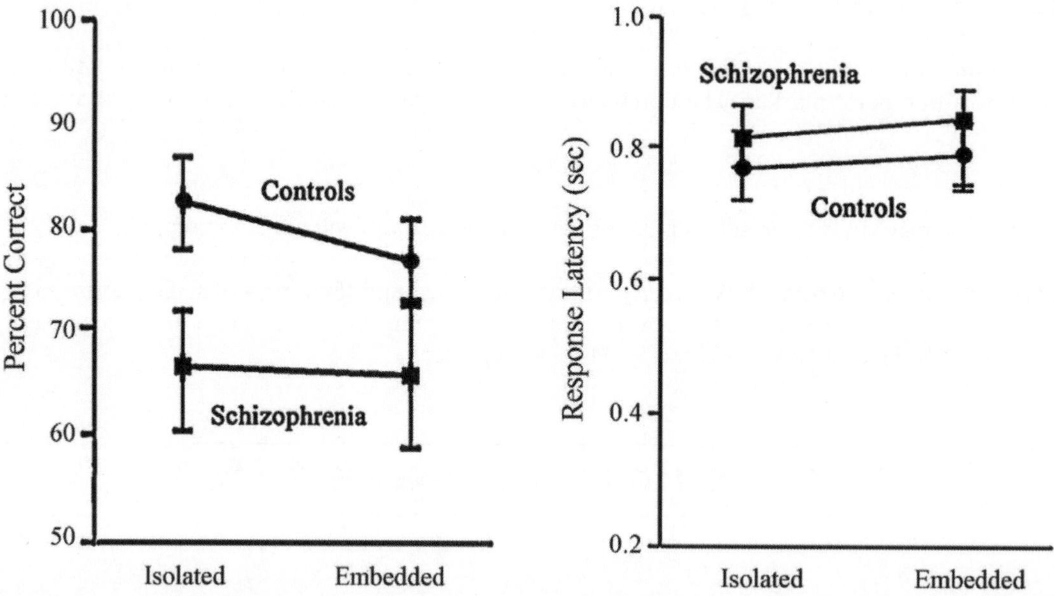

Figure 1 Accuracy and reaction time data by condition, by group. Error bars reflect standard error of measurement.

Sources: Adapted from K.F. McCarthy, E.H. Ondaatje, L. Zakaras, and A. Brooks, "Gifts of the Muse: Reframing the Debate about the Benefits of the Arts." Copyright 2004 RAND Corporation; J. Wagemans, J.H. Elder, M. Kubovy et al., "A Century of Gestalt Psychology in Visual Perception: I. Perceptual Grouping and Figure–Ground Organization." Copyright 2012 Psychological Bulletin; S.M. Silverstein, S. Berten, B. Essex et al., "Perceptual Organization and Visual Search Processes during Target Detection Task Performance in Schizophrenia, as Revealed by fMRI." Copyright 2010 Neuropsychologia.

Question 1

Which of the following conclusions is supported by the data presented in Figure 1?

- ○ **A.** There is a wider standard deviation for the schizophrenia group than for the control group.
- ○ **B.** Both groups have longer reaction times for the isolated than for the embedded condition.
- ○ **C.** The control group has apparently fewer perceptual organization difficulties because, for this group, latency is shorter and their accuracy is higher.
- ○ **D.** The schizophrenia group's accuracy is lower than the control group's accuracy because its participants' reaction times are longer.

Question 2

Which of the following illusions helps to demonstrate the phi phenomenon, described by Wertheimer and mentioned in the passage?

- ○ **A.** Two slim rectangles of equal dimensions are placed one above the other in between two convergent parallel-appearing lines. At a certain disposition of lines and rectangles, one of the rectangles seems to be considerably bigger than the other.
- ○ **B.** The stationary image of a white grid placed on a black background is shown. Small white circles are placed at the intersections of the grid. At a certain level of contrast and attention, the circles seem to both scintillate and contain a dark circle inside.
- ○ **C.** Two similar images composed of stationary dots are shown in succession. At a certain combinations of dot spacing and timing of images' exposition, the dots seem to be moving from one place to the other and/or around their localizations.
- ○ **D.** Two small squares of equal sizes and shades of gray are placed inside two larger squares, one white and one black, of equal sizes with a joint edge. At a certain level of contrast between the colors, the gray square in the black background seems darker than the one in the white background.

Question 3

The author described how people with autism suffered from perceptual organization difficulties. According to the *Diagnostic and Statistical Manual of Mental Disorders V* (*DSM-V*), which of the following symptoms does NOT help to characterize autistic spectrum disorder?

- ○ **A.** Verbal communication difficulties
- ○ **B.** Loss of interest or pleasure in daily activities
- ○ **C.** Limited and repetitive patterns of behavior
- ○ **D.** Nonverbal social interaction difficulties

Question 4

Which of the following quantitative social measures could help to assess the intrinsic value of arts?

- ○ **A.** Comparing the number of Facebook friends of people who have an interest in or past experience with the arts with the number of Facebook friends of those who do not
- ○ **B.** Constructing a closed-ended question survey about people's current health condition and their interest in or past experience with the arts
- ○ **C.** Comparing the unemployment levels in cities with university art courses with the unemployment levels in cities without such courses
- ○ **D.** Randomly selecting participants, presenting them with a well-known painting, and assessing their endorphin levels

Passage 2 (Questions 5–9)

Money is at the heart of economic activity. As much as we like to think we are rational beings, more often than not we make financial decisions based on our heart versus our mind. Studies have shown that if subjects were offered \$15 in cash today or \$25 in a month, more subjects would select the \$15. In other studies, functional magnetic resonance imaging scans were done as subjects made such decisions. When subjects had the choice of an immediate reward or a delayed option and they chose the delayed option, the "rational" regions of the brain were more activated than the part of the brain that is linked to emotions.

Money is also a leading contender in stress. According to the American Psychological Association, which conducted a survey in August 2014 with more than 3,000 adult Americans, 72% indicated feeling stressed about money and finances at some period during the past month. Money is especially a source of stress for parents, millennials (18- to 35-year-olds), and Gen Xers (36- to 49-year-olds).

Some say money is the root of all evil. It seems to weaken social relationships. Some studies show that research subjects primed with the word money are more likely to disclose that they would engage in unethical behavior than unprimed participants. In an interesting study, the manner in which money was acquired also affected how money was perceived and used. Specifically, research subjects were recruited and randomly assigned to the control or experimental group. The control group participants were told that they had found a winning lottery ticket on the street (moral condition). The experimental group participants were told that they had found the winning ticket after observing the winner, who knew having won, drop it on the street (immoral condition). Subjects were asked how they felt about the money, what they would do with it, and how much they would spend on a much desired vacation. Figure 1 shows how subjects felt more guilt and would spend less of it in the immoral than in the moral condition. Researchers concluded that experimental subjects felt that they had "dirty money" on their hands.

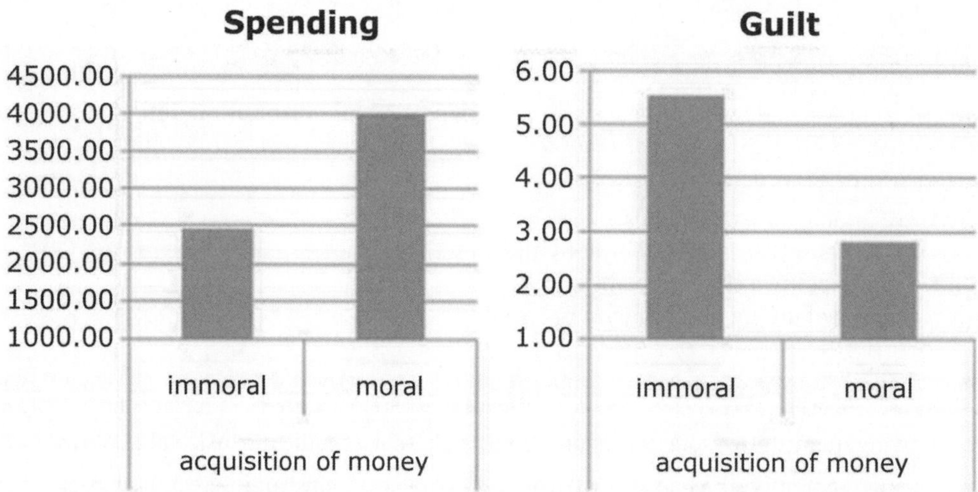

Figure 1 Level of spending and guilt emotions as a function of immoral or moral procurement of money

Source: Adapted from P. Kardos and E. Castano, "Money Doesn't Stink. Or Does It? The Effect of Immorally Acquiring Money on Its Spending," Copyright 2012 Current Psychology.

Question 5

Which phenomenon best explains the findings in Figure 1?

- ○ **A.** Magical law of contagion
- ○ **B.** Implicit memory
- ○ **C.** Anchoring bias
- ○ **D.** Distributive justice

Question 6

To evaluate how Lawrence Kohlberg's first stage of the "conventional morality" level affected the findings of the study about moral versus immoral procurement of money, participants in the immoral condition could be split in half randomly, and one half would be further told that:

- ○ **A.** the person who had dropped the winning lottery ticket was a friend of theirs. The other half would be told that the person who dropped the ticket was a stranger.
- ○ **B.** their actions would be rewarded or punished, in accordance with their ethical rightness.
- ○ **C.** observers would judge whether they were a good or a bad person in the light of their actions.
- ○ **D.** their principles of justice and equality were paramount.

Question 7

'Throwing good money after bad money' is an expression used to describe the continuous re-investment on what resulted originally from a bad financial decision, as if in the hope of 'fixing' the past mistake. Which of the following psychological mechanisms may be actively affecting an investor who thinks highly of himself but keeps throwing good money after bad money?

- ○ **A.** Diffusion of responsibility
- ○ **B.** Availability heuristic
- ○ **C.** Group polarization
- ○ **D.** Cognitive dissonance

Question 8

Given what is known about narcissistic personality disorder, what hypothesis might researchers, interested in the relationship between low vs. high narcissistic personality survey scores and patterns of financial investments, formulate?

- ○ **A.** Subjects who score low on narcissism are more likely to feel they belong to the group of high-powered and successful investors than those who score high on narcissism.
- ○ **B.** Subjects who score high on narcissism are more likely to invest in stocks that exhibit high volatility (i.e., large price fluctuations) than those who score low on narcissism.
- ○ **C.** Subjects who score low on narcissism are more likely to multiply their investments without great evidence of viability than those who score high on narcissism.
- ○ **D.** Subjects who score high on narcissism are more likely to seek conservative investments with a stable rate of return than those who score low on narcissism.

Question 9

Which characteristic below does NOT describe the phenomenon of groupthink?

- ○ **A.** Members are extremely optimistic.
- ○ **B.** Members are pressured not to dissent.
- ○ **C.** The group perceives majority views as biased.
- ○ **D.** Members who have some doubts do not bring them up.

The following questions are NOT based on a descriptive passage (Questions 10–13).

Question 10

Smoking raises the level of a "feel-good" chemical in the body called:

- O **A.** melatonin.
- O **B.** cortisol.
- O **C.** oxytocin.
- O **D.** dopamine.

Question 11

Which of the following senses is NOT used to send communicative signals to other organisms?

- O **A.** Vestibular sense
- O **B.** Seismic sense
- O **C.** Haptic sense
- O **D.** Bioluminescence

Question 12

Which of the following statements about consciousness is correct?

- O **A.** Consciousness has but one state or level. A person is either conscious or not.
- O **B.** There is a well-known neural region responsible for an individual's consciousness.
- O **C.** Consciousness is a non-controversial construct, measurable with simple standard procedures.
- O **D.** Consciousness can be defined as awareness of internal and/or external stimuli.

Question 13

At a bus stop, a male confederate placed a bag down. In condition 1, he left immediately. In conditions 2, 3, and 4, he said he would be right back when asking a female subject, vs. a group of subjects, and vs. the subject who was most similar to him in terms of demographics (gender, race, and age), respectively, to watch his bag. The step which followed across conditions was a male confederate picking the bag up, and quickly walking away, while subjects' reactions were registered. Which condition measured for diffusion of responsibility with greater reliability?

- O **A.** Condition 1
- O **B.** Condition 2
- O **C.** Condition 3
- O **D.** Condition 4

Note: This page is left blank so that the passage would be visible without turning pages while assessing the passage-based questions.

Passage 3 (Questions 14–17)

One may be thrilled with one's creative achievements, while knowing one is not Mozart or Einstein. Indeed, there are two kinds of creativity: the little c (or "mini-C") and the big C. Both types bring to existence something new, original, functional, future oriented, and appropriate. Both involve relating and applying existing knowledge in a novel manner. Differences exist between the two: the little c is useful for everyday problem solving and adaptation to change, thus having great individual value and being more widespread. The big C involves generating outstanding ideas that make significant intellectual and cultural contributions, like Mozart's and Einstein's. It has a major social impact and is rarer.

The creative process is believed to rely on two distinct modes of thought: associative or divergent, and analytical or convergent. Associative thought is unstructured, "defocused, suggestive, and intuitive, revealing remote or subtle connections between items." Analytical thought is critical, structured, "focused and evaluative, more conducive to analyzing relationships of cause and effect." Scientific innovation is often associated with convergent thinking, artistic innovation with divergent thinking. Yet whatever the field, both processes are useful for generating innovative output.

Creativity is often regarded as individually and socially beneficial. Since interindividual differences exist, this ability is sometimes targeted in training courses. Tasks that enhance creativity include thinking aloud, brainstorming, bubble mapping, journal writing, artwork creation, and free writing. Figure 1 illustrates the results obtained with three types of training sessions (creative ideation, general ideation, and rule switching) on a divergent-thinking task for two age groups (adolescents and adults).

The widespread belief that creativity is associated with psychopathology has gathered limited empirical support and fueled such positive takes on creativity. Yet a recent Swedish large-scale study concluded that patients with schizophrenia or bipolar disorder and their relatives were overrepresented in creative occupations (i.e., artistic and scientific). In the second large-scale study, with the exception of bipolar disorder, individuals in overall creative professions were not more likely to suffer from investigated psychiatric disorders. With writers, the likelihood of schizophrenia, bipolar disorder, unipolar depression, anxiety disorders, substance abuse, and suicide for them and their first-degree relatives was higher.

In light of these studies, a change in paradigm can be claimed. Some psychiatric diagnoses may simultaneously be diseases and gateways to innovation and change. Beneficial and prejudicial aspects must be negotiated prior to treatment choice.

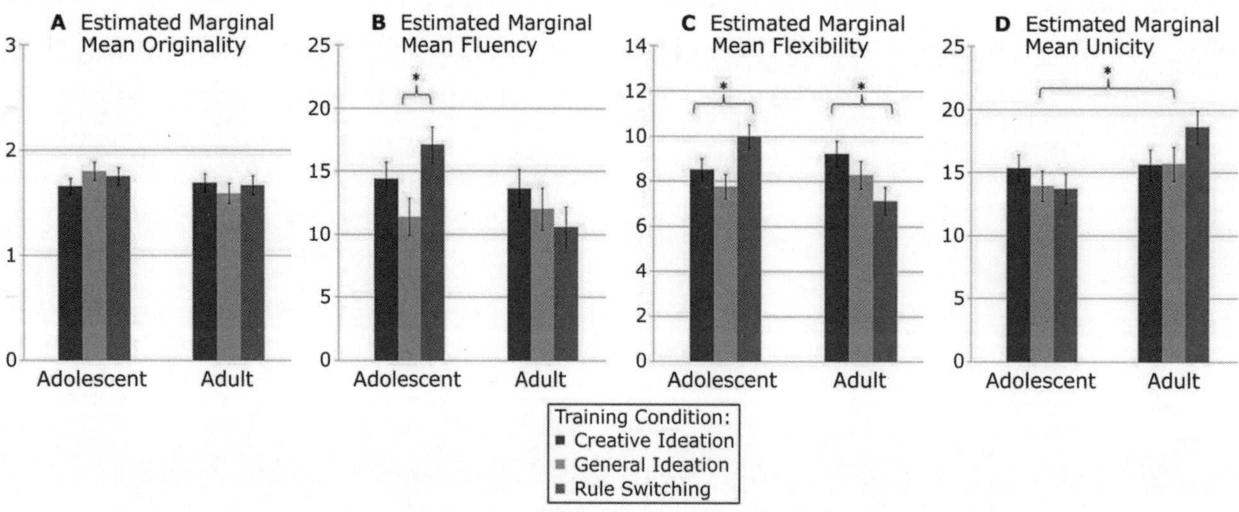

Figures 1A, 1B, 1C, and 1D Post-test performance for adults and adolescents per training condition on measures (A) originality (1 = "not original" to 5 = "highly original"), (B) fluency (number of solutions), (C) flexibility (number of categories used in solutions), and (D) unicity (inverse of uniqueness, i.e., mean frequency of provided solution in data set)

Source: Adapted from R.L. DeHaan, "Teaching Creativity and Inventive Problem Solving in Science." Copyright 2009 The American Society for Cell Biology; S. Kyaga, M. Landén, M. Boman et al., "Mental Illness, Suicide and Creativity: 40-year Prospective Total Population Study." Copyright 2013 Journal of Psychiatric Research; C.E. Stevenson, S.W. Kleibeuker, C.K.W. de Dreu, and E.A. Crone, "Training Creative Cognition: Adolescence as a Flexible Period for Improving Creativity." Copyright 2014 Frontiers Human Neuroscience.

Question 14

Which of the following conclusions CANNOT be drawn from the findings in Figures 1A, 1B, 1C, and 1D?

- ○ **A.** The adolescents performed statistically significantly better on the fluency measure for the rule-switching training condition.
- ○ **B.** Flexibility was statistically significantly and differently affected by the different types of training across age groups.
- ○ **C.** The adults' performance was statistically significantly better in the unicity measure.
- ○ **D.** Originality was statistically significantly better on the general ideation training condition for the adolescent group.

Question 15

The passage noted that thinking out loud can enhance creativity. If, during a workshop, participants are shown an image and asked to say out loud whatever crosses their mind, what type of thinking is being aimed at with such a task?

- ○ **A.** Inductive
- ○ **B.** Bottom-up
- ○ **C.** Divergent
- ○ **D.** Convergent

Question 16

The passage described two Swedish studies. From the information provided, what is the most reliable conclusion that can be drawn from both studies, and what seems to be the type of statistical analysis performed (conclusion; statistical test, respectively)?

- ○ **A.** People who suffer from psychopathological disorders and/or their relatives more often have creative occupations; correlations.
- ○ **B.** Patients with bipolar disorder and/or their relatives more often have creative occupations; correlations.
- ○ **C.** There are significant differences between creative and non-creative occupations in regard to the frequency of schizophrenia; group differences.
- ○ **D.** There are significant differences between creative and non-creative occupations in regard to the frequency of bipolar disorder; group differences.

Question 17

The passage claims that the little c is useful for everyday problem solving. Which type of problem-solving obstacle is a girl experiencing if she wants to open a glass bottle with a bottle opener for being thirsty, and keeps looking for one for two hours, getting thirstier by the minute?

- ○ **A.** Confirmation bias
- ○ **B.** Mental set
- ○ **C.** Functional fixedness
- ○ **D.** Insight

Passage 4 (Questions 18–22)

In Western contemporary society, childhood is viewed as a distinct stage of the developmental life cycle; however, this was not always the case. In the Middle Ages, for example, children were regarded simply as miniature adults. In the Reformation in the 16th century, people believed children were to be protected but also that they were sinful creatures.

In some countries, particularly in developing countries where poverty is prevalent, children are often perceived as commodities that can be exchanged or sold for money or goods. Gender inequalities in some Asian countries have placed young girls at high risk for child sex trafficking. In some countries where arranged marriages are still prevalent, poor families are promised a dowry or a bride price, and then the girl is forced into a marriage and may be later recruited for forced sex and/or labor. In some countries in Africa, young children are kidnapped and conscripted to be soldiers and terrorized into submission so that they participate in brutal killings.

In the United States in 2009, the rate of child abuse and neglect was 9.3 per 1000 children. Furthermore, racial minority children are overrepresented in the child protective services system. When child maltreatment is reported, incidences involving children of color are more likely to be substantiated than those cases involving white children. See Table 1 for a breakdown of incidences of child maltreatment by race.

Abused children and children who have been rescued from trafficking have displayed a wide range of physical, psychological, social, and emotional symptoms including fear, difficulty sleeping, repeated nightmares, affective disorders, behavioral disorders such as aggression and delinquency, and social, relational, and academic issues. Studies have shown that foster children with maltreatment histories also experience a range of neurocognitive functioning such as poor memory skills, less developed language skills, and lower scores on intelligence tests.

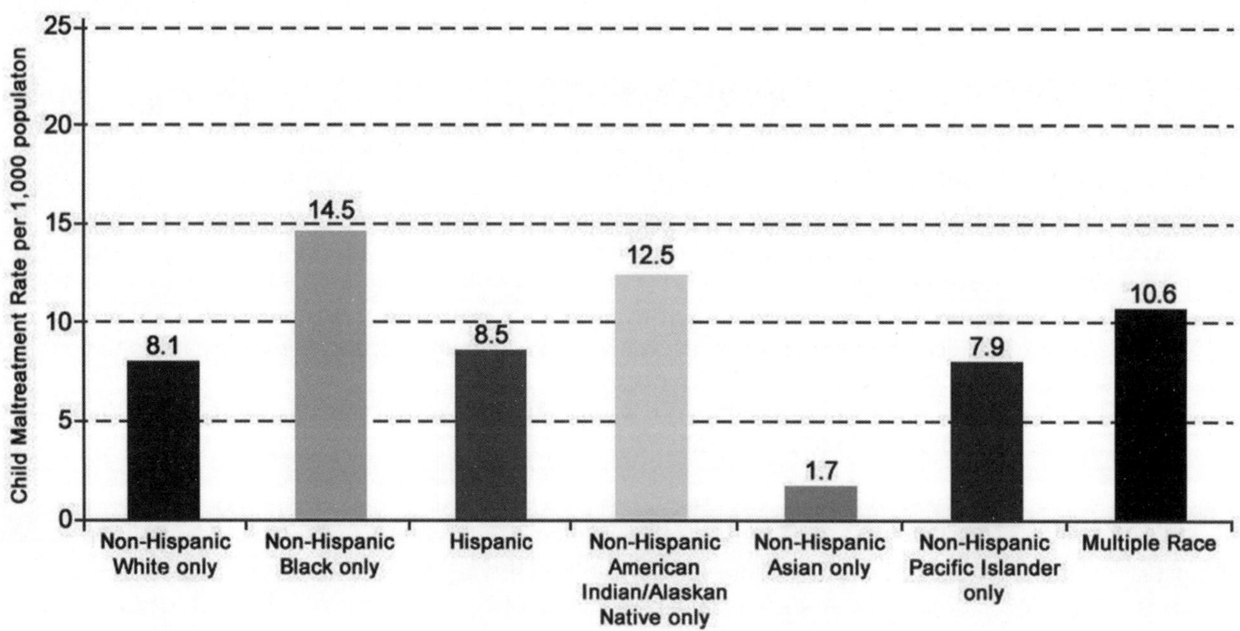

Figure 1 Child maltreatment rate (unique victims per 1,000 population) by race and Hispanic origin, 2013. Estimates for specific race groups have been revised to reflect the new OMB race definitions, and include only those who are identified with a single race. Hispanics may be of any race.

Source: Adapted from Child Trends DataBank & U.S. Department of Health and Human Services, "Child Maltreatment." Copyright 2012/2015 U.S. Government Printing Office/ http://www.childtrends.org.

Question 18

Which well-known psychological experiment would best help in understanding child soldiers and the social dynamics involved in their participation in brutal killings?

- ○ **A.** Stanley Milgram's experiment
- ○ **B.** Ivan Pavlov's experiment
- ○ **C.** Sherif's Robbers Cave experiment
- ○ **D.** Harry Harlow's experiment

Question 19

In a qualitative study that explores how former child soldiers were kidnapped and what they witnessed during their time in combat, which potential ethical issue would most likely become paramount for the ethical approval of the study?

- ○ **A.** Ensuring that the sample size is large enough that the findings are meaningful and generalizable; otherwise the study will inconvenience the research participants
- ○ **B.** Ensuring the trustworthiness of the responses obtained by implementing an audit trail and member checks during data collection to bolster the overall credibility of the study
- ○ **C.** Protecting participants' identities so that traffickers cannot locate and harm them as well as implementing mechanisms to reduce any emotional distress as a result of talking about their experiences
- ○ **D.** Ensuring that the study documents (e.g., flyers, informed consent forms, and other study materials) are written at an eighth-grade reading level so that all participants understand the nature of the study as well as their right to withdraw at any time without giving a reason

Question 20

Which concept or theory is the most relevant for explaining how a boy who has experienced trauma from sexual abuse by his father ends up with a distorted mental representation of the world, others, and self?

- ○ **A.** Surrounding mesosystem
- ○ **B.** Attachment with primary caregiver
- ○ **C.** Archetypes of mother and child
- ○ **D.** Anomie

Question 21

What factor is the LEAST likely to explain the race-related disparities illustrated in Figure 1?

- ○ **A.** Practitioners' professional ethnocentrism
- ○ **B.** False positives stemming from lack of understanding of cultural norms
- ○ **C.** Having chosen to sample clinics from areas with greater incidence of racial minorities, poverty, and unemployment
- ○ **D.** Medical and health care providers' practice of cultural relativism when dealing with racial and ethnic minority groups

Question 22

An adult female survivor of sexual child abuse started therapy. Within a month, she began to unconsciously reenact the dynamics of her abusive relationship with her male therapist, whom felt silenced, as if he had minimal options or solutions for problems. What phenomenon best classifies the therapist's experience?

- ○ **A.** Bystander effect
- ○ **B.** Dissociation
- ○ **C.** Countertransference
- ○ **D.** Transference

Passage 5 (Questions 23–27)

Lobotomy was often used during the 1950s for the treatment of psychiatric disorders. Temporal lobotomy in particular was the last resource when treating epileptic disorders. This involved making an incision in the medial temporal lobe, severing its neural connections.

William Scoville performed quite a few of these surgeries; however, in two particular cases, he bilaterally damaged the hippocampus. He observed that these patients' memory had been impaired. In particular, the patient H.M. was unable to create new memories, yet his working memory and the memories that were formed long before the surgery remained intact. The patient underwent an MRI scan in 1997, which confirmed that the amygdala, the hippocampus, and their surrounding areas were extensively damaged. Scoville further noticed in other patients that the bilateral removal of only the uncus and amygdala did not seem to cause such memory impairment. Scoville concluded that physiology (damage to the hippocampus) and psychology (the ability to create memories) were related. Furthermore, he concluded there were different types of memory. The hippocampus specifically seemed to be responsible for the passage of new information into long-term memory storage. Moreover, short- and long-term memory seemed to rely on different psychological processes and neural substrates.

Recently the idea that short- and long-term memory do not share the same physiological processes and neuronal areas has been challenged. Yet the study of certain psychiatric neurodegenerative disorders further supports some of Scoville's conclusions. For example, Alzheimer's patients have temporally graded amnesia, as well as short-term and semantic memory impairment. Similar physiological markers are found.

Memory also decays naturally with aging. Older people have been shown to perform only slightly worse when required to memorize, for short periods of time, strings of random digits. However, they have drastically poorer performance when asked to recall a longer set of unrelated words or objects (instead of numbers), and when asked to both hold and manipulate information. Moreover, in comparison with recognition tasks, their performance is found to be worse for cued-recall and free-recall tasks.

To compensate for memory decay, some strategies can be adopted. Given the effects of sleep deprivation on people's working memory, the adoption of sleep hygiene techniques is recommended. There are also a few encoding strategies that improve memorization: reorganizing information into higher-order groups; representational and mnemonic imagery or semantic associations; generating and answering questions; conceptualization; the activation of prior knowledge; similarity of encoding and retrieval contexts; and recall strategies for memorization. In short, the more similar the study and the testing contexts, and the more the information is processed during encoding, inclusive of how to retrieve it, the better one's recall performance will be.

Sources: Adapted from W.B. Scoville and B. Milner, "Loss of Recent Memory after Bilateral Hippocampal Lesions." Copyright 1957 Journal of Neurology and Neurosurgical Psychiatry; M.W. Eysenck (ed.), The Blackwell Dictionary of Cognitive Psychology. *Copyright 1997 Blackwell Publishers Ltd.*

Question 23

As described in the passage, the patient H.M. was subjected to an incision in the medial temporal lobe. His hippocampus was affected. In addition to their memory-related functions, which other functions have been associated with these physiological structures (temporal lobe; hippocampus, respectively)?

- O **A.** Visual perception and interpretation; emotional behavior and motivation
- O **B.** Reasoning and motor skills; sleep/wake cycle regulation and posture
- O **C.** Speech perception and interpretation; learning and stress regulation
- O **D.** Tactile and somatosensory perception; breathing and sneezing

Question 24

According to the information provided in the passage, a comparison between the patient H.M. and Alzheimer's patients shows that both had/have:

- O **A.** anterograde amnesia.
- O **B.** retrograde amnesia.
- O **C.** episodic memory problems.
- O **D.** difficulty accessing newer information.

Question 25

According to the information provided in the passage, which type of memory shows great decline with age?

- O **A.** Working memory
- O **B.** Long-term memory
- O **C.** Semantic memory
- O **D.** Episodic memory

Question 26

Which of the following is the type of memory test being used when showing briefly a battery of faces to participants, then showing a second battery of faces, composed of the same and different faces, while asking participants to identify the faces that had already been shown to them in the first round?

- O **A.** Free-recall test
- O **B.** Cued-recall test
- O **C.** Recognition test
- O **D.** Relearning test

Question 27

The passage described a set of strategies that can be used to facilitate memorization and recall. These include conceptualization, prior knowledge activation, and semantic associations. These types of cognitive processes are examples of:

- O **A.** maintenance rehearsal.
- O **B.** elaborative rehearsal.
- O **C.** shallow processing.
- O **D.** priming.

The following questions are NOT based on a descriptive passage (Questions 28–31).

Question 28

What three colors is each of the three receptors in the retina responsible for, so that in combination they produce the perception of any color in the spectrum?

- O **A.** Purple, red, and blue
- O **B.** Green, red, and blue
- O **C.** Yellow, green, and orange
- O **D.** White, orange, and blue

Question 29

Research subjects were asked upon arrival to read media summaries about a postal worker who did not get a promotion, shot his boss, and then killed himself. Which items below might have been part of a survey about the likelihood of various dispositional causes for the murderer's behavior, which was subsequently presented to participants?

- O **A.** History of child abuse, violent environment, and personality disorders
- O **B.** Poverty, mental illness, and shame
- O **C.** Homelessness, economic recession, and family issues
- O **D.** Mental illness, personality disorders, and controlling tendencies

Question 30

Studies have shown that downward comparison is correlated with affect. How might researchers go about testing this hypothesis?

- O **A.** Ask research subjects to select the shortest string and arranging for a confederate to select the longest string. Then administer an instrument to measure personality disorders.
- O **B.** Have research subjects read vignettes about someone who recently won a grand prize worth several hundred dollars. Then administer an instrument to measure self-efficacy.
- O **C.** Describe, to research subjects who have recently received a diagnosis about their chronic illness, someone worse off than they are. Then administer an instrument to measure for mood.
- O **D.** Ask research subjects to rate their willingness to help people in distress, including strangers, friends and family members. Then administer an instrument to measure well-being.

Question 31

The "tip of the tongue" phenomenon can be explained by:

- O **A.** loss of memory due to temporally graded retrograde amnesia.
- O **B.** interruption in the encoding process while the memory is being formed.
- O **C.** cue failure that is affecting metacognition processes.
- O **D.** failure of the retrieval component of memory.

Note: This page is left blank so that the passage would be visible without turning pages while assessing the passage-based questions.

Passage 6 (Questions 32–35)

In 2007, a leading tobacco company in the United States targeted adolescent girls by producing cigarette packaging in shiny black boxes with hot-pink borders. They gave out free hot-pink products such as purses, cell phone jewelry, and wristbands to match the cigarette box. This type of advertising is not necessarily novel: back in the 1920s, tobacco companies also targeted women, linking smoking to maintaining a slim figure by using the slogan "Reach for a Lucky instead of a sweet." Studies as conducted as recently as the late 2000s show that adolescents and young adults still believe that smoking helps with weight control, and females are more likely to believe this perception.

Smoking includes more than just tobacco cigarette smoking. E-cigarettes, for example, are very popular. Data for 2011–2012 estimated that 160,000 youths who had used e-cigarettes had never smoked before. Flavored cigarettes have also enhanced the initiation of smoking or induced the occasionally smoking youth to become a daily smoker. This is in part because the flavored cigarettes mask some of the harsh odor and taste of the tobacco.

Hookah smoking is another popular phenomenon in the U.S., particularly among adolescents. Hookahs are water-based pipes and are generally perceived as less noxious than cigarette smoking, which is one reason for the popularity of hookah smoking among adolescents. Another reason is that hookah smoking is a social activity, with many hookah cafes and restaurants emerging. Adolescents and young adults like to hang out sharing the bowl and passing the pipe around. In an online survey with 943 university students recruited, the reasons for smoking hookahs included socializing, the taste, relaxation, the smell, perceived lesser risk, and a way of dealing with boredom. In another study examining websites of hookah-smoking establishments, researchers found that 16% of the 144 websites in the sample included explicit statements that hookah smoking was safe. Almost three-quarters (72%) of the websites described the range of flavors offered, and 71% talked about the relaxation offered by hookah smoking.

Question 32

A young woman gained aversion to regular cigarettes after having become violently ill within two hours of smoking one. She started smoking bubblegum-flavored cigarettes instead, even though she knew intellectually that what had caused her illness had been a stomach virus. What phenomenon best explains her new taste aversion?

- ○ **A.** The young woman is a supertaster, with a heightened sense of flavor nuances. The harsh taste of regular cigarettes triggers the avoidance of the tobacco cigarettes, whereas the bubblegum-flavored cigarettes suit her supertaste.
- ○ **B.** The neutral stimulus (cigarette) was paired with an unconditioned stimulus (illness). This led to an unconditioned response (feeling sick). The cigarettes are now a conditioned stimulus that elicits a conditioned response (avoiding normal-flavored cigarette smoking).
- ○ **C.** The positive reinforcement (smoking pleasure) turned into a negative reinforcer (becoming violently ill), and thus she reduced the frequency of the behavior of regular cigarettes' smoking (response).
- ○ **D.** The young woman was primed due to simultaneous exposure to cigarette smoking and illness, which then resulted in a biased cognitive schema linking the two stimuli—smoking and illness.

Question 33

Early studies on the effectiveness of using fear appeals to curb smoking indicated an inverted U–shaped relationship between the strength of the threat and the effectiveness of the appeal. How should this finding be interpreted?

- O **A.** There is an optimal level of fear that would produce a maximum level of the desired behavioral response. However, below this level, the fear arousal is not sufficient to initiate an action such as ceasing smoking, while above this level, the fear appeal interferes with acceptance of the message and potentially indicates denial.
- O **B.** Fear arousal serves as a cue to initiate some sort of action (e.g., steps to stop smoking). The motivation to continue the positive behavior continues at an incremental and constant level but then tapers off at a pace that is similar to the movement of the positive behavior.
- O **C.** It demonstrates that there is a monotonic trend that shows a gradually increasing sequence of frequency of the targeted behavior that is greater than the preceding event. Gradually it flattens out and continues with this trend.
- O **D.** It demonstrates a linear trend between the independent variable (fear appeal) and the dependent variable (frequency of the smoking behavior) along with a covariate that takes into account confounding variables.

Question 34

What would Jean Piaget maintain is the reason why adolescents smoke hookahs despite warnings about how they are just as dangerous as cigarette smoking?

- O **A.** Their superego is not fully developed, and therefore they cannot fully evaluate the merits and limitations of their decision. Instead, they are focused on the immediate gratification of hookah smoking, which has a social component. Consequently the id is driving their decision.
- O **B.** Their basic needs for self-worth, identity, security, attachment, and belonging have not yet been attained. As a result, they are not seeking to meet their needs for self-actualization, that is, to improve themselves health wise.
- O **C.** Because they have not personally experienced the long-term negative effects of hookah smoking, they are not able to extrapolate from the abstract concept that hookah smoking has deleterious effects.
- O **D.** At the developmental stage in which they are asking themselves "Who am I?" adolescents are attempting to solidify their identity and what others think of them. Consequently they are not concerned with any negative health ramifications of hookah smoking.

Question 35

Researchers conducted a study that compared 50 smokers with brain damage to the insula and 50 smokers who did not have any brain damage to find out how brain damage to the insula affected smoking cessation. What would the data most likely indicate?

- O **A.** Smokers without brain damage to the insula were more likely to have more intense sleep cycles, and therefore they were able to "sleep off" the withdrawal effects of smoking.
- O **B.** Smokers with brain damage involving the insula were more likely to quit smoking more easily and immediately without persistence of the urge to smoke than smokers without any brain damage.
- O **C.** Smokers with brain damage in the insula region were more likely to have more intense sleep cycles, and therefore they were able to "sleep off" the withdrawal effects of smoking.
- O **D.** Smokers without any brain damage to the insula were more likely to quit smoking more easily and more quickly without persistence of the urge to smoke than smokers with brain damage to the insula.

Passage 7 (Questions 36–40)

Eric Turkheimer's laws of behavioral genetics state that the factors affecting people's phenotypes and their interindividual differences, in decreasing order of importance or weight, consist of genetic factors, idiosyncratic factors (unaccounted for by the other two variables, e.g., diseases and traumas), and child-rearing factors. These laws affect both physical and psychological attributes.

Turkheimer's claims stand against the core assumption of the founders of behavioral psychology, and have gathered some empirical support in favor of the greater influence of genetic factors on people's phenotypes than of parenting and idiosyncratic factors. Twin studies are particularly revealing, principally when they involve the study of monozygotic twins reared apart. Overall, the correlations between monozygotic twins tend to be higher across measures of intelligence, physical attributes (e.g., weight), and/or personality than those found for dizygotic twins. For example, according to some studies, twins' "openness to experience" (a personality trait evaluated by the NEO Personality Inventory) seems to be mainly determined by their genotypes. The same is not observed for the "agreeableness" trait. Table 1 illustrates the intraclass correlations between monozygotic and dizygotic twins, reared either apart or together, regarding a personality test.

Turkheimer's laws and conclusions have been criticized. First, variability is greater than usually stated. For example, intelligence heritability, estimated at around 50%, can vary between 50% and 80%. These differences can also arise from the type of measures, the sample, or the statistical methods utilized. It has even been noted that unlike animal behavioral models, human behavioral models "have failed to reveal even one bona fide, replicable gene effect pertinent to the normal range of variation in intelligence and personality. . . . For several psychiatric disorders, including autism and schizophrenia . . . the disorders are heterogeneous; different cases with the same diagnosis have different causes." That is, some reviews of existing evidence contradict Turkheimer's elegant model and supporting research.

Moreover, some genetic studies also posit that parents' "regard" of their children affects how intensely the adolescents manifest their genotypes, whether or not they are adopted. When such regard is absent, interindividual differences attributable to genetic factors seem to dilute. That is, parenting style (e.g., with more or less regard of each child) may mediate the relationship between genetics and phenotype, principally in later life.

Table 1 Intraclass Correlations for Three Higher-order Scales of the Multidimensional Personality Questionnaire for Four Kinship Groups

Scale	MZA	DZA	MZT	DZT
Primary				
Well-Being	.48	.18	.58	.23
Social Potency	.56	.27	.65	.08
Achievement	.36	.07	.51	.13
Social Closeness	.29	.30	.57	.24
Stress Reaction	.61	.27	.52	.24
Alienation	.48	.18	.55	.38
Aggression	.46	.06	.43	.14
Control	.50	.03	.41	−.06
Harm Avoidance	.49	.24	.55	.17
Traditionalism	.53	.39	.50	.47
Absorption	.61	.21	.49	.41
Higher order				
Positive Emotionality	.34	−.07	.63	.18
Negative Emotionality	.61	.29	.54	.41
Constraint	.57	.04	.58	.25

Note. MZA = Monozygotic twin pairs reared apart (n = 44), DZA = dizygotic twin pairs reared apart (n = 27), MZT = monozygotic twin pairs reared together (n = 217), and DZT = dizygotic twin pairs reared together (n = 114).

Sources: Adapted from R.F. Krueger, S. South, W. Johnson, and W. Iacono, "The Heritability of Personality Is Not Always 50%: Gene-Environment Interactions and Correlations between Personality and Parenting." Copyright 2009 Journal of Personality; M.H.M. de Moor, P.T.

Costa, A. Terracciano et al., "Meta-analysis of Genome-Wide Association Studies for Personality." Copyright 2012 Molecular Psychiatry; D. Wahlsten, "The Hunt for Gene Effects Pertinent to Behavioral Traits and Psychiatric Disorders: From Mouse to Human." Copyright 2012 Wiley Periodicals Inc.; A. Tellegen, D.T. Lykken, T.J. Bouchard et al., "Personality Similarity in Twins Reared Apart and Together." Copyright 1988 Journal of Personality and Social Psychology.

Question 36

The author claims that the evidence gathered within the field of behavioral genetics goes against the core assumption of the founders of behavioral psychology. What is this belief or assumption, and what is the main assumption of behavioral genetics (behavioral psychology; behavioral genetics, respectively) that replaces it?

- O **A.** Behavior is intelligent; behavior is random.
- O **B.** Behavior is learned; behavior is inherited.
- O **C.** Behavior is inherited; behavior is modeled.
- O **D.** Behavior is emotional, behavior is intelligent.

Question 37

What is the difference between monozygotic and dizygotic twins?

- O **A.** The zygote undergoes mitosis for monozygotic twins, whereas dizygotic twins do not undergo this process.
- O **B.** The zygote undergoes mitosis for dizygotic twins, whereas monozygotic twins result from two zygotes.
- O **C.** Monozygotic twins result from two ova, whereas dizygotic twins result from one single ovum.
- O **D.** The zygote undergoes a split for monozygotic twins, whereas dizygotic twins result from two ova.

Question 38

Why did the author claim that "twin studies are particularly revealing, principally when they involve the study of monozygotic twins reared apart," in discussing behavioral genetics?

- O **A.** They illuminate the relative importance of nature as opposed to nurture in what concerns psychological attributes.
- O **B.** They show how adoption is the best solution for the social and psychological development of twins.
- O **C.** They prove that genes are more important than child rearing in determining behavior.
- O **D.** They allow for a comparison between genetically related and non–genetically related twins.

Question 39

Which of the following personality traits shows greater heritability, as based on the results presented in Table 1 and identified below in parentheses?

- O **A.** Positive emotionality ($r = 0.63$)
- O **B.** Positive emotionality ($r = -0.07$)
- O **C.** Negative emotionality ($r = 0.61$)
- O **D.** Negative emotionality ($r = 0.41$)

Question 40

The author described how parental regard interacted with the offspring's genetic material and influenced which genes became a phenotype. What is the personality theory that explores the influence of the parents' positive regard on the offspring's development?

- O **A.** Psychoanalysis
- O **B.** Humanistic theory
- O **C.** Behaviorism
- O **D.** Social cognitive theory

Passage 8 (Questions 41–44)

Food has symbolic meaning, conveying history, tradition, culture, and values. Family meals are inextricably linked to family and individual identity, and food is often the vehicle for the transmission and socialization of values. Food is also embedded in everyday language. Consider the use of food metaphors: "Isn't she sweet?" It has also been observed that the emotion of disgust is another example of how food has been co-opted as a metaphor. Disgust stems from the rejection of food, that is, the rejecting food from the mouth based on a negative oral experience such as taste, flavor, and/or texture.

Many individuals eat because they are bored, stressed, or depressed. In two parallel experiments, subjects were recruited for experiment to test (1) whether induced boredom predicted eating of chocolate and (2) whether subjects were more inclined to self-administer electric shocks due to boredom. Subjects were randomly assigned to the boredom condition, which involved watching a repetitive clip from a documentary for an hour, or the neutral condition, which consisted of watching the whole hourlong documentary. During the first experiment, the subjects were given as many M&Ms as they wanted, and in the second experiment, they could freely administer electrical shocks to themselves. Findings showed that subjects consumed more M&Ms in the bored condition and administered more electrical shocks to themselves than in the neutral condition. Consequently, the researchers concluded that eating is sometimes driven by the need to escape monotony.

The term "comfort food" refers to food that triggers a positive, nostalgic feeling or that serves to mitigate negative feelings such as stress. In a study, 30 healthy female subjects were recruited and were administered a stress questionnaire. While viewing in random order photos of foods such as pies, cake, candy bars, and other high-caloric items; photos of healthy foods such as vegetables, black beans, and fruit; and photos of neutral items like phones, baseball, tables, and chairs, they were given brain scans. On viewing the high-calorie food photos, high-chronic-stress women showed different patterns of brain activity compared with low-chronic-stress women, as shown in Figure 1.

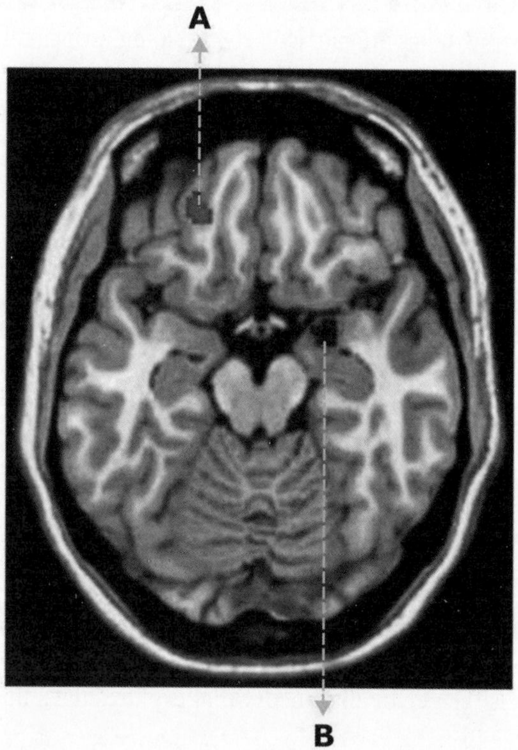

Figure 1 Brain scan of high-stress women when viewing photos of high-caloric food items

Source: Adapted from M. Wood, "Your Brain and Comfort Foods: Neuroimages Capture Effects." Copyright 2014 Agricultural Research.

Question 41

In Figure 1, the brain scan of the high-stress women showed diminished activity in the area associated with the letter A, which shows the:

- O **A.** medulla.
- O **B.** prefrontal cortex.
- O **C.** pons.
- O **D.** amygdala.

Question 42

Which option below best describes the style of communication of a non-Hispanic White family that is described by others as utterly gregarious, loud, and enthusiastic, and as rarely making any long pauses, or going straight to the point of a story when holding family conversations?

- O **A.** Low-context culture communication
- O **B.** Hierarchical communication
- O **C.** High-context culture communication
- O **D.** Paralanguage-reliant communication

Question 43

What sequence of events would best be exemplified in using the James–Lange theory to explain a man's emotion of disgust toward artichokes?

- O **A.** He places artichokes in his mouth. He chews and feels like vomiting. He looks around at others at the dinner table and observes that everyone else is grimacing. He assumes this is disgust and feels the same way.
- O **B.** He places artichokes in his mouth. He chews and feels like vomiting. He reasons that he does not like the color or smell of this vegetable. Therefore, he experiences the emotion of disgust.
- O **C.** He places artichokes in his mouth. He chews and feels like vomiting; simultaneously, he experiences disgust.
- O **D.** He puts artichokes in his mouth. He chews and begins to feel like vomiting. He interprets the physical reaction as disgust.

Question 44

In the boredom, M&Ms, and electrical shock study, if the subjects were not randomly assigned to the two conditions but instead the assignment was on a first-come, first-served basis—in other words, the first 15 subjects to arrive were placed in the boredom condition—what would be a concern when interpreting the results?

- O **A.** Higher attrition rates in the boredom group versus the neutral group
- O **B.** Confounding variables such as personality and individual differences affecting the results
- O **C.** The ethical integrity of the design of the study, specifically the justice principle
- O **D.** The face validity and split-half reliability of the measures would be threatened, which would adversely affect the validity of the results.

The following questions are NOT based on a descriptive passage (Questions 45–48).

Question 45

When teaching a psychology of gender class, the teacher takes on the perspective of essentialism in regard to gender. Consequently, what is the main theme that runs through the class?

- ○ **A.** Gender serves an important purpose so that a variety of social functions can be maintained and reinforced. These social functions include common ideology, purpose of life, and belonging.
- ○ **B.** Gender is an essential, socially constructed concept and has specific meaning for individuals as they live out their gender; the meanings are culturally laden.
- ○ **C.** Gender is an unchangeable characteristic that resides in an individual. All women share the same psychological characteristics, which are different from men's psychology.
- ○ **D.** Cross-cultural research is at the heart of essentialism, as gender and other psychological traits are not universal but culturally specific.

Question 46

If the research subjects in a study experience acute pain during cold pressor activity, what part of the brain is likely being activated?

- ○ **A.** Parietal lobe of the cerebral cortex
- ○ **B.** Cerebellum
- ○ **C.** Hippocampus of the limbic system
- ○ **D.** Medulla oblongata

Question 47

Which one of the following explanations pertains to the cocktail party effect?

- ○ **A.** Someone named Robert is engaged in a conversation. A person standing at the other end of the room who is engaged in a different conversation mentions Robert's name. Although Robert was not listening to the conversation before, he now shifts his attention to attend to it. This brain feature is called selective attention and explains our ability to cope with a variety of stimuli that are simultaneously present.
- ○ **B.** Participants in an experiment are asked to watch a video and count the frequency of interaction between two groups of people. The video shows a man in a gorilla costume entering the scene, staying in the middle of the groups, and leaving. About half the participants do not see the gorilla. At a cocktail party, this mechanism, which is called perceptual blindness, works in our favor and helps us tune out irrelevant conversations.
- ○ **C.** Research has found that people's skills and values correspond with the kinds of people they like to surround themselves with, for example, at social gatherings. Those six principal people environments have been described as realistic, investigative, artistic, social, enterprising, and conventional. The fact that we like to surround ourselves with similar people explains why it is easier to listen to the most stimulating conversation at a social gathering and tune out less relevant conversations.
- ○ **D.** Research has shown that people are able to store auditory information in their memory for longer amounts of time than visual information. This brain capability helps us to perform a delayed selection of information that allows us to focus on one conversation while several other auditory and visual stimuli are simultaneously present.

Question 48

A fish tank distributes food from two stations at an equal rate. After some time, one tank doubles the amount of distributed food. The ideal free distribution theory predicts that the six fish living in the tank will:

- ○ **A.** consume resources in proportion to the available resources. Hence a change in rate will provoke a change in the amount consumed.
- ○ **B.** distribute themselves per food station in proportion to the available resources. Hence a change in rate will provoke a change in the fishes' distribution.
- ○ **C.** consume resources in proportion to the existing food needs. Hence a change in rate will not provoke a change in the amount consumed.
- ○ **D.** distribute themselves per food station in proportion to the existing population. Hence a change in rate will not provoke a change in the amount consumed.

Passage 9 (Questions 49–52)

Seemingly minor developments and contentions in statistics can have a huge impact upon individual and social decision-making processes and research conclusions. For example, it was found that political moderates, compared with political extremists, literally perceive more shades of gray (N = 1979 people; p = 0.01). However, while replicating the study before publishing, the same researchers found that the *p*-value had changed drastically (p = 0.056); that is, there were no differences in the shades of gray perceived by moderates compared with extremists. This disparity, the fruit of a type I *p*-value error, poses no immediate threats to anyone. However, the same does not apply to certain mistakes occurring in the field of medicine.

In 2006 Anil Potti and colleagues published their "revolutionary" approach to cancer screening and treatment. They argued that laboratory cell lines could be used to predict patients' lung cancer progression as well as which chemotherapy treatment would be most effective for each particular cancer case (personalized medicine). Cell lines are gene expression arrays, or colorful registries of the activity patterns of the many genes in a tissue sample. Potti and colleagues went on to organize clinical trials, which should follow strict ethical guidelines. However, when another team of researchers attempted to replicate their findings, they failed. Slowly Potti's work came under scrutiny. Potti was found to have lied about his academic credentials, and as a result, the article summarizing the research results was corrected and then retracted. The clinical trials were temporarily halted, and then ceased.

These pitfalls can be minimized by performing sensitivity and specificity analyses. Sensitivity (or true positive rate) establishes the proportion of positives that are correctly identified as such, e.g., the number of sick patients who have been correctly diagnosed. Specificity (or true negative rate) establishes the proportion of negatives that are correctly identified as such, for example, the number of healthy people who have been correctly diagnosed. In association, a positive or negative predictive value (likelihood of replicating the findings for each of the tested individuals) can be further calculated. Table 1 compares three methods for detection of dentin caries and their performance on these indicators.

Ideally, tests should have high sensitivity and high specificity; sometimes, however, trade-offs must be made. Moreover, these are complementary indicators that rely on population incidence. Hence population-related cutoff points are used and influence the results. Often used in medical clinical trials, these analyses are a necessity, not a statistician's fancy. Mistakes such as Potti's can have disastrous consequences.

Table 1 Sensitivity (Se), Specificity (Sp), Positive Predictive Value (PPV), and Negative Predictive Value (NPV) of the Methods for Detection of Dentin Caries

Methods	Se %	Sp %	PPV %	NPV %
Visual Inspection	0.50	0.95	0.83	0.80
Bitewing Radiography	0.26	0.94	0.69	0.73
Laser Fluorescence	0.93	0.75	0.63	0.96

Sources: Adapted from B.A. Nosek, J.R. Spies, & M. Motyl, "Scientific Utopia: II. Restructuring Incentives and Practices to Promote Truth over Publishability." Copyright 2012 http://www.motyl.people.uic.edu; A. Potti, H.K. Dressman, A. Bild et al., "Genomic Signatures to Guide the Use of Chemotherapeutics." Copyright 2006 Nature Medicine; "An Array of Errors." Copyright 2011 The Economist; A.G. Glaros and R.B. Kline, "Understanding the Accuracy of Tests with Cutting Scores: The Sensitivity, Specificity, and Predictive Value Model." Copyright 1988 Journal of Clinical Psychology; A.M. Costa, L.M. de Paula, and A.C.B. Bezerra. "Use of Diagnodent for Diagnosis of Non-cavitated Occlusal Dentin Caries." Copyright 2008 Journal of Applied Oral Science.

Question 49

If a dentist was aware of the implications of specificity and sensitivity and was shown Figure 1, what would be the best dentin caries diagnostic method he could choose to employ in his practice?

- ○ **A.** Visual inspection
- ○ **B.** Bitewing radiography
- ○ **C.** Laser fluorescence
- ○ **D.** Combining visual inspection and laser fluorescence

Question 50

The author mentioned that clinical trials should follow strict ethical guidelines. Why should the guidelines be stricter for clinical trials than for other types of studies?

- ○ **A.** Human volunteers must be protected from unknown and potentially harmful effects of tested treatments or interventions.
- ○ **B.** Clinical researchers are more often ill intended and want to obtain direct gain from pharmaceutical companies and other interested parties.
- ○ **C.** Health research is more important than any other type of research. The guidelines assure that the field is given proper attention by society.
- ○ **D.** Clinical researchers are more often ignorant about statistics. The guidelines assure that statistical errors are prevented.

Question 51

The measures of sensitivity, specificity, and negative and positive predictive values are more likely related to which one of the following research-trustworthiness aspects?

- ○ **A.** Predictive values are validity measures, whereas sensitivity and specificity are reliability measures.
- ○ **B.** Sensitivity and specificity are validity measures, whereas predictive values are reliability measures.
- ○ **C.** Sensitivity is a measure of validity, whereas specificity and predictive values are a measure of reliability.
- ○ **D.** Specificity is a measure of validity, whereas sensitivity and predictive values are a measure of reliability.

Question 52

The passage described how a study investigated whether the perception of shades of gray was related to people's political views. Which are the sensory receptors and the main lobe responsible for the perception of color (cells, lobe, respectively)?

- ○ **A.** Free nerve endings, parietal lobe
- ○ **B.** Meissner corpuscles, parietal lobe
- ○ **C.** Cones, occipital lobe
- ○ **D.** Rods, occipital lobe

Passage 10 (Questions 53–56)

Schools perform a variety of functions within society. They provide social integration for a diverse population. It has been argued that education increases meritocracy because it rewards talent and hard work. This helps to increase upward mobility. Furthermore, it provides child care for people who work and brings together people who are of marriageable age.

Structural functionalists such as Robert Merton have divided educational institutions into different functions, namely latent and manifest. There has been ongoing discussion in various disciplines about what the school curriculum should consist of. This discussion expands beyond explicit, conscious, formally planned content that is taught in schools (manifest curriculum). Research that is rather critical toward the traditional education system, such as radical pedagogy, points out that the hidden curriculum in schools strongly influences students' attainment and facilitates social inequalities, rather than eradicating them.

This criticism is supported by various studies confirming the existence of racial disparities in educational attainment and access to education. Many political programs try to address this issue, for example, through affirmative action programs and stipends for students from minority ethnic backgrounds. Still, the gap persists. Figure 1 shows these disparities in higher education, comparing different racial groups' share of the population with their share of degrees earned. Women earned more degrees in every racial/ethnic category.

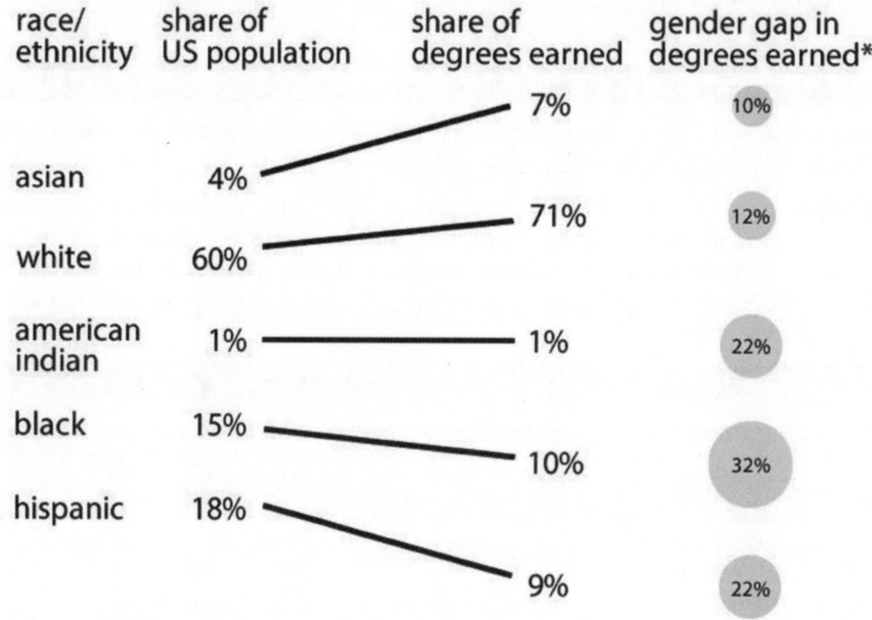

Figure 1 Bachelor's degrees granted in 2009/2010 by race/ethnicity

Source: Adapted from L. Norén, "Race and Gender in Higher Education: Who Gets Degrees?" Copyright 2012 http://www.thesocietypages.org.

Question 53

Which one of the options below is NOT a latent function of schooling?

O **A.** Socializing students into commonly shared values that are expressed in curricula and school manifestos
O **B.** Legitimizing existing class structure
O **C.** Providing child care for parents who are at work
O **D.** Serving as a meeting place for romantic relationships by bringing together people of similar background and age

Question 54

Figure 1 displays and connects data about race/ethnicity, gender, and educational attainment. What is the most probable behind this choice of illustrating data?

O **A.** It indicates gender inequality in educational attainment.
O **B.** It shows racial inequality in educational attainment.
O **C.** It shows the intersectionality of social inequalities.
O **D.** It indicates that there is more gender equality than racial equality in society.

Question 55

How would the Thomas theorem explain the findings from Figure 1 in relation to race?

O **A.** A common stereotype about Black youth is that they are educational underachievers. This perpetuates their and their teachers' expectations, and they underperform when taking tests.
O **B.** White people have fewer stereotypes to face than Black people. Furthermore, they automatically enjoy greater social status and more cultural affirmation of their identities. This affects their educational performance and leads to better educational attainment.
O **C.** White people acquire an accumulated advantage over the course of their educational careers. This advantage leads to higher achievements in relation to degrees.
O **D.** Black people have less access to goods, services, and opportunities during the course of their education. The underlying reason for this lies in the way educational systems, policies, programs, and interactions are planned and conducted.

Question 56

A functionalist perspective would argue that the hidden curriculum:

O **A.** is a system of rules the student can either fully accept, partially accept, partially refuse, or fully refuse.
O **B.** promotes middle-class values and reproduces social inequality.
O **C.** enhances social mobility because it provides a shared value base for students from different social backgrounds.
O **D.** consists of socially accepted values and beliefs and serves the interests of larger society.

The following questions are NOT based on a descriptive passage (Questions 57–59).

Question 57

How would a salesperson at an organic pre-made meals company use the door-in-the-face technique to persuade people who do not want to subscribe to purchase the meals?

- O **A.** Ask individuals if they want to subscribe to the meals for two years, and then later scale it down to a month.
- O **B.** Ask individuals if they want to subscribe to the meals, and if they are interested, say that they should do so immediately because the 15% discount will end within two days.
- O **C.** Ask individuals if they want to subscribe to the meals using a trial basis of one week. Once they agree, she would then ask if they want a six-month subscription.
- O **D.** Ask individuals if they want to subscribe to the meals and then hand out a flyer of endorsements given by famous chefs.

Question 58

What is the name and frequency of the majority of the electromagnetic waves produced during non–rapid eye movement (NREM) sleep stage 4 (name, frequency, respectively)?

- O **A.** Delta, <4 Hz
- O **B.** Theta, 4–7 Hz
- O **C.** Alpha, 8–12 Hz
- O **D.** Beta, 13–24 Hz

Question 59

A subset of retinal ganglion cells detects light changes. The information is then sent toward the pineal gland. Which hormone or neurotransmitter is released by this gland in proportion to levels of darkness?

- O **A.** Adenosine
- O **B.** Testosterone
- O **C.** Epinephrine
- O **D.** Melatonin

Full-length MCAT Practice Test GS-3

Periodic Table of the Elements

You may consult this page anytime you wish during the following exam sections:

- Section I: Chemical and Physical Foundations of Biological Systems
- Section III: Biological and Biochemical Foundations of Living Systems

On the real exam, the computer-based shortcut to see the periodic table is Alt + T.

1 **H** 1.0																	2 **He** 4.0
3 **Li** 6.9	4 **Be** 9.0											5 **B** 10.8	6 **C** 12.0	7 **N** 14.0	8 **O** 16.0	9 **F** 19.0	10 **Ne** 20.2
11 **Na** 23.0	12 **Mg** 24.3											13 **Al** 27.0	14 **Si** 28.1	15 **P** 31.0	16 **S** 32.1	17 **Cl** 35.5	18 **Ar** 39.9
19 **K** 39.1	20 **Ca** 40.1	21 **Sc** 45.0	22 **Ti** 47.9	23 **V** 50.9	24 **Cr** 52.0	25 **Mn** 54.9	26 **Fe** 55.8	27 **Co** 58.9	28 **Ni** 58.7	29 **Cu** 63.5	30 **Zn** 65.4	31 **Ga** 69.7	32 **Ge** 72.6	33 **As** 74.9	34 **Se** 79.0	35 **Br** 79.9	36 **Kr** 83.8
37 **Rb** 85.5	38 **Sr** 87.6	39 **Y** 88.9	40 **Zr** 91.2	41 **Nb** 92.9	42 **Mo** 95.9	43 **Tc** (98)	44 **Ru** 101.1	45 **Rh** 102.9	46 **Pd** 106.4	47 **Ag** 107.9	48 **Cd** 112.4	49 **In** 114.8	50 **Sn** 118.7	51 **Sb** 121.8	52 **Te** 127.6	53 **I** 126.9	54 **Xe** 131.3
55 **Cs** 132.9	56 **Ba** 137.3	57 **La*** 138.9	72 **Hf** 178.5	73 **Ta** 180.9	74 **W** 183.9	75 **Re** 186.2	76 **Os** 190.2	77 **Ir** 192.2	78 **Pt** 195.1	79 **Au** 197.0	80 **Hg** 200.6	81 **Tl** 204.4	82 **Pb** 207.2	83 **Bi** 209.0	84 **Po** (209)	85 **At** (210)	86 **Rn** (222)
87 **Fr** (223)	88 **Ra** (226)	89 **Ac**** (227)	104 **Unq**** (261)	105 **Unp** (262)	106 **Unh** (263)	107 **Uns** (262)	108 **Uno** (265)	109 **Une** (267)									
			*	58 **Ce** 140.1	59 **Pr** 140.9	60 **Nd** 144.2	61 **Pm** (145)	62 **Sm** 150.4	63 **Eu** 152.0	64 **Gd** 157.3	65 **Tb** 158.9	66 **Dy** 162.5	67 **Ho** 164.9	68 **Er** 167.3	69 **Tm** 168.9	70 **Yb** 173.0	71 **Lu** 175.0
			**	90 **Th** 232.0	91 **Pa** (231)	92 **U** 238.0	93 **Np** (237)	94 **Pu** (244)	95 **Am** (243)	96 **Cm** (247)	97 **Bk** (247)	98 **Cf** (251)	99 **Es** (252)	100 **Fm** (257)	101 **Md** (258)	102 **No** (259)	103 **Lr** (260)

CANDIDATE'S NAME ______________________________

RAW SCORE AND SCALED SCORE ______________________

GS-3
Mock Exam 3 of 7
Solutions at MCAT-prep.com

GS-3 Section I: Chemical and Physical Foundations of Biological Systems

Questions: 1-59
Time: 95 minutes

INSTRUCTIONS: Of all the questions on this test, most are organized into groups preceded by a passage. After evaluating the passage, select the best answer to each question in the group. Fifteen questions are independent of any descriptive passage or each other. Similarly, select the best answer to these questions. If you are unsure of an answer, eliminate the alternatives that you know to be incorrect and select an answer from the remaining alternatives. To indicate your selection, use a pencil to blacken the corresponding circle next to the answer choice and/or you can use the answer document at the back of this book. No marks are deducted for wrong answers.

The computer-based real MCAT has an on-screen highlighter function and ~~STRIKEOUT~~ function. These tools help to spotlight text or assist in the process of elimination. You may use a yellow highlighter for this paper-based exam and/or a pen (or preferably a pencil to make it easier should you change your mind) to mark text. At the time of publishing, both highlighting and strikeout functions can be used for passages, questions and answer choices. You can also flag a question to review later should time remain.

For the real exam, you will be provided with a dry erase board which is a white laminated noteboard booklet accompanied by a fine point marker. The noteboard includes 9 graph-lined pages for you to write though you cannot erase. You can simulate the experience with a fine point marker on a noteboard or with 8" x 14" plain graph paper.

You may consult the periodic table at any point during the science subtests.

Please note: For the real MCAT, a small number of field-tested questions will remain unscored.

This practice test has been designed exclusively to test knowledge and thinking skills. This exam may contain hypothetical statements and/or express controversial ideas. Statements contained herein do not necessarily reflect the policy, position, or view of RuveneCo Inc. or MCAT-prep.com.

START EXAM ONLY WHEN TIMER IS READY.

Passage 1 (Questions 1–4)

A student studied the mechanisms of the reactions of 2-bromohexane with sodium t-butoxide and with sodium ethoxide.

In Reaction I, the treatment of 2-bromohexane with sodium t-butoxide at 40 °C gave almost exclusively one product. The reaction yielded Compound A which had the general molecular formula C_nH_{2n}. The ^{1}HNMR spectrum of compound A revealed the presence of vinylic protons. The kinetic rate expression indicated second order kinetics for the reaction.

In Reaction II, the treatment of 2-bromohexane with sodium ethoxide (Na^+EtO^-) at 30 °C yielded an ether (Compound B) and Compound A. Compound B accounted for only 20% of the total product. The remainder consisted of Compound A. The student was able to separate the two compounds using the technique of fractional distillation.

After having been isolated, Compound B was found to be stable to base, dilute acid and most reducing agents. The infrared spectrum of Compound B revealed a strong band at 1100 cm^{-1} and the absence of stretching absorptions at 1730 cm^{-1} was noted.

Compound A was readily oxidized by a neutral solution of cold dilute potassium permanganate. During the oxidation process, the characteristic purple color of the permanganate ion (MnO_4^-) disappeared and was replaced by a brown precipitate indicating the formation of manganese dioxide (MnO_2).

Question 1

Which of the following best describes the reaction mechanisms that led to the formation of products A and B?

- ○ **A.** A is the S_N1 product.
- ○ **B.** B is the S_N1 product.
- ○ **C.** A is the S_N2 product.
- ○ **D.** B is the S_N2 product.

Question 2

Compound A belongs to which of the following classes of organic compounds?

- ○ **A.** Alcohol
- ○ **B.** Ketone
- ○ **C.** Alkene
- ○ **D.** Ester

Question 3

Which of the following most accurately represents the activated complex formed in Reaction II and that subsequently led to Compound A? (note: methoxide was used to replace ethoxide in this repeat of Reaction II)

○ **A.**

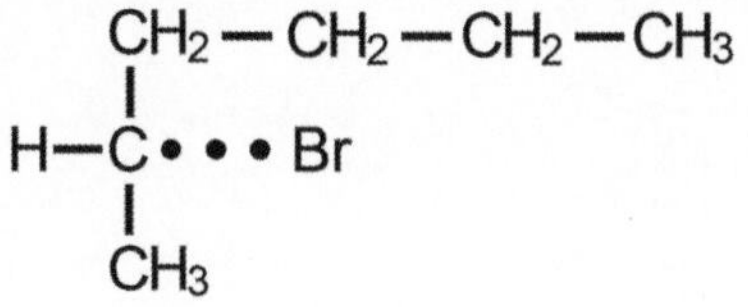

$CH_2-CH_2-CH_2-CH_3$
|
$H-C\bullet\bullet\bullet Br$
|
CH_3

○ **B.**

$CH_2-CH_2-CH_2-CH_3$
|
$H-C \oplus$
|
CH_3

○ **C.**

$CH_2-CH_2-CH_3$
|
H CH_2
| |
δ^- δ^-
$CH_3-O\bullet\bullet\bullet H\bullet\bullet\bullet C\overset{\bullet\bullet\bullet}{=}C\bullet\bullet\bullet Br$
| |
H H

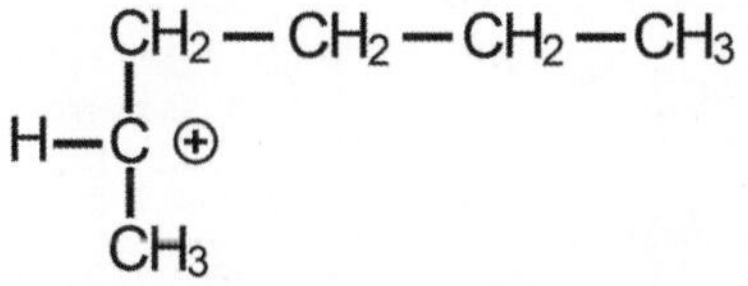

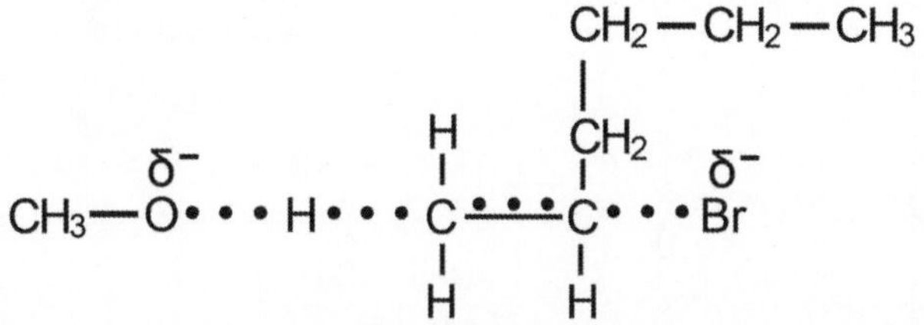

○ **D.**

$CH_2-CH_2-CH_3$
|
CH_2
δ^- | δ^-
$CH_3-O\bullet\bullet\bullet C\bullet\bullet\bullet Br$
(wedge) CH_3, (hashed) H

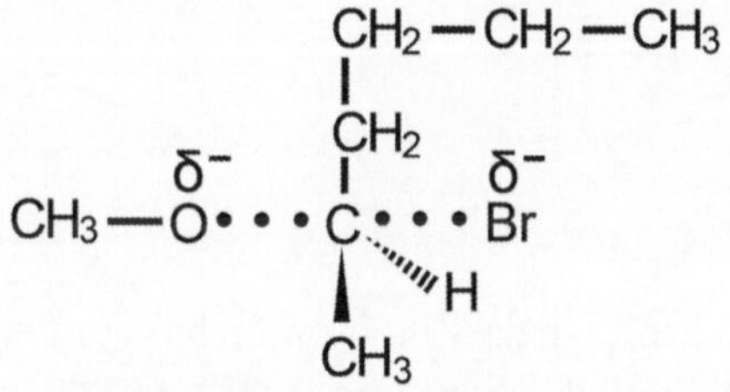

Question 4

Which of the following compounds is an accurate representation of Compound B?

○ **A.** CH_3OCH_3
○ **B.** $C_2H_5OC_2H_3$
○ **C.** $(CH_3)_2CHOCH_3$
○ **D.** $CH_3CH_2OC_6H_{13}$

Passage 2 (Questions 5–8)

Jacques Charles was a French scientist who became interested in the relationship between volume changes in a gas in response to a change in temperature. To obtain quantitative measurements, Charles designed an apparatus demonstrated in Figure 1.

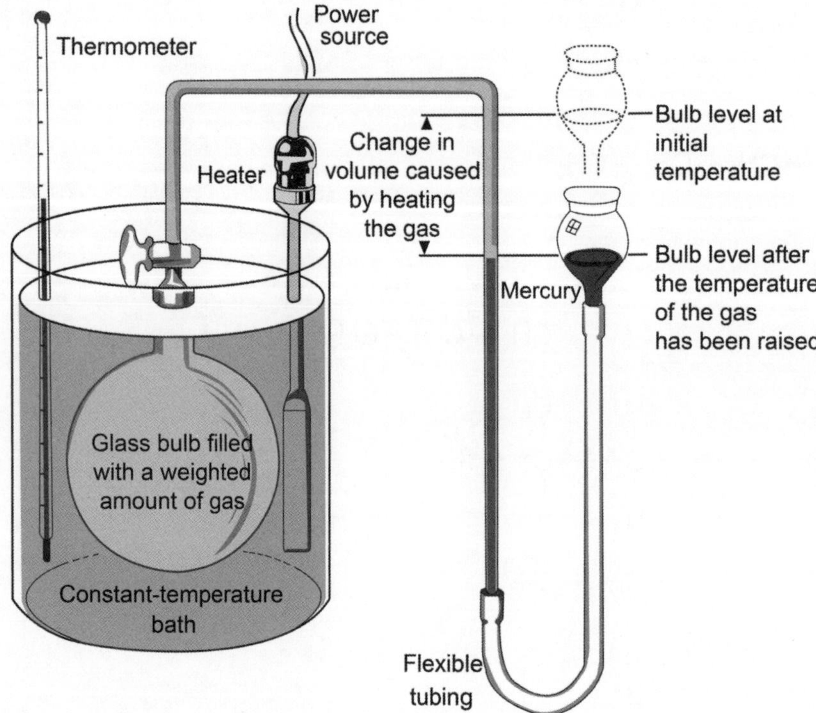

Figure 1 Charles' law measurements. The flexible tubing is attached to a glass tubing which is continuous with the glass bulb containing the gas. The glass bulb containing mercury is open to the air.

Other experiments by scientists would clarify the relationships between pressure, temperature and volume of gases. Because of the work of Charles, Boyle, Dalton, Gay-Lussac and others, the ideal gas law was developed which created a new constant of proportionality R, as in $PV/T = nR$. The ideal (or *universal*) gas law is expressed more commonly as follows:

$$PV = nRT$$

where P is the pressure, V is the volume, n is the number of moles, T is the temperature in kelvin and R is the universal gas constant.

Question 5

The apparatus used by Charles, as demonstrated in Figure 1, is designed to maintain which of the following constant?

I. Volume
II. Temperature
III. Pressure
IV. Number of moles

- **A.** I only
- **B.** I and II
- **C.** II and III
- **D.** III and IV

Question 6

The likely explanation for choosing flexible tubing in the apparatus in Figure 1 is so that:

- ○ **A.** the gas will experience varying pressure while the change of volume can be measured in the glass tubing.
- ○ **B.** the gas will experience varying pressure while the change of volume can be measured in the glass bulb containing mercury.
- ○ **C.** the gas will be maintained at atmospheric pressure while the change of volume can be measured in the glass tubing.
- ○ **D.** the gas will be maintained at atmospheric pressure while the change of volume can be measured in the glass bulb containing mercury.

Question 7

Consider the following model that demonstrates the basic aspects of lung function. Note that the bell jar is sealed except for inlet/outlet of the rubber tube. The 'thoracic' space represents the area between the balloon and the bell jar/diaphragm.

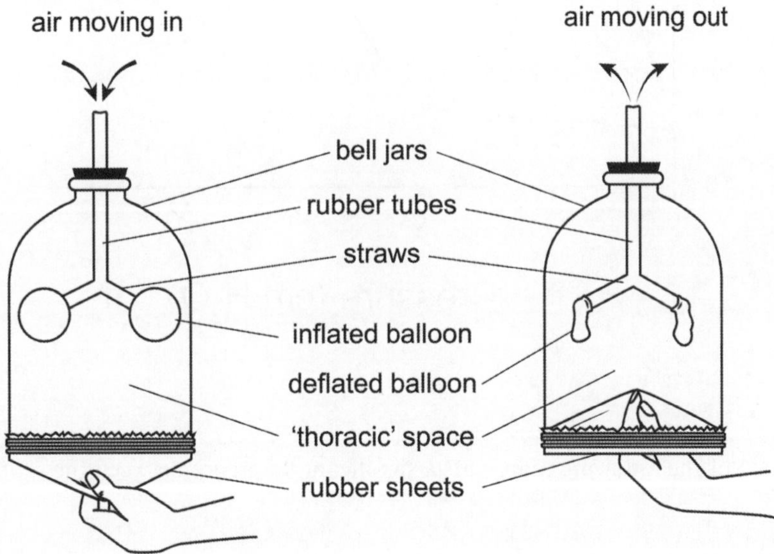

Of the following events, which one occurs first in the sequence preceding the inflation of the balloon?

- ○ **A.** The volume of air inside the balloon increases.
- ○ **B.** The volume of 'thoracic' air increases.
- ○ **C.** Pressure decreases in the 'thoracic' space.
- ○ **D.** Pressure decreases inside of the balloon.

Question 8

Consider Figure 2 below which was created using data from a realistic artificial lung model. The dark dots represent expiration (deflation) and the light dots represent inspiration (inflation).

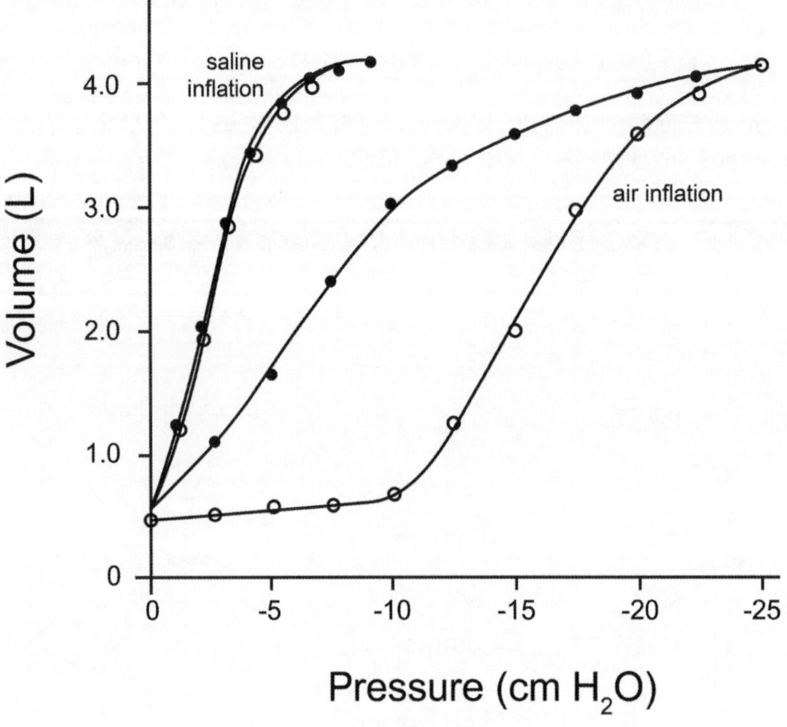

Figure 2

Based on Figure 2, which of the following represents a significant difference between the saline and air inflation of the lungs?

- O **A.** Maximum volume
- O **B.** Minimum volume
- O **C.** Work done
- O **D.** None of the above

The following questions are NOT based on a descriptive passage (Questions 9–12).

Question 9

Recent experimental evidence has shown that laser pulses tuned to the right frequency can kill certain viruses. If a virus is made to resonate, which of the following properties would NOT have become its maximum?

- O **A.** Power
- O **B.** Energy
- O **C.** Amplitude
- O **D.** Speed

Question 10

Extracorporeal shock wave lithotripsy (ESWL) is a treatment option that uses sound waves (ultrasound) to break up simple kidney stones. Consider two ESWL mechanical waves of the same frequency passing through the same kidney stone. The range of amplitudes possible when the two waves pass through the medium is between four and eight units. Which of the following best describes the possible amplitudes of the two waves?

- O **A.** 6 units and 2 units
- O **B.** 8 units and 4 units
- O **C.** 12 units and 4 units
- O **D.** 10 units and 2 units

Question 11

Consider the following statement: A burn from steam at 100 °C is more severe than a burn from boiling water at 100 °C. Is the preceding statement valid?

- O **A.** No, because it is an isothermal process.
- O **B.** No, because there is no difference in the sum of kinetic and potential energy of the molecules.
- O **C.** Yes, because steam is hotter than the boiling water.
- O **D.** Yes, because the steam will give off a large amount of heat as it condenses.

Question 12

Lactone rings are cyclic esters that occur widely as building blocks in nature, such as in ascorbic acid and hormones, in addition to many medications. Which of the following compounds is capable of forming a delta-lactone?

- O **A.** HO_2C … CO_2H
- O **B.** MeO_2C … OH
- O **C.** HO_2C … OH
- O **D.** HO_2C … OMe

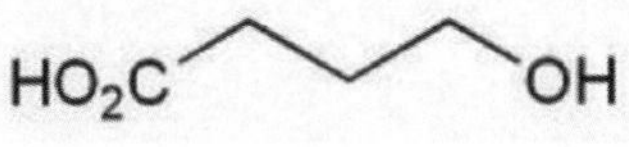

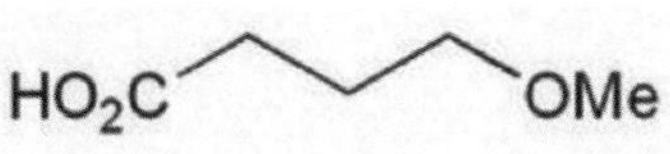

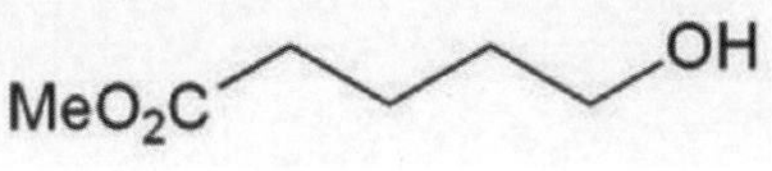

Passage 3 (Questions 13–16)

Researchers are currently trying to develop materials which could be used to replace damaged or destroyed human muscle tissue. One of the more promising avenues of research involves the use of substances that contract with the application of a small electric current.

Two physicists published an article relating to their work with Substance Q42, a material which contracts with the application of very small electric currents.

The atomic structure of the substance, they report, is designed so that the magnetic fields from each atom maintain a certain distance between adjacent atoms. With the application of an electrical current, the atoms' magnetic fields are dampened slightly, causing them to draw closer together. The extent to which it contracts is dependent upon the strength of the current passing through it , but will at any rate never exceed a 20% reduction in length.

Moreover, the physicists report, Substance Q42 essentially operated like a spring — but one which can compress itself. The force generated by a spring, F_s, is given by the following equation:

$$F_s = -kx$$

where k is the spring of constant in N/m, and x is the distance of compression (or expansion, but that is irrelevant for this example, since Substance Q42 only compresses).

With this in mind, it is possible to calculate the feasibility of using Substance Q42 as a replacement for human muscle tissue. Assume a section of test Substance Q42 is hooked to a scalable electrical source. The section is 10 cm long at its fully extended state, and 8 cm long when fully compressed due to an electrical current.

Question 13

A force-meter is attached to one end of a section of Substance Q42; the other end of the section is secured to a non-moving surface. When fully compressed, the force-meter registers a force exerted by the section of 250 N. What is the spring constant?

○ **A.** 12 500 N/m
○ **B.** 12 800 N/m
○ **C.** 16 700 N/m
○ **D.** 20 500 N/m

Question 14

How much force does the section apply when it compresses from rest state to 9.5 cm in length?

k = 40 000 N/m

- ○ **A.** 100 N
- ○ **B.** 200 N
- ○ **C.** 500 N
- ○ **D.** 1000 N

Question 15

Substance Q42 is fully expanded and then contracts in response to a 5.0 amp current. Which of the following best represents the conversion of energies in the process described?

- ○ **A.** Potential → kinetic → mechanical
- ○ **B.** Potential → mechanical → kinetic
- ○ **C.** Electrical → mechanical → potential
- ○ **D.** Potential → mechanical → electrical

Question 16

If an artificial arm muscle must be capable of doing 8 J work in 0.5 seconds time in order to efficiently substitute for human tissue, what average power must the section of Substance Q42 be capable of?

- ○ **A.** 16 Watts
- ○ **B.** 22 Watts
- ○ **C.** 32 Watts
- ○ **D.** 36 Watts

Passage 4 (Questions 17–20)

Vitamin C, or L-ascorbate, is an essential nutrient. L-ascorbate is a cofactor in at least eight enzymatic reactions, including several collagen synthesis reactions that, when dysfunctional, cause the most significant symptoms of scurvy. Ascorbate can also act as an antioxidant against oxidative stress.

L-ascorbate is synthesized naturally by many plants and animals from glucose. Humans, however, along with many other animals including higher primates, cannot synthesize ascorbate, due to an inability to make L-gulonolactone oxidase, and therefore must consume dietary vitamin C.

Below is a simplified diagram of the synthesis of L-ascorbate from glucose-6-phosphate in plants. Researchers analyzed *Arabidopsis thaliana* mutants deficient for VTC1, VTC2, and VTC4 (notated as VTC1m, VTC2m, and VTC4m). Each plant was found to be deficient in L-ascorbate.

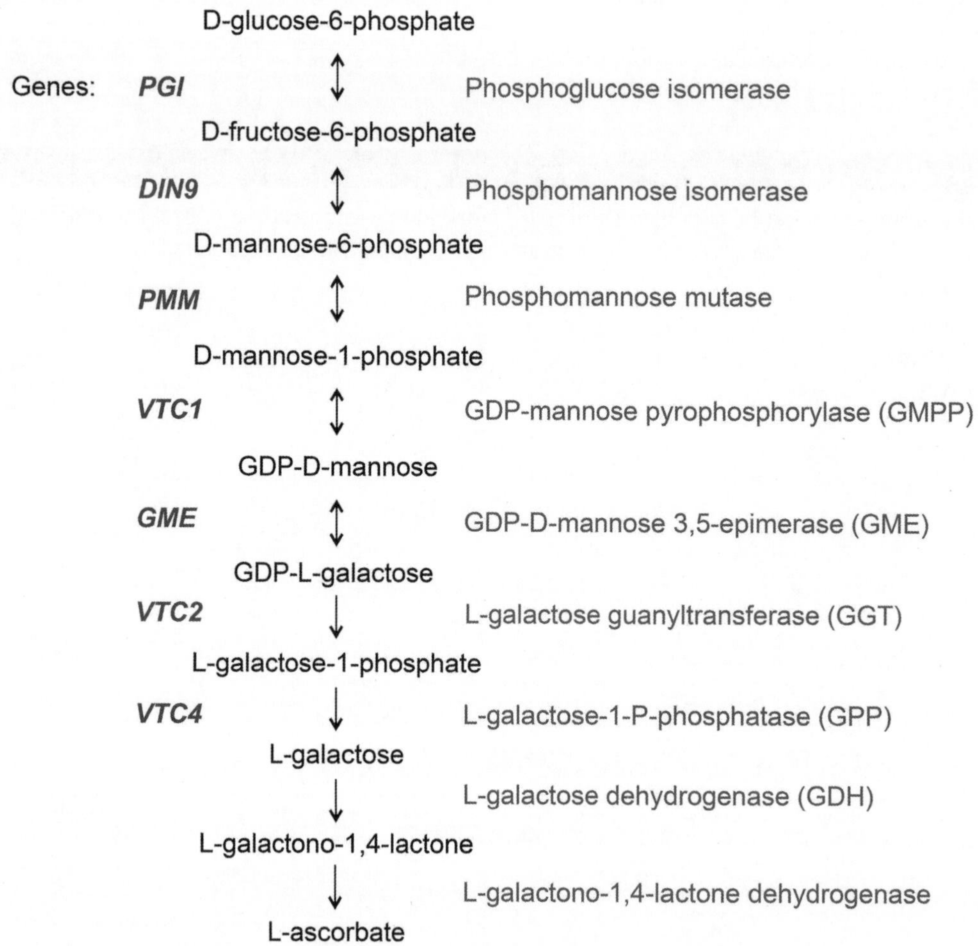

Figure 1 Synthesis of L-ascorbate from glucose-6-phosphate. Each step is catalyzed by the enzyme listed in lighter gray in the right column, with the related gene listed in darker gray in the left column.

Question 17

Figure 1 shows that the gene residing at the VTC1 locus encodes GDP-mannose pyrophosphorylase which catalyzes the synthesis of GDP-D-mannose from D-mannose-1-phosphate. The category of biological molecules which best describes GDP would be which of the following?

- O **A.** Lipids
- O **B.** Amino acids
- O **C.** Carbohydrates
- O **D.** Nucleotides

Question 18

Cell cultures described in the passage that are given additional supplements of GDP-L-galactose would be expected to show:

- O **A.** increased vitamin C production in VTC1m only.
- O **B.** increased vitamin C production in both VTC1m and VTC2m.
- O **C.** increased vitamin C production in VTC4m only.
- O **D.** increased vitamin C production in all three mutants.

Question 19

Seedlings of all three plant populations were given a mixture of supplements containing two pathway intermediates. All of the plants yielded vitamin C production. After maturation, the leaves were crushed, and the lysates from the ruptured cells were examined using Western blot analysis, with the following results (where X represents protein detection):

	GMPP	GME	GGT	GPP	GDH
VTC1m		X	X	X	X
VTC2m	X	X			X
VTC4m	X	X	X		X

Assuming a positive feedback system where genes are not transcribed unless activated by an increased concentration of the prior intermediate, the results show that the supplement mixture contained which of the following?

- O **A.** GDP-L-galactose, L-galactose
- O **B.** D-mannose-1-phosphate, L-galactose
- O **C.** GDP-D-mannose, L-galactose
- O **D.** GDP-D-mannose, GDP-L-galactose

Question 20

The enantiomer of Vitamin C is D-ascorbate which is not found in nature. D-ascorbate has identical antioxidant activity to L-ascorbate, yet far less vitamin activity. Which of the following reactions is likely NOT stereospecific?

I. Conversion of the procollagen to collagen by oxidizing proline residues to hydroxyproline
II. Neutralization of hydrogen peroxide and associated free radicals

- O **A.** I only
- O **B.** II only
- O **C.** Both I and II
- O **D.** Neither I nor II

Passage 5 (Questions 21–24)

The enthalpy of solution (ΔH_{soln}) of a salt depends on two other quantities: the energy released when free gaseous ions of the salt combine to give the solid salt (lattice energy: ΔH_{latt}) and the energy released when free gaseous ions of the salt dissolve in water via solute-solvent interactions to yield the solvated ions (enthalpy of hydration: ΔH_{solv}). The relationship between these quantities is given by Equation I.

Equation I

$\Delta H_{soln} = \Delta H_{solv} - \Delta H_{latt}$

From the formal definition of the quantities, it can be seen that both ΔH_{latt} and ΔH_{solv} are exothermic. Although these values seem to be in competition, the factors that affect ΔH_{latt} and ΔH_{solv} do so in the same way. Firstly, the smaller the ion, the closer the association of the ion with either other ions in the crystal lattice, or, with water molecules and thus the more negative ΔH_{latt} and ΔH_{solv} become. Also, the greater the charge on the ion, the greater the increase in electrostatic forces of attraction between itself and other ions or water molecules, and the more negative ΔH_{latt} and ΔH_{solv} become.

Although ΔH_{latt} and ΔH_{solv} undergo similar changes, the change in ΔH_{solv} up or down a group is much more profound than that of ΔH_{latt}. A good example of this is seen in the solubility changes of the Group II carbonates (*see* Table 1).

However, there is one exception to these general rules. If the cation of the salt is approximately the same size as the anion, the arrangement of ions in the crystal lattice is more uniform and hence the lattice is more stable and ΔH_{latt} is more negative. This would in turn make the salt less soluble.

Table 1

Group II Carbonate	Solubility (mol L^{-1} H_2O)
$MgCO_3$	1.30 x 10^{-3}
$CaCO_3$	0.13 x 10^{-3}
$SrCO_3$	0.07 x 10^{-3}
$BaCO_3$	0.09 x 10^{-3}

Question 21

The solubility product for $MgCO_3$ is:

- ○ **A.** 1.3 x 10^{-4}
- ○ **B.** 2.6 x 10^{-4}
- ○ **C.** 1.7 x 10^{-6}
- ○ **D.** 6.7 x 10^{-8}

Question 22

$Ca(OH)_2$ has approximately the same K_{sp} as $CaSO_4$. Which of them has the greater solubility in terms of mol L^{-1}?

- ○ **A.** They both have the same solubility.
- ○ **B.** $Ca(OH)_2$
- ○ **C.** $CaSO_4$
- ○ **D.** It depends on the temperature at the time.

Question 23

The CO_3^{2-} anion is approximately the same size as:

- ○ **A.** Mg^{2+}.
- ○ **B.** Ca^{2+}.
- ○ **C.** Sr^{2+}.
- ○ **D.** Ba^{2+}.

Question 24

A solution of $SrCO_3$ in water boils at a higher temperature than pure water. Why is this?

- O **A.** $SrCO_3$ increases the density of water.
- O **B.** $SrCO_3$ decreases the vapor pressure of the water.
- O **C.** $SrCO_3$ has a low solubility in water.
- O **D.** $SrCO_3$ decreases the surface tension of the water.

The following questions are NOT based on a descriptive passage (Questions 25–28).

Question 25

Which of the following is consistent with a disulfide bridge?

I. cys-cys
II. cys-met
III. met-met

- O **A.** I only
- O **B.** III only
- O **C.** I and III only
- O **D.** I, II and III

Question 26

Oxidative phosphorylation is best described as:

- O **A.** the process in which ATP is formed as electrons are transferred from electron carriers to oxygen.
- O **B.** the process in which ATP is formed as glucose is converted into pyruvate.
- O **C.** the process in which ATP is formed as pyruvate is converted into acetyl CoA.
- O **D.** the process in which ATP is formed as acetyl CoA is completely oxidized to carbon dioxide.

Question 27

Which of the following best identifies the following organic compound?

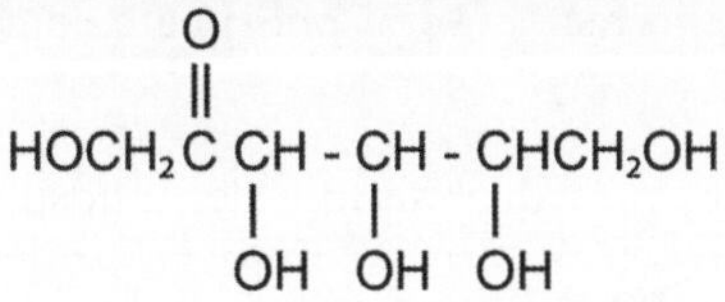

$$HOCH_2\overset{\overset{\displaystyle O}{\|}}{C}\,\underset{\underset{\displaystyle OH}{|}}{CH}-\underset{\underset{\displaystyle OH}{|}}{CH}-\underset{\underset{\displaystyle OH}{|}}{CH}CH_2OH$$

- O **A.** Hydroxy-nucleotide
- O **B.** Triacyl glyceride
- O **C.** Aldehyde
- O **D.** Carbohydrate

Question 28

Morphine, a chiral compound, is illustrated below. How many stereogenic carbon centers are there in morphine?

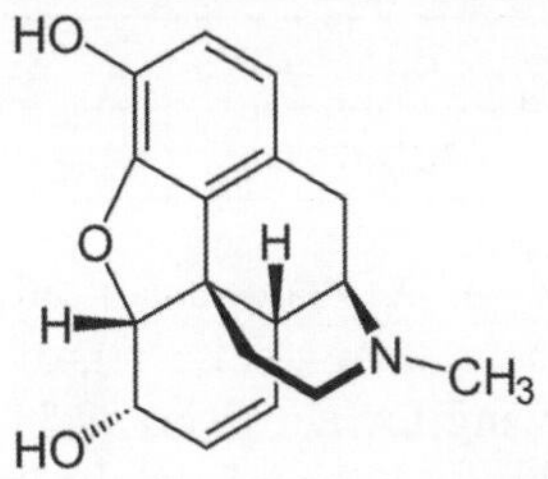

HO, O, H, H, N–CH_3, HO

- O **A.** 5
- O **B.** 6
- O **C.** 7
- O **D.** More than 7

Passage 6 (Questions 29–33)

ATP, or adenosine triphosphate, is often referred to as the energy currency of the cell. The 'high-energy' molecule stores and transports chemical energy within cells, and is present in both the cytoplasm and the nucleoplasm. Energy is released when ATP undergoes hydrolysis, and one of its 'high-energy' phosphate bonds is severed to form ADP, adenosine diphosphate, and inorganic phosphate, P_i (Figure 1).

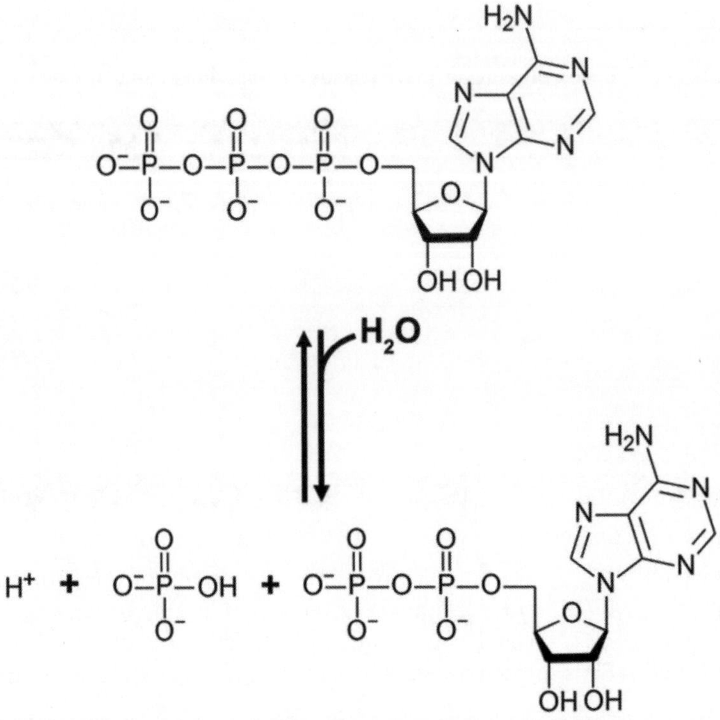

H_2O

H^+ + ADP + P_i

Figure 1 Hydrolysis of ATP into ADP and P_i

This reaction is not limited to ATP, and in fact, several phosphate compounds are capable of releasing energy upon hydrolysis.

Table 1 The free energy of hydrolysis for select phosphorylated compounds

Compound	ΔG° (kJ·mol^{-1})
Phosphoenolpyruvate	-61.9
Phosphocreatine	-43.1
Phosphoarginine	-32.0
ATP (to ADP)	-30.5
Pyrophosphate	-19.3
Glucose-6-phosphate	-13.8
Glycerol-3-phosphate	-9.0

Despite the body's reliance on ATP, hydrolysis of ATP alone can only supply enough energy for a few seconds of activity. In contrast, the ATP-phophocreatine system (ATP-PC), or phosphogen system, can be used to extend this burst of energy to 10-12 seconds, allowing for activities such as a brief sprint, or lifting a heavy object. Phosphocreatine is hydrolyzed to form creatine and phosphate, the latter of which is used to regenerate ATP. The reaction is modeled with the formula:

$$\text{Phosphocreatine} + \text{ADP} + P_i \leftrightharpoons \text{Creatine} + \text{ATP} + P_i \qquad \textbf{Reaction 1}$$

Over prolonged periods of exercise, the source of ATP changes, shifting eventually to the aerobic metabolic pathway, where ATP is regenerated through other means (see Figure 2).

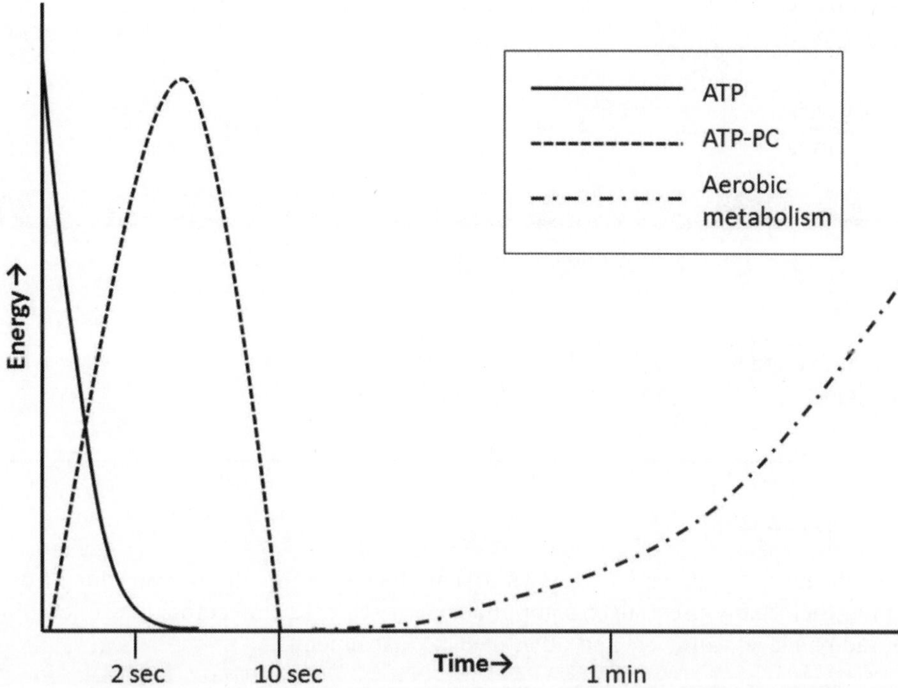

Figure 2 The body's source of energy over various periods of activity

Question 29

A runner sprints at maximum intensity for exactly one minute. If the muscles involved were tested afterward, it would reveal a build up of:

- ○ **A.** ADP.
- ○ **B.** phosphocreatine.
- ○ **C.** glucose.
- ○ **D.** lactate.

Question 30

Which of the following can NOT be inferred from the information provided in the passage?

- ○ **A.** The phosphocreatine reserve is depleted after approximately 10 seconds.
- ○ **B.** After 1 minute, the rate of reaction per molecule of substrate would be greater than the main energy-generating processes at any point under 10 seconds.
- ○ **C.** ATP-PC is associated with more power at any given time in the first 2 seconds than during aerobic metabolism at any given time within the first 60 seconds.
- ○ **D.** The hydrolysis of phosphocreatine indirectly supplies energy to muscles.

Question 31

Phosphoenolpyruvate is hydrolyzed to generate one molecule of pyruvate and one phosphate group. Based on the information provided in the passage, how much energy is released when a phosphate group is transferred from phosphoenolpyruvate to ADP to form ATP?

- ○ **A.** $-31.4\ kJ \cdot mol^{-1}$
- ○ **B.** $-38.6\ kJ \cdot mol^{-1}$
- ○ **C.** $-61.9\ kJ \cdot mol^{-1}$
- ○ **D.** $-92.4\ kJ \cdot mol^{-1}$

Question 32

The hydrolysis of phosphoenolpyruvate in the presence of ADP releases energy. The preceding is a necessary step in which metabolic process?

- O **A.** Pentose phosphate pathway
- O **B.** Oxidative phosphorylation
- O **C.** Glycolysis
- O **D.** Citric acid cycle

Question 33

In humans, phosphagens, or 'high-energy' phosphate compounds, are mostly found in:

- O **A.** the kidneys.
- O **B.** the liver.
- O **C.** the circulatory system.
- O **D.** muscle tissue.

Passage 7 (Questions 34–38)

Silver is still one of the most versatile metals known to man, being used in almost everything from electrical wires to jewellery. Among their many uses, silver compounds are used as disinfectants and microbiocides, added to wound dressings and bandages, catheters and other medical instruments.

Silver is quite unreactive, and is resistant to attack by common agents such as acid and oxygen. Needless to say, the mining of this precious metal is the mainstay of the economy of many countries. Unfortunately, silver does not occur in its elemental state in nature. It is mined as argentite (Ag_2S containing ore) and horn silver (AgCl containing ore).

The main method used in industry for separating silver from its ores involves complexation and the cyanide ligand (CN-). The cyanide ligand is used to produce the soluble silver cyanide complex according to Reaction I and Reaction II.

Reaction I

$Ag_2S + 4CN^- \rightarrow 2[Ag(CN)_2]^- + S^{2-}$

Reaction II

$AgCl + 2CN^- \rightarrow [Ag(CN)_2]^- + Cl^-$

The silver metal in its elemental form is then precipitated by adding zinc dust to the solution as shown in Reaction III.

Reaction III

$2[Ag(CN)_2]^- + Zn \rightarrow [Zn(CN)_4]^{2-} + 2Ag(s)$

Silver complexes provide one of the most fascinating demonstrations of the relative strengths of different ligands for a particular cation. This is a common occurrence with most complexes of this nature but what makes silver unique is that many of its complexes differ in color. Table 1 is a list of a few of the silver complexes and their colors.

Table 1

Complex	Color
$[Ag(CN)_2]^-$	Clear solution
AgI	Yellow precipitate
$[Ag(EDTA)]^-$	Clear solution
Ag_2S	Black precipitate

One will notice that precipitates are listed in the table. These can be regarded as neutral complexes and as is often the case with neutral complexes, they are quite insoluble and hence precipitate out of solution.

Question 34

The ability of silver ions to form complexes of many different colors identifies it as being a:

- O **A.** univalent metal.
- O **B.** Group IB element.
- O **C.** Period V element.
- O **D.** transition metal.

Question 35

Given that $K_{a1}(H_2S) = 9.1 \times 10^{-8}$ and $K_{a2}(H_2S) = 1.2 \times 10^{-15}$, what would be the effect on Reaction I if protons were added to the reaction mixture at equilibrium?

(note: the effect of protons on CN^- is relatively negligible).

- O **A.** The equilibrium would shift to the left.
- O **B.** The equilibrium would shift to the right.
- O **C.** There would be no change in the equilibrium position of the reaction.
- O **D.** The change in the equilibrium position cannot be determined from the information given.

Question 36

12 grams of silver was extracted from a sample of an ore from which the only source of silver was Ag_2S. How many grams of Ag_2S were in the original sample?

- O **A.** 27.6 grams
- O **B.** 13.8 grams
- O **C.** 8.6 grams
- O **D.** 5.2 grams

Question 37

One of the complexes formed by silver is silver bromide, AgBr. Why would you expect it to be insoluble?

- O **A.** Because it is a neutral complex.
- O **B.** Because Br^- is a large anion.
- O **C.** Because the relative molecular mass of AgBr is large.
- O **D.** Because most bromides are insoluble.

Question 38

From the following data, which of the following ligands would you add to a clear silver complex in solution to determine which of the clear complexes in Table 1 was present?

In order of decreasing affinity for silver ions:

EDTA > S^{2-} > CN^- > I^-

- O **A.** EDTA
- O **B.** S^{2-}
- O **C.** CN^-
- O **D.** I^-

Passage 8 (Questions 39–43)

To determine whether or not an alpha-amino acid was present in solution, a student designed a series of reactions which result in a color change if the amino acid is primal. The following represents the initial steps in the reaction mechanism.

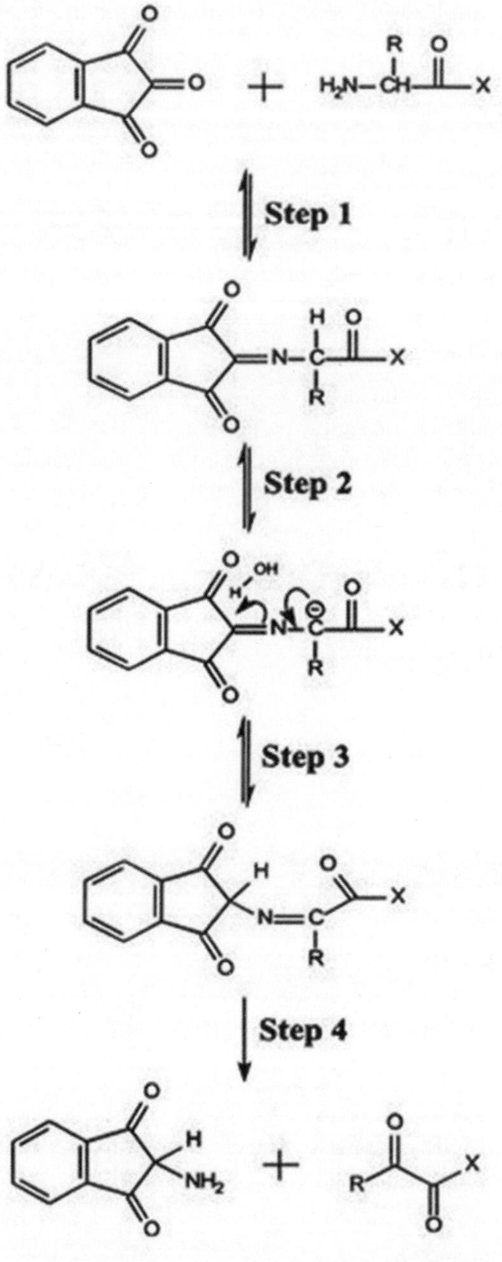

Step 1

Step 2

Step 3

Step 4

Question 39

In order for Step 2 to proceed as illustrated, the student added which of the following to the reaction mixture?

- O **A.** A Lewis base
- O **B.** A Lewis acid
- O **C.** A Bronsted base
- O **D.** A Bronsted acid

Question 40

Which of the following compounds would have infrared spectra which indicate strong peaks at 3,350 cm^{-1} and 1,740 cm^{-1}?

O A.

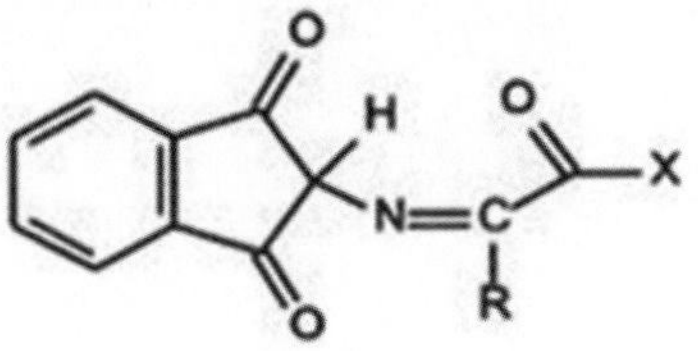

O B.

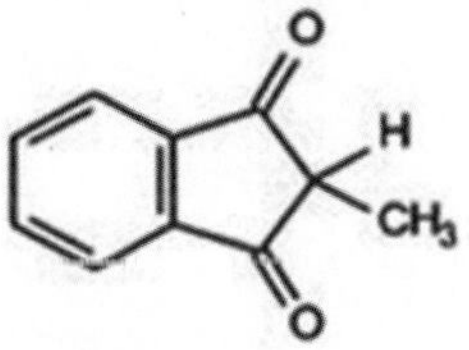

O C.

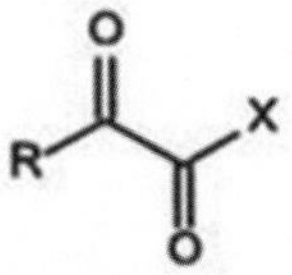

O D.

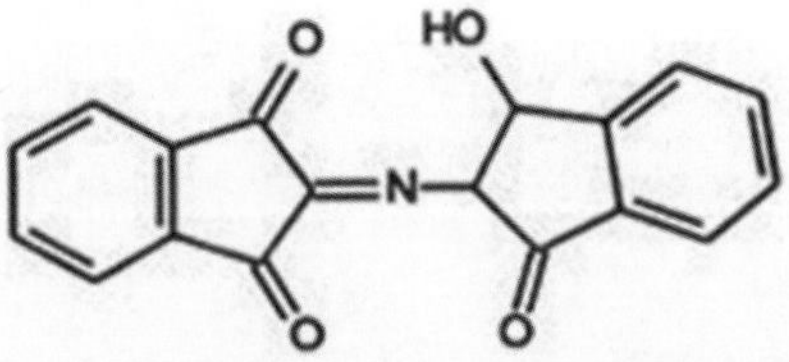

Question 41

The inorganic reactant used in Step 4 of the reaction mechanism must have been which of the following?

O A. HCl
O B. CO_2
O C. H_2O
O D. H_2O_2

Question 42

The first step in the reaction mechanism is most consistent with which of the following?

O A. S_N1
O B. S_N2
O C. Decarboxylation
O D. Oxidation

Question 43

Which of the following is NOT consistent with the reaction mechanism provided?

O A. The reaction is designed to remove the amino group from the amino acid.
O B. If X represents the hydroxyl functional group (OH), and R is the ligand $(CH_2)_4(NH_2)$, then the alpha-amino acid lysine was present in solution.
O C. If Step 2 of the reaction was blocked, the reaction would still proceed to completion if there was an added supplement containing the reactants from Step 3.
O D. If Step 3 of the reaction was blocked, the reaction would still proceed to completion if there was an added supplement containing an alpha-amino acid.

The following questions are NOT based on a descriptive passage (Questions 44–47).

Question 44

Consider the following molecular structure where 5 protons are labeled: A, B, C, D and E.

Which of the following is NOT true regarding the relative acidity of the labeled protons?

- O **A.** Proton E is more acidic than proton D.
- O **B.** Proton C is more acidic than proton B.
- O **C.** Proton B is more acidic than proton A.
- O **D.** Proton E and proton C have a similar magnitude of acidity.

Question 45

Consider the substrate (S) to product (P) reaction S $\leftrightarrow$ P which can be catalyzed by two enzymes, Q and R. The reaction coordinate diagrams for these two enzymes are shown below.

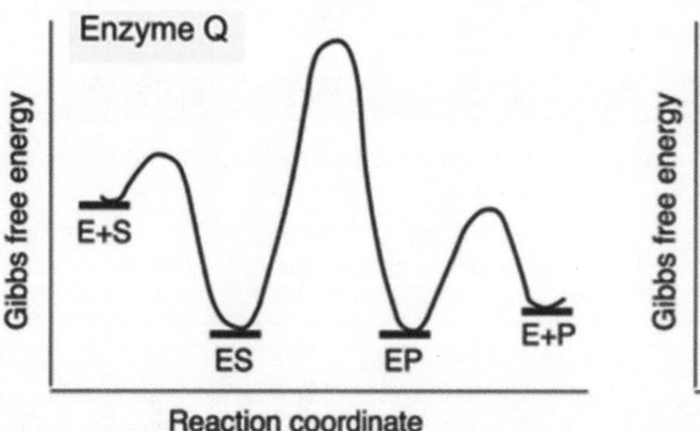

Which of the following is NOT consistent with the data summarized by the 2 diagrams?

- O **A.** Both reactions are equally exergonic.
- O **B.** The rate-limiting step for both reactions involves: ES $\rightarrow$ EP
- O **C.** Enzyme R binds more tightly to the substrate.
- O **D.** Enzyme R is the better of the two catalysts.

Question 46

The equilibrium constant Ka is also called the acid dissociation constant and Kb is the base dissociation constant. If the value of Ka is relatively low, this would mean that, relatively, its:

- O **A.** pKa is low and the pKb of its conjugate base is high.
- O **B.** pKa is high and the pKb of its conjugate base is low.
- O **C.** pKa is low and the pKb of its conjugate base is low.
- O **D.** pKa is high and the pKb of its conjugate base is high.

Question 47

Atherosclerosis and thrombosis can partially occlude an artery as material adheres to the arterial walls over a small portion of its length. What happens to the pressure and the velocity of blood in the partially occluded region as compared to just prior to the partial occlusion?

- O **A.** Velocity decreases, pressure decreases
- O **B.** Velocity decreases, pressure increases
- O **C.** Velocity increases, pressure increases
- O **D.** Velocity increases, pressure decreases

Passage 9 (Questions 48–51)

The viscosity of a fluid, that is, a gas, a pure liquid or a solution, is an index of its resistance to flow. The viscosity of a fluid in a cylindrical tube of radius R and length L is given by Equation I.

Equation I

$n = \pi \Delta P R^4 t/(8VL)$

where n = viscosity of fluid, π = pi, ΔP = change in pressure, t = time, V = volume of fluid and V/t = rate of flow of fluid.

Equation I can be applied to the study of blood flow in the human body. The heart pumps blood through the various vessels in our bodies to supply all of its tissues. At rest, the rate of blood flow is about 80 $cm^3\ s^{-1}$ and this is maintained in all blood vessels. However, the radii of the blood vessels decreases the further away blood moves from the heart. Therefore, in order to maintain the rate of blood flow, a pressure drop occurs as one moves from one blood vessel to another of smaller radius.

A great number of physiological conditions can be explained using Equation I, for example, hypertension.

Question 48

Hypertension involves the decrease in the radius of certain blood vessels. If the radius of a blood vessel is halved, by what factor must the pressure increase to maintain the normal rate of blood flow, all other factors being constant?

- ○ **A.** 2
- ○ **B.** 4
- ○ **C.** 8
- ○ **D.** 16

Question 49

The equation for the rate of flow of a fluid (from Equation I) has often been compared to Ohm's law. Given that P can be likened to the voltage and flow rate can be likened to the current, which of the following can be likened to resistance?

- O **A.** πR^4
- O **B.** $\pi R^4/(8Ln)$
- O **C.** $8Ln/(\pi R^4)$
- O **D.** 8Ln

Question 50

What would be the pressure drop per cm of the blood in the first blood vessel leaving the heart if the blood vessel is of unit radius and the body is at rest? $n_{blood} = 0.04$ dyn s cm^{-3}

- O **A.** $25.6/\pi$ dyn cm^{-3}
- O **B.** $16000/\pi$ dyn cm^{-3}
- O **C.** $\pi/25.6$ dyn cm^{-3}
- O **D.** $\pi/16000$ dyn cm^{-3}

Question 51

Which of the following has the greatest effect on the viscosity of a fluid per unit change in its value?

- O **A.** Volume of the fluid
- O **B.** Length of the tube
- O **C.** Pressure of the fluid
- O **D.** Radius of the tube

Passage 10 (Questions 52–56)

Amino acids are carboxylic acids that contain an amine function. Under certain conditions the amine group of one amino acid and the carboxyl group of a second can react, uniting the two amino acids by an amide bond, also known as a peptide bond. All of the amino acids from which proteins are derived are α (alpha) amino acids.

The feature that differentiates one amino acid from another is the side chain attached to the α carbon. The side chains of the 20 amino acids that are normally present in proteins categorize the amino acids into four types: acidic, basic, hydrophobic, and hydrophilic.

The physical properties of typical amino acids suggest that they are very polar. These properties are attributed to the fact that they often exist as zwitterions (i.e., having both a positive and negative element). The isoelectric point is the pH at which the amino acid bears no net charge; it corresponds to the pH at which the concentration of zwitterion is at a maximum.

The relative strength of the carboxylic acid in an amino acid can be expressed in terms of the acid dissociation constant, K_a or the pK_a.

Question 52

The side chain of an amino acid affects the acidity of the carbonyl group of an amino acid in which of the following ways?

- ○ **A.** If the side chain is an electron donor, the amino acid is more acidic.
- ○ **B.** If the side chain is an electron acceptor, the amino acid is more acidic.
- ○ **C.** If the side chain is hydrophilic, the amino acid is less acidic.
- ○ **D.** If the side chain is hydrophobic, the amino acid is less acidic.

Question 53

Which of the carbons below is an α carbon?

$$NH_2CH_2CH_2CH_2COOH$$

1 2 3 4

- ○ **A.** 1
- ○ **B.** 2
- ○ **C.** 3
- ○ **D.** 4

Question 54

At pH 14, what is the charge on lysine

[NH_2-$(CH_2)_4$-$CH(NH_2)$-$COOH$]?

- ○ **A.** -1
- ○ **B.** +1
- ○ **C.** -2
- ○ **D.** +2

Question 55

The following is a list of the acid–base properties of some amino acids with ionizable side chains. Which amino acid has the greatest isoelectric point?

Amino acid	pKa_1	pKa_2	pKa_3
Aspartic acid	1.88	3.65	9.60
Glutamic acid	2.19	4.25	9.67
Tyrosine	2.20	9.11	10.07
Cysteine	1.96	8.18	10.28

- ○ **A.** Aspartic acid
- ○ **B.** Glutamic acid
- ○ **C.** Tyrosine
- ○ **D.** Cysteine

Question 56

Consider the following pentapeptide: Ser-Asp-Phe-Arg-Lys. What is its net charge at pH = 7?

- ○ **A.** -1
- ○ **B.** 0
- ○ **C.** +1
- ○ **D.** Greater than +1

The following questions are NOT based on a descriptive passage (Questions 57–59).

Question 57

A biochemical reaction at constant temperature and pressure in a cellular environment is at equilibrium when the absolute temperature is equal to which of the following?

- ○ **A.** 0
- ○ **B.** $-(\Delta H)(\Delta S)$
- ○ **C.** -RT log Keq
- ○ **D.** $\Delta H/\Delta S$

Question 58

The ideal gas equation is given by PV = nRT where P is the pressure, V is the volume, n is the number of moles, R is the gas constant and T is the absolute temperature. Given the ideal gas equation, determine which of the following is consistent with the units of the gas constant R.

- ○ **A.** Joules/mole/K
- ○ **B.** (Joules)(mole)/K
- ○ **C.** (Pa)(mole)(K)
- ○ **D.** Pa/mole/K

Question 59

A student used a distillation apparatus to separate ethyl acetate from 1-butanol because of the difference in boiling points of these 2 compounds. This difference is most likely attributed to which of the following factors?

- ○ **A.** Hydrogen bonding
- ○ **B.** Bond hybridization
- ○ **C.** Temperature scanning
- ○ **D.** Resonance stabilization

CANDIDATE'S NAME ______________________________

RAW SCORE AND SCALED SCORE ______________________

GS-3
Mock Exam 3 of 7
Solutions at MCAT-prep.com

GS-3 Section II: Critical Analysis and Reasoning Skills (CARS)

Questions: 1-53
Time: 90 minutes

INSTRUCTIONS: This test contains nine passages, each of which is followed by several questions. After reading the passage, select the best answer to each question. If you are unsure of the answer, eliminate the alternatives you know to be false then select an answer from the remaining alternatives. To indicate your selection, use a pencil to blacken the corresponding circle next to the answer choice and/or you can use the answer document at the back of this book. No marks are deducted for wrong answers.

The computer-based real MCAT has an on-screen highlighter function and ~~STRIKEOUT~~ function. These tools help to spotlight text or assist in the process of elimination. You may use a yellow highlighter for this paper-based exam and/or a pen (or preferably a pencil to make it easier should you change your mind) to mark text. At the time of publishing, both highlighting and strikeout functions can be used for passages, questions and answer choices. You can also flag a question to review later should time remain.

For the real exam, you will be provided with a dry erase board which is a white laminated noteboard booklet accompanied by a fine point marker. The noteboard includes 9 graph-lined pages for you to write though you cannot erase. You can simulate the experience with a fine point marker on a noteboard or with 8" x 14" plain graph paper.

Please note: For the real MCAT, a small number of field-tested questions will remain unscored.

This practice test has been designed exclusively to test knowledge and thinking skills. This exam may contain hypothetical statements and/or express controversial ideas. Statements contained herein do not necessarily reflect the policy, position, or view of RuveneCo Inc. or MCAT-prep.com.

START EXAM ONLY WHEN TIMER IS READY.

Passage 1 (Questions 1–6)

"Deconstruction" is the name of a currently influential movement in American literary criticism. The underlying theory was developed not by literary critics but by a French professor of philosophy, Jacques Derrida, and many of his ideas are in turn indebted to Nietzsche and Heidegger. In his book *On Deconstruction*, Jonathan Culler writes as a disciple of Derrida, and his primary aim is to expound his master's philosophy and show how it "bears on the most important issues of literary theory."

What exactly is deconstruction, and why has it become so influential in American literary criticism while largely ignored by American philosophers? I think if you asked most practicing deconstructionists for a definition, they would not only be unable to provide one, but would regard the very request as a manifestation of that "logocentrism" which it is one of the aims of deconstruction to, well, deconstruct. By "logocentrism" they mean roughly the concern with truth, rationality, logic, and "the word" that marks the Western philosophical tradition. I think the best way to get at it, which would be endorsed by many of its practitioners, is to see it, at least initially, as a set of methods for dealing with texts, a set of textual strategies aimed in large part at subverting logocentric tendencies. One of the several merits of Culler's book is that he provides a catalog of these strategies and a characterization of their common aims: "To deconstruct a discourse is to show how it undermines the philosophy it asserts, or the hierarchical oppositions on which it relies, by identifying in the text the rhetorical operations that produce the supposed ground of argument, the key concept or premise."

First, and most important, the deconstructionist is on the lookout for any of the traditional binary oppositions in Western intellectual history, e.g., speech/writing, male/female, truth/fiction, literal/metaphorical, signified/signifier, reality/appearance. In such oppositions, the deconstructionist claims that the first or left-hand term is given a superior status over the right-hand term, which is regarded "as a complication, a negation, a manifestation, or a disruption of the first." These hierarchical oppositions allegedly lie at the very heart of logocentrism, with its obsessive interest in rationality, logic, and the search for truth.

The deconstructionist wants to undermine these oppositions, and so undermine logocentrism, by first reversing the hierarchy, by trying to show that the right-hand term is really the prior term and that the left-hand term is just a special case of the right-hand term; the right-hand term is the condition of possibility of the left-hand term. This move gives some very curious results. It turns out that speech is really a form of writing, understanding a form of misunderstanding, and that what we think of as meaningful language is just a free play of signifiers or an endless process of grafting texts onto texts.

When asked "What is deconstruction?" Derrida replied, "I have no simple and formalizable response to this question. All my essays are attempts to have it out with this formidable question." Derrida believes that the term deconstruction is necessarily complicated and difficult to explain since it actively criticizes the very language needed to explain it.

Derrida's defenders argue that in giving this reply, Derrida was simply being consistent: the word "deconstruction" is as slippery as any other word in the dictionary. Others criticize Derrida for being unable to define the discipline that he himself created, and for being evasive about it. Still, Rebecca Goldstein, a professor of philosophy, asserts, "In deconstruction, the critic claims there is no meaning to be found in the actual text, but only in the various, often mutually irreconcilable, 'virtual texts' constructed by readers in their search for meaning."

Reproduced in part from: Searle, J. R. (1983, October 27). The World Turned Upside Down. *The New York Review of Books*, 307.

Question 1

The practice of deconstruction is best understood as an activity in which a textual critic focuses on:

- ○ **A.** concepts that the author of a text frames as opposites which are really identical or versions of each other.
- ○ **B.** terms that the author of a text sees as having a single meaning which really have plural or multiple meanings.
- ○ **C.** terms and concepts that seem to have stable meanings but are really ambiguous.
- ○ **D.** the way that a text has been interpreted and reinterpreted throughout history.

Question 2

Suppose that a deconstructionist critic was analyzing a text about the ideal qualities of a "real man." The deconstructionist would likely argue that masculinity:

- O **A.** has been defined too narrowly and is whatever a given man wants it to be.
- O **B.** is an abstract ideal that no real-world man can actually live up to.
- O **C.** has no inherent meaning, but is defined in opposition to femininity.
- O **D.** is an unhelpful concept because men are not very different from women.

Question 3

In deconstruction, the meaning of a text is found:

- O **A.** in the interplay of the text itself and all its variations.
- O **B.** in structural relations among textual elements that are brought out through careful reading.
- O **C.** in the logocentric structures of political ideology and hegemonic practices.
- O **D.** among the readers' various interpretations.

Question 4

Based on passage information, one potentially valid critique of deconstruction is that:

- O **A.** it is really no different from deductive analysis.
- O **B.** it is apolitical and does not critique harmful ideologies.
- O **C.** it cannot be defined with any critical rigor.
- O **D.** it does not produce original readings of texts.

Question 5

Derrida would probably inform other scholars and academicians that hierarchal oppositions in society and textuality are:

I. the underlying premise for the claims made by most texts.
II. seemingly real, but likely to unravel if examined closely.
III. based on an individual author's unique view of the world.

- O **A.** I, II, III
- O **B.** I only
- O **C.** I and II only
- O **D.** III only

Question 6

Based on passage information, deconstructionists would likely most strongly agree with which of the following claims?

- O **A.** The Western philosophical tradition is flawed because it mis-identifies which issues are important to discuss.
- O **B.** It is important to have a concrete understanding of your critical stance before using it to analyze a text.
- O **C.** Only if a writer understands rhetoric will they be able to write a text that means what they intend it to say.
- O **D.** Many concepts that people believe are natural are actually products of human culture.

Passage 2 (Questions 7–13)

In the modern era, one of the most active metaphors for the spiritual project is "art." The activities of the painter, the musician, the poet, the dancer et al., once they were grouped together under that generic name (a relatively recent move), have proved to be a peculiarly adaptable site on which to stage the formal dramas besetting consciousness, each individual work of art being a more or less astute paradigm for regulating or reconciling these contradictions. Of course, the site needs continual refurbishing. Whatever goal is set for art eventually proves restrictive, matched against the widest goals of consciousness. Art, itself a form of mystification, endures a succession of crises of demystification; older artistic goals are assailed and, ostensibly, replaced; outgrown maps of consciousness are redrawn. But what supplies all these crises with their energy—an energy held in common, so to speak—is the very unification of numerous, quite disparate activities into a single genus. At the moment at which "art" comes into being, the modern period of art begins. From then forward, any of the activities therein subsumed becomes a profoundly problematic activity, each of whose procedures and, ultimately, whose very right to exist, can be called into question.

Following on the promotion of the arts into "art" comes the leading myth about art, that of the "absoluteness" of the artist's activity. In its first, more unreflective version, this myth considered art as an expression of human consciousness, consciousness seeking to know itself. (The critical principles generated by this myth were fairly easily arrived at: some expressions were more complete, more ennobling, more informative, richer than others.) The later version of the myth posits a more complex, tragic relation of art to consciousness. Denying that art is mere expression, the newer myth, ours, rather relates art to the mind's need or capacity for self-estrangement. Art is no longer understood as consciousness-expressing and therefore, implicitly, affirming itself. Art is not consciousness per se, but rather its antidote — evolved from within consciousness itself. (The critical principles generated by this myth were much harder to get at.)

The newer myth, derived from a post-psychological conception of consciousness, installs within the activity of art many of the paradoxes involved in attaining an absolute state of being described by the great religious mystics. As the activity of the mystic must end in a via negativa [negative way], a theology of God's absence, a craving for the cloud of unknowingness beyond knowledge and for the silence beyond speech, so art must tend toward anti-art, the elimination of the "subject" (the "object," the "image"), the substitution of chance for intention, and the pursuit of silence.

In the early, linear version of art's relation to consciousness, a struggle was held to exist between the "spiritual" integrity of the creative impulses and the distracting "materiality" of ordinary life, which throws up so many obstacles in the path of authentic sublimation. But the newer version, in which art is part of a dialectical transaction with consciousness, poses a deeper, more frustrating conflict: The "spirit" seeking embodiment in art clashes with the "material" character of art itself. Art is unmasked as gratuitous, and the very concreteness of the artist's tools (and, particularly in the case of language, their historicity) appears as a trap. Practiced in a world furnished with second-hand perceptions, and specifically confounded by the treachery of words, the activity of the artist is cursed with mediacy. Art becomes the enemy of the artist, for it denies him the realization, the transcendence, he desires.

Therefore, art comes to be estimated as something to be overthrown. "A new element enters the art-work and becomes constitutive of it: the appeal (tacit or overt) for its own abolition—and, ultimately, for the abolition of art itself.

Sontag, S. (2009). *Styles of radical will* (Aesthetics of Silence). London: Penguin Books.

Question 7

It can be inferred from the final two paragraphs that:

I. art should be overthrown.
II. art carries its own contradiction within it.
III. art's abolition is an end in itself.

- ○ **A.** I and II
- ○ **B.** II only
- ○ **C.** III only
- ○ **D.** I and III

Question 8

The artist could expand her argument by exploring which of the following?

- O **A.** What separates our era of art from earlier ones
- O **B.** The tools or materials the artist uses
- O **C.** Artists' reasons for expressing themselves through art
- O **D.** Whether audiences seek art that expresses an "aesthetic of silence"

Question 9

Based on passage information, the titular "Aesthetics of Silence" can be inferred to refer to:

- O **A.** art becoming focused on anti-art and the pursuit of what it is not.
- O **B.** minimalist art that includes as few materials and details as possible.
- O **C.** a form of art in which the silences or blank spaces mean as much as the notes, words or images.
- O **D.** a form of art that directs attention to "silence" and blankness to show that even seeming nothingness is filled with beauty.

Question 10

Which of the following ideas within the passage best exemplifies the author's assertion that "art becomes something to be overthrown"?

- O **A.** "The creative impulse leads to a number of artistic paradoxes."
- O **B.** "The conscious act of art becomes a self-conscious trap."
- O **C.** "The mystical dimension of art will always be at odds with the material aspect."
- O **D.** "The mediacy of the artist's tools interferes with a quest for spiritual transcendence."

Question 11

In context, what does the author likely mean in paragraph 4 by the "historicity" of language?

- O **A.** Language is a part of history because it is preserved for a long time.
- O **B.** Language is determined by a historical and cultural milieu, and is not specific to the individual.
- O **C.** Language contains outdated ideas from history and has trouble expressing new ones.
- O **D.** Language is an outdated form of expression, while art must find new ones.

Question 12

The author's argument would be most undermined by an article showing that:

- O **A.** the qualities of art have changed so much over history that it is misleading to call them all by the same name.
- O **B.** art always expresses the author's consciousness, even if the artist feels estranged from that consciousness.
- O **C.** many artists are increasingly embracing the materiality of their craft and rejecting the ideal of "transcendence."
- O **D.** the life of a mystic is inherently paradoxical because a conscious human can never experience "unknowingness."

Question 13

According to the author, a key turning point in cultural history was when:

- O **A.** art's original goal became demystified because it was too restrictive.
- O **B.** consciousness united disparate activities together as "art."
- O **C.** consciousness wished to know and express itself.
- O **D.** art became a mystical act imbued with spiritualism.

Passage 3 (Questions 14–18)

The problem of consciousness remains with us. What exactly is it and why is it still with us? The single most important question is: How exactly do neurobiological processes in the brain cause human and animal consciousness? Related problems are: How exactly is consciousness realized in the brain? That is, where is it and how does it exist in the brain? Also, how does it function causally in our behavior?

To answer these questions we have to ask: What is it? Without attempting an elaborate definition, we can say the central feature of consciousness is that for any conscious state there is something that it feels like to be in that state, some qualitative character to the state. For example, the qualitative character of drinking beer is different from that of listening to music or thinking about your income tax. This qualitative character is subjective in that it only exists as experienced by a human or animal subject. It has a subjective or first-person existence (or "ontology"), unlike mountains, molecules, and tectonic plates that have an objective or third-person existence. Furthermore, qualitative subjectivity always comes to us as part of a unified conscious field. At any moment you do not just experience the sound of the music and the taste of the beer, but you have both as part of a single, unified conscious field, a subjective awareness of the total conscious experience. So the feature we are trying to explain is qualitative, unified subjectivity.

Now it might seem that is a fairly well-defined scientific task: just figure out how the brain does it. In the end I think that is the right attitude to have. But our peculiar history makes it difficult to have exactly that attitude—to take consciousness as a biological phenomenon like digestion or photosynthesis, and figure out how exactly it works as a biological phenomenon. Two philosophical obstacles cast a shadow over the whole subject. The first is the tradition of God, the soul, and immortality. Consciousness is not a part of the ordinary biological world of digestion and photosynthesis: it is part of a spiritual world. It is sometimes thought to be a property of the soul and the soul is definitely not a part of the physical world. The other tradition, almost as misleading, is a certain conception of Science with a capital "S." Science is said to be "reductionist" and "materialist," and so construed there is no room for consciousness in Science. If it really exists, consciousness must really be something else. It must be reducible to something else, such as neuron firings, computer programs running in the brain, or dispositions to behavior.

There are also a number of purely technical difficulties to neurobiological research. The brain is an extremely complicated mechanism with about a hundred billion neurons in humans, and most investigative techniques are, as the researchers cheerfully say, "invasive." That means you have to kill or hideously maim the animal in order to investigate the operation of the brain. Noninvasive research techniques, such as brain imaging, are useful, but they have so far not given us the sort of detailed understanding of the workings of the conscious mind that we would like.

Searle, J. R. (2013, January 10). Can Information Theory Explain Consciousness? *The New York Review of Books*, 181.

Question 14

According to the passage, what is the problem of consciousness?

- o **A.** The problem of coping with the often painful experience of being a conscious organism.
- o **B.** The problem of conducting research on conscious test subjects without harming or killing them.
- o **C.** The problem of understanding why humans and animals are conscious, but other entities are not.
- o **D.** The difficulty of understanding how the experience of consciousness arises from mechanical processes.

Question 15

Which of the following would be most consistent with the main purpose of the passage?

- O **A.** To define consciousness as a unified, subjective experience
- O **B.** To set out the problems involved in trying to explain consciousness
- O **C.** To explain why research into consciousness has progressed so slowly
- O **D.** To critique views of consciousness that equates it with spiritual entities like the soul

Question 16

The author would likely reject all of the following EXCEPT:

- O **A.** a behaviorist account of human and animal actions that attempts to explain them through the relationship between stimulus and response.
- O **B.** a neurological account explaining that the concept of "consciousness" is flawed because this phenomenon is reducible to electrical activity.
- O **C.** a biological account of consciousness discussing the evolutionary reasons that could have made it beneficial for organisms to develop consciousness.
- O **D.** a theological account arguing that consciousness is beyond the reach neurobiology because it is not reducible to biological operations.

Question 17

How might Searle respond to an author who argued that machines are becoming conscious because they are capable of holding intelligent conversations and carrying out complex operations?

- O **A.** He would disagree, because consciousness is a biological mechanism that only biological organisms can experience.
- O **B.** He would disagree, because the ability to do tasks does not indicate that machines have the subjective experience of consciousness.
- O **C.** He would agree, because the "problem of consciousness" remains the same whether the processes that produce consciousness are organic or inorganic.
- O **D.** He would disagree, because machines cannot match the extreme complexity of the human brain.

Question 18

The author's use of "cheerfully" in paragraph 4 can be described as:

- O **A.** critical.
- O **B.** admiring.
- O **C.** paradoxical.
- O **D.** curious.

Passage 4 (Questions 19–24)

The "broken windows" theory and application of policing in New York purportedly became a "miracle" in reduction of crime, particularly homicide, within the city of New York. The interpretations of this idea became conflated with the ideas of "zero tolerance" practices in a number of cities, as well as in institutional contexts, such as education.

The idea behind "broken windows" is to make public space hospitable for everyone by eliminating incivilities that keep people off the streets. It's designed with policing communities, not people, in mind. Zero tolerance policing, by contrast, aggressively targets people—with results that even broken windows proponents agree can be disastrous. George Kelling, one of broken windows' original theorists, is a vigorous defender of New York's policing. But even he points out that the theory as he originally conceived it was intended not to justify aggressive police stops, but to reinforce neighborhood cohesion. "What's going on is the restoration of public spaces," says Kelling. "In some places, it's done wonderfully, and in some places, it's done terribly." So how did the broken windows theory turn into zero-tolerance policing—and can it be salvaged?

Kelling and James Q. Wilson made criminological history in 1982, when they argued in Atlantic Monthly that public disorder—panhandling, graffiti, and groups of unsupervised youth — were signals to would-be criminals that no one is watching. Disorder makes citizens withdraw from public places, they wrote, ceding those areas to disorderly people who feel little restraint from committing crimes. Wilson and Kelling believed disorder and its message of tolerance for crime was contagious, spreading from citizen to citizen and neighborhood to neighborhood—a kind of domestic domino theory.

There's one major problem: a significant lack of evidence that disorder encourages crime. Several recent studies have blown apart "disorder policing" research from the early 1990s, showing instead that the contribution of disorder to crime rates has been small at best. University of Chicago sociologist Robert Sampson found that many of the factors that produce disorder in neighborhoods—poverty, inequality, poor housing—also produce crime. In Baltimore, Temple University criminologist Ralph Taylor found that disorder and crime are loosely connected, but without a causal relationship. And in 1998, University of Arizona law professor Bernard Harcourt reanalyzed data from six cities, joining the chorus that found no evidence of a solid connection between disorder and crime.

But the influential theory survives in the public imagination as proven fact—and as the justification for zero-tolerance policing. When N.Y. Mayor Giuliani hired Bratton as police commissioner, he applied the broken windows theory to a range of minor crimes: jaywalking, panhandling, open bottles. Bratton even worked with Kelling, as head of New York's transit police, to target turnstile jumpers—whom he would later call "the biggest broken window in the transit system." Later dubbed "zero tolerance," Bratton's method of policing swept the nation, earning praise and emulation from departments nationwide.

But zero tolerance wasn't just an experiment that didn't pan out. Instead of building community confidence in public space, such policing undermined it by aggressively policing poor people in poor places. Studies by the state attorney general and the Civilian Complaint Review Board, as well as newspaper accounts, all tally with what citizens already knew: that police stops were often accompanied by verbal and physical abuse. In the city's poorest neighborhoods, and especially among African-American and Latino citizens, zero tolerance left a bitter aftertaste of citizen distrust of the police.

A growing body of evidence shows that citizens are more likely to comply with the law and cooperate with law enforcement when they feel they have been treated fairly by the police and the courts.

George L. Kelling, James Q. Wilson, The Atlantic Monthly Group. (2018, May 04). Broken Windows. Retrieved from https://www.theatlantic.com/magazine/archive/1982/03/broken-windows/304465/

Question 19

According to passage information, the connection between "broken windows" and "zero tolerance" is that:

- O **A.** the broken windows theory provided a false justification for zero tolerance policing.
- O **B.** the success of "broken windows" led to public use of zero tolerance policing.
- O **C.** broken windows focuses on individual criminals, while zero tolerance focuses on communities.
- O **D.** broken windows was successful, while zero tolerance has no scientific basis.

Question 20

The passage describes the causal link between disorder and crime as:

- O **A.** well-established and valid.
- O **B.** based on an over-generalization.
- O **C.** tenuous to nonexistent.
- O **D.** probable, but it is unclear which way the link runs.

Question 21

The author would likely support an initiative in large cities to:

- O **A.** replace zero-tolerance policing with more humane broken-windows policing.
- O **B.** institute zero-tolerance policing only in areas rife with disorder.
- O **C.** persuade law-abiding citizens not to withdraw from public life.
- O **D.** alter police behavior to gain the trust of citizens by being less aggressive.

Question 22

It can be inferred from the passage that:

- O **A.** zero tolerance policing led to the idea of "broken windows."
- O **B.** "broken windows" led to the public's rejection of zero tolerance policing.
- O **C.** zero tolerance policing and "broken windows" were offshoots of the same sociological theory
- O **D.** zero tolerance policing was incorrectly associated with the earlier concept of "broken windows"

Question 23

Which of the following ideas best represents the theme of "broken windows" policing?

- O **A.** Preventing breakages by arresting the small-time thugs and thieves
- O **B.** Targeting disordered acts to discourage more serious crime
- O **C.** Using small crimes like broken windows as clues to larger crimes
- O **D.** Targeting small-time criminals to prevent larger crime

Question 24

Zero tolerance policing in New York:

I. appeared to lead to a gradual proliferation in crime.
II. led to physical and verbal abuse often directed towards minorities.
III. would even focus on small crimes, such as "turnstile jumping" on transit systems.

- O **A.** I, II, III
- O **B.** III only
- O **C.** II and III
- O **D.** I and II

Passage 5 (Questions 25–29)

I have often heard people wonder what Shakespeare would say, if he could see Mr. Irving's production of his *Much Ado About Nothing*, or Mr. Wilson Barrett's setting of his *Hamlet*. Would he take pleasure in the glory of the scenery and the marvel of the colour? Would he be interested in the Cathedral of Messina, and the battlements of Elsinore? Or would he be indifferent, and say the play, and the play only, is the thing?

Speculations like these are always pleasurable, and in the present case happen to be profitable also. For it is not difficult to see what Shakespeare's attitude would be; not difficult, that is to say, if one reads Shakespeare himself, instead of reading merely what is written about him.

Speaking, for instance, directly, as the manager of a London theatre, through the lips of the chorus in *Henry V*, he complains of the smallness of the stage on which he has to produce the pageant of a big historical play, and of the want of scenery which obliges him to cut out many of its most picturesque incidents, apologises for the scanty number of supers who had to play the soldiers, and for the shabbiness of the properties, and, finally, expresses his regret at being unable to bring on real horses.

In the *Midsummer Night's Dream*, again, he gives us a most amusing picture of the straits to which theatrical managers of his day were reduced by the want of proper scenery. In fact, it is impossible to read him without seeing that he is constantly protesting against the two special limitations of the Elizabethan stage—the lack of suitable scenery, and the fashion of men playing women's parts, just as he protests against other difficulties with which managers of theatres have still to contend, such as actors who do not understand their words; actors who miss their cues; actors who overact their parts; actors who mouth; actors who gag; actors who play to the gallery, and amateur actors.

And, indeed, a great dramatist, as he was, could not but have felt very much hampered at being obliged continually to interrupt the progress of a play in order to send on someone to explain to the audience that the scene was to be changed to a particular place on the entrance of a particular character, and after his exit to somewhere else; that the stage was to represent the deck of a ship in a storm, or the interior of a Greek temple, or the streets of a certain town, to all of which inartistic devices Shakespeare is reduced, and for which he always amply apologises.

Besides this clumsy method, Shakespeare had two other substitutes for scenery—the hanging out of a placard, and his descriptions. The first of these could hardly have satisfied his passion for picturesqueness and his feeling for beauty, and certainly did not satisfy the dramatic critic of his day. But as regards the description, to those of us who look on Shakespeare not merely as a playwright but as a poet, and who enjoy reading him at home just as much as we enjoy seeing him acted, it may be a matter of congratulation that he had not at his command such skilled machinists as are in use now at the Princess's and at the Lyceum.

For had Cleopatra's barge, for instance, been a structure of canvas and Dutch metal, it would probably have been painted over or broken up after the withdrawal of the piece, and, even had it survived to our own day, would, I am afraid, have become extremely shabby by this time. Whereas now the beaten gold of its deck is still bright, and the purple of its sails still beautiful; its silver oars are not tired of keeping time to the music of the flutes they follow, nor the Nereid's flower-soft hands of touching its silken tackle; the mermaid still lies at its helm, and still on its deck stand the boys with their coloured fans.

Yet lovely as all Shakespeare's descriptive passages are, a description is in its essence undramatic. Theatrical audiences are far more impressed by what they look at than by what they listen to; and the modern dramatist, in having the surroundings of his play visibly presented to the audience when the curtain rises, enjoys an advantage for which Shakespeare often expresses his desire.

Reproduced in part from: Wilde, Oscar. A Critic in Pall Mall: Shakespeare on Scenery. *The Literature Network: Online Classic Literature, Poems, and Quotes. Essays & Summaries*, Jalic Inc. Retrieved from www.online-literature.com/wilde/a-critic/4/.

Question 25

What is this passage's main argument about Shakespeare's attitude to scenery?

- ○ **A.** Shakespeare would have disapproved of the elaborate scenery because it detracts from the poetry of descriptions.
- ○ **B.** Shakespeare would have approved of the elaborate scenery of the author's day because it made plays more dramatic and vivid.
- ○ **C.** Shakespeare would have been ambivalent about elaborate scenery because it adds to the visuals but detracts from the language.
- ○ **D.** Shakespeare lovers should spend less time debating about hypothetical questions and more time reading his work.

Question 26

The author's main point would be most weakened by the existence of:

- ○ **A.** a theater review from Shakespeare's time showing that Elizabethan sets were not always as minimal as once believed.
- ○ **B.** a modern production of a Shakespeare play which used no sets, props or costumes, but was hailed as brilliant.
- ○ **C.** a quote from Shakespeare in which he praised the way a person's imagination can conjure up an image more beautiful than any reality.
- ○ **D.** a quote from Shakespeare in which he criticized other dramatists for failing to describe the imagined settings of their plays in enough detail.

Question 27

In ancient Greece, productions of plays used only one or two actors to portray all the characters. Imagine the author was asked to consult on an upcoming production of an ancient Greek tragedy by Sophocles. The author would most likely recommend:

- ○ **A.** staging the play in exactly the same way as the ancient Greeks would have in order to stay true to Sophocles' vision.
- ○ **B.** staging the play with a different actor for each character in order to update it for modern times and conform to modern viewers' expectations.
- ○ **C.** using elaborate costumes to clarify the difference between characters.
- ○ **D.** using more than two actors if necessary in order to make the production as dramatic as possible.

Question 28

The author's main point in paragraph 6 is that:

- ○ **A.** Shakespeare's verbal descriptions are a perfect guide for how to stage his scenes.
- ○ **B.** unlike physical scenery, Shakespeare's verbal descriptions are still here for us to enjoy.
- ○ **C.** unlike physical scenery, Shakespeare's verbal descriptions are static and cannot be updated for new eras.
- ○ **D.** Shakespeare's physical scenery would have been destroyed or neglected because he was not revered as he is in our time.

Question 29

Which piece of evidence within the passage most strongly supports the claim that "it is not difficult to see what Shakespeare's attitude would be"?

- ○ **A.** "Shakespeare had two other substitutes for scenery—the hanging out of a placard, and his descriptions."
- ○ **B.** "The mermaid still lies at its helm, and still on its deck stand the boys with their coloured fans."
- ○ **C.** "In the *Midsummer Night's Dream*, again, he gives us a most amusing picture of the straits to which theatrical managers of his day were reduced by the want of proper scenery."
- ○ **D.** "He protests against other difficulties with which managers of theatres have still to contend, such as actors who do not understand their words; actors who miss their cues; actors who overact their parts."

Passage 6 (Questions 30–34)

Inferiority feelings and compensation originated with Adler's early studies of organ inferiority and compensation. In his book *Study of Organ Inferiority and Its Physical Compensation* (1907), Adler described the process of compensation for physical disabilities or limitations. Depending on the attitude taken toward his defects, a person's compensation for disabilities or limitations will be satisfactory or unsatisfactory. Favorite examples for Adler were Demosthenes, who became a great speaker in compensation for an early defect in speech; Annette Kellerman, who became a champion swimmer not as much despite as because of bodily weakness; and the limping Nurmi, who become a famous runner. Others with similar problems did not compensate by excelling, but used their defect as an excuse to preserve their fantasy that they would have gained prestige had they not had the defect.

From his understanding of organ inferiority, Adler began to see each individual as having a feeling of inferiority. Adler wrote, "To be a human being means to feel oneself inferior. The child comes into the world as a helpless little creature surrounded by powerful adults. A child is motivated by his feelings of inferiority to strive for greater things. When he has reached one level of development, he begins to feel inferior once more, and the striving for something better begins again which is the great driving force of mankind."

Every person has inferiority feelings, whether he will or can admit it. Adler says that since the feeling of inferiority is regarded as a sign of weakness and as something shameful, there is naturally a strong tendency to conceal it. Indeed, the effort of concealment may be so great that the person himself ceases to be aware of his inferiority as such, being wholly preoccupied with the consequences of the feeling and with all the objective details that subserve its concealment. So effectively may an individual train his whole mentality for this task that the entire current of his psychic life flows ceaselessly from below to above, that is, from feeling of inferiority to that of superiority. This occurs automatically and escapes his own notice. It is not surprising that we often receive a negative reply when we ask persons whether they have a feeling of inferiority. It is better not to press the point, but to observe their psychological movements, in which the attitude and individual goal can always be discerned.

The negative responses to these feelings of inferiority become the inferiority complex or the superiority complex. Both reflect feelings of inferiority, for they are two sides of the same coin. There are those who act and feel inferior and those who feel inferior but in denial try to lord it over others. The interesting thing is that they are both symptoms of a poor self-image. Individuals with a superiority complex are more concerned with attaining selfish goals than with social interest. They may express this selfishness through a need to dominate, or a refusal to cooperate, or they may want to take and not to give. Feelings of inferiority activate some to strive upward so that normal feelings of inferiority impel the human being to solve their problems successfully. On the other hand, the inferiority complex and/or the superiority complex impede or prevent them from doing so.

These feelings of inferiority lead to a striving for superiority. The striving for superiority is innate and carries individuals from one stage to the next. This striving can and does manifest itself in many different ways, and each person has his own way of attempting to achieve perfection. This idea progressed through three stages. Adler first came to the conclusion that aggression is more important than sexuality. The aggressive impulse was followed by the "will to power" and finally "striving for superiority." Many people reading Adler come to the false conclusion that striving for superiority is equated with "striving for power." Adler described the striving for power as a source of neurosis and crime. He pointed out that striving for power drives people in useless directions. Power-lust is a mental disorder or disease.

Reproduced in part from: Durbin, P.G. (2005, May). Alfred Adler's Understanding of Inferiority. *Subconsciously Speaking*. Retrieved from connection.ebscohost.com/c/articles/17270928/alfred-adlers-understanding-inferiority, Accession #17270928.

Question 30

The passage implies that, according to Adler, a person with a healthy self-image would likely engage in which of the following behaviors?

- ○ **A.** Develop a superiority complex
- ○ **B.** Strive for success but not for power
- ○ **C.** Strive successfully for power
- ○ **D.** Conceal his or her negative feelings

Question 31

Adler develops a number of famous examples of physical overcompensation including Demosthenes and Annette Kellerman. Which of the following famous personalities would NOT be an example of such overcompensation?

- ○ **A.** Nijinski, a famous dancer born with bird-like bone structure in his feet
- ○ **B.** Mel Tillis, a famous country singer afflicted with uncontrollable stuttering
- ○ **C.** John F. Kennedy, an asthma sufferer and great American politician and orator
- ○ **D.** Einstein, a great scientist afflicted with Asperger's syndrome and lack of social skills

Question 32

According to passage information, which of the following types of evidence would most strongly disprove Adler's theories?

- ○ **A.** Information from psychological assessments showing that there are far more people with an inferiority complex than a superiority complex
- ○ **B.** Information from confidential psychological assessments and clinical reports showing that some people never suffer feelings of inferiority
- ○ **C.** Evidence showing that some people with congenital diseases and disabilities are completely average in their career performance
- ○ **D.** Evidence from sociological studies showing that an inferiority complex is more harmful to career prospects than a superiority complex

Question 33

According to passage information, which of the following is true of inferiority feelings?

I. They have a positive aspect in spurring people to achieve more.
II. They can be overcome with effective therapy.
III. They produce harmful results if a person denies having them.

- ○ **A.** I only
- ○ **B.** I and III
- ○ **C.** II only
- ○ **D.** II and III

Question 34

Freud famously argued that a person's psychological development is dominated by the Oedipus complex, a child's unconscious desire to have sexual relations with the opposite-sex parent. Adler would likely:

- ○ **A.** disagree, because emotions and motives that are important to a person's psyche tend to take place at the conscious level.
- ○ **B.** disagree, because aggression is more important to the psyche than sexuality.
- ○ **C.** disagree, because theories about psychological development must be backed up by experimental data.
- ○ **D.** agree, because unconscious motives are crucial to human psychological life.

Passage 7 (Questions 35–41)

Every schoolboy knows that the Middle Ages arose on the ruins of the Roman Empire. The decline of Rome preceded and in some ways prepared the rise of the kingdoms and cultures which composed the medieval system. Yet in spite of the self-evident truth of this historical proposition we know little about life and thought in the watershed years when Europe was ceasing to be Roman but was not yet medieval. We do not know how it felt to watch the decline of Rome; we do not even know whether the men who watched it knew what they saw, though we can be quite certain that none of them foretold, indeed could have foreseen, the shape which the world was to take in later centuries.

Yet the tragic story, its main themes and protagonists were for all to see. No observer should have failed to notice that the Roman Empire of the fourth and fifth centuries was no longer the Roman Empire of the great Antonine and Augustan age; that it had lost its hold over its territories and its economic cohesion and was menaced by the barbarians who were in the end to overwhelm it. The territory of the Roman Empire had at its height stretched from the lands bordering the North Sea to the lands on the northern fringes of the Sahara, and from the Atlantic coast of Europe to the central Asiatic Steppes; it comprised most of the regions of the former Hellenic, Iranian, and Phoenician empires, and it either ruled or kept in check great clusters of peoples and principalities beyond its Gallic and north African frontiers. From these farthest frontiers Rome of the fourth century had retreated and was still retreating.

What then did it feel like to live at a time when civilization was going down before the forces of barbarism? Did people realize what was happening? Did the gloom of the Dark Ages cast its shadow before? It so happens that we can answer these questions very clearly if we fix our eyes on one particular part of the Empire, the famous and highly civilized province of Gaul. We can catch the decline at three points because in three consecutive centuries, Gallo-Roman writers have left us a picture of their life and times. In the fourth century we have Ausonius, in the fifth Sidonius Apollinarius, in the sixth Gregory of Tours and Fortunatus, a stranger from Italy, who made his home in Poitiers. They show us Auvergne and the Bordelais in the evening light. The fourth, the fifth, and the sixth centuries--going, going, gone!

Going! This is the world of Ausonius, south-western France in the latter half of the fourth century, "an Indian summer between ages of storm and wreckage." Ausonius himself is a scholar and a gentleman, the friend alike of the pagan Symmachus and of St Paulinus of Nela. He is for thirty years professor of rhetoric in the university of Bordeaux, for some time tutor to a prince, praetorian prefect of Gaul, consul, and in his last years just an old man contentedly living on his estates. His most famous poem is a description of the Moselle, which for all its literary affectations evokes most magically the smiling countryside which was the background of his life. High above the river on either bank stand the villas and country houses, with their courts and lawns and pillared porticos, and the hot baths from which, if you will, you can plunge into the stream.

Equally peaceful, equally pleasant is life on Ausonius' own estate in the Bordelais, his little patrimony (he calls it) although he had a thousand acres of vineyard and tillage and wood. Here he tends his roses and sends his boy round to the neighbours to bid them to luncheon, while he interviews the cook. Six, including the host, is the right number—if more it is not a meal but a mêlée. Then there are all his relatives to be commemorated in verse, his grandfather and his grandmother and his sisters and his cousins and his aunts (especially his aunts).

Such is the world depicted for us by Ausonius. But while this pleasant country house and senior common room life was going calmly on, what do we find happening in the history books? Ausonius was a man of nearly fifty when the Germans swarmed across the Rhine in 357, pillaging forty-five flourishing cities, and pitching their camps on the banks of the Moselle. He had seen the great Julian take up arms ("O Plato, Plato, what a task for a philosopher") and in a series of brilliant campaigns drive them out again. Ten years later when he was tutor to Gratian he had himself accompanied the emperor Valentinian on another campaign against the same foes. While he was preening himself on his consulship ten years later still, he must have heard of the disastrous battle of Adrianople in the east, when the Goths defeated a Roman army and slew an emperor. He died in 395 and within twelve years of his death the host of Germans had burst across the Rhine, "all Gaul was a smoking funeral pyre," and the Goths were at the gates of Rome. And what have Ausonius and his correspondents to say about this? Not a word. Ausonius and Symmachus and their set ignore the barbarians as completely as the novels of Jane Austen ignore the Napoleonic wars.

Power, Eileen Edna. *Medieval People*. Tredition Classics, 2013.

Question 35

What is the implied significance of the detail "Six, including the host, is the right number—if more it is not a meal but a mêlée"?

- ○ **A.** Life in 4th century Auvergne was governed by rigid codes of conduct, including for meals
- ○ **B.** People in 4th century Auvergne had lost the ability to hold peaceful large gatherings like those at the height of Roman civilization
- ○ **C.** Ausonius was an urbane man with a sophisticated outlook on every aspect of life
- ○ **D.** Ausonius was an elitist who liked to have as little contact as possible with most of his neighbors

Question 36

What is the main purpose of this passage?

- ○ **A.** To portray the 4th through 6th centuries as an unusual time period and explore what it was like to live through it
- ○ **B.** To portray the complex character of a man who was unique for his time because of his urbanity
- ○ **C.** To criticize other historians who have failed to answer the crucial question of what the 4th through 6th centuries were like
- ○ **D.** To lament the terrible loss to culture and civilization that took place when the Roman empire fell

Question 37

The author's main point in this passage would be most strongly contradicted by which of the following pieces of evidence?

- ○ **A.** An historical account showing that some aspects of Roman civilization persisted until the end of the 6th century
- ○ **B.** An account from the 4th century explaining why Germans resented the Roman empire and felt justified in occupying Roman land
- ○ **C.** A firsthand account from a 6th century Gallic landowner agonizing over the decline of civilization he was witnessing
- ○ **D.** A firsthand account from another 4th century Gallic author agonizing over the potential effects of Gothic invasion

Question 38

Which of the following types of scholars would likely find parallels between the historical account in the passage and our own time?

- ○ **A.** A historian who argues that present-day worries about the "dumbing down" of the American populace are overblown because people are actually performing better in IQ tests.
- ○ **B.** A historian who argues that the US's wars with Iraq and Afghanistan are a fluke in a greater trend toward ongoing peace between nations.
- ○ **C.** A scholar who believes "the American century" has ended and the U.S. is beginning to decline from the role of first-rate democracy.
- ○ **D.** A historian who argues that America continues to repeat the same mistakes because we are governed by the mythos of "American exceptionalism."

Question 39

A potential weakness of the passage is its lack of which of the following types of evidence?

- ○ **A.** Archaeological evidence demonstrating when the Barbarian invasions actually took place
- ○ **B.** Quotations from and analysis of Ausanius' poetry
- ○ **C.** A description of what the Middle Ages were like and how they differed from the Roman empire
- ○ **D.** Accounts from middle or lower-class citizens expressing their attitudes to political changes taking place

Question 40

Which of the following is NOT an implication of the passage?

- O **A.** Art, education and social graces are all marks of advanced civilization.
- O **B.** A way of life can be in decline for a long time before members of a society notice things are changing.
- O **C.** The decline of Roman civilization was able to take place because citizens like Ausanius were apathetic and did nothing to prevent it.
- O **D.** The lives of individuals are as important to the story of history as wars and political dynasties.

Question 41

How does the passage suggest the author views Ausonius' situation?

- O **A.** As poignant, because he did not realize how soon his way of life would disappear
- O **B.** As immoral, because he enjoyed a lavish lifestyle while other citizens suffered from the invasions
- O **C.** As banal, because he was a typical bourgeois estate holder
- O **D.** As significant, because Ausonius' household was indicative of changes to come

---

Passage 8 (Questions 42–46)

The most influential factor in Inca architecture was undeniably religion, which, along with the customs they practiced, depended largely on the climate of the region the Incas lived in. Evidently, in regions where the sun was oppressive during the day and night offered a pleasant coolness, the people worshiped the stars and moon instead. However, on the Peruvian Plateau where heat is not retained because of the high altitude of the Andes and the nights are extremely cold, it would be expected for the cult of the sun to be practiced. The adoration of the sun is also explained by the second story of the origin, which claims that the Sun spoke to his two children and proclaimed his greatness, which all the Incas acknowledged thereafter:

> I give men warmth when they are cold; I cause their fields to fructify and their cattle to multiply; each day that passes I go all around the world in order to have a better knowledge of men's needs and to satisfy these needs: follow my example.

Therefore, the Incas' general belief that their survival depended on the Sun, without which crops could not grow and their lives were generally intolerable, clearly explains and justifies the construction of one of the most beautiful structures in Cuzco, the Temple of the Sun. Periods of the year when the sun went farther north and the shadows became longer and longer were especially feared, for the people thought that it would eventually disappear and leave them to freeze and starve. Therefore, there is no doubt that the Temple of the Sun was erected as a sign of worship of the sun, a place where sacrifices were made and ceremonies were held to seek the favor of the Sun and ensure the prosperity of the Empire. It is associated with the Inca Yupanqui, the grandfather of Huaina Capac, not because he built it, for it existed from the time of the first Inca, but because he completed its decoration and lavished upon it the state of wealth and majesty in which the Spaniards found it. The Temple of the Sun was located on the site where stands today the Church of San Dominique and where the body of Manco Capac was believed to have turned into stone upon his death.

The temple's altar was situated on the east side, and over what was the high altar could be found the image of the Sun on a gold plate twice as thick as the wall-plates. This image, where the sun was represented with a round face and beams and flames of fire all in one piece, was so large that it stretched from wall to wall over the entire side of the temple. Metal in the Andes had a special status, and was a symbol of power holding religious significance. So the sole gigantic representation of their god using such rich materials clearly illustrates the importance of the worship of the Sun in the Inca religion, as well as the capital role of religion in the society.

Vega, G., et al. (2006). *Royal Commentaries of the Incas and General History of Peru: Abridged.* Hackett Pub. Co.

Question 42

The passage implies which of the following general statements?

- ○ **A.** Metal is a sign of reverence and power in all pre-state societies.
- ○ **B.** The Temple of the Sun still stands and is studied by archaeologists today.
- ○ **C.** A society's religious beliefs are the key to understanding their values.
- ○ **D.** A society's material circumstances will influence their beliefs.

Question 43

Based on passage information, it is likely that Huaina Capac was:

- ○ **A.** an Inca ruler who was revered for his achievements.
- ○ **B.** a Spanish adventurer who lived among the Incas.
- ○ **C.** a mythological figure and descendant of the first Inca.
- ○ **D.** an Inca holy man believed to be in favor with the Sun god.

Question 44

According to the passage, metal, particularly gold, was considered a "symbol of power holding religious significance." Based on this context, what does gold connote?

- ○ **A.** Luminescence
- ○ **B.** Monetary worth
- ○ **C.** Endurability
- ○ **D.** Propriety

Question 45

The author primarily discusses the temple as:

- ○ **A.** a magnificent structure that inspires awe and reverence in all who enter.
- ○ **B.** an example of the ways different societies express their beliefs.
- ○ **C.** proof of the size and vast wealth of Inca society.
- ○ **D.** evidence of Inca religious faith and reverence for the sun.

Question 46

Which of the following types of evidence would NOT weaken the author's claims in this passage?

- ○ **A.** Evidence that the Incas worshiped the moon and stars, although to a lesser extent than the sun
- ○ **B.** Evidence of a society that lived in a hot climate, but worshiped the sun
- ○ **C.** Evidence of an Inca building as magnificent as expensive as the Sun temple, but built for secular purposes
- ○ **D.** Evidence that metal was plentiful in the Andes, and gold was used for a variety of practical purposes

Passage 9 (Questions 47–53)

Noisy explosions, fast-paced editing that will most probably give you a headache, manly men saving Planet Earth from ridiculously terrifying enemy attackers, numerous scenes filled with violence, car chases and plenty of fighting of epic proportions. Sound familiar? These characteristics of the high-budget action blockbuster constitute Hollywood's quite possibly most overused generic formula in the last four decades—always poised for success and guaranteed to make a splash. The blockbuster film appears to satisfy viewers and fulfill their perhaps most primitive motive to go to the movies in the first place: to be entertained.

Blockbusters prove to be relatively accessible as they are a little bit of everything, which brings the issue of genre into discussion. Genre often helps us determine our expectations prior to viewing films. In the case of Hollywood blockbusters, which are dominated by the action and adventure genres, these expectations are often met, since film companies are fully conscious of what the audience wishes to see on the screen, of which they make use to do well at the box-office. It is, therefore, safe to say that one of genre's many functions is to lead filmmakers and film companies so their films can make profit by using conventions the audience is already familiar with. As pointed out by Steve Neale, genres "serve as basic and 'convenient' categories in which to organize capital assets so as to ensure that their capacity will be utilized to the maximum." To that end, genres have been known to be mingled to appeal to all kinds of audiences. Rick Altman states "At every turn, we find that Hollywood labours to identify its pictures with multiple genres, in order to benefit from the increased interest that this strategy inspires in diverse demographic groups."

Altman's categorization of genres may also come in handy at this point. He divides genres into three categories in relation to their appeal to various audiences: male, female, and tertium quid [third thing] genres, exemplified by the Western, romantic comedy, and fantasy respectively. The aforementioned action genre, characterized by never-ending adventure that keeps the audience on the edge of their seat, is inherently male, featuring almost exclusively male protagonists. Male genres, as a result, are more inclined to be targeted at male audiences. To attract female audiences as well, however, these mainstream films traditionally incorporate female characters and romance subplots into the mix.

This strategy has long been used, as made evident by Leo A. Handel's study titled "Hollywood Looks at Its Audience: A Report of Film Audience Research." Even though the survey was conducted back in 1942, it seems relevant to this today. Richard Maltby touches upon the survey in his article:

> Women expressed strong dislikes for mystery and horror pictures, gangster and G-men movies, war movies and Westerns. Their greatest enthusiasms were for love stories, which was the category most strongly disliked by men, whose strongest preference was for war movies. Hollywood's logic was to combine the two.

The aforementioned romance subplot seldom intersects with the primary storyline at hand and is often separated from it, not forwarding the main action of the film in any way. Female characters are usually left out from the venture taking place, or are present in the film for the entertainment of men. They tend to be portrayed as worrying about the male characters while they do all the work. Nevertheless, I would not go so far as to call their existence in these films utterly pointless, as they provide what I like to call "romantic relief."

The term is derived from "comic relief"—a device that functions as a getaway for the audience to relax in films otherwise deemed serious or heavy. I have coined this term to refer to any romance scene in a given film that features the male lead and his love interest.

Kartal, E. (2014). It Is a Man's World: Romantic Relief in The Hollywood Blockbuster. *CINEJ Cinema Journal*, *3*(6), 165–174. doi:10.5195/cinej.2014.89.

Question 47

The main purpose of this passage can be described as:

- ○ **A.** critiquing the Hollywood action blockbuster as sexist and formulaic.
- ○ **B.** analyzing the differences between male and female taste in movies.
- ○ **C.** analyzing the reasons the Hollywood action blockbuster appeals to primarily male audiences.
- ○ **D.** explaining why Hollywood movies make use of genre mixing and "romantic relief."

Question 48

Which of the following arguments could NOT be used to effectively question the need for studios to use "romantic relief"?

- ○ **A.** Women dislike genres such as action because they are typically made in a sexist way, and not because of the lack of romance.
- ○ **B.** Male viewers also enjoy the romance subplots in action movies.
- ○ **C.** The study "Hollywood Looks at Its Audiences" is too dated to apply well to today's viewers.
- ○ **D.** "Romantic relief" may be popular because it introduces relateable female characters, not because it uses romance plots.

Question 49

Why does the passage suggest that popular movies have so many formulaic elements?

- ○ **A.** Audiences are more satisfied by movies that contain familiar elements.
- ○ **B.** Hollywood writers and directors are unimaginative.
- ○ **C.** Hollywood writers and directors' stereotypical views of men and women prevents them from creating original characters.
- ○ **D.** Hollywood writers and directors must work within genres that are rigidly defined and do not evolve.

Question 50

We can infer from the passage that if Hollywood producers did not have to worry about how much money they would make from a given production, which of the following might happen?

- ○ **A.** There would be more romantic comedies and fewer mystery and horror movies.
- ○ **B.** Romance plots would be more integrated with movies' main plotlines.
- ○ **C.** Movies would appeal to more narrow segments of the viewing audience.
- ○ **D.** There would be fewer romance elements in movies.

Question 51

Which of the following assertions is LEAST supported by evidence in the passage?

- ○ **A.** "Film companies are fully conscious of what the audience wishes to see on the screen."
- ○ **B.** "This strategy has long been used."
- ○ **C.** "Genres have been known to be mingled to appeal to all kinds of audiences."
- ○ **D.** "Their perhaps most primitive motive to go to the movies in the first place [is] to be entertained."

Question 52

Which of the following hypothetical pieces of information would most strengthen the author's argument?

- ○ **A.** In a review of popular movies from the past ten years, over 70 percent featured a male lead character.
- ○ **B.** In test screenings, women reacted more favorably to an action movie when it was altered to feature a prominent romance subplot.
- ○ **C.** A study on box office ratings from the past ten years found that among single-genre movies, romantic comedies fared better than action movies.
- ○ **D.** A study of movies released in the past ten years showed that the vast majority of all releases featured some romance elements.

Question 53

Which of the following best describes the way that the author views the Hollywood establishment's attitude to women?

- ○ **A.** Female audience members are "separate but equal" because they watch different movies, but are considered just as important to cater to.
- ○ **B.** Female audience members are ignored in most genres.
- ○ **C.** Female audience members are a secondary consideration in most genres.
- ○ **D.** Hollywood has historically tried to attract female audience members, but largely failed.

 END OF EXAM SECTION.

CANDIDATE'S NAME ______________________________

RAW SCORE AND SCALED SCORE ______________________

GS-3
Mock Exam 3 of 7
Solutions at MCAT-prep.com

GS-3 Section III: Biological and Biochemical Foundations of Living Systems

Questions: 1-59
Time: 95 minutes

INSTRUCTIONS: Of all the questions on this test, most are organized into groups preceded by a passage. After evaluating the passage, select the best answer to each question in the group. Fifteen questions are independent of any descriptive passage or each other. Similarly, select the best answer to these questions. If you are unsure of an answer, eliminate the alternatives that you know to be incorrect and select an answer from the remaining alternatives. To indicate your selection, use a pencil to blacken the corresponding circle next to the answer choice and/or you can use the answer document at the back of this book. No marks are deducted for wrong answers.

The computer-based real MCAT has an on-screen highlighter function and ~~STRIKEOUT~~ function. These tools help to spotlight text or assist in the process of elimination. You may use a yellow highlighter for this paper-based exam and/or a pen (or preferably a pencil to make it easier should you change your mind) to mark text. At the time of publishing, both highlighting and strikeout functions can be used for passages, questions and answer choices. You can also flag a question to review later should time remain.

For the real exam, you will be provided with a dry erase board which is a white laminated noteboard booklet accompanied by a fine point marker. The noteboard includes 9 graph-lined pages for you to write though you cannot erase. You can simulate the experience with a fine point marker on a noteboard or with 8” x 14” plain graph paper.

You may consult the periodic table at any point during the science subtests.

Please note: For the real MCAT, a small number of field-tested questions will remain unscored.

This practice test has been designed exclusively to test knowledge and thinking skills. This exam may contain hypothetical statements and/or express controversial ideas. Statements contained herein do not necessarily reflect the policy, position, or view of RuveneCo Inc. or MCAT-prep.com.

START EXAM ONLY WHEN TIMER IS READY.

Passage 1 (Questions 1–4)

Neuroblastoma, a cancer that develops from immature nerve cells, is the most prevalent cancer in infancy, with nearly half of all cases occurring in children younger than the age of two. A group of scientists are particularly interested in Gli1, a transcription factor that tends to be amplified in cancerous cells, although the exact mechanism by which Gli1 affects neuroblastoma growth remains unclear.

Gli1 is downstream of the AKT signaling pathway, a signal transduction pathway that promotes cell growth and survival in response to extracellular signals. Stimulation by a variety of growth factors can trigger the pathway, leading to the activation of AKT. The overexpression of AKT's many isoforms, including AKT2, have been linked to the progression of several cancers such as neuroblastoma.

Experiment 1

To examine Gli1 transcriptional activity, human neuroblastoma cell lines BE(2)-C and BE(2)-M17 were co-transfected with His-GLI1, as well as plasmids containing either constitutively active AKT2 (Myr-AKT2) or empty plasmid (pcDNA). His-GLI1 contains a luciferase reporter gene, which is transcribed alongside Gli1 upon transcriptional activation. Luciferase reacts with a substrate to produce luminescence, which can be quantified as a measurement of transcriptional activity.

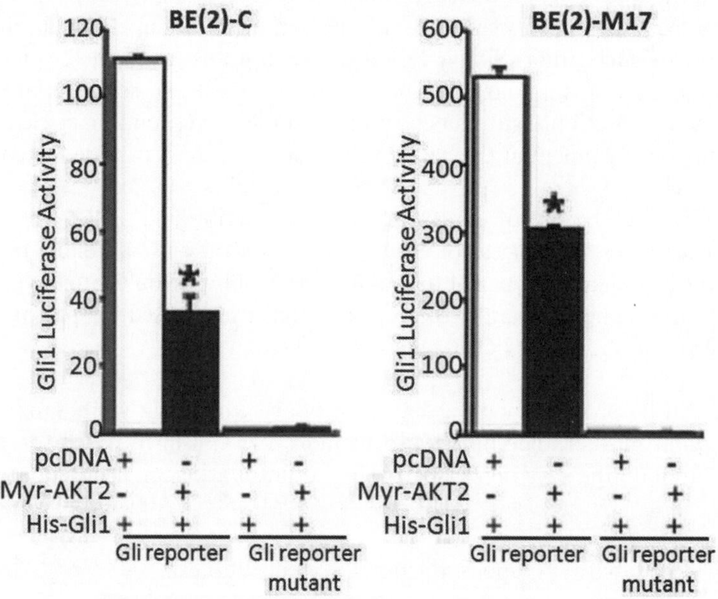

Figure 1 Effects of AKT2 overexpression on Gli1 transcriptional activity. A Gli reporter mutant was used as a negative control to establish a baseline for luciferase activity.

Experiment 2

In a separate experiment, the scientists discovered that silencing the expression of AKT2 significantly increased Gli1 transcriptional activity. However, silencing a different isoform, AKT1, had no significant effect on Gli1.

Adapted from P. Paul et al, "Gli1 Transcriptional Activity is Negatively Regulated by AKT2 in Neuroblastoma," *Oncotarget* (2013).

Question 1

Which of the following is most consistent with the relationship between AKT2 and Gli1?

- O **A.** Transcription of Gli1 causes AKT2 to be constitutively activated.
- O **B.** AKT2 overexpression increases Gli1 transcriptional activity.
- O **C.** All isoforms of AKT2 have an inhibitory effect on Gli1 transcription.
- O **D.** The activation of AKT2 negatively regulates Gli1.

Question 2

An enzyme known as GSK3β has been shown to negatively regulate AKT2. If Experiment 1 were repeated such that Myr-AKT2 is replaced with a plasmid (Myr-GSK3β) that leads to an overexpression of GSK3β, what would researchers expect to see?

- O **A.** Baseline luciferase activity would significantly increase.
- O **B.** There would be an increase in reporter luciferase activity in cells co-transfected with Myr-GSK3β.
- O **C.** The experiment results would closely mirror those conducted with Myr-AKT2.
- O **D.** Gli1 transcriptional activity would be significantly compromised.

Question 3

Active Gli1 likely accumulates in the:

- O **A.** nucleus.
- O **B.** mitochondria.
- O **C.** endoplasmic reticulum.
- O **D.** cytoplasm.

Question 4

Mouse embryos engineered to selectively overexpress Gli1 in the epidermis develop skin tumors that express endogenous Gli1. Analysis of the tumors show that the cells test negative for any of the known gene mutations that often typically lead to cancer. This suggests that:

- O **A.** an over-abundance of Gli1 alone is sufficient to drive tumor growth.
- O **B.** mice are an ineffective cancer modeling system.
- O **C.** Gli1 may have DNA repair functions that can correct oncogene mutations.
- O **D.** AKT2 is not expressed in epidermal cells.

Passage 2 (Questions 5–9)

Tryptophan is an essential amino acid in the human diet. Plants and microorganisms commonly synthesize tryptophan.

Sydney Brenner isolated *Salmonella typhimurium* mutants that were implicated in the biosynthesis of tryptophan and would not grow on minimal medium. When these mutants were tested on minimal medium to which one of four compounds had been added, the growth responses shown in Table 1 were obtained.

Table 1 Growth response on minimum unsupplemented medium and with indicated supplements.

Mutant	Minimal medium	Anthranilate	Indole-3-glycerol-phosphate	Indole	Tryptophan
trp-2	–	–	+	+	+
trp-3	–	–	–	+	+
trp-1	–	–	–	–	+
trp-8	–	+	+	+	+

Figure 1 Proposed biosynthetic pathway for naturally occurring tryptophan. There are 4 steps being considered and enumerated below from 1 to 4.

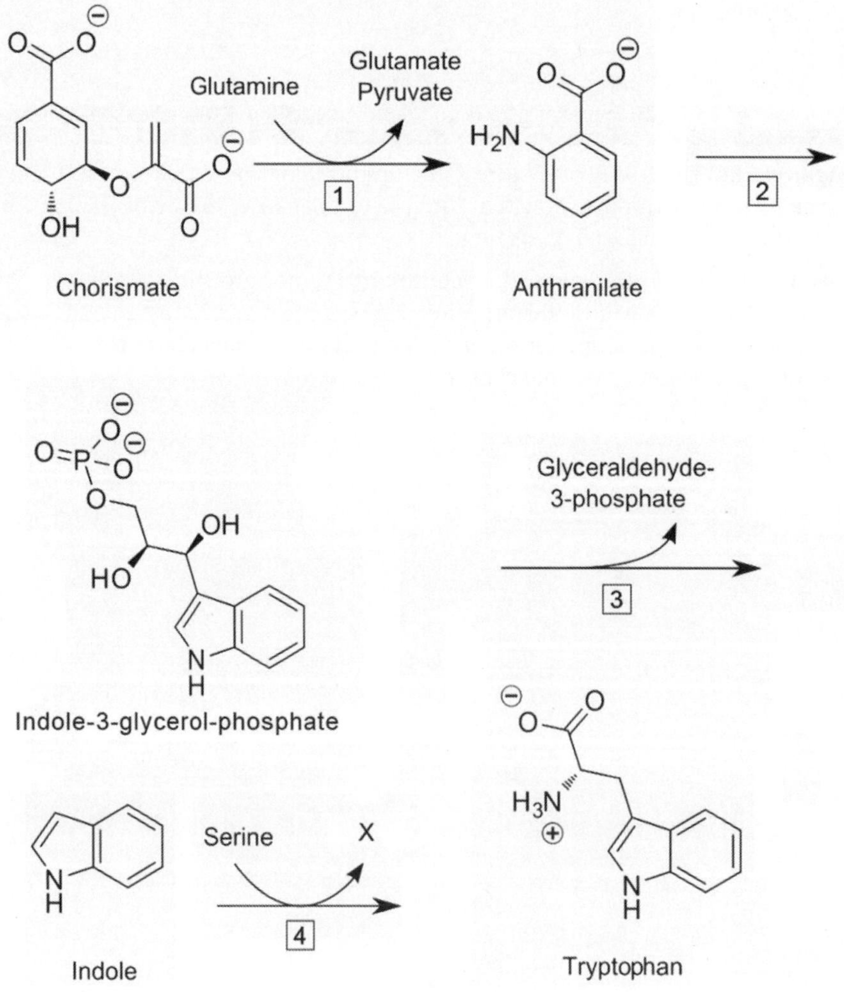

Glutamine
Glutamate
Pyruvate
1
2
Chorismate
Anthranilate
Glyceraldehyde-3-phosphate
3
Indole-3-glycerol-phosphate
Serine
X
4
Indole
Tryptophan

Question 5

Which of the following is NOT an accurate description of naturally occurring tryptophan?

- **A.** A cyclic enamine
- **B.** *L*-Configuration
- **C.** α-Amino acid
- **D.** *R*-Configuration

Question 6

The accumulation of indole-3-glycerol phosphate in cells would most immediately be associated with which of the following mutants?

- **A.** *trp*-2
- **B.** *trp*-3
- **C.** *trp*-1
- **D.** *trp*-8

Question 7

According to the information provided, a *trp*-1 mutant would only directly affect which of the following steps?

- **A.** Step 1
- **B.** Step 2
- **C.** Step 3
- **D.** Step 4

Question 8

In the biosynthetic pathway presented in Figure 1, in Step 4, what does the letter X represent?

- **A.** Hydroxide
- **B.** Water
- **C.** Ammonia
- **D.** Carbon dioxide

Question 9

Serotonin is a neurotransmitter biochemically derived from tryptophan. Consider the structure of serotonin below.

NH_2

HO

N
H

The most likely enzyme(s) involved in the biosynthesis of serotonin from tryptophan is (are) which of the following?

I. Isomerase
II. Hydroxylase
III. Decarboxylase

- **A.** I only
- **B.** II only
- **C.** II and III only
- **D.** I, II and III

The following questions are NOT based on a descriptive passage (Questions 10–13).

Question 10

Pyrimidines differ from purines in that they:

- O **A.** contain nitrogen.
- O **B.** are polar.
- O **C.** are smaller.
- O **D.** are found in DNA but not RNA.

Question 11

Which of the following can initiate the completion of the second meiotic division in oogenesis?

- O **A.** Estrogen
- O **B.** Progesterone
- O **C.** FSH
- O **D.** Fertilization

Question 12

All chordates possess a:

- O **A.** hollow dorsal nerve cord.
- O **B.** vertebral column.
- O **C.** cranium.
- O **D.** heart with a closed vascular system.

Question 13

All of the following are in the correct anatomic order EXCEPT:

- O **A.** trachea → larynx → bronchus.
- O **B.** nose → nasal cavity → nasopharynx.
- O **C.** alveolar ducts → alveolar sacs → alveolus.
- O **D.** bronchus → bronchioles → alveolar ducts.

Note: This page is left blank so that the passage would be visible without turning pages while assessing the passage-based questions.

Passage 3 (Questions 14–17)

Sweat is a watery fluid containing between 0.1 and 0.4% sodium chloride, sodium lactate and urea. It is less concentrated than blood plasma and is secreted by the activity of sweat glands under the control of pseudomotor neurons. These neurons are part of the sympathetic nervous system and they relay impulses from the hypothalamus.

When sweat evaporates from the skin surface, energy as latent heat of evaporation is lost from the body and this reduces body temperature. Experiments have now confirmed that sweating only occurs as a result of a rise in core body temperature. Blood from the carotid vessels flows to the hypothalamus and these experiments have indicated its role in thermoregulation. Inserting a thermistor against the eardrum gives an acceptable estimate of hypothalamic temperature.

Consider Figure 1.

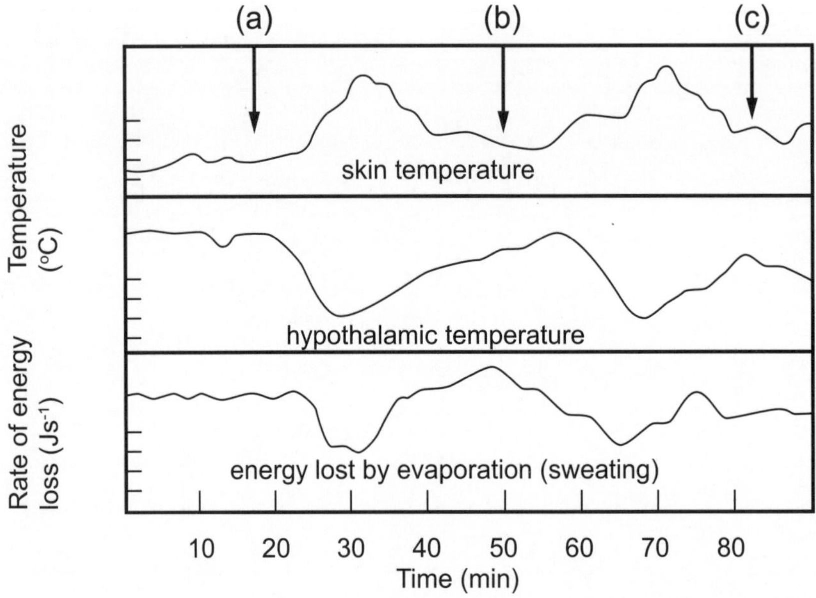

Figure 1 The relation between skin temperature, hypothalamic temperature and rate of evaporation for a human in a warm chamber (45 °C). Iced water is swallowed at points labeled (a), (b) and (c).

Question 14

The movement of electrolytes from blood plasma to the sweat glands would most reasonably be explained by which of the following processes?

- O **A.** Osmosis
- O **B.** Diffusion
- O **C.** Active transport
- O **D.** All of the above

Question 15

Drinking iced water results in a lowering of core body temperature. Thus, a trial exposing the skin to heat while drinking iced water would result in which of the following according to the passage?

- ○ **A.** If the person had been sweating prior to exposure to the trial then there would be an increase in sweating.
- ○ **B.** If the person had been sweating prior to exposure to the trial then there would be a decrease in sweating.
- ○ **C.** Irrespective of whether the person had been sweating prior to the trial, there would be an increase in sweating followed by a decrease in sweating.
- ○ **D.** Irrespective of whether the person had been sweating prior to the trial, there would be no change in sweat production.

Question 16

Based on the information provided, the relationship between hypothalamic temperature and rate of sweating could be best described as:

- ○ **A.** direct, suggesting that the rate of sweating is controlled by hypothalamic activity.
- ○ **B.** direct, suggesting that hypothalamic activity is controlled by the rate of sweating.
- ○ **C.** inverse, suggesting that changes in the rate of sweating occur in the opposite direction to changes in hypothalamic temperature.
- ○ **D.** independent, suggesting that the rate of sweating and hypothalamic activity change independently of each other.

Question 17

According to Figure 1, shortly after ingestion of the iced water, skin temperature rises. This can best be explained by which of the following?

- ○ **A.** As the evaporation rate falls, latent heat is no longer being lost front the skin, causing a rise in skin temperature.
- ○ **B.** The unusually high temperature of the chamber over the 30 minute period caused the rise in temperature.
- ○ **C.** The skin temperature rose to counteract the disturbance in body temperature caused by ingestion of the iced water.
- ○ **D.** Change in skin temperature always occurs in the opposite direction to change in hypothalamic temperature.

Passage 4 (Questions 18–21)

β-carotene, a pre-cursor of vitamin A, is a highly-pigmented terpenoid naturally found in many plants and algae. It is the main dietary source of provitamin A worldwide, with each molecule of β-carotene able to synthesize two molecules of vitamin A.

One natural, abundant source for β-carotene is the halophilic green algae, *Dunaliella salina*, which is cultivated for its over-production of carotenoids, which also causes the algae to appear orange. Because of the ease in which the organisms can be cultured, *D. salina* are also widely studied as a model system for carotenogenesis, the biosynthesis of carotenoids.

Researchers interested in studying the carotenogenesis pathway in *D. salina* chose to examine the effects of two possible carotenogenesis inhibitors: mevinolin, a fungal metabolite used as an anti-cholesterol drug, and fosmidomycin, an antibiotic that has also been used to treat malaria. Mevinolin functions by inhibiting HMG-CoA reductase, which catalyzes the conversion of HMG-CoA to mevalonate, while fosmidomycin inhibits DXP reductoisomerase (DXR).

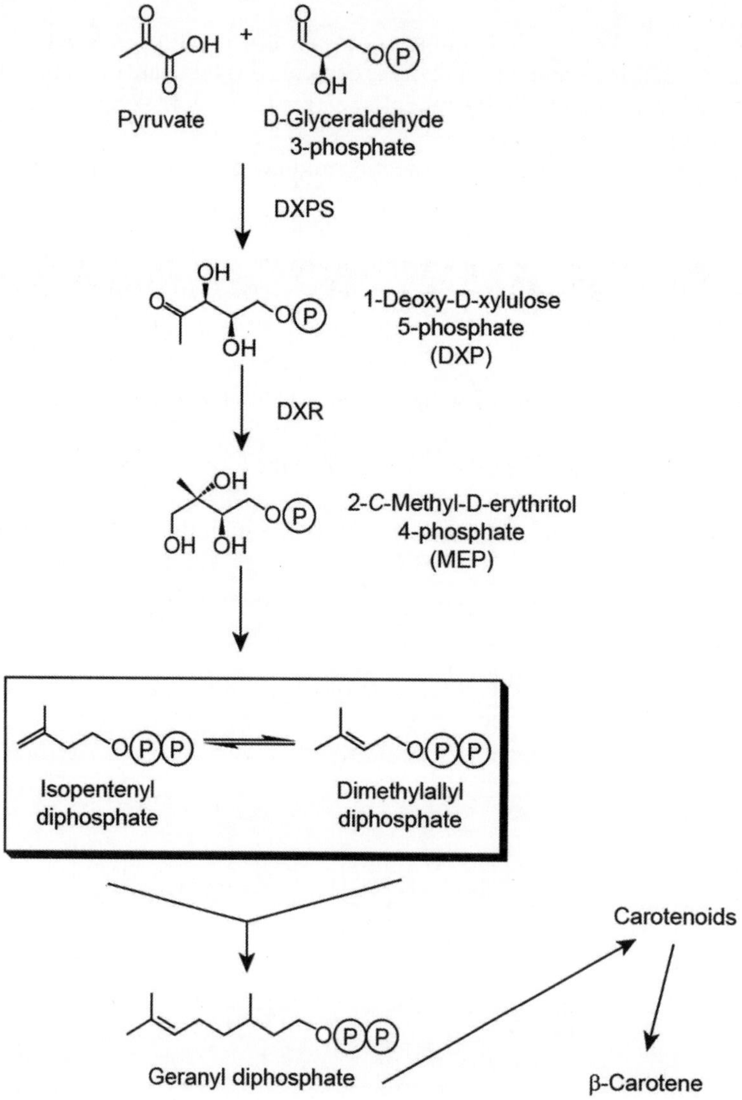

Pyruvate + D-Glyceraldehyde 3-phosphate

↓ DXPS

1-Deoxy-D-xylulose 5-phosphate (DXP)

↓ DXR

2-C-Methyl-D-erythritol 4-phosphate (MEP)

↓

Isopentenyl diphosphate ⇌ Dimethylallyl diphosphate

↓

Geranyl diphosphate → Carotenoids → β-Carotene

Figure 1 Simplified pathway showing the early steps of carotenogenesis and eventual β-carotene accumulation in *D. salina*. The conversion of pyruvate and D-glyceraldehyde-3-phosphate to DXP, catalyzed by DXPS, is the rate-limiting step.

Experiment 1

Three cultures of *D. salina* were grown simultaneously under conditions which enhance carotenoid production. Samples were taken every day for four days, and measured for β-carotene, which was normalized against cell numbers to account for any decreases in cell growth or viability.

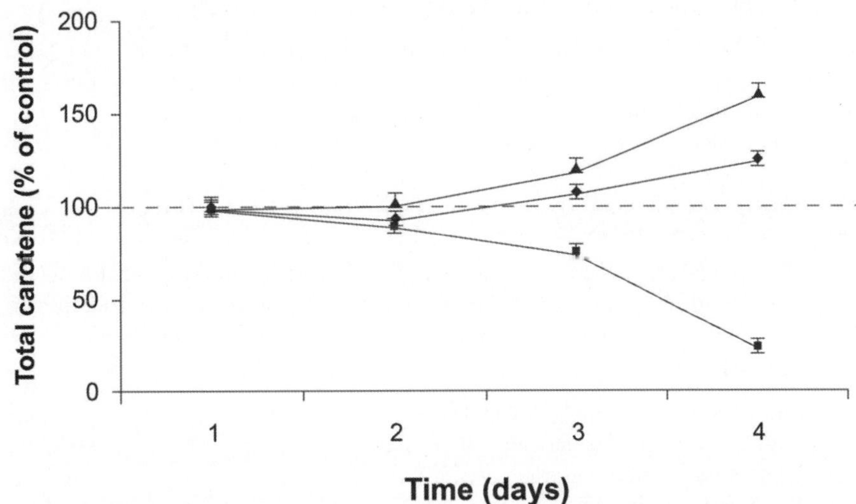

Figure 2 Change in total β-carotene percentage over time in *D. salina* with or without inhibitor. Total quantities of β-carotene were measured from samples taken from control *D. salina* without inhibitors (triangles), *D. salina* with 1 μM mevinolin (diamonds), and *D. salina* with 200 μM fosmidomycin (squares), and compared against fresh cultures. Data points are means ± SD, with each point representing n=3.

Adapted from J. Paniagua-Michel et al. *Mar Drugs*. Mar 2009; 7(1): 45–56.

Question 18

After four days, D. salina cultures with 200 μM fosmidomycin showed:

- O **A.** a 1.5-fold decrease in total β-carotene.
- O **B.** a 4-fold decrease in total β-carotene.
- O **C.** a 6.5-fold decrease in total β-carotene.
- O **D.** a 10-fold increase in total β-carotene.

Question 19

Plant and algae products that contain a significantly greater quantity of chlorophyll – as compared to β-carotene – appear green, while those that produce lower quantities of chlorophyll, such as carrots and mature pumpkins, appear orange. After five days of growing, spectrophotometric measurements of the *D. salina* cultures with inhibitors, compared to fresh cultures, would reveal:

- O **A.** increased absorption of green wavelengths in *D. salina* + fosmidomycin.
- O **B.** increased absorption of orange wavelengths in *D. salina* + fosmidomycin.
- O **C.** increased absorption of green wavelengths in *D. salina* + mevinolin.
- O **D.** decreased absorption of orange wavelengths in *D. salina* + mevinolin.

Question 20

Geranyl diphosphate is an intermediate in the HMG-CoA reductase pathway and is used in the biosynthesis of terpenoids such as β-carotene. When researchers performed Western blot analysis using the lysates from identical quantities of *D. salina*, with or without inhibitor, they found that both control algae and algae with mevinolin had similar amounts of geranyl diphosphate, while algae with fosmidomycin showed a moderate decrease. All of the following could be possible explanations for the findings, EXCEPT:

- O **A.** the inhibition of DXR decreases the rate of geranyl diphosphate synthesis.
- O **B.** mevinolin's mechanism of inhibition acts on intermediates downstream of geranyl diphosphate.
- O **C.** mevinolin is an inefficient inhibitor of HMG-CoA reductase in *D. salina*.
- O **D.** fosmidomycin completely blocks synthesis of geranyl diphosphate.

Question 21

Two mutant strains of *D. salina* (strains: A, B) were generated, each with defective carotenogenesis pathways marked by significantly decreased β-carotene production. An excess of pyruvate was added to both cultures. Strain A showed no effects, while Strain B showed a moderate increase in β-carotene production. What is a possible explanation for these results?

- O **A.** Pyruvate is not necessary for β-carotene synthesis.
- O **B.** A is deficient in DXR, while B is deficient in DXPS.
- O **C.** Only A has a defective carotenogenesis pathway.
- O **D.** Both A and B are deficient in DXPS.

Passage 5 (Questions 22–25)

A mutation is a change in the base sequence of DNA. The most common type of mutation involving single base pairs is "base substitution" or "point mutation," where a single base at one point in the DNA is replaced with a different base.

One method for detecting mutants involves selecting for an altered phenotype. Positive selection entails the detection of mutant cells by rejecting non-mutated parent cells. For example, a mutation for a particular antibiotic resistance in bacterial cells can be selected for by plating bacterial cells on a medium containing the particular antibiotic. Only the bacterial cells which have a mutant gene giving them resistance to the antibiotic are able to grow on the medium.

Negative selection entails "replica plating." This technique requires plating nearly 100 bacterial cells on a non-selective rich medium. After incubating, a sterile velvet pad is then applied to the colonies which form.

The pad is then applied to two different plates of media, one containing the same type of rich media from which the cells were lifted, the other a minimal media on which non-mutant bacteria can grow. Mutant colonies which grow on the rich media, but not the minimal media, are selected against.

Question 22

Which of the following best accounts for the reason a researcher would choose to perform a negative selection as opposed to a positive selection test?

- O **A.** The researcher wants to characterize the genome of a non-mutant wild type bacteria.
- O **B.** The researcher wants to characterize the genome of mutant bacteria.
- O **C.** The researcher wants to isolate non-mutant wild type bacteria.
- O **D.** The researcher wants to isolate mutant bacteria.

Question 23

As mentioned in the passage, point mutations are relatively common compared to other types of mutations. Which of the following represents a genetic mutation in which bases are added or deleted in numbers other than multiples of three?

- O **A.** Inversion
- O **B.** Duplication
- O **C.** Frame shift
- O **D.** Translocation

Question 24

Consider the following diagram:

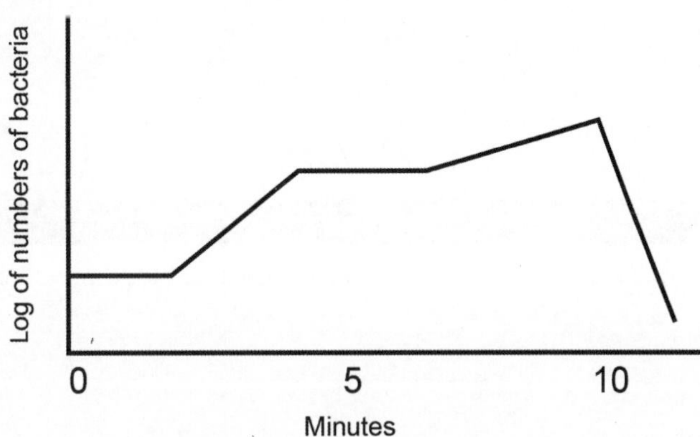

Figure 1 Bacterial Growth Curve

Which of the following is LEAST likely to account for the data presented in Figure 1?

- O **A.** The media contains two different carbohydrates, one of which serves as a more optimal growth source.
- O **B.** The temperature was increased 5 minutes into the test.
- O **C.** The pH of the medium was lowered 5 minutes into the test.
- O **D.** The bacterial cells lie dormant 10 minutes into the test.

Question 25

An effect of UV radiation on DNA is the formation of harmful covalent bonds among bases. For example, adjacent thymines form thymine dimers. Which of the following is most likely true of the bonds which create the dimers?

- O **A.** They consist of two carbon-carbon bonds between purines.
- O **B.** They consist of two carbon-carbon bonds between pyrimidines.
- O **C.** They consist of one carbon-carbon bond and one oxygen-sulfur bond between pyrimidines.
- O **D.** They consist of one carbon-carbon bond and one nitrogen-sulfur bond between pyrimidines.

The following questions are NOT based on a descriptive passage (Questions 26–29).

Question 26

Acid catalysts such as phosphoric acid are often used to dehydrate alcohols. The role of the acid catalyst is to:

- O **A.** lower $\Delta G°$ and increase the activation energy for the dehydration reaction.
- O **B.** increase $\Delta G°$ and lower the activation energy for the dehydration reaction.
- O **C.** maintain $\Delta G°$ at the same value and lower the activation energy for the dehydration reaction.
- O **D.** increase $\Delta G°$ and increase the activation energy for the dehydration reaction.

Question 27

All of the following are closely associated with microtubules EXCEPT:

- O **A.** cilia.
- O **B.** flagella.
- O **C.** villi.
- O **D.** centrioles.

Question 28

The structure in the brain responsible for maintaining homeostasis (i.e. blood pressure, body temperature, etc.) is the:

- O **A.** cerebellum.
- O **B.** pituitary.
- O **C.** hypothalamus.
- O **D.** thalamus.

Question 29

When electrons flow along the electron transport chain of a mitochondrion, which of the following changes occur?

- O **A.** The pH of the matrix increases.
- O **B.** ATP synthase pumps protons by active transport.
- O **C.** The electrons gain free energy.
- O **D.** The cytochromes of the chain phosphorylate ADP to form ATP.

Note: This page is left blank so that the passage would be visible without turning pages while assessing the passage-based questions.

Passage 6 (Questions 30–35)

β sheets are the second most common of the many possible secondary structures in proteins, behind alpha helices. β sheets are made up of laterally connected β strands, which are held together by hydrogen bonds, and can be arranged in parallel, or in anti-parallel configurations (Figure 1).

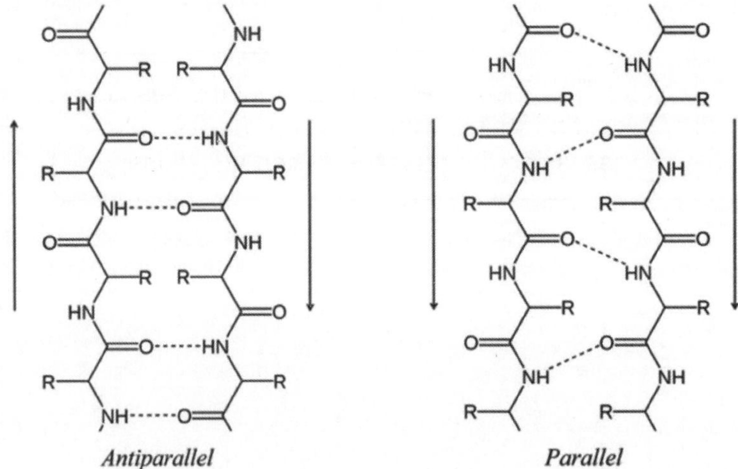

Figure 1 Hydrogen bonds between β strands. Dashed lines represent hydrogen bonds, while the arrows denote the direction of the peptide sequences (C → N).

Such β sheet structures are also commonly found in amyloids, insoluble fibrous protein aggregates that can arise as the product of misfolded proteins and other polypeptides found in the body. Often, these misfolded proteins inadvertently interact with each other, resulting in fibrils. Amyloids have been implicated in several neurodegenerative disorders, including Alzheimer's disease, the onset of which is associated with the formation of amyloid β (Aβ), the primary component of the amyloid plaques found in the brains of Alzheimer's patients. In addition to plaque formation, increased levels of Aβ can induce neuronal apoptosis, which can lead to the neurodegeneration seen in Alzheimer's disease.

Studies have shown that estrogen may be able to shield neuronal cells from Aβ-induced apoptosis by regulating certain mitochondrial proteins, such as the anti-apoptotic protein Bcl-2, and Bax, a protein that has been shown to promote cell death.

Experiment 1

Rat hippocampal neurons were pre-treated with either 10 ng/mL estradiol (E_2) or a control, and then exposed to Aβ for 72 hours. Cells were assessed for apoptosis using TUNEL staining, an assay that detects DNA fragmentation by labeling the terminal ends of nucleic acids.

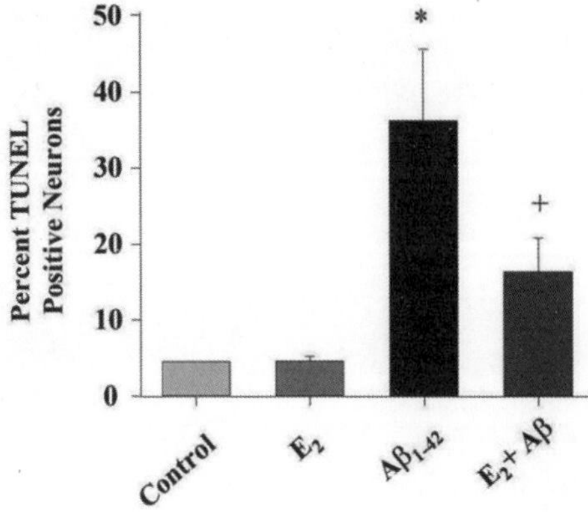

Figure 2 Counts of TUNEL-positive neurons normalized to total nuclei. Cells were treated with E_2 or control prior to 72-hour incubation with Aβ. (the symbols * and + = $p < 0.05$)

To establish how E_2 works to regulate Bcl-2 and Bax, two experiments were set up to show its effects on the expression of both proteins, and the translocation of Bax.

Experiment 2

Rat hippocampal neurons were pre-treated with either 10 ng/mL E_2 or control for 48 hours, then exposed to Aβ for 24 hours. Mitochondrial fractions were assessed for Bcl-2 expression by Western blot analysis.

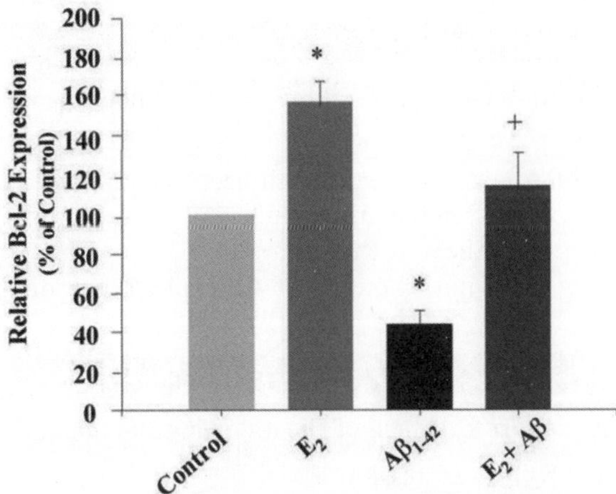

Figure 3 Western blot analysis of Bcl-2 expression in cells pre-treated with E_2 or control, and exposed to Aβ for 24 hours. (* = $p < 0.05$ as compared to control; + = $p < 0.05$ as compared to Aβ alone)

Experiment 3

One cause of neurotoxicity as a result of apoptosis results from the translocation of Bax from the cytosol to the mitochondria, where it can mediate the release of certain apoptotic factors. Rat hippocampal neurons were pre-treated with E_2 or control for 48 hours, then exposed to Aβ for 24 hours. Both mitochondrial and cytosolic fractions were assessed by Western blot analysis for Bax expression, as well as Bax localization.

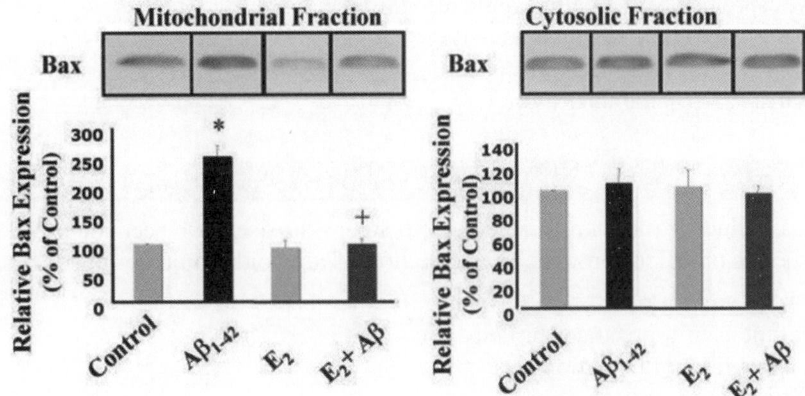

Figure 4 Western blot analysis of Bax expression in mitochondrial and cytosolic fractions in cells pre-treated with E_2 or control prior to Aβ exposure. (* = $p < 0.05$ as compared to control; + = $p < 0.05$ as compared to Aβ alone)

Adapted from Nilsen et al, "Estrogen protects neuronal cells from amyloid beta-induced apoptosis via regulation of mitochondrial proteins and function," BMC Neuroscience, 2006.

Question 30

Which arrangement of beta strands yields the most stable secondary structure?

- O **A.** Parallel
- O **B.** Antiparallel
- O **C.** Both are equal
- O **D.** Cannot be determined

Question 31

Considering the data presented, the pre-treatment of rat hippocampal neurons with E_2 provides evidence for all of the following EXCEPT:

- O **A.** lowering the percentage of Aβ-exposed neurons subject to apoptosis.
- O **B.** increasing the expression of Bcl-2 in the mitochondria of Aβ-exposed neurons.
- O **C.** promoting Bax translocation to the mitochondria.
- O **D.** decreasing Bax expression in the mitochondria of Aβ-exposed neurons.

Question 32

The experiments provide the most support for which of the following statements?

- O **A.** Aβ formation is triggered by Bax expression.
- O **B.** Overexpression of Bcl-2 leads to apoptosis.
- O **C.** Bax expression is induced by Aβ formation.
- O **D.** E_2 increases mitochondrial Bcl-2 expression.

Question 33

During apoptosis, the cell undergoes karyorrhexis, wherein the nucleus is fragmented, and chromatin is distributed throughout the cytoplasm. During this process, DNA is cleaved by an enzyme called caspase-activated-DNase (CAD), which cuts the DNA into fragments of roughly 180 base pairs. What is a likely explanation for this phenomenon?

- O **A.** CAD cleaves specifically at a palindromic recognition site.
- O **B.** CAD cleaves at internucleosomal linker sites.
- O **C.** CAD inhibits DNA repair mechanisms.
- O **D.** CAD activates nearby endonucleases.

Question 34

Over a dozen amyloids, including those implicated in Alzheimer's disease, have been identified to date. Each one is a by-product of a specific precursor protein. The formation of amyloids could be caused by:

- O **A.** hydrophobic interactions.
- O **B.** random mutations of a precursor protein.
- O **C.** significant temperature fluctuations.
- O **D.** all of the above.

Question 35

Mutations introducing proline into the middle of a β sheet often disrupt the protein's secondary structure. Proline is not favored in beta sheet structures because:

- O **A.** it exists in both *trans* and *cis* configurations.
- O **B.** its negative charge disrupts the H-bonding network.
- O **C.** its side chain is too bulky.
- O **D.** it cannot complete the H-bonding network.

Passage 7 (Questions 36–39)

Following blastula formation the developing embryo undergoes gastrulation, a tremendous reshaping with little or no additional cell growth. Since the blastulas vary in shape between different animals, the geometry of the reshaping also varies. Regardless of the type of animal, gastrulation results in the same fundamental cell layers: the ectoderm, the endoderm and the mesoderm. These three tissue types or *primordial layers* will form every organ in the developing embryo.

Research has recently shed light on the cells responsible for the continuation of the life cycle - the gametes. Early in the development of all animals, certain cells undergo determination producing primordial germ cells. Experiments have demonstrated an area in the egg cytoplasm of some animals which appears to be responsible for the determination of the primordial germ cell. This special region is the *germ plasm*.

To clarify the importance of the germ plasm, experiments have been carried out using microinjection of the developing fruit fly *Drosophila melanogaster*. Under normal conditions, pregametic cells arise from the posterior end of the syncytial blastoderm. Irradiation of this end of the egg produces a sterile fly. If cytoplasmic material from the posterior part of the developing egg is suctioned with a micropipette and injected into the anterior part of another developing egg, germ cells are formed at this abnormal site as well as the normal position. No nuclei are transferred in this experiment thus the evidence points to non-genetic material in the germ plasm of the egg being responsible for germ cell formation.

Question 36

Damage to the ectoderm during gastrulation will result in an embryo with an underdeveloped:

- ○ **A.** reproductive system.
- ○ **B.** nervous system.
- ○ **C.** excretory system.
- ○ **D.** digestive system.

Question 37

Immediately prior to gastrulation, which of the following events take place?

- ○ **A.** The sperm penetrates the corona radiata and zona pellucida so that fusion of the gametes occurs.
- ○ **B.** The secondary oocyte becomes a mature ovum by completing its second meiotic division.
- ○ **C.** Implantation in the endometrium occurs.
- ○ **D.** Rapid mitotic divisions result in daughter cells, smaller than their parent cells, being formed.

Question 38

After sexual maturation, the primordial germ cells in the testes are initially called:

- ○ **A.** spermatids and are haploid.
- ○ **B.** primary spermatocytes and are haploid.
- ○ **C.** primary spermatocytes and are diploid.
- ○ **D.** spermatogonia and are diploid.

Question 39

Which of the following experimental results would contradict the conclusion made from the experiment in the passage?

- ○ **A.** The only subunits detected after digesting the germ plasm were non-uracil containing nucleotides.
- ○ **B.** Microinjection of the midportion of a developing egg with germ plasm resulted in germ cell production at an abnormal site.
- ○ **C.** Microinjection of proteases into the posterior end of the syncytial blastoderm inhibited the production of germ cells.
- ○ **D.** The irradiated egg which produced a sterile fly demonstrated no post-radiation genetic abnormalities.

Passage 8 (Questions 40–43)

Much of the study of evolution of interspecific interactions had focused on the results rather than the process of coevolution. In only a few cases has the genetic bases of interspecific interactions been explored. One of the most intriguing results has been the description of "gene-for-gene" systems governing the interaction between certain parasites and their hosts. In several crop plants, dominant alleles at a number of loci have been described that confer resistance to a pathogenic fungus; for each such gene, the fungus appears to have a recessive allele for "virulence" that enables the fungus to attack the otherwise resistant host. Cases of character displacement among competing species are among the best evidence that interspecific interactions can result in genetic change.

Assuming that parasites and their hosts coevolve in an "arms race," we might deduce that the parasite is "ahead" if local populations are more capable of attacking the host population with which they are associated than other populations. Whereas the host may be "ahead" if local populations are more resistant to the local parasite than to other populations of the parasite.

Several studies have been done to evaluate coevolutionary interactions between parasites and hosts, or predators and prey. In one, the fluctuations in populations of houseflies and of a wasp that parasitized them were recorded. The results of the experiment are shown in Figure 1.

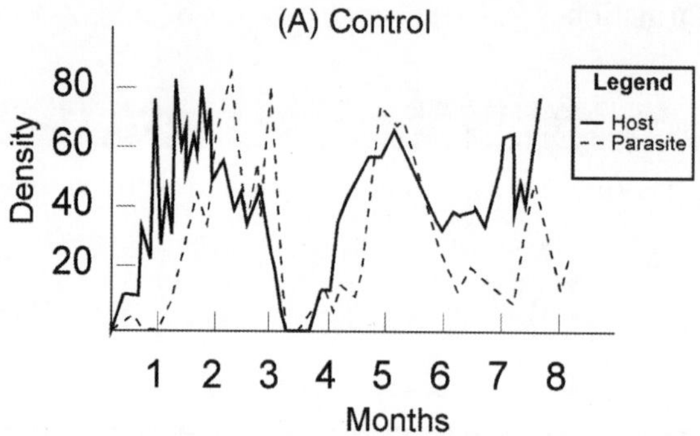

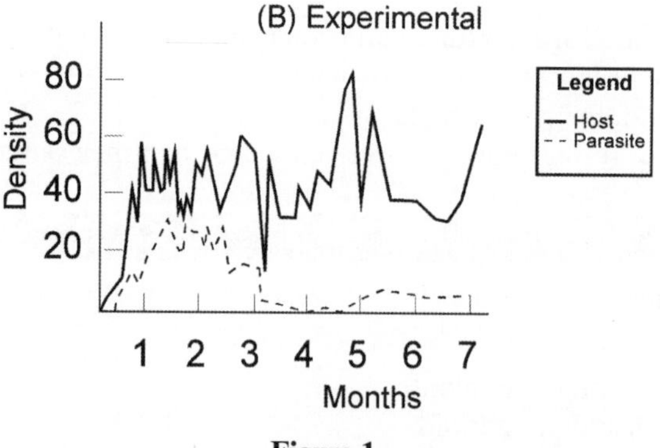

Figure 1

Question 40

A pathogenic fungus is more capable of growth and reproduction on its native population of its sole host, the wild hog peanut, than on plants from other populations of the same species. It is reasonable to conclude that:

- ○ **A.** the fungus, in this instance, was capable of more rapid adaptation to its host than vice versa.
- ○ **B.** the fungus, in this instance, was capable of more rapid adaptation to all populations of the host species than vice versa.
- ○ **C.** the host, in this instance, was capable of more rapid adaptation to the fungus than vice versa.
- ○ **D.** all populations of the host species were capable of more rapid adaptation to the fungus than vice versa.

Question 41

The passage suggests that one result of interspecific interactions might be:

- **A.** genetic drift within sympatric populations.
- **B.** genetic drift within allopatric populations.
- **C.** genetic mutations within sympatric populations.
- **D.** genetic mutations within allopatric populations.

Question 42

The control in the experiment likely consisted of:

- **A.** members from different populations of the host and parasite species used in the experimental group, that had a short history of exposure to one another.
- **B.** members of the host and parasite species used in the experimental group, that had a long history of exposure to one another.
- **C.** members of the host and parasite species used in the experimental group that had no history of exposure to one another.
- **D.** members from different populations of the host and parasite species used in the experimental group, that had a long history of exposure to one another.

Question 43

Penicillin is an antibiotic which destroys bacteria by interfering with cell wall production. Could the development of bacterial resistance to Penicillin be considered similar to coevolution?

- **A.** Yes, a spontaneous mutation is likely to confer resistance to Penicillin.
- **B.** No, an organism can only evolve in response to another organism.
- **C.** Yes, as antibiotics continue to change there will be a selective pressure for bacterial genes which confer resistance.
- **D.** No, bacteria have plasma membranes and can survive without cell walls.

The following questions are NOT based on a descriptive passage (Questions 44–47).

Question 44

During strenuous exercise, the NADH formed in the glyceraldehyde-3-phosphate dehydrogenase reaction in skeletal muscle must be reoxidized to NAD^+ if glycolysis is to continue. The key reaction involved in the reoxidation of NADH is most clearly outlined by which of the following?

- **A.** glucose 6-phosphate → fructose 6-phosphate
- **B.** dihydroxyacetone phosphate → glycerol 3-phosphate
- **C.** isocitrate → α-ketoglutarate
- **D.** pyruvate → lactate

Question 45

The biosynthesis of a pentasacharide of the monomer D-glucose ($C_6H_{12}O_6$) would be expected to have a molecular formula consistent with which of the following?

- **A.** $C_{30}H_{52}O_{26}$
- **B.** $C_{30}H_{58}O_{29}$
- **C.** $C_{30}H_{50}O_{25}$
- **D.** $(C_6H_{12}O_6)_5$

Question 46

When a dilute solution of formaldehyde is dissolved in ^{18}O-labeled water and allowed to equilibrate, ^{18}O incorporation occurs thus indicating the existence of the primary product. Which of the following compounds best represents the product of this ^{18}O exchange?

○ **A.** 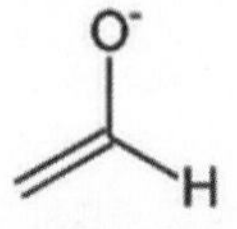 O^- ... H

○ **B.** 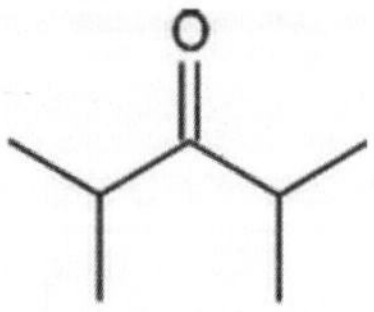 O

○ **C.** 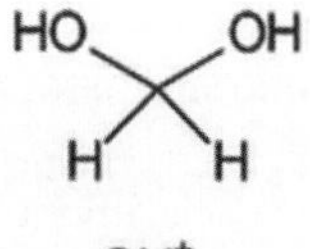 HO OH / H H

○ **D.** 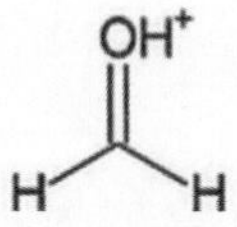 OH^+ / H H

Question 47

Which of the following is the first step in the polymerase chain reaction (PCR)?

○ **A.** Denaturation
○ **B.** Cooling
○ **C.** Primer extension
○ **D.** Annealing

Passage 9 (Questions 48–52)

E. coli is a bacterial cell which contains a single circular chromosome and three DNA polymerase enzymes - Pol I, Pol II, and Pol III. Replication of DNA in *E. coli* leads to the formation of a replication eye at which point, the replicating chromosome is referred to as the theta structure.

It is reasonable to conclude that the replication eye contains two partially separated parental DNA strands and two newly synthesized DNA strands. It was not clear for a long time, however, whether or not replication occurred in one direction or both directions about the origin of replication. Eventually, convincing evidence of bidirectional replication was obtained by measuring gene frequencies during replication.

Continuous synthesis on both strands of a replication fork requires synthesis in the 5' to 3' direction on one strand and in the 3' to 5' direction on the other strand. Since Pol I only adds nucleotides in the 5' to 3' direction, it was proposed that Pol I could not be the enzyme responsible for DNA replication in *E. coli*. In order to prove this and determine the role of Pol I in *E. coli*, the following experiments were performed.

Experiment 1

The Pol A Mutant of *E. coli*, which lacks Pol I enzyme activity was grown on agar for several generations and then exposed to ultraviolet light.

Result:

The Pol A Mutants grew in the agar successfully for several generations, but died when they were exposed to ultraviolet light.

Experiment 2

The temperature sensitive type mutants (TS type) of *E. coli*, which contains a mutant gene that codes for a Pol III enzyme that does not work at high temperatures, were grown on two separate agar dishes. The dishes were incubated at 30 °C and 42 °C, respectively, and left to grow for several generations.

Result:

The TS type *E. coli*, incubated at 42 °C, did not grow, but the TS type *E. coli*, incubated at 30 °C, grew successfully for several generations.

Question 48

If replication occurred in a bidirectional manner, then shortly after initiation:

- ○ **A.** each gene in the *E. coli* genome would be represented only once.
- ○ **B.** each gene in the *E. coli* genome would be represented twice.
- ○ **C.** DNA duplication would begin on both sides of the origin of replication.
- ○ **D.** gene frequencies should be very high for regions symmetrically disposed about the origin.

Question 49

In Experiment 1, if the researcher wanted to prove that the ultraviolet light had killed the bacteria, she would simultaneously:

- ○ **A.** grow TS type *E. coli* and expose to ultraviolet light.
- ○ **B.** grow Pol A Mutants and irradiate.
- ○ **C.** grow Pol A Mutants without ultraviolet light.
- ○ **D.** not run an experiment since the conclusion is obvious.

Question 50

The strongest evidence that Pol I was not the main replicating enzyme in *E. coli* was given by the fact that:

- ○ **A.** Pol A Mutants grew successfully.
- ○ **B.** Pol A Mutants died from exposure to ultraviolet radiation.
- ○ **C.** TS type *E. coli* grew successfully at 30 °C, but not at 42 °C.
- ○ **D.** the Pol III enzyme does not work at temperatures over 42 °C.

Question 51

The passage suggests that the main reason that TS type *E. coli* cannot grow above 42 °C, is that:

- ○ **A.** the TS mutant gene causes dehydration of the cell contents at high temperatures.
- ○ **B.** high temperatures cause DNA mutations that cannot be repaired because of the dysfunctional Pol III.
- ○ **C.** the TS mutant gene causes the cell to stop producing Pol III at high temperatures.
- ○ **D.** the TS mutant gene causes the tertiary structure of Pol III to be lost at high temperatures.

Question 52

In a separate experiment, wild-type *E. coli* was allowed to replicate in the presence of ^{3}H-thymidine. During the second round of replication, what would an autoradiograph, which detects irradiation, show if the replication was semi-conservative?

- ○ **A.** A uniformly unlabeled structure
- ○ **B.** A uniformly labeled structure
- ○ **C.** One branch of the growing replication eye would be half as strongly labeled as the remainder of the chromosome
- ○ **D.** One branch of the growing replication eye would be twice as strongly labeled as the remainder of the chromosome

Passage 10 (Questions 53–56)

Viral hepatitis type B (serum hepatitis) is an infection of humans that primarily damages the liver. The causative agent is a virus called HBV, which is transmitted in much the same way as the HIV virus.

If HBV could be cultivated in the laboratory in unlimited amounts, it could be injected into humans as a vaccine to stimulate immunity against hepatitis type B. Unfortunately, it is not yet possible to grow HBV in laboratory culture. However, the blood of chronically infected people contains numerous particles of a harmless protein component of the virus. This protein, called HBsAg, can be extracted from the blood, purified, and treated chemically to destroy any live virus that might also be present. When HBsAg particles are injected into humans, they stimulate immunity against the complete infectious virus.

Of late, a new source of HBsAg particles have become available. Thanks to genetic engineering, a technique for cloning the gene for HBsAg into cells of the common bread yeast *Saccharomyces cerevisiae* has been developed. The yeast expresses the gene and makes HBsAg particles that can be extracted after the cells are broken. Since yeast cells are easy to propagate, it is now possible to obtain unlimited amounts of HBsAg particles.

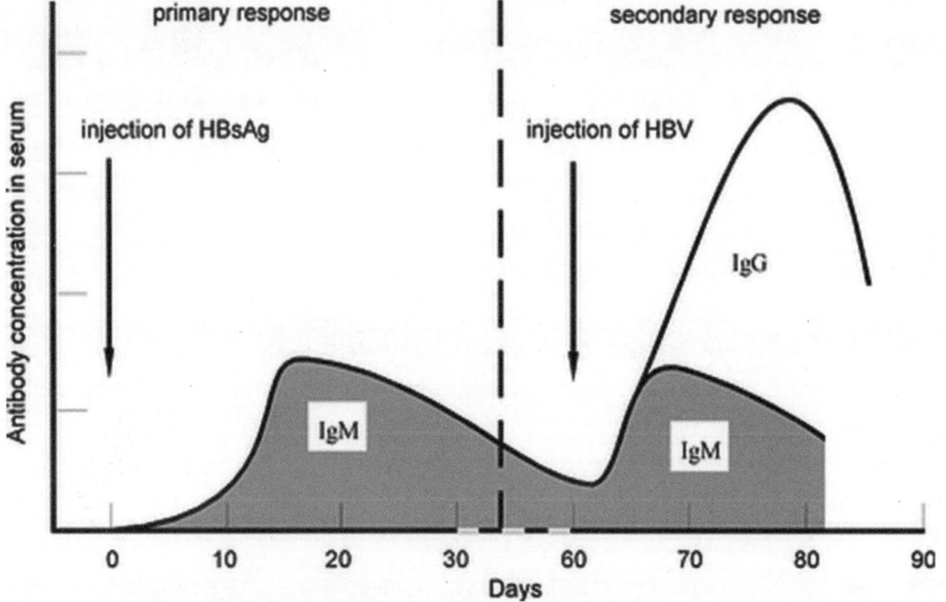

Figure 1 Mammalian animal model of immune response *in vivo* in response to an initial injection of HBsAg and a subsequent injection of the HBV virus

Question 53

Before being injected into humans, the HBV virus would first have to:

- O **A.** be cloned in yeast cells to ensure that enough of the virus had been injected to elicit an immune response.
- O **B.** have its protein coat removed.
- O **C.** be purified.
- O **D.** be inactivated.

Question 54

HBsAg is likely a component of:

- O **A.** the capsid of the virus.
- O **B.** the nucleic acid core of the virus.
- O **C.** the tail of the virus.
- O **D.** the slimy mucoid-like capsule on the outer surface of the virus.

Question 55

Consider the response to the initial injection of HBsAg and the subsequent injection of the HBV virus as shown in Figure 1. Which of the following best explains the differences in the two responses?

- O **A.** During the initial response, the immune response was carried out primarily by macrophages and B-lymphocytes.
- O **B.** During the secondary response, T-cells possessing membrane receptors, recognized and attacked the viral antigens.
- O **C.** Memory cells produced by T- and B-cells during the first exposure made the second response faster and more intense.
- O **D.** Memory cells produced by red blood cells during the first infection recognized the viral antigens more quickly during the second infection, causing antibody production to be increased.

Question 56

Yeast cells used for cloning the gene for HBsAg could be propagated by all but which of the following methods?

- O **A.** Budding
- O **B.** Transduction
- O **C.** Fusion
- O **D.** Meiotic division

The following questions are NOT based on a descriptive passage (Questions 57–59).

Question 57

Gene loci A, B, H and J are in the same linkage group but not necessarily in that order. Test crosses were done with each cross involving two of the gene loci. A percent recombination was obtained for each pair of gene loci.

Pair of Loci	A and B	A and J	B and H	J and H
Recombination	16%	10%	11%	5%

What is the order of the loci?

- ○ **A.** B, H, J, A
- ○ **B.** A, J, B, H
- ○ **C.** B, J, H, A
- ○ **D.** A, J, H, B

Question 58

Consider the structure of the following tetrapeptide.

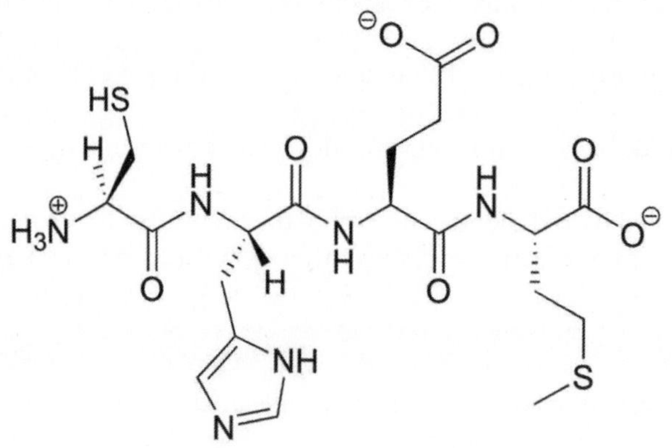

Which of the following is NOT accurate regarding the structure of the tetrapeptide provided?

- ○ **A.** At a higher pH, at least one carboxylate group would eventually be protonated.
- ○ **B.** The primary structure can be represented as CHEM.
- ○ **C.** There is no potential for an intramolecular disulfide bond.
- ○ **D.** There is potential to receive and donate hydrogen bonds.

Question 59

The concept of "induced fit" is most closely related to which of the following?

- ○ **A.** Enzyme specificity is induced by enzyme-substrate binding.
- ○ **B.** Enzyme-substrate binding induces movement following the reaction coordinate to the transition state.
- ○ **C.** Substrate binding can induce a conformational change in the enzyme, which subsequently brings catalytic groups into proper orientation.
- ○ **D.** When a substrate binds to an enzyme, the enzyme induces desolvation, or water loss, from the active site for optimal binding.

CANDIDATE'S NAME ____________________________________

RAW SCORE AND SCALED SCORE ____________________________

GS-3
Mock Exam 3 of 7
Solutions at MCAT-prep.com

GS-3 Section IV: Psychological, Social, and Biological Foundations of Behavior

Questions: 1-59
Time: 95 minutes

INSTRUCTIONS: Of all the questions on this test, most are organized into groups preceded by a passage. After evaluating the passage, select the best answer to each question in the group. Fifteen questions are independent of any descriptive passage or each other. Similarly, select the best answer to these questions. If you are unsure of an answer, eliminate the alternatives that you know to be incorrect and select an answer from the remaining alternatives. To indicate your selection, use a pencil to blacken the corresponding circle next to the answer choice and/or you can use the answer document at the back of this book. No marks are deducted for wrong answers.

The computer-based real MCAT has an on-screen highlighter function and ~~STRIKEOUT~~ function. These tools help to spotlight text or assist in the process of elimination. You may use a yellow highlighter for this paper-based exam and/or a pen (or preferably a pencil to make it easier should you change your mind) to mark text. At the time of publishing, both highlighting and strikeout functions can be used for passages, questions and answer choices. You can also flag a question to review later should time remain.

For the real exam, you will be provided with a dry erase board which is a white laminated noteboard booklet accompanied by a fine point marker. The noteboard includes 9 graph-lined pages for you to write though you cannot erase. You can simulate the experience with a fine point marker on a noteboard or with 8” x 14” plain graph paper.

Please note: For the real MCAT, a small number of field-tested questions will remain unscored.

This practice test has been designed exclusively to test knowledge and thinking skills. This exam may contain hypothetical statements and/or express controversial ideas. Statements contained herein do not necessarily reflect the policy, position, or view of RuveneCo Inc. or MCAT-prep.com.

START EXAM ONLY WHEN TIMER IS READY.

Passage 1 (Questions 1–4)

The way we work and perceive our work has changed significantly. A diversification of working arrangements has been observed. Working remotely from home is a trend that is growing, especially for women. A review conducted in 2010 found empirical evidence about generational differences in work attitudes. There is a trend for men to work longer, past retirement age. Self-employment is very common for those working past retirement age, and they often work in industries that are less physically demanding. The 2006 American Community Survey found that men working past retirement age are most likely to work in the management and professional sectors. They are more likely to be in a relationship and well educated than people who are not working and are older than 65 years.

Furthermore, working patterns are influenced by social and economic events such as the most recent recession in 2008 and 2009. Men especially were hit by the economic downturn, finding it harder to obtain a new job as well as to stay in their current job. One of the reasons for this finding is that male-dominated fields such as the construction sector were affected worse than female-dominated fields such as nursing. Figure 1 shows the impact that recessions from 1975 onward had on the number of workers who were working full time.

It is not only working patterns that have been subjected to changes but attitudes toward work as well. Recent reviews of the literature on work attitudes have shown that the younger generation places more value on leisure time and has a weaker work ethic than the baby-boomer generation. It has been argued that the current generation is more interested in intrinsic values such as finding meaning and interest in work than the previous one. This is not confirmed by J.M. Twenge's study, in which intrinsic values seem to remain the same while the new generation expresses a stronger interest in extrinsic values.

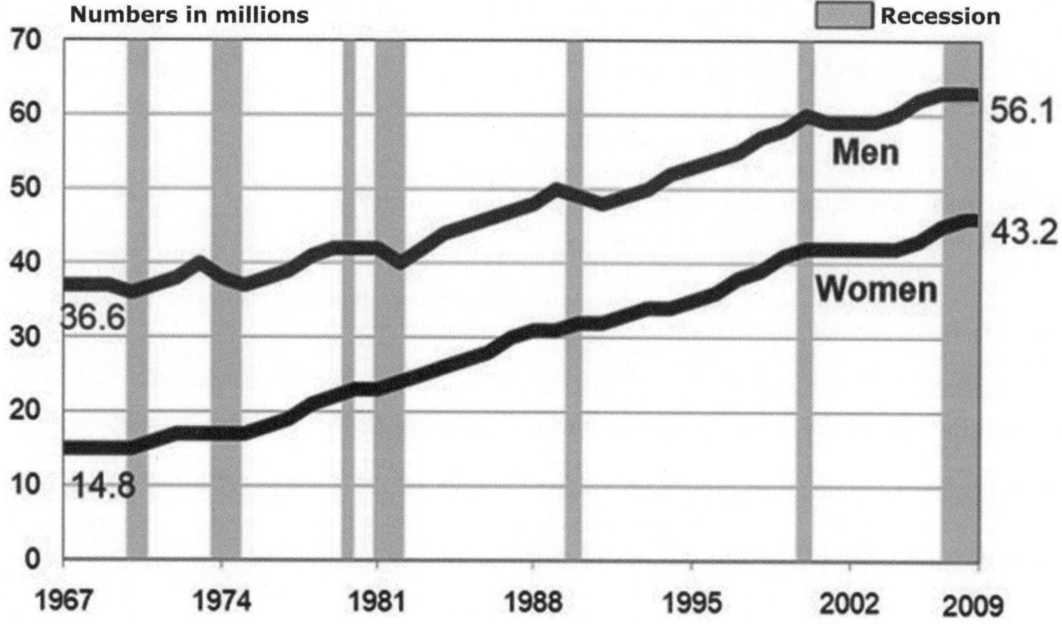

Figure 1 Number of full-time, year-round workers by sex, 1967–2009

Sources: Adapted from United States Census Bureau, "Women in the Workforce," Copyright 2010 www.census.gov; J.M Twenge, "A Review of the Empirical Evidence on Generational Differences in Work Attitudes," Copyright 2010 Journal of Business and Psychology.

Question 1

What does Figure 1 suggest in relation to the observation that recessions bring more women into the workforce?

- O **A.** It does not support the statement, because the graph shows no impact of recessions on the female workforce.
- O **B.** It supports the statement, because the graph shows that at the beginning of each recession the number of female workers tends to stay stable or grows.
- O **C.** It does not support the statement, because the graph shows that the number of male workers tends to keep growing faster than the number of female workers, despite recessions.
- O **D.** It supports the statement, because after each recession the number of female workers tends to keep stable.

Question 2

In accordance with incentive theory, what approach would probably increase the productivity of the current workforce?

- O **A.** Helping employees find more meaning in their work
- O **B.** Paying a bonus for every week that workers reach their target
- O **C.** Reducing tension by providing free food
- O **D.** Cutting workers' pay if they do not reach the yearly target

Question 3

What specific advantage do time-lag study designs provide to researcher investigating changes in work attitudes?

- O **A.** It examines data of people of different ages collected at one point in time.
- O **B.** It examines the strength of the changes in work attitudes.
- O **C.** It examines data on people of the same age at different points in time.
- O **D.** It examines data gathered at the exact time when changes occur.

Question 4

If the Yerkes–Dodson law is taken into account, how would working from home alone, as opposed to working in a shared office, most likely influence performance?

- O **A.** Well-known routine tasks would be performed better.
- O **B.** Complex accomplishable tasks would be performed better.
- O **C.** The absence of distractions would boost performance.
- O **D.** The lower levels of arousal would cause performance declines.

Passage 2 (Questions 5–9)

Sleep is essential for health and well-being. While asleep, people go through a set of sleep cycles per night, each with alternating REM (rapid eye movement) and NREM (non-rapid eye movement) phases. Both phases are important for different memory consolidation processes. Total or partial REM sleep deprivation can affect the processing of procedural memory, while NREM sleep seems tightly connected with declarative memory. It has also been shown that changes in the sequence and progression of cycles (via selective sleep deprivation) can affect various memory functions, including procedural and declarative memory.

It is common among many people to have a glass of wine or beer in order to fall asleep more easily. Even small amounts of alcohol before going to sleep can affect sleep and its known functions. Figures 1a shows the normal sleep cycles' progression and duration throughout the night sleep schedule, and 1b show how this habit affects the progression and duration of REM and NREM sleep during the same schedule.

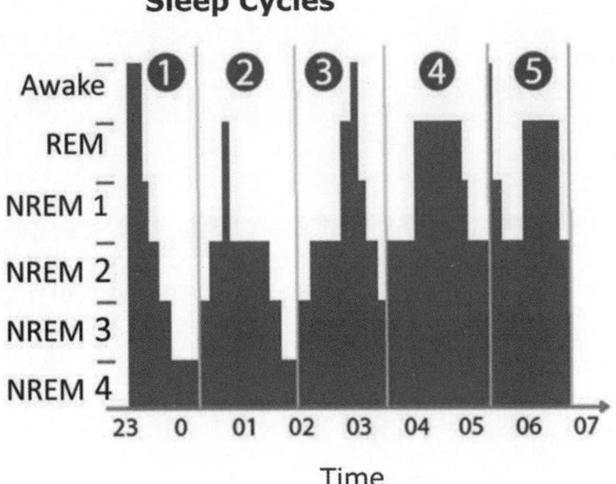

Figure 1a Hypnogram of normal healthy adult

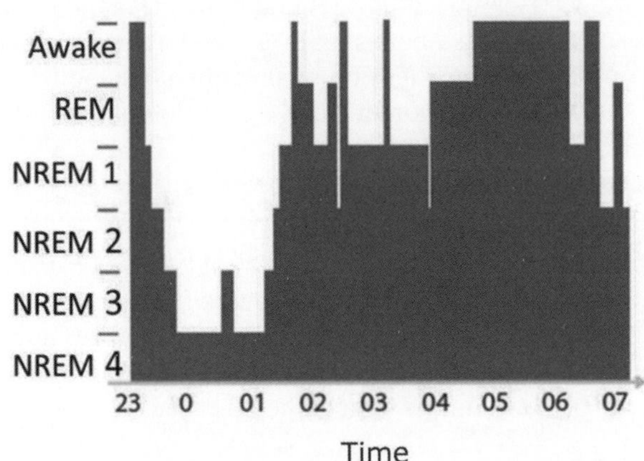

Figure 1b Hypnogram of adult after 0.5 liters of red wine

Recently it has been found that being an early bird or a night owl is strongly determined by genetically inherited circadian rhythms. Although sleep is strongly tied to biological processes such as this, it is also shaped by social interactions and conventions. One example is when falling asleep and waking up times are no longer determined by the natural day-night light cycle or circadian rhythms, but regulated through electric light, alarm clocks, social life, work schedules, and social norms instead.

Sleeping well is difficult in a society that demands high productivity. Material factors such as income influence how sleep is negotiated. Napping in the workplace is becoming more acceptable as an efficient way to deal with the need to sleep. Furthermore, it can serve as proof of hard work. In Japan, inemuri ("sleeping while present") refers to the common practice of napping during work time in order to show one's commitment.

Sources: R. Meadows, "The 'Negotiated Night': an Embodied Conceptual Framework for the Sociological Study of Sleep." Copyright 2005 The Sociological Review; figure adapted from Rainer Wild-Stiftung, http://www.gesunde-ernaehrung.org.

Question 5

Taking into account the effect alcohol consumption has on sleep cycles (Figure 1b), how would having two glasses of wine before going to sleep most likely affect the memory functions of a person the next morning?

- O **A.** It would mainly affect procedural memory.
- O **B.** It would affect declarative and procedural memory.
- O **C.** It would not affect memory function; the amount of alcohol is too small.
- O **D.** It would mainly affect declarative memory.

Question 6

Which argument mentioned in the passage can be seen as a proof of commodification of sleep?

- O **A.** Sleep deprivation can negatively affect memory functions.
- O **B.** Sleeping times are regulated through alarm clocks rather than through the availability of daylight.
- O **C.** Material factors such as income influence how we negotiate sleep with ourselves and others.
- O **D.** Japanese workers practice inemuri in order to show commitment.

Question 7

If a research study sought to test whether sleep has become what George Ritzer would name a McDonaldized good, what categories would have to be considered in the study?

- O **A.** Normative, pragmatic, experiential, and visceral forms
- O **B.** Individual expectations, desires, and social roles
- O **C.** Efficiency, calculability, predictability, and control
- O **D.** Ideas, meanings, and values

Question 8

How would a researcher following the thinking of Erving Goffman probably interpret the behavior of Japanese workers who just pretend to sleep when their managers or coworkers are around, rather than actually practicing inemuri? Their behavior is:

- O **A.** front-stage work that seeks to control how the audience of managers and coworkers perceives them.
- O **B.** evidence of peer pressure exercised in the workplace.
- O **C.** a sign of nonverbal communication that shows the worker's commitment to his or her work.
- O **D.** the outcome of a power relation between workers and managers that forces the workers to pretend they are napping.

Question 9

What might one observe about the sleeping pattern of someone who, having the weekend off, drinks heavily on Friday night? That person:

- O **A.** falls asleep quickly. However, REM sleep is disrupted. Thus, emotional regulation, memory retrieval processes, and concentration difficulties are experienced the following day.
- O **B.** has difficulty falling asleep. However, REM sleep is not affected. The following day, positive emotionality and ease of concentrating and memory recall are experienced.
- O **C.** experiences insomnia, pacing back and forth in a lethargic manner and stumbling about. Physical exhaustion is experienced the following day.
- O **D.** sleeps extremely well throughout the night due to alcohol's sedative effects. The following day there is a feeling of being refreshed and a willingness to work.

The following questions are NOT based on a descriptive passage (Questions 10–13).

Question 10

Which type of impression management technique is being used by a nice-looking woman who decides to wear glasses, do her hair up, and borrow formal unimpressive clothes for a job interview?

- O **A.** Other-enhancement
- O **B.** Self-enhancement
- O **C.** Self-serving bias
- O **D.** Actor–observer effect

Question 11

Which of the following scenarios best represents the planning fallacy? University students, being given three weeks to produce a paper, start by:

- O **A.** working on the paper as soon as assigned by going to the library and beginning the library research. At that point, they realize that they are not at all familiar with the topic, and fine-tune their time management approach.
- O **B.** working on the paper two days prior to the deadline. As they begin doing the library research, they realize that there is a massive amount of literature that needs to be reviewed and they will not be able to achieve a high quality paper on time.
- O **C.** working on the paper early because they feel good about themselves and in control of the situation. This allows them to manage their time very well.
- O **D.** rehearsing in their minds all that is needed to get the paper done a week before the due date. In doing this, they are able to form a visual representation of all the concrete tasks and steps that are required.

Question 12

A healthy 18-year-old was brought to the ER because he exhibited signs of confusion in the absence of substance abuse history. During the hospitalization period, doctors saw how he kept forgetting where the bed was, what he had just read, with whom he had just talked to, or even what he had just said. He also had no memory of the previous day. It sounds like he might have:

- O **A.** fugue amnesia.
- O **B.** retrograde amnesia.
- O **C.** anterograde amnesia.
- O **D.** dissociative amnesia.

Question 13

What tactic is a beauty salon owner using when initially offering a cut and color package deal of $75 and, when the person is about to start the haircut, coming up to say having made a mistake and that the actual package deal costed $85?

- O **A.** Lowball technique
- O **B.** Foot-in-the-door technique
- O **C.** Scarcity technique
- O **D.** Deadline technique

Note: This page is left blank so that the passage would be visible without turning pages while assessing the passage-based questions.

Passage 3 (Questions 14–17)

The technological world is evolving at a bewildering pace. Newly created and marketed inventions become obsolete and outdated increasingly fast. Moore's Law, formulated in 1965 and revised in 1975, was based on this observation. It stated that the number of transistors doubled every two years and was expected to continue to grow at such exponential rate. The same type of growth can be observed in regard to technological aspects such as quality-adjusted microprocessor prices, memory capacity, sensors, and the number and size of pixels in digital cameras.

Especially when affecting people's daily habits, society should keep track of technological changes and their impacts and side effects. This is the most adequate way to enact damage control and swift interventions. These studies require ethical and reliable research designs that monitor self-confirmatory and other biases. Such studies are lengthy and time-consuming, hardly keeping pace with the exponential growth of technological change. For example, cell phones emit a non-ionizing electromagnetic radiation that has been identified as a possible risk factor for cancer. However, even before solid evidence of their health effects has been gathered, cell phones' usage became wide spread.

Some researchers are rather more interested in psychosocial effects. For example, they looked into whether the generation born into a digital world was different from the preceding generation, and in what ways. Terms such as digital natives, the Net generation, Generation Y, the Google generation, and millennials have been used to refer to the young, technologically literate avid consumers. These are often contrasted to "digital immigrants," who consist of older people who use technologies but were not born into a digital world. Some researchers have argued that each generation is "thinking and processing information in fundamentally different ways" and have hypothesized intergenerational neuronal changes. In a somehow panicked and rushed manner, they began to advocate radical and immediate educational system reforms.

It has also been found that the recently developed social media and smartphones technologies have, as Oulasvirta and colleagues noted in their 2012 research paper, "a pervasive, habit-forming" quality. This is partly because they can be used for multiple purposes, while allowing people to be more diversely and frequently socially connected. Yet they also have disadvantages. For example, attention deficits have been reported; phone addiction (a "constant" preoccupation with one's phone) can develop; face-to-face non-casual conversations can decrease in quality; and antisocial behaviors can be reinforced.

To the left of Figure 1 the smartphone addiction risk across two age groups (teenagers and adults) and between 2011 and 2013 is illustrated. To the right, these age groups' different smartphone uses is compared.

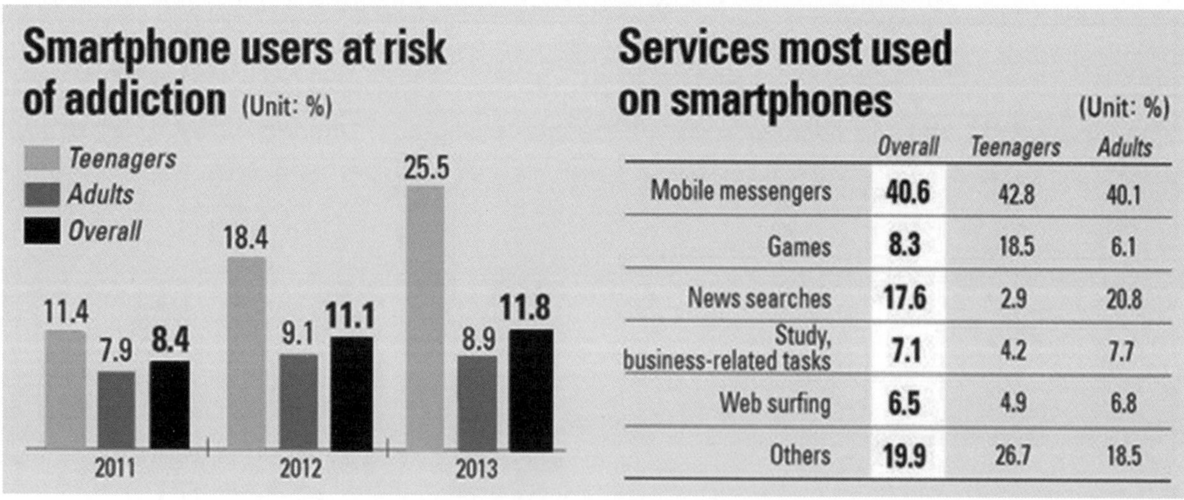

Services most used on smartphones (Unit: %)

	Overall	Teenagers	Adults
Mobile messengers	**40.6**	42.8	40.1
Games	**8.3**	18.5	6.1
News searches	**17.6**	2.9	20.8
Study, business-related tasks	**7.1**	4.2	7.7
Web surfing	**6.5**	4.9	6.8
Others	**19.9**	26.7	18.5

Figure 1 Risk of smartphone addiction and smartphone usage per age group

References/sources after Question 17.

Question 14

What would be the most correct and evidence-based conclusion about phone addiction that could be drawn from the information described in the passage and the findings in Figure 1?

- ○ **A.** Smart phone addiction is growing exponentially in the younger group.
- ○ **B.** Digital immigrants have a higher risk of phone addiction.
- ○ **C.** Digital natives have a higher risk of phone addiction.
- ○ **D.** Smartphone addiction risk has a rising tendency.

Question 15

In a study about the social impact of new technologies, which of the following research designs would be most effective at reducing the odds of the occurrence of self-confirmatory and self-fulfilling prophecy biases?

- ○ **A.** Longitudinal
- ○ **B.** Randomized
- ○ **C.** Double-blind
- ○ **D.** Controlled

Question 16

How could Figure 1 serve as evidence of Moore's Law also explaining smartphones' usage? Figure 1 illustrates:

- ○ **A.** the most frequently used smartphone services. This diversity supports the claims of Moore's Law.
- ○ **B.** differences between teenagers and adults' phone addiction risk. These support the claims of Moore's Law.
- ○ **C.** the rise in smartphone addiction. This could at most serve as indirect evidence of Moore's Law.
- ○ **D.** the rise in smartphone addiction. This could serve as direct evidence of Moore's Law.

Question 17

The passage described advantages and disadvantages associated with smartphone use. Which of the following LESS likely represents a disadvantage associated with interpersonal aspects?

- ○ **A.** Attentional split
- ○ **B.** Social interaction anxiety
- ○ **C.** Incivility
- ○ **D.** Social accessibility

Sources: Adapted from G. Kennedy et al., "Immigrants and Natives: Investigating Differences between Staff and Students' Use of Technology." Copyright 2008 Proceedings ascilite Melbourne 2008; E. Helsper and R. Enyon, "Digital Natives: Where Is the Evidence?" Copyright 2009 British Educational Research Journal; S.P. Walsh, K.M. White, S. Cox, and R.M. Young, "Keeping in Constant Touch: The Predictors of Young Australians' Mobile Phone Involvement." Copyright 2011 Computers in Human Behavior; A. Oulasvirta, T. Rattenbury, L. Ma, and E. Raita, "Habits Make Smartphone Use More Pervasive." Copyright 2012 Pers Ubiquit Comput; figure adapted from National Information Society Agency, "Smartphones." Copyright 2014 Korea Internet Security Agency.

Passage 4 (Questions 18–22)

The term "community" has been defined as a network whose members can rely on each other for support. Communities can be based on geography or physical locale such as neighborhoods, towns, or city blocks. Communities do not have to be restricted to geography; they can also be relational, characterized by interpersonal relationships. As a matter of fact, in 1974 Seymour Sarason, a psychologist, maintained that we should take into account a "psychological sense of community." Subsequently McMillan and Chavis in 1986 more concisely labeled Sarason's concept as a "sense of community." They defined it as "a feeling that members have of belonging, a feeling that members matter to one another and to the group, and a shared faith that members' needs will be met through their commitment to be together." See Figure 1 for Canadians' perceptions of their sense of belonging.

The need for belonging ranks high with human beings. Humans are social creatures. Researchers have proposed that human beings' need to belong and feel connected to a social group is a fundamental need and even has a physiological basis. The antithesis of belonging is social rejection, and some studies have found that social rejection is processed in the same manner as physical pain in the neural pathways.

Because of human beings' need to belong, we see the formation of social groups, whether they be face-to-face or online on a regular basis. Social groups are formed based on vocational or avocational interests, religious/spiritual affiliations, age/developmental life cycle, and/or specific needs. An example of groups based on an avocational interest is alternative sports groups such as skateboarding groups. Groups of skateboarders often convene at skate parks, where they establish new friendships, bond as a group, and formulate a unique identity in part defined by a skateboarding subculture. Their members find a sense of self-worth and social identity as they gain peer acceptance and status based on their skateboarding prowess.

Skateboarders can also connect and build community online. In a women's skateboarding online forum, researchers found that female skateboarders built a sense of group affiliation and developed both an individual and a collective identity. This website consisted of blogs, photos, and videos of the female skateboarders' experiences, skateboarding tips, and promotion of other female skateboarders and their experiences. They provided support and encouragement to each other.

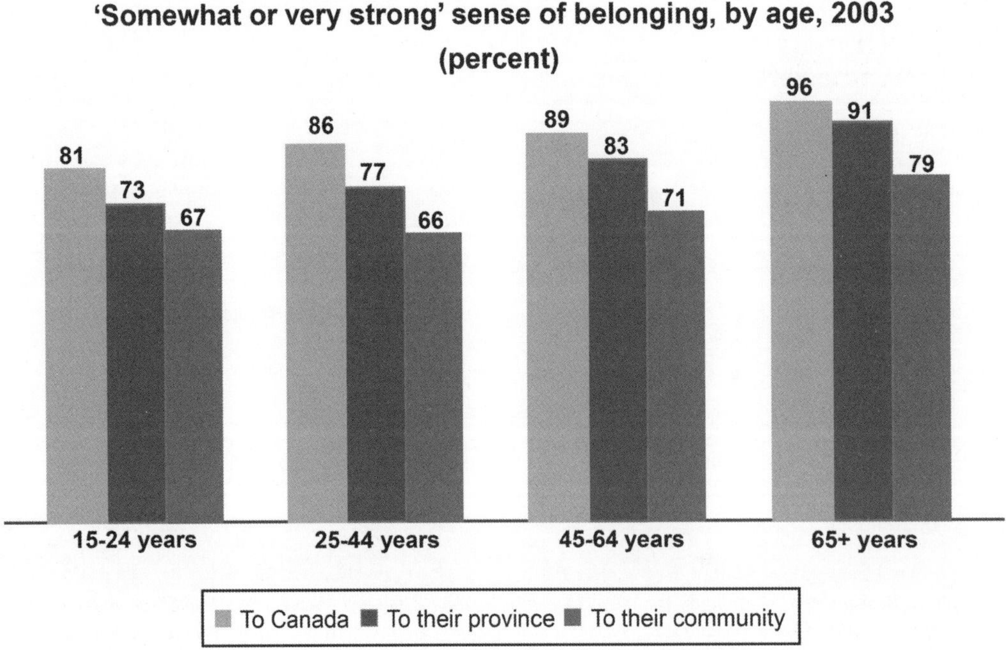

Figure 1 Canadians' perception of their sense of belonging by age group

Source: Statistics Canada. *2003 General Social Survey on Social Engagement, Cycle 17: An overview of Findings.* Ottawa, Statistics Canada, 2004 (Cat. No.89-598-XIE). http://hrsdc.gc.ca.

Question 18

How would a researcher employing activity theory formulate a hypothesis to test the trends displayed in Figure 1?

- O **A.** Adolescents and young adults, as compared to older groups, are more likely to disengage from their roles and activities, and consequently feel less connected to and part of their community.
- O **B.** Individuals aged 65 years and older embark on the grief and mourning developmental stage, begin to "let go" of their social roles, and get increasingly detached from their community.
- O **C.** Individuals aged 65 years and older are embarking on the grief and mourning process and beginning to "let go." As a result, they feel less connected to their community.
- O **D.** Middle-aged people, as compared to older groups, are more likely to focus on their work activities and to engage in political activities, and consequently feel less connected to and part of their community.

Question 19

In an ethnographic study of a skateboarding group, a researcher conducting observations heard some members of the group make the following comments: "We are skateboarders and not rollerbladers. We are a bit like rebels. Skateboarders have more prowess than rollerbladers." How would social identity theory explain what this researcher heard?

- O **A.** Individuals tend to mingle with in-group members to learn their skills and passions. They end up holding for themselves the opinions of the group.
- O **B.** Individuals' social identities are enhanced by placing labels and descriptors on social groups. They then eventually conform to the labels and descriptors of their in-group, and assume roles that mirror the labels.
- O **C.** People tend to categorize themselves and others into social categories and groups. They adopt the identity of the group they belong to, and tend to regard it as superior to that of outgroups.
- O **D.** Individual, social, and collective identities are rooted in nationality, ethnicity, religion, and social class. Ethnocentrism is triggered when someone compares oneself and one's group to outgroups and their members.

Question 20

Psychologists following on the Diagnostic and Statistical Manual of Mental Disorders, Fifth Edition (DSM-5), might describe delinquent skateboarders, involved in activities such as graphitting, as holding a:

- O **A.** schizotypal personality disorder.
- O **B.** avoidant personality disorder.
- O **C.** deviant personality disorder.
- O **D.** antisocial personality disorder.

Question 21

Which theorist did NOT discuss concepts of belonging or affiliation in his theory?

- O **A.** Erich Fromm
- O **B.** Abraham Maslow
- O **C.** Henry Murray
- O **D.** Burrhus Skinner

Question 22

A neuroscientific study using MRIs to find out how ostracism or social rejection affects brain structures speculated that social rejection is linked to physical pain. MRIs would thus be expected to show activation in ostracized people's:

- O **A.** right ventral prefrontal cortex.
- O **B.** occipital lobe.
- O **C.** central flocculonodular lobes of the cerebellum.
- O **D.** corpus callosum.

Passage 5 (Questions 23–27)

Aristotle called pain a passion of the soul, and consequently it was previously thought of as an emotion. Today the International Association for the Study of Pain defines pain as "an unpleasant sensory and emotional experience associated with actual or potential tissue damage, or described in terms of such damage." As such, pain has biological and psychological components.

The gate-control theory of pain was formulated in 1965 by Ronald Melzack and Patrick Wall. The model incorporated physiological and psychological mechanisms. It maintained that neural impulses from the spinal cord modulated noxious impulses through a "gatelike" mechanism. Pain-related impulses would not travel toward the brain if simultaneously occurring non-painful stimuli closed the gate. In their absence, the experience of pain continued to the central nervous system, where it would be further modulated by the individual's past experiences, cognitive state, and emotions. Some researchers maintain that pain also has a sociocultural dimension, because although pain is universal, the meanings, experiences, expressions, whether one seeks formal or informal help, and coping with pain are colored by culture.

Music, for example, is believed to relieve pain. In an experimental study, researchers first hypothesized that music would help to relieve pain, more so for women than men. Then they hypothesized that the type of music would also have an impact, and therefore the two conditions of music were Iranian folk music and music the research subjects selected themselves. A total of 50 healthy Iranian medical students were recruited and asked to report their pain tolerance via pain ratings while being given a cold pressor test. Participants were randomized into the no-music control group, the Iranian folk music group, and the self-selected preferred music group. Figure 1 displays their pain ratings per gender and music condition.

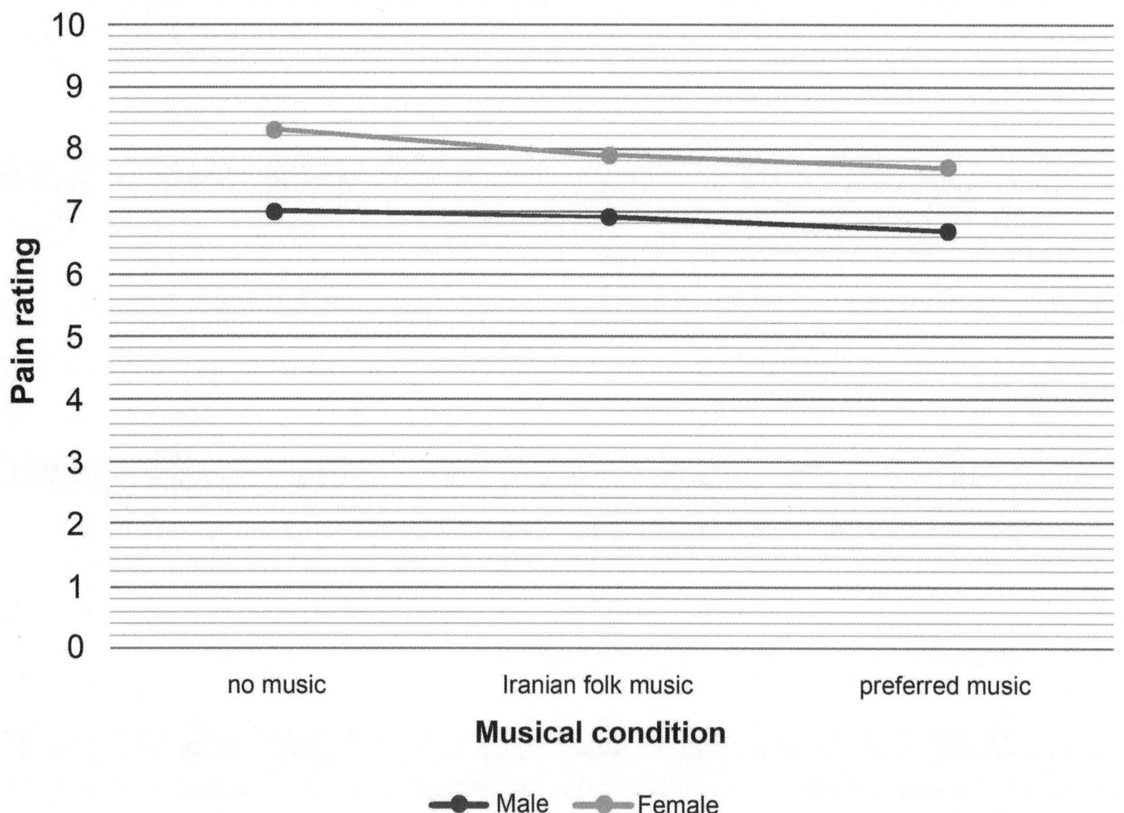

Figure 1 Average pain rating scores in three musical conditions by gender

Source: S. Ghaffaripou, H. Mahmoudi, M.A. Sahmeddini et al., "Music Can Effectively Reduce Pain Perception in Women Rather Than Men." Copyright 2013 Pakistan Journal of Medical Sciences.

Question 23

If researchers found that vivid memories of pleasant childhood experiences were re-experienced while listening to Iranian folk music but not while listening to other types of music, then the Iranian folk music:

- ○ **A.** cued an emotional memory.
- ○ **B.** was a repressed memory.
- ○ **C.** was a positive reinforcement.
- ○ **D.** cued a reflective response.

Question 24

Which of the following mechanisms UNLIKELY explains the findings from the study illustrated in Figure 1?

- ○ **A.** Nociceptors are stimulated by the cold pressor. The information travels along the nervous system into the brain. The parietal lobe receives and processes the information so that pain ratings can be made.
- ○ **B.** Music modulates the release of stress hormones and the activation of the opioid system.
- ○ **C.** Not hearing music frees up attentional resources that can be used to control and minimize the pain experience.
- ○ **D.** Not hearing music leads to an overall greater hypoactivation of neurophysiological systems that is commonly experienced as relaxation.

Question 25

An additional sample was submitted to the same procedures utilized in the study in Figure 1. It was composed of non-Hispanic White Americans. The aim was to study the effects of race, gender, and music on pain ratings. How would this change the study?

- ○ **A.** It would no longer be an experimental design.
- ○ **B.** One additional independent variable would be included in the design.
- ○ **C.** One mediating variable would be included in the regression model.
- ○ **D.** It would decrease the possibility of attrition and increase the internal validity of the study.

Question 26

From the perspective of believers, to what explanative model of pain are they most likely adhering to when arguing that pain is the testing of one's religious faith?

- ○ **A.** Biopsychosocial
- ○ **B.** Semiotics of culture
- ○ **C.** Cultural congruence
- ○ **D.** Biopsychosocial-spiritual

Question 27

In addition to music listening, which of the following therapeutic interventions would LEAST likely relieve the pain experienced by chronic pain patients?

- ○ **A.** Moderate physical exercise
- ○ **B.** Daily meditation
- ○ **C.** Hypnosis
- ○ **D.** Catharsis

The following questions are NOT based on a descriptive passage (Questions 28–31).

Question 28

Research has demonstrated that the Sami language of Norway, Sweden, and Finland has around 180 snow- and ice-related words and as many as 1,000 different words for reindeer. This particular idea could be of use for investigating which notion below?

- ○ **A.** The Sapir–Whorf hypothesis
- ○ **B.** The James–Langer theory
- ○ **C.** The Schechter–Singer theory
- ○ **D.** The cultural variance model

Question 29

What did R.D. Walk and E.J. Gibson (1960) observe during their visual cliff experiment, while infants approached the deep end of the cliff? Seven months-old infants:

- ○ **A.** crawled rapidly to their mothers as their heart rates accelerated because they had developed deep attachments to them.
- ○ **B.** infallibly continued crawling until they reached their mothers because they had yet to develop depth perception at that age.
- ○ **C.** were reluctant to continue crawling because they used depth cues and were fearful of approaching the deep end.
- ○ **D.** waited to obtain additional informational cues so as to make a decision about continuing or ceasing to crawl toward the deep end.

Question 30

Someone sleeping in a dorm was suddenly woken up while in stage 3 of sleep. They would likely be:

- ○ **A.** alert and keen to talk. They would even maybe comment that they had just been resting their eyes.
- ○ **B.** very disoriented and sluggish. They would take a long while to react to the noise appropriately.
- ○ **C.** rested, but their eyes would be bloodshot because of all the rapid eye movement they were experiencing at that sleep stage.
- ○ **D.** bundled up and claiming to be cold. This is typical because one's body temperature decreases at this stage of sleep.

Question 31

A psychodynamic therapist interpreted the distressing dream of his under-treatment, young, anorectic female client, where the client's female dog nursed the puppies and ignored the client's interaction attempts, as suggestive that her relationship with her mother was behind her eating disorder. According to Freudian dream analysis theory, such interpretation would relate to what type of dream content?

- ○ **A.** Latent
- ○ **B.** Manifest
- ○ **C.** Archetypal
- ○ **D.** Symbolic

Note: This page is left blank so that the passage would be visible without turning pages while assessing the passage-based questions.

Passage 6 (Questions 32–35)

There has been increased demand for quantitative research and evidence-based practices, yet some academics have complained about the misuse of quantitative statistical methods in a variety of research fields.

Even experts in statistics sometimes make mistakes. For example, John Ioannidis alarmed the scientific community when statistically demonstrating that "it was more likely for a research claim to be false than true." Specifically, the probability of arriving at correct conclusions via statistical methods could be as low as 1%. The highest correctness probabilities (around 50%) derived from large, randomized controlled trials and their meta-analyses. However, such "dramatic" conclusions were soon shown to be incorrect, derived from circular thinking, and based upon questionable statistical assumptions.

Nevertheless, Stephen Goodman correctly identified a common problem with existing research. For him, "biological plausibility and prior evidence" were being neglected to the benefit of the "p-value fallacy"—in which case, the p-value, obtained via the application of some statistical test, was embraced as the single and sufficient reason for accepting of the truthfulness of some claim. Since then, the use of p-values has been under heated discussion and intense scrutiny.

Several statistical and non-statistical measures, targeted at reducing type I (false positive), type II (false negative), and other common statistical liabilities have been developed since then. An example is the power of the test measure (see Table 1). It evaluates the likelihood of making incorrect statistics-based conclusions in two areas: specificity (false negatives, or the odds of incorrectly judging the hypothesis as untrue) and sensibility (false positives, or the odds of incorrectly determining the hypothesis as true). Whenever the results for one area increase, the results for the other decrease. Hence, the best statistics-based decisions show a compromise between specificity and sensibility.

When compared with a simplistic p-value use, the power of the test is one of the (albeit few) better and less error-prone ways of answering scientific questions. Even so, past research is always valuable for comparison and corroboration purposes.

Table 1 Type I and Type II Error Description

Veracity of H_0	H_0 is true	H_0 is false
p-value based decision		
Reject H_0	Type I error $p=\alpha$ Incorrect rejection of H_0 False negative*	$p=1-\beta \rightarrow$ Power of the test Correct decision
Accept H_0	$p=1-\alpha$ Correct decision	Type II error $p=\beta$ Incorrect acceptance of H_0 False positive*

*Sometimes, the terms false negatives and false positives are used in the literature as being associated with errors type II and error type I, respectively (the logical opposite of what is here defined).

Source: Adapted from S. Goodman and S. Greenland, "Why Most Published Research Findings Are False: Problems in the Analysis." Copyright 2007 PLoS Medicine; S. N. Goodman, "Toward Evidence-Based Medical Statistics.1: The P Value Fallacy." Copyright 1999 American College of Physicians–American Society of Internal Medicine D.C.; J.P.A. Ioannidis, "Why Most Published Research Findings Are False." Copyright 2005 PLoS Medicine; D.C. Howell, "Statistical Methods for Psychology." Copyright 1997/2007 Thompson Wadsworth.

Question 32

What criticism was raised in the passage about current research procedures?

- ○ **A.** Some authors are impolite to each other and do not respect each other's opinions and conclusions.
- ○ **B.** Investigators are performing qualitative studies rather than quantitative ones.
- ○ **C.** Research conclusions are not guiding the implementation of practices.
- ○ **D.** Published papers sometimes contain quantitative data analysis errors and disseminate erroneous conclusions.

Question 33

Which of the following best describes the randomized controlled trials mentioned in the passage?

- ○ **A.** There are at least two groups constituted by chance. Both groups are unaware of whether they are being subjected to the independent variable(s).
- ○ **B.** There are at least two groups being studied over time. One group does not possess (a) certain characteristic(s) under study.
- ○ **C.** There are at least two groups constituted by chance. One group is not subjected to the independent variable(s).
- ○ **D.** There are at least two variables. One or more is controlled by the investigator, whereas the other(s) is (are) not.

Question 34

A group of experts reviewed and listed existing evidence on health care disparities in the US. Which of the following would UNLIKELY be included?

- ○ **A.** Insurance status, income, and age are some of the factors that create health care disparities.
- ○ **B.** Bias, stereotyping, prejudice, and clinical uncertainty contribute to existing health care disparities.
- ○ **C.** Racial and ethnic minority patients are slightly more likely than white patients to accept treatment.
- ○ **D.** Racial and ethnic minorities more often suffer from cancer, heart disease, infant mortality, mother mortality, end-stage renal disease, and diabetes.

Question 35

In a study, participants were requested to do a problem-solving task, and demographic data was collected. The correlational test results between age and problem-solving were $r=-0.308$; $p=0.019$. The p-value significance was set at the 0.05 level. Which of the following conclusions about the obtained p-value could be offered in a way that would demonstrate the p-value fallacy?

- ○ **A.** Given that $p=0.019 \leq p=0.05$, age and problem-solving are significantly negatively correlated variables. Therefore older people are not as good at problem-solving as younger people.
- ○ **B.** Given that $p=0.019 \leq p=0.05$, age and problem-solving are not significantly negatively correlated variables. Therefore another distinguishing variable should be selected.
- ○ **C.** Given that $p=0.019$, there is a 98.1% level of confidence that age and problem-solving are significantly correlated.
- ○ **D.** Given that $p=0.019$, there is a 98.1% level of confidence that age and problem-solving are significantly negatively correlated.

Passage 7 (Questions 36–39)

The Centers for Disease Control and Prevention recommends that adults should be involved in 150 minutes per week of moderate or 75 minutes per week of vigorous physical activity. The World Health Organization recommends that older adults who have poor mobility should also be engaged in physical activity at least three or more days per week in order to help with their balance so as to prevent falls. Children are not exempt from physical exercise. The American Heart Association recommends that children participate in at least 60 minutes of moderate to vigorous physical activity every day.

Studies have found that specific inflammatory biomarkers are elevated among overweight children; however, in one study after a six-month physical activity intervention, some of these inflammatory biomarkers were reduced. Exercise also appears to affect the cognitive and affective arenas. Physical activity appears to release chemicals in the brain that positively affect memory and mood. In a study that involved 49 children who were screened as being "fit" or "not fit," the researchers used magnetic resonance imaging (MRI) and found size differences in certain brain structures among the fit and unfit children.

Aerobic exercise has been shown to be just as effective as antidepressant medications. Biologically, exercising increases beta endorphins, and psychologically it increases a sense of self-efficacy—both of which can reduce depressive symptoms. In a pilot study that examined the efficacy of a vigorous endurance regimen (i.e., mountain hiking) on high-risk suicidal individuals, research subjects responded to a flyer about the study. Then 10 individuals who had attempted suicide at least once were randomly placed in one group that began with the nine-week hiking phase followed by nine weeks of assessments, or in a second group of seven individuals who began with the nine-week assessment phase followed by the nine-week mountain hiking regimen. Table 1 shows the findings.

Table 1 Comparison of Levels of Hopelessness, Depression and Suicide Ideation in Hiking Phase and Assessment Phase

	9-week hiking phase (n = 17)				9-week assessment phase (n = 17)				Change in hiking vs. change in assessment
	Pre	Post	Change	P	Pre	Post	Change	p	P
BHS	31 ± 5	26 ± 5	-5.3	< .0001	28 ± 5	29 ± 5	1	0.135	< .0001
BDI	27 ± 11	14 ± 11	-13	< .0001	19 ± 14	23 ± 12	3.5	0.040	< .0001
BSI	1.9 ± 0.5	6 ± 8	-4.4	0.005	10 ± 9	8 ± 8	-1.8	0.212	0.25
Sense of belonging	2.2 ± 0.9	2.8 ± 0.8	0.6	0.03	2.3 ± 1	2.1 ± .09	-0.3	0.292	0.04

BHS = Beck Hopelessness Scale

BDI = Beck Depression Inventory

BSI = Beck Scale of Suicidal Ideation

Source: J. Sturm, M. Plöderl, C. Fartacek et al., "Physical Exercise through Mountain Hiking in High-Risk Suicide Patients. A Randomized Crossover Trial." Copyright 2012 Acta Psychiatrica Scandinavica.

Question 36

Researchers interested in examining the role of physical activity on the size of brain structures related to memory and learning would likely focus on the:

- O **A.** medulla.
- O **B.** hippocampus.
- O **C.** pons.
- O **D.** midbrain.

Question 37

In the mountain hiking study, why did the researchers implement two different phases and change their temporal order, ending up with two groups, one in which assessment was given at the beginning and another in which assessment was given at the end?

- O **A.** The assessment phases served as a control group.
- O **B.** The assessment phases served as mechanisms to reduce attrition.
- O **C.** The assessment phases served as a way to keep the researchers blind.
- O **D.** The assessment phases served as a way to increase external validity.

Question 38

Which theory would NOT explain the findings in Table 1?

- O **A.** Emile Durkheim's anomie theory
- O **B.** Henry Murray's theory of psychogenic needs
- O **C.** Carl Rogers' person-centered theory
- O **D.** Martin Seligman's learned helplessness theory

Question 39

What concept related to sampling might contribute to the limitations of the mountain hiking and suicide study?

- O **A.** Self-selection bias
- O **B.** Probability sampling design
- O **C.** Confounding spillover effect of the intervention into the assessment phase in Group 1
- O **D.** Double blind procedures

Passage 8 (Questions 40–44)

Some studies have examined the health effects of discrimination. Discrimination is a behavioral outcome of prejudice. It entails hidden actions that are carried out by members of a dominant group against members of a subordinate group. Discrimination apparently affects health outcomes (e.g., cardiovascular disease and hypertension). Some have further suggested that discrimination is a mediating variable of stress on health. Yet measuring the effects of discrimination on health is challenging. Discrimination may be a chronic stressor, and it is also contingent on how individuals perceive it. In other words, some may have become accustomed to discrimination and simply perceive it in the form of typical day-to-day occurrences. Even so, such habituation does not necessarily mean there will be no negative health consequences.

Some argue that discrimination is pervasive. For example, looking at the gender composition of the military, men make up the predominant portion of the Department of Defense's Active Duty at 85.6% and women comprise the remaining 14.4%. In the Selected Reserves, over the last 10 years the percentage of women has increased. In 2000, 17.5% of the officers and 16.4% of enlisted were female. By 2010, the gender gap was decreasing as 18.2% officers were male and 17.8% enlisted were female.

The "Don't Ask, Don't Tell" policy implemented by the Department of Defense in 1994 was an attempt to combat discrimination in the military. The premise of the regulation was that sexual orientation is a private and personal matter among gay and lesbian military personnel unless it is expressed in a form of homosexual conduct. For example, it is no longer a private issue if someone openly and verbally expresses it ("I am gay") or inadvertently says the name of their same-sex partner. The implicit goal of the policy was to promote inclusion of homosexuals in the enlistment of military personnel as long as they do not reveal their sexual orientation. Public sentiments in the United States have changed in recent years.

Source: B. D. Rostker, S. D. Hosek, and M. E. Vaiana, "Gays in the Military: Eventually, New Facts Conquer Old Taboos." Copyright 2011 http://www.rand.org.

Question 40

What type of intervention would the contact hypothesis propose to reduce levels of prejudice among adults who do not favor allowing homosexuals, who openly announce their orientation, in the military?

- O **A.** Promoting cooperation by bringing individuals together to work out their differences and identify common goals.
- O **B.** Reducing fears and anxieties by reducing the frequency and intensity of contact between the two groups.
- O **C.** Bringing together the two groups so that they can learn about each other's experiences, backgrounds, and goals.
- O **D.** Decreasing levels of aggression by congregating the two groups and allowing them to jointly identify another scapegoat for their aggression.

Question 41

Which statement best describes the role of discrimination as a mediating variable in the study of stress, health, and psychological outcomes?

- O **A.** When the variable discrimination is introduced, it helps to explain the relationship between stress and health.
- O **B.** When the variable discrimination is introduced, it strengthens the relationship between stress and health.
- O **C.** When the variable discrimination is introduced, it biases the relationship between stress and health.
- O **D.** When the variable discrimination is introduced, it causes a regression toward the mean between stress and health.

Question 42

If researchers want to study singlism, how might they set up the study?

- O **A.** Ask research subjects to answer survey questions about gender stereotypes
- O **B.** Have research subjects ascribe traits to single people and married people
- O **C.** Have research subjects discuss ethnocentrism in focus groups
- O **D.** Ask research subjects to link their implied associations to ingroups and outgroups

Question 43

Which would be illustrative of a study that examines the relationship of phenotype to prejudice?

- O **A.** A study that examines the relationship of authoritarian personality structure and adherence to gender stereotypes
- O **B.** A study that examines internal justifications for economic gaps between various social classes
- O **C.** A study that examines how age groups evoke different emotional responses
- O **D.** A study that examines dark-skinned, vs. light-skinned men and frequency of profiling and police harassment

Question 44

What well-known factor aids people to legitimize discrimination against an immigrant group?

- O **A.** Perceived threat
- O **B.** Perceived sense of contentment
- O **C.** Breakdown of social norms
- O **D.** Diffusion of responsibility

The following questions are NOT based on a descriptive passage (Questions 45–48).

Question 45

Which concept is demonstrated when a 6-year-old boy uses nearby known written words as contextual cues and figures out the meaning of an unknown written word?

- O **A.** Recency recall
- O **B.** Selective attention
- O **C.** Semantic priming
- O **D.** Automatic processing

Question 46

Which scenario below would increase more the odds of someone remembering all the items on a verbalized shopping list? The person verbalizing the items should:

- O **A.** discuss unrelated topics after adding a new item to the list.
- O **B.** limit the number of items to seven.
- O **C.** place the most important items at the beginning or at the end of the list.
- O **D.** clearly identify the beginning and end of the list.

Question 47

Some sociologists would say that the melting pot in society has been achieved when:

- O **A.** there is no more violence.
- O **B.** interracial marriages are commonplace.
- O **C.** reverse discrimination occurs.
- O **D.** more ethnic radio and TV programs are offered.

Question 48

It was observed that research subjects tended to select answer C in a series of multiple-choice questions. The researchers decided to randomly vary the serial position of the correct answer in order to:

○ **A.** prevent a response set.
○ **B.** provide a rationale for conducting a pilot study.
○ **C.** increase face validity.
○ **D.** increase ecological validity.

Passage 9 (Questions 49–52)

The definition of risk is complex and multifaceted. Some researchers define risk as the appraised probability of a negative outcome, and risk-taking behavior as controllable behavior that ignores such estimates. However, others question the extent to which someone can tolerate negative appraised consequences relative to what other rewards might be gained. In this case, risk-taking behaviors are associated with a perceived uncertainty about the benefits and costs for oneself and/or others. If this definition is employed, then a range of behaviors might be considered risky behaviors, such as smoking, driving under the influence of alcohol, unprotected sex, not wearing a helmet when skiing or snowboarding, not wearing a seatbelt, and the list goes on indefinitely.

Risk compensation theory maintains that people will generally modify their behavior based on the perceived risk level. Therefore, those who wear a helmet may sense they are more protected and less at risk and consequently will be less careful and engage in more risk. Some assert that this is a possible reason why some public health programs' efforts to reduce HIV by distributing condoms are not effective. In a survey study with experienced skiers and snowboarders, a range of variables, including demographic, personality, and helmet usage were examined to see what would predict risk taking when skiing and snowboarding. Again not surprisingly, males, high sensation seekers, and those who scored high on impulsivity were more likely to demonstrate risky behaviors. Helmet use was also a statistically significant predictor for increased risky behaviors, a finding that could be explained by risk compensation theory.

Sexting may also be considered a risky behavior. Sexting involves sending sexually explicit photos via cell phone. An individual could send a sexually explicit photo to his/her partner or to individuals with whom one is not romantically involved. Studies have been conducted in an attempt to understand what factors predict sexting. In a study with 88 undergraduate students who completed an anonymous survey, three-fifths (61%) reported sexting. Not surprisingly, the researchers found that having unprotected sex predicted sexting. Those who had had unprotected sex were 4.5 times more likely to sext, and those who had video chatted previously with a stranger were 2.4 times more likely to sext.

In a study about a program offering HIV testing in a hospital in Uganda and how it affected subsequent behaviors, the researchers found that unmarried individuals who participated in the program and who scored high on risky sex behaviors were more likely to behave more safely and begin 100% condom use compared with married/cohabitating participants. Figure 1 compares the findings of the two groups.

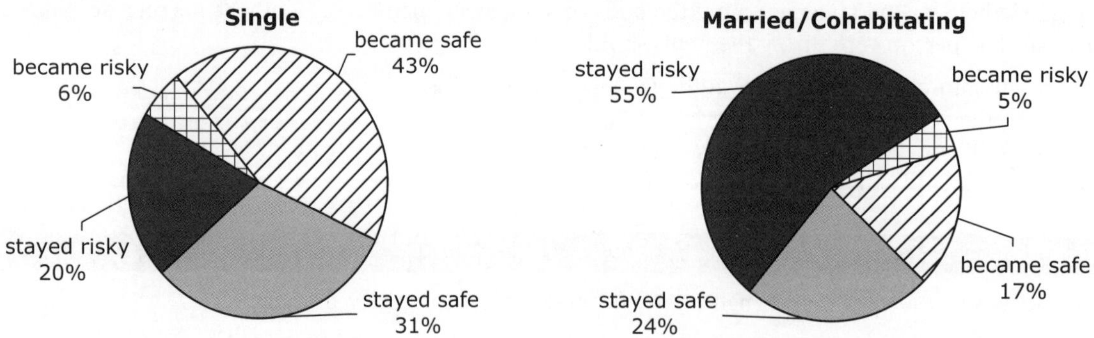

Figure 1 Comparing risky and safe behaviors between single and married/cohabiting individuals

Source: Adapted from S.M. Kiene, M. Bateganya, R. Wanyenze et al., "Initial Outcomes of a Provider-Initiated Routine HIV Testing and Counseling During Outpatient Care at a Rural Ugandan Hospital: Risk Sexual Behavior, Partner HIV Testing, Disclosure, and HIV Care Seeking." Copyright 2010 AIDS Patient Care & STDs.

Question 49

If, in a study about sexting and adolescents, the researchers wanted to examine how brain structures affected sensation seeking and reward processing, what would they incorporate into the design of the study?

- ○ **A.** An MRI to look at the occipital cortex
- ○ **B.** An MRI to examine the extent of thinning in regions of the prefrontal cortex
- ○ **C.** An MRI to examine the convolution of Broca
- ○ **D.** An MRI to investigate the medulla oblongata

Question 50

If a cross-cultural study about risk-taking aimed at inspecting the role of collectivism in risk aversion in two groups described as collectivistic-oriented (Asians and Hispanics), which of the following hypotheses would relate to collectivism?

- ○ **A.** Larger family and extended networks will predict lower risk aversion among Asian and Hispanic adults compared with their U.S.-born White counterparts.
- ○ **B.** High-context cultural orientation will predict higher risk aversion among Asian and Hispanic adults compared with their U.S.-born White counterparts.
- ○ **C.** Stricter adherence to traditional ideologies about hierarchies will predict lower risk aversion among Asian and Hispanic adults compared with their U.S.-born White counterparts.
- ○ **D.** Greater adherence to respect to elders will predict lower risk aversion among Asian and Hispanic adults compared with their U.S.-born White counterparts.

Question 51

How would Robert Agnew's general strain theory explain the findings of the study conducted in Uganda about the differences in single and married/cohabiting individuals' decisions to be safe and use condoms?

- ○ **A.** Single individuals experience greater autonomy and freedom. Consequently, they engage more in risk-taking taking behaviors.
- ○ **B.** Married/cohabiting individuals are more likely to experience greater disillusionment of their dream of the perfect mate and will engage in more risks in their sexual encounters in order to find the right person.
- ○ **C.** Married/cohabiting individuals experience greater levels of stress in relationships, which evoke a negative emotional state that then leads to greater risk-taking.
- ○ **D.** Single individuals experience greater social pressure in finding the right mate, and consequently they are more likely to take more risks in sexual encounters.

Question 52

Which of the items below is the LEAST useful for assessing Jean Piaget's concept of egocentrism, in a survey being developed for the helmet usage study?

- ○ **A.** "Everyone knows that I fell down just now."
- ○ **B.** "The person staring at me sees the same as I do."
- ○ **C.** "Although I like it, others might not."
- ○ **D.** "I give presents to all of my friends."

Passage 10 (Questions 53–56)

Typically, the age marker of 65 years is employed for the definition of old age, particularly in developing countries. In the United States, the time frame of when one can receive social security is the marker of what is considered "old age." We also think of retirement as another social marker. However, in many undeveloped countries, this does not make sense because of the importance of continuing work due to the economic ramifications for family systems. Overall, these social and chronological markers are arbitrary. In the United States, the elderly can be classified into various groups: the young-old, defined as 65 to 74 years of age; middle-old, defined as 75 to 84 years of age; and the oldest-old, defined as 85 years of age and older.

The elderly population of the United States is growing, partly due to technological advances. According to the U.S. Census Bureau in 2013, it is estimated that by 2060 there will be 92 million adults 65 years of age and older, which reflects 20% of the U.S. population. As this population grows, there is also concern that they will outlive their financial resources. According to the U.S. Census, in 2011, 8.7% of Americans 65 years of age or older lived in poverty. See Figure 1 for data breaking down by race/ethnicity and gender. Other studies have demonstrated that for Asian American elders, the issue of poverty might be masked. Asian elders are more likely to reside with family members, and this might be a response to poverty rather than personal or familial presence. Some scholars remark that poverty among Asian elders might be invisible due to the "model minority myth."

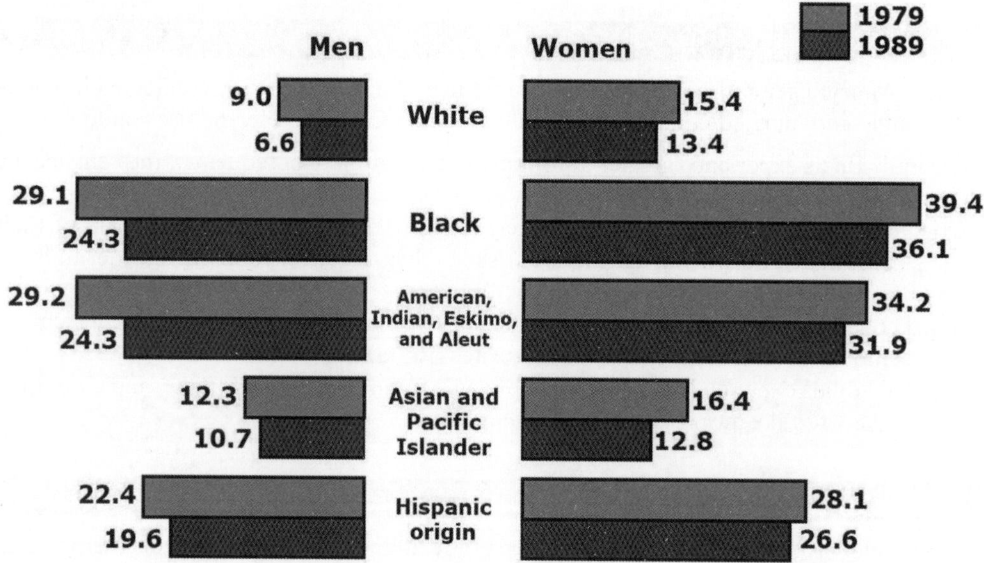

Figure 1 Racial/ethnic and gender differences in poverty rates in 1979 and 1989

Source: Adapted from U.S. Census, "Sixty-Five Plus in the United States" Copyright 1995 U.S. Census Bureau.

Question 53

What might be a quite probable reason for the large projected growth of the elderly population around 2030?

- ○ **A.** Aging of the baby boomers
- ○ **B.** Urbanization increase
- ○ **C.** Chronic disease mortality decrease
- ○ **D.** Increase in the fertility rates of women in their 40s

Question 54

What theory could explain the poverty patterns illustrated by Figure 1?

- ○ **A.** Culture of poverty
- ○ **B.** The "undeserving poor" theory
- ○ **C.** Feminization of poverty
- ○ **D.** Strain theory

Question 55

Before conducting a research study with elders about well-being, the Institutional Review Board (IRB) asked the principal investigators to screen out those participants who might be diagnosed with dementia. The IRB was concerned because:

- ○ **A.** dementia might be a confounding variable.
- ○ **B.** an adequate literature review exploring the role of dementia and psychological well-being should have been conducted.
- ○ **C.** elders with dementia might disclose sensitive information, thereby failing to respect privacy and confidentiality clauses.
- ○ **D.** elders with dementia may not have the cognitive capacity to make an informed decision about participation in the study.

Question 56

Which of the following theories was developed to understand the stages of grief for elder and otherwise populations?

- ○ **A.** Alfred Adler's theory
- ○ **B.** Apoptosis theory
- ○ **C.** Kübler-Ross theory
- ○ **D.** Locus of control theory

The following questions are NOT based on a descriptive passage (Questions 57–59).

Question 57

Which of the following topics would most interest family ecology theory researchers?

- ○ **A.** The different types and levels of needs of family members, and how the members' goals meet these needs
- ○ **B.** Women's domestic work in families and how the allocation of tasks influences power in the family structure
- ○ **C.** The effect of neighborhoods on family interdependence and on family resources
- ○ **D.** The family life cycle and how adopting children affects the family's connection with social institutions

Question 58

Which is the most accurate definition of Wernicke–Korsakoff syndrome?

- ○ **A.** It is a neurodegenerative disease mainly characterized by resting tremor.
- ○ **B.** It is a mood disorder mainly characterized by feelings of grandeur, irritability, or extreme happiness.
- ○ **C.** It is a neurodegenerative disease mainly characterized by memory loss.
- ○ **D.** It is a mood disorder mainly characterized by feelings of sadness, emptiness, or irritability.

Question 59

Which of the following short-memory related constructs could have inspired the hypothesis that people are able to recall recent information more quickly than older information?

- ○ **A.** Ecological validity
- ○ **B.** Cues and triggering
- ○ **C.** Regression
- ○ **D.** Recency

Full-length MCAT Practice Test GS-4

Periodic Table of the Elements

You may consult this page anytime you wish during the following exam sections:

- Section I: Chemical and Physical Foundations of Biological Systems
- Section III: Biological and Biochemical Foundations of Living Systems

On the real exam, the computer-based shortcut to see the periodic table is Alt + T.

1 **H** 1.0																	2 **He** 4.0
3 **Li** 6.9	4 **Be** 9.0											5 **B** 10.8	6 **C** 12.0	7 **N** 14.0	8 **O** 16.0	9 **F** 19.0	10 **Ne** 20.2
11 **Na** 23.0	12 **Mg** 24.3											13 **Al** 27.0	14 **Si** 28.1	15 **P** 31.0	16 **S** 32.1	17 **Cl** 35.5	18 **Ar** 39.9
19 **K** 39.1	20 **Ca** 40.1	21 **Sc** 45.0	22 **Ti** 47.9	23 **V** 50.9	24 **Cr** 52.0	25 **Mn** 54.9	26 **Fe** 55.8	27 **Co** 58.9	28 **Ni** 58.7	29 **Cu** 63.5	30 **Zn** 65.4	31 **Ga** 69.7	32 **Ge** 72.6	33 **As** 74.9	34 **Se** 79.0	35 **Br** 79.9	36 **Kr** 83.8
37 **Rb** 85.5	38 **Sr** 87.6	39 **Y** 88.9	40 **Zr** 91.2	41 **Nb** 92.9	42 **Mo** 95.9	43 **Tc** (98)	44 **Ru** 101.1	45 **Rh** 102.9	46 **Pd** 106.4	47 **Ag** 107.9	48 **Cd** 112.4	49 **In** 114.8	50 **Sn** 118.7	51 **Sb** 121.8	52 **Te** 127.6	53 **I** 126.9	54 **Xe** 131.3
55 **Cs** 132.9	56 **Ba** 137.3	57 **La*** 138.9	72 **Hf** 178.5	73 **Ta** 180.9	74 **W** 183.9	75 **Re** 186.2	76 **Os** 190.2	77 **Ir** 192.2	78 **Pt** 195.1	79 **Au** 197.0	80 **Hg** 200.6	81 **Tl** 204.4	82 **Pb** 207.2	83 **Bi** 209.0	84 **Po** (209)	85 **At** (210)	86 **Rn** (222)
87 **Fr** (223)	88 **Ra** (226)	89 **Ac**** (227)	104 **Unq**** (261)	105 **Unp** (262)	106 **Unh** (263)	107 **Uns** (262)	108 **Uno** (265)	109 **Une** (267)									
			*	58 **Ce** 140.1	59 **Pr** 140.9	60 **Nd** 144.2	61 **Pm** (145)	62 **Sm** 150.4	63 **Eu** 152.0	64 **Gd** 157.3	65 **Tb** 158.9	66 **Dy** 162.5	67 **Ho** 164.9	68 **Er** 167.3	69 **Tm** 168.9	70 **Yb** 173.0	71 **Lu** 175.0
			**	90 **Th** 232.0	91 **Pa** (231)	92 **U** 238.0	93 **Np** (237)	94 **Pu** (244)	95 **Am** (243)	96 **Cm** (247)	97 **Bk** (247)	98 **Cf** (251)	99 **Es** (252)	100 **Fm** (257)	101 **Md** (258)	102 **No** (259)	103 **Lr** (260)

CANDIDATE'S NAME ______________________________

RAW SCORE AND SCALED SCORE ______________________

GS-4 Section I: Chemical and Physical Foundations of Biological Systems

Questions: 1-59
Time: 95 minutes

INSTRUCTIONS: Of all the questions on this test, most are organized into groups preceded by a passage. After evaluating the passage, select the best answer to each question in the group. Fifteen questions are independent of any descriptive passage or each other. Similarly, select the best answer to these questions. If you are unsure of an answer, eliminate the alternatives that you know to be incorrect and select an answer from the remaining alternatives. To indicate your selection, use a pencil to blacken the corresponding circle next to the answer choice and/or you can use the answer document at the back of this book. No marks are deducted for wrong answers.

The computer-based real MCAT has an on-screen highlighter function and ~~STRIKEOUT~~ function. These tools help to spotlight text or assist in the process of elimination. You may use a yellow highlighter for this paper-based exam and/or a pen (or preferably a pencil to make it easier should you change your mind) to mark text. At the time of publishing, both highlighting and strikeout functions can be used for passages, questions and answer choices. You can also flag a question to review later should time remain.

For the real exam, you will be provided with a dry erase board which is a white laminated noteboard booklet accompanied by a fine point marker. The noteboard includes 9 graph-lined pages for you to write though you cannot erase. You can simulate the experience with a fine point marker on a noteboard or with 8" x 14" plain graph paper.

You may consult the periodic table at any point during the science subtests.

Please note: For the real MCAT, a small number of field-tested questions will remain unscored.

This practice test has been designed exclusively to test knowledge and thinking skills. This exam may contain hypothetical statements and/or express controversial ideas. Statements contained herein do not necessarily reflect the policy, position, or view of RuveneCo Inc. or MCAT-prep.com.

START EXAM ONLY WHEN TIMER IS READY.

Passage 1 (Questions 1–5)

Carnitine is an important molecule related to fatty acid metabolism. Carnitine is biosynthesized from the amino acids lysine and methionine. Consider the structure of carnitine below, followed by Figure 1 which displays the key pathway that involves carnitine, followed by Experiment 1 which explores the effect of L-aminocarnitine (L-AC) and malonyl-CoA on CPT I (CPT 1) and CPT II (CPT 2) activity.

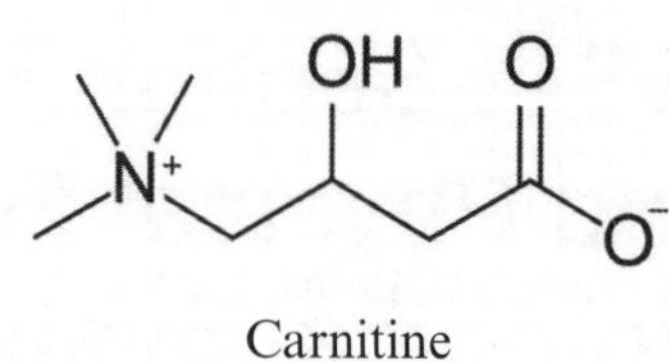

Carnitine

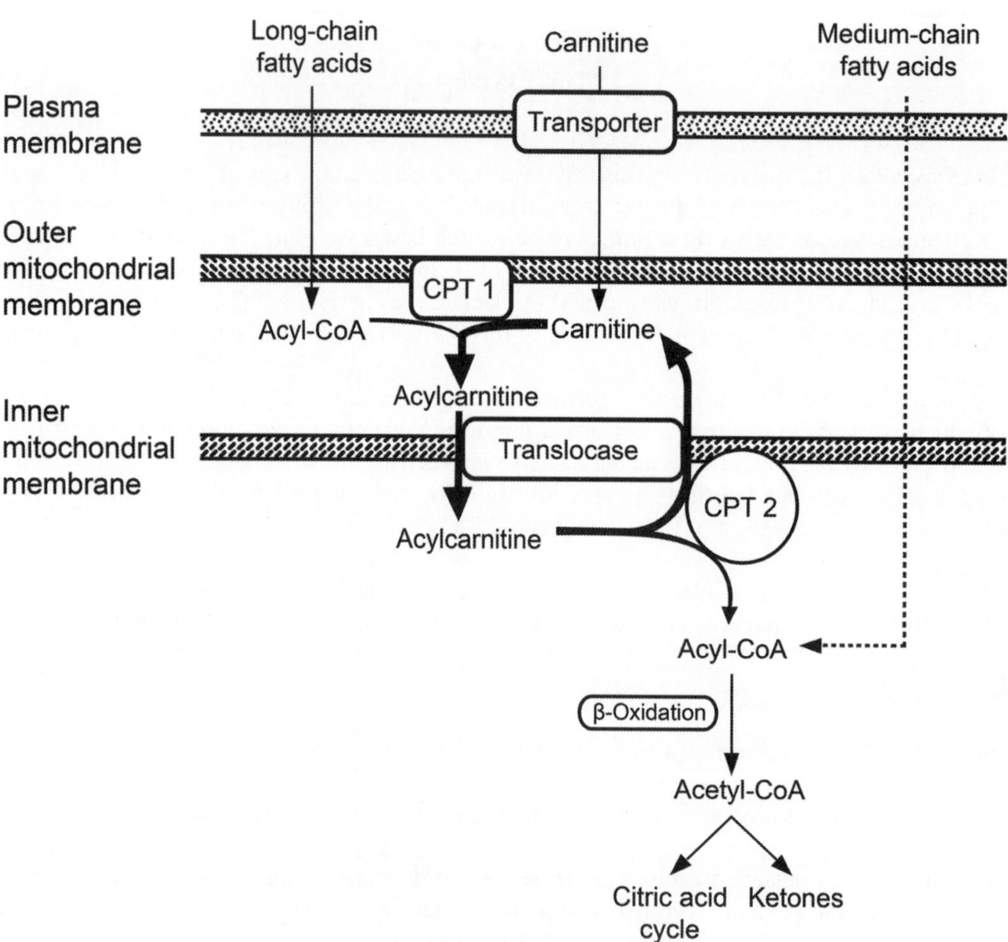

Figure 1 The Role of Carnitine—Acylcarnitine Translocase in the Carnitine Cycle of Mitochondrial Oxidation of Long-Chain Fatty Acids. CPT – carnitine palmitoyltransferase; IMM – inner mitochondrial membrane (ref. N Engl J Med 1992; 327:19-23)

Experiment 1

Human skeletal muscle homogenates were incubated with 1% Tween 20, which is known to release CPT from mitochondrial membranes. After ultracentrifugation, the supernatant was incubated either with 0.5 mM L-AC, with 0.4 mM malonyl-CoA, or with neither. To these incubations, the second reagent was added in increasing concentrations as indicated.

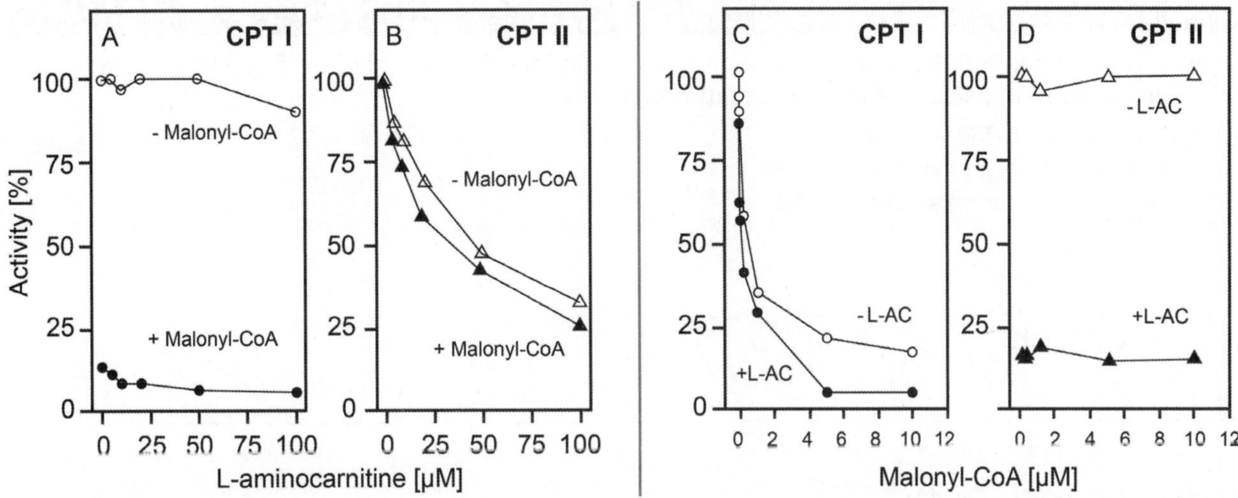

Figure 2 Individual percent activity curves showing the kinetics of CPT I and CPT II +/- malonyl-CoA and +/- L-aminocarnitine (L-AC) in the presence of increasing concentrations of L-aminocarnitine (A, B) or in the presence of increasing concentrations of malonyl-CoA (C, D). [ref: Biochimica et Biophysica Acta, 15(2004), pp. 149–154]

Question 1

Which of the following is NOT an accurate description of carnitine?

- O **A.** It is a quaternary ammonium compound.
- O **B.** It is a beta-hydroxy-gamma-aminocarboxylate.
- O **C.** It has a maximum of 4 enantiomers.
- O **D.** It is a zwitterion.

Question 2

According to Figure 1, carnitine is:

- O **A.** a membrane transporter.
- O **B.** active in the cytosol.
- O **C.** a fatty acid transporter.
- O **D.** active in the intercellular space.

Question 3

CPT I and CPT II are likely necessary because:

- O **A.** acyl CoA cannot cross the IMM.
- O **B.** they both must catalyze the same reaction.
- O **C.** of synergies in the TCA cycle.
- O **D.** they both produce acylcarnitine.

Question 4

Which of the following is NOT indicated by the data presented in Experiment 1?

- O **A.** Almost 90% of CPT I activity can be inhibited by malonyl-CoA in the absence of L-AC.
- O **B.** L-AC is a far more powerful inhibitor of CPT II as compared to CPT I.
- O **C.** L-AC potentiates the inhibitory effect of malonyl-CoA on CPT I.
- O **D.** Malonyl-CoA has a statistically significant inhibitory effect on CPT II.

Question 5

Drawing from your knowledge of the β-oxidation of fatty acids, which of the following is (are) true of the oxidation of 1 mole of palmitate (a 16-carbon saturated fatty acid)?

I. 8 moles of acetyl-CoA are formed.
II. 1 mole of $FADH_2$ is produced per cycle.
III. There is no direct involvement of NAD^+.

- O **A.** I only
- O **B.** II and III only
- O **C.** I and II only
- O **D.** I, II and III

Passage 2 (Questions 6–10)

Carbon is the second most abundant element by mass in the human body, after oxygen. This abundance, along with the unique diversity of organic compounds and their atypical polymer-forming ability at the temperatures commonly encountered on Earth, make carbon the chemical basis of all known life.

It is well known that there are two major forms of carbon, that is, carbon has two main allotropes: graphite and diamond. These differ greatly from each other with respect to their physical properties as shown in Table 1. The physical properties of silicon are also shown in Table 1 for comparison as carbon and silicon belong to the same group in the periodic table.

Table 1

Physical properties	Graphite	Diamond	Silicon
Density (g cm^{-3})	2.26	3.51	2.33
Enthalpy of combustion to yield oxide (ΔHc) kJ mol^{-1}	-393.3	-395.1	-910
Melting point (°C)	2820	3730	1410
Boiling point (°C)		4830	2680
Conductivity (electrical)	Fairly good	Non-conductor	Good
Conductivity (thermal)	Fairly good	Non-conductivity	Good

Graphite possesses what is commonly known as a layer structure: carbon atoms form three covalent bonds with each other to yield layers of carbon assemblies parallel with each other. These layers are held together via weak Van der Waals' forces which permit some movement of the layers relative to one another.

The most common compound of carbon is carbon dioxide which makes up 0.03% of the atmosphere. The triple point of carbon dioxide occurs at 217 K and 515 kPa.

One of the unique properties of carbon is that it can form multiple bonds between itself and other atoms, including other carbon atoms. Thus, large polymers involving carbon atoms are possible.

Question 6

Which of the following is a correct representation of the phase diagram for carbon dioxide?

○ **A.** 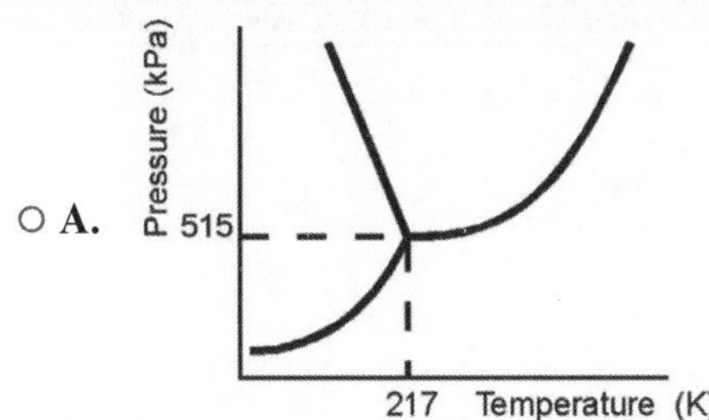

○ **B.** 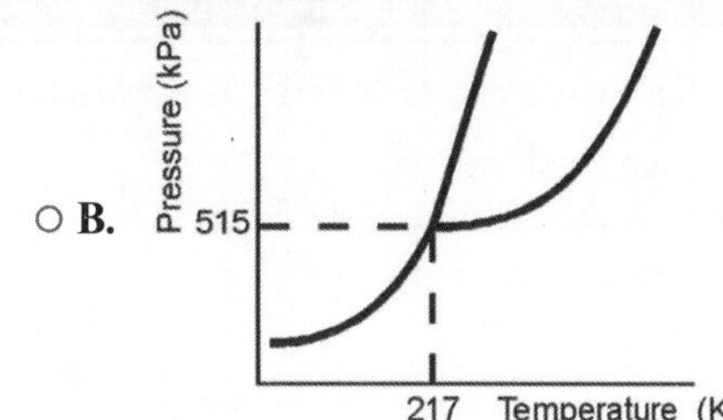

○ **C.** 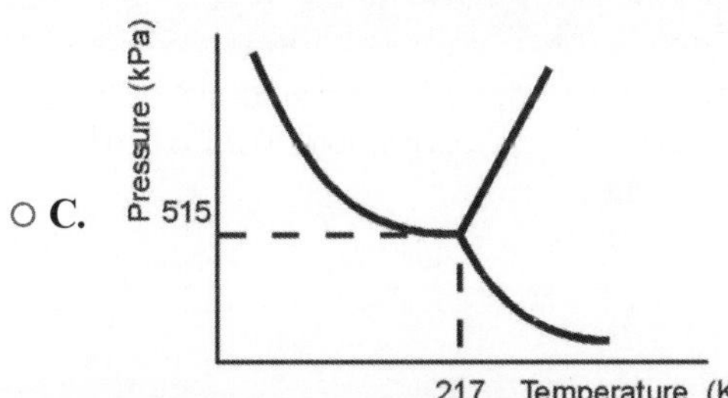

○ **D.** 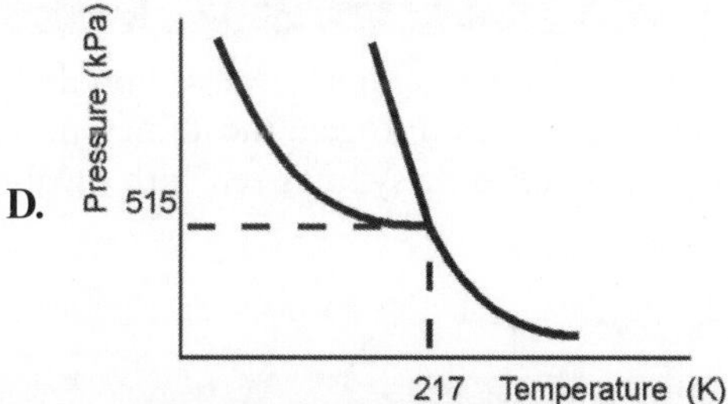

Question 7

Using the information in the table, calculate the enthalpy change for the following process:

$$C_{graphite} \rightarrow C_{diamond}$$

○ **A.** 1.8 kJ mol^{-1}.
○ **B.** -1.8 kJ mol^{-1}.
○ **C.** 1.0 kJ mol^{-1}.
○ **D.** -1.0 kJ mol^{-1}.

Question 8

It is possible to convert graphite into diamond via various chemical processes. Based on the information in the passage, which of the following would facilitate increased amounts of diamond assuming that the system is in equilibrium?

○ **A.** Higher pressures
○ **B.** Lower temperatures
○ **C.** A catalyst
○ **D.** None of the above

Question 9

Diamond consists of tetrahedral arrangements of carbon atoms, with each atom covalently bound to four others to yield a giant molecular structure. What is the hybridization state of carbon in diamond?

○ **A.** It is not hybridized.
○ **B.** sp
○ **C.** sp^2
○ **D.** sp^3

Question 10

Carbon is in Group IV of the periodic table, along with such elements as silicon. However, compared with silicon, carbon forms more stable covalent bonds with itself. Why is a C-C bond stronger than a Si-Si bond?

○ **A.** Because carbon is not as good an electrical conductor.
○ **B.** Because carbon has a smaller atomic number.
○ **C.** Because carbon has a smaller atomic radius.
○ **D.** Because carbon has a smaller relative atomic mass.

The following questions are NOT based on a descriptive passage (Questions 11–14).

Question 11

Water droplets on skin tend to resemble spheres as opposed to other shapes so as to:

- O **A.** minimize surface tension.
- O **B.** maximize the area to volume ratio.
- O **C.** minimize cohesive forces.
- O **D.** maximize adhesive forces.

Question 12

Addition reactions with primary amines give, essentially, stable imines. However, with an aryl group or certain stabilizing alkyl substituents on nitrogen, the imine - now called a *Schiff base* - is *truly* stable. Which of the following represents a Schiff base synthesized with the use of an acid halide?

O A.

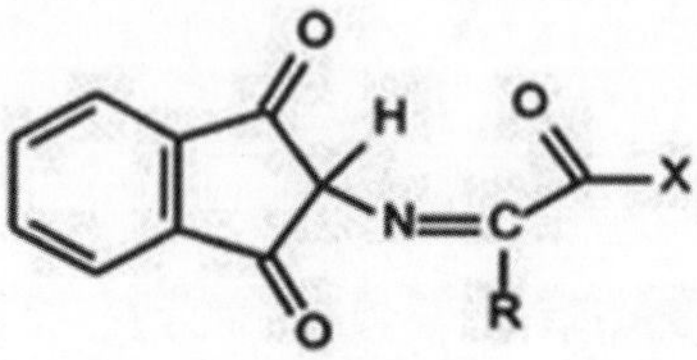

O B.

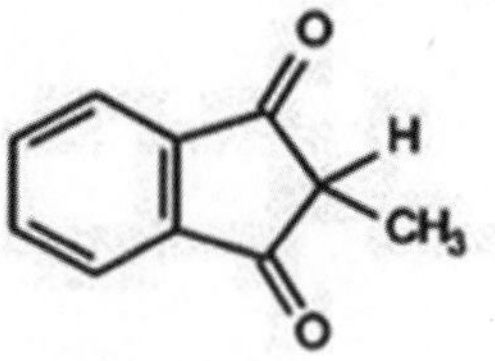

O C.

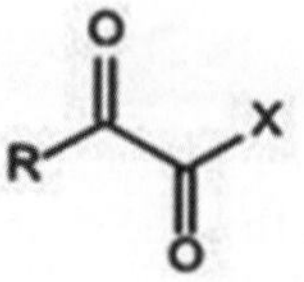

O D.

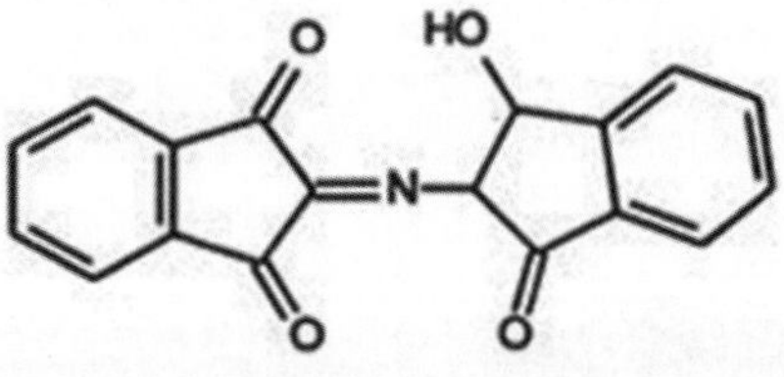

Question 13

What would be the expected rotation of plane polarized light for the product of the following reaction?

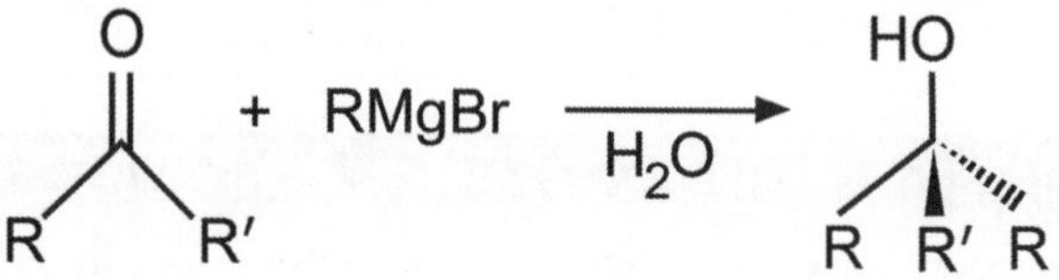

$$RC(=O)R' + RMgBr \xrightarrow{H_2O} R_2C(OH)R'$$

- O **A.** 30°
- O **B.** 60°
- O **C.** 0°
- O **D.** -30°

Question 14

The digestion of the disaccharide sucrose is a hydrolysis reaction resulting in the production of the monomers glucose and fructose. Consider the data in Table 1 which was determined for the hydrolysis of sucrose in 0.20 M HCl at body temperature.

Table 1

Concentration of Sucrose (M)	Initial Rate (M / min)
0.500	1.80×10^{-3}
0.400	1.46×10^{-3}
0.200	7.32×10^{-4}

Which of the following would be most consistent with the rate law for the acid-catalyzed hydrolysis of sucrose at body temperature?

- ○ **A.** rate = $(1.46 \times 10^{-3}\ min^{-1}M^{-1})[sucrose]^2$
- ○ **B.** rate = $(3.66 \times 10^{-3}\ min^{-1})[sucrose]$
- ○ **C.** rate = $(1.46 \times 10^{-4}\ min^{-1})[sucrose]$
- ○ **D.** rate = $(3.66 \times 10^{-4}\ min^{-1}M^{-1})[sucrose]^3$

Passage 3 (Questions 15–18)

Sulfurous acid is a colorless liquid commonly used as a fruit and vegetable preservative, as well as a medical antiseptic.

The essential stages in the manufacture of H_2SO_3 involve the burning of sulfur or roasting of sulfide ores in air to produce SO_2. This is then mixed with air, purified and passed over a vanadium catalyst (either VO_3^- or V_2O_5) at 450 degrees Celsius. Thus the following reaction occurs.

Reaction I

$2SO_2(g) + O_2(g) \leftrightarrow 2SO_3(g)$ $\Delta H = -197\text{ kJ mol}^{-1}$

If the SO_2 is very carefully dissolved in water, sulfurous acid (H_2SO_3) is obtained. The first proton of this acid ionizes as if from a strong acid while the second ionizes as if from a weak acid.

Reaction II

$H_2SO_3 + H_2O \rightarrow H_3O^+ + HSO_3^-$

Reaction III

$HSO_3^- + H_2O \leftrightarrow H_3O^+ + SO_3^{2-}$ $K_a = 5.0 \times 10^{-6}$

The concentration of H_2SO_3 in cleaning fluid was determined by titration with 0.10 M NaOH (strong base) as shown in Figure 1. Two equivalence points were determined using 30 ml and 60 ml of NaOH respectively:

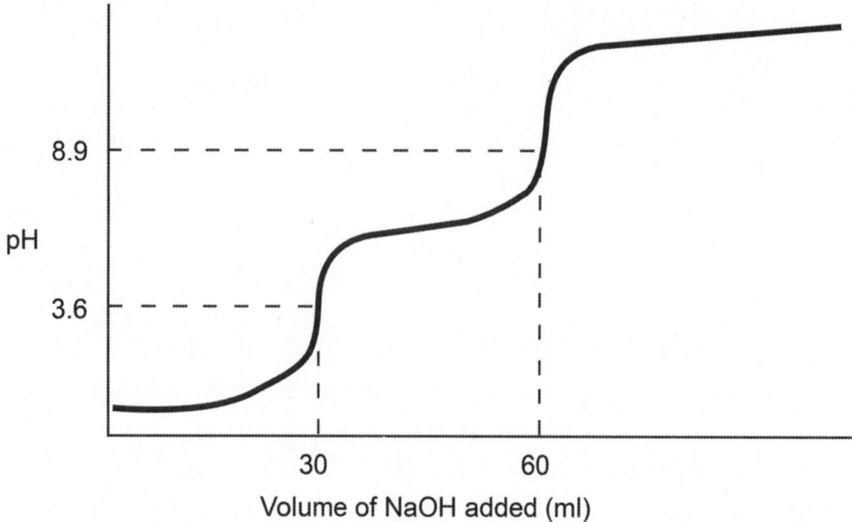

Figure 1

Question 15

If no catalyst was used in Reaction I, which of the following would experience a change in its partial pressure when the same system reaches equilibrium?

○ **A.** There will be no change in the partial pressure of any of the reactants.
○ **B.** SO_3 (g)
○ **C.** SO_2 (g)
○ **D.** O_2 (g)

Question 16

If the temperature was decreased in Reaction I, which of the following would experience an increase in its partial pressure when the same system reaches equilibrium?

○ **A.** There will be no change in the partial pressure of any of the reactants.
○ **B.** SO_3 (g)
○ **C.** SO_2 (g)
○ **D.** O_2 (g) and SO_2 (g)

Question 17

Reaction I is usually carried out at atmospheric pressure. During the reaction, before equilibrium was reached, the mole fractions of SO_2 (g) and SO_3 (g) were 1/2 and 1/6, respectively. What was the partial pressure of O_2 (g)?

○ **A.** 0.66 atm
○ **B.** 0.16 atm
○ **C.** 0.50 atm
○ **D.** 0.33 atm

Question 18

What is the pH of 0.01 M H_2SO_3?

○ **A.** 1.0
○ **B.** 2.0
○ **C.** 3.0
○ **D.** 4.0

Passage 4 (Questions 19–22)

Ordinary chemical reactions consist simply of rearrangements of the electrons in atoms and molecules. In these changes, the atomic nuclei involved are not affected. In the phenomenon of radioactive disintegration, both nuclei and electrons can be involved. A chemical reaction of this kind is referred to as a *nuclear reaction.*

Transmutations (producing nuclear alteration) occur naturally through radioactive decay, or artificially by bombarding the nucleus of a substance with various kinds of high speed subatomic particles (*see* Figure 1).

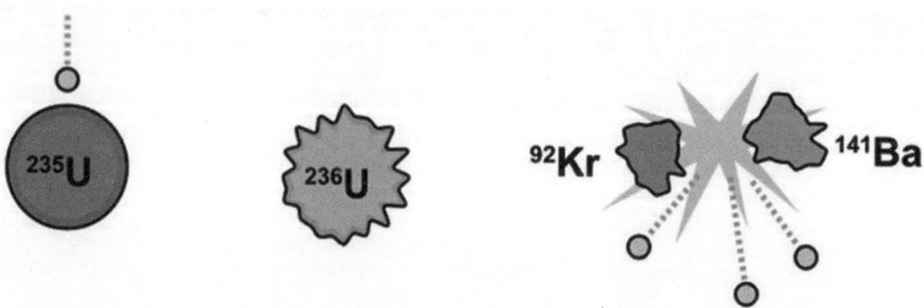

Figure 1 The artificial nuclear transmutation of uranium to krypton, barium and other particles

The possibility of artificial transmutation was first suggested when it was discovered that different kinds of atoms are composed of the same fundamental units: protons, electrons and neutrons. Essentially, the problem is in how the number of each of these types of particles could be changed. Rutherford first suggested that alpha particles, which could be easily obtained from radium, could be used. He thought that a few of the particles might make direct hits and either combine with the nuclei or break them up. His theory was proven when he used these particles to transmute ^{14}N to ^{17}O, and the chemical community was shocked. Since then, protons (p), photons (γ-rays in particular), neutrons (n), electrons (e or $^{0}_{-1}e$) and positrons (e^+ or $^{0}_{+1}e$) have been used in these types of reactions.

As an example of natural transmutation, radioactive cobalt-60 undergoes beta decay in radiation therapy for cancer treatment.

Question 19

What is the nuclear reaction for the transmutation of ^{14}N to ^{17}O ?

- O **A.** $^{14}_{7}N + \alpha \text{-->} n + {}^{17}_{8}O$
- O **B.** $^{14}_{7}N + \alpha \text{-->} p + {}^{17}_{8}O$
- O **C.** $^{14}_{7}N + \alpha \text{-->} e + {}^{17}_{8}O$
- O **D.** $^{14}_{7}N + \alpha \text{-->} e^+ + {}^{17}_{8}O$

Question 20

The larger the bombarding particle and the greater its charge, the more difficult it is to use in artificial transmutation. Which of the following represents the order of particles in terms of increasing ability to be used in these types of reactions given that charge is the more important factor?

- O **A.** $n < p < e < \alpha$
- O **B.** $n < e < p < \alpha$
- O **C.** $\alpha < e < p < n$
- O **D.** $\alpha < p < e < n$

Question 21

A radioactive form of phosphorus undergoes β - decay. What would the radioactivity level (R) versus time graph for the decay process look like?

○ A.

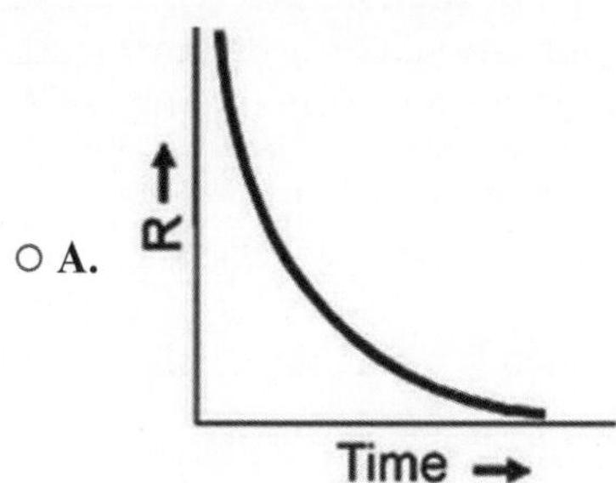

○ B.

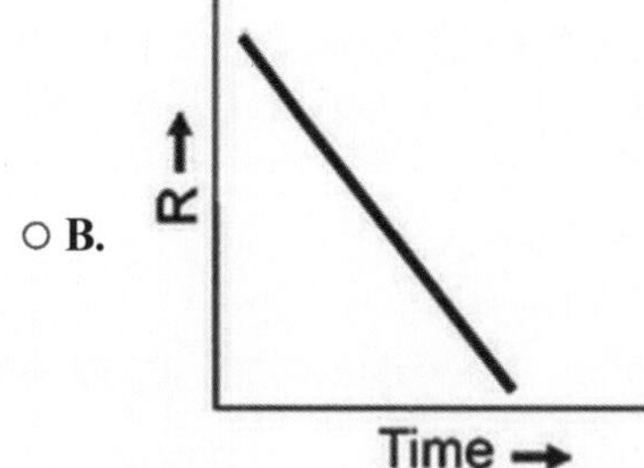

○ C.

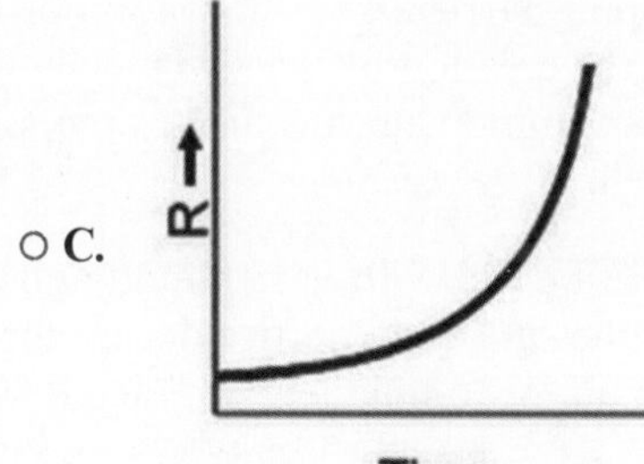

○ D.

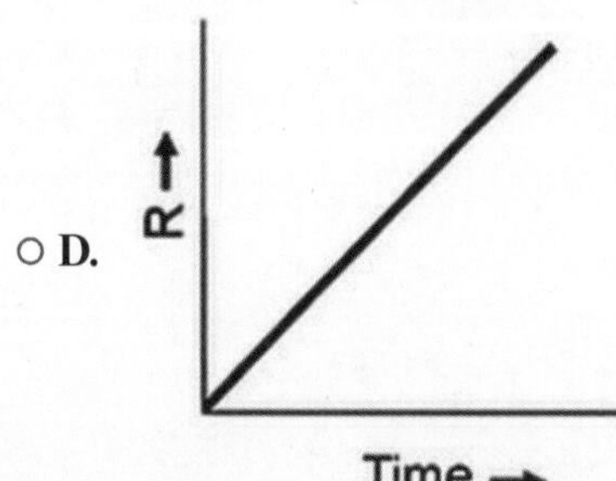

Question 22

Given that a particular β particle has a kinetic energy of 2.275×10^{-15} J, what is the velocity of this particle?

Speed of light in free space = 3.0×10^{8} m s^{-1}

Mass of an electron = 9.1×10^{-31} kg

○ **A.** 1.0×10^{8} m s^{-1}
○ **B.** 2.5×10^{7} m s^{-1}
○ **C.** 7.1×10^{7} m s^{-1}
○ **D.** 1.4×10^{7} m s^{-1}

Passage 5 (Questions 23–28)

Statins are medications that are HMG-CoA reductase (HMGR) inhibitors. Since HMGR is involved in a rate-limiting step in cholesterol formation, use of statins can dramatically reduce blood cholesterol levels. Statins are similar in structure to HMG-CoA and their development stands as a triumph for rational drug design. Generally, statins bind to HMGR with a Ki of between 0.1 and 2.3 nM while the Michaelis constant Km for HMG-CoA is approximately 4 μM.

Certain statins are given to patients in an inactive form and subsequently activated in the body. One such example is simvastatin. The conversion of the inactive form of simvastatin to the active form is catalyzed by a group of enzymes known as carboxylesterases, which break the ring structure to form the active metabolite as shown below.

Figure 1 Simvastatin and an active metabolite

Carboxylesterases are present in the small intestines, liver, and the blood-brain barrier. Thus activation of the simvastatin molecule can happen before it enters the liver. This is similar to the creation of inactive metabolites of simvastatin by the enzyme cytochrome P450 3A4 (abbreviated CYP3A4) a common enzyme in the processing of many therapeutic drugs, which has distribution in the small intestines as well.

Once the active metabolite is in circulation, the medication is highly protein bound with 95% bound and 5% unbound. This protein binding is taken into consideration when calculating the safe and effective dosage for its use as a cholesterol-lowering medication. The unbound metabolite is thus available to interact with the HMGR active site.

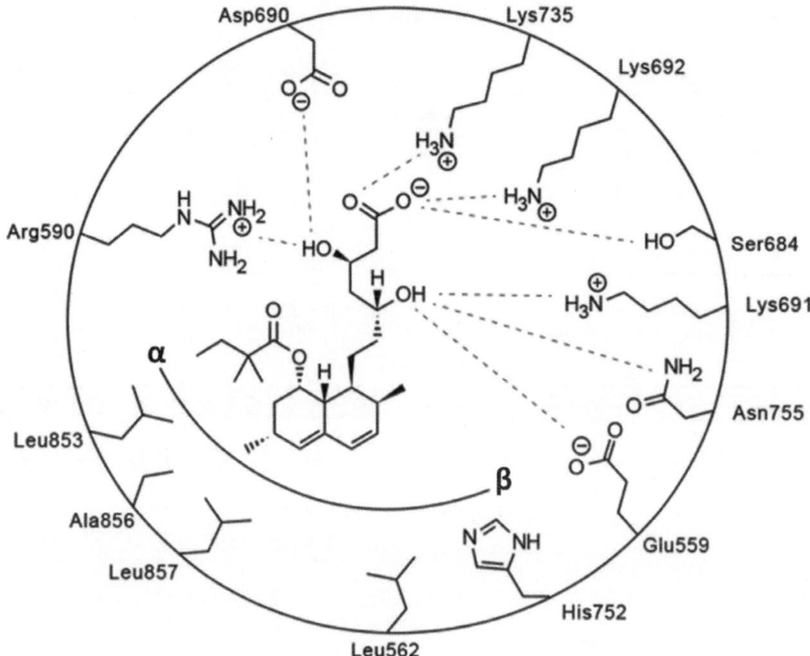

Figure 2 Binding of the active metabolite of simvastatin to the HMGR active site highlighting key amino acids. Dashed lines and the curvilinear line between **α** and **β** represent various interactions between the metabolite and the active site.

Question 23

Simvastatin, as a cholesterol-lowering agent given to patients, would be best described as which of the following?

- O **A.** Agonist with high affinity to the HMGR active site
- O **B.** Antagonist with similar affinity to HMGR as compared to HMG-CoA
- O **C.** Antagonist that significantly outcompetes HMG-CoA in binding to HMGR
- O **D.** Catalyst that lowers the activation energy for HMG-CoA synthesis

Question 24

Which of the following does NOT accurately describe the conversion of simvastatin to its active metabolite?

- O **A.** Produces one additional chiral center
- O **B.** Doubles the number of donatable H-bonds at physiological pH
- O **C.** Converts a hydroxy-delta-lactone to a beta-hydroxy acid
- O **D.** Produces a compound with greater HMG-CoA similarity

Question 25

Carboxylesterase is best described as which of the following?

- O **A.** Hydroxylase
- O **B.** Hydrolase
- O **C.** Oxireductase
- O **D.** Decarboxylase

Question 26

In individuals with liver disease, the concentration of the blood protein albumin may be decreased. Given that there was no change in the patient's medication dosage, how would advanced liver disease be expected to affect the free concentration of the active metabolite of simvastatin within the bloodstream?

- O **A.** No net change in free/unbound concentration due to equilibrium effects
- O **B.** Increase in free/unbound concentration
- O **C.** Decrease in free/unbound concentration
- O **D.** No net changes due to unaltered binding effects

Question 27

Conventional high performance liquid chromatography (HPLC), with a polar stationary phase and a non-polar mobile phase, was used to separate simvastatin and its metabolite. Which statement accurately describes the process?

- O **A.** Decreasing simvastatin's affinity to the stationary phase will increase its relative retention time as compared to its metabolite.
- O **B.** Simvastatin will elute first because it is more hydrophilic than its metabolite.
- O **C.** Simvastatin will elute first because it does not interact as favorably with the stationary phase as its metabolite.
- O **D.** Increasing the polarity of the stationary phase would increase the relative retention of simvastatin as compared to its metabolite.

Question 28

Considering Figure 2, which of the following statements is true?

I. The dashed lines represent electrostatic interactions involving hydrogen bonding.
II. The curvilinear line between **α** and **β** represents van der Waals interactions within a hydrophobic pocket.
III. An A856W mutant would be unlikely to significantly affect the Ki for the simvastatin metabolite.

- O **A.** I only
- O **B.** II only
- O **C.** I and II only
- O **D.** I, II and III

The following questions are NOT based on a descriptive passage (Questions 29–32).

Question 29

Consider the following schematic of a ^{1}HNMR:

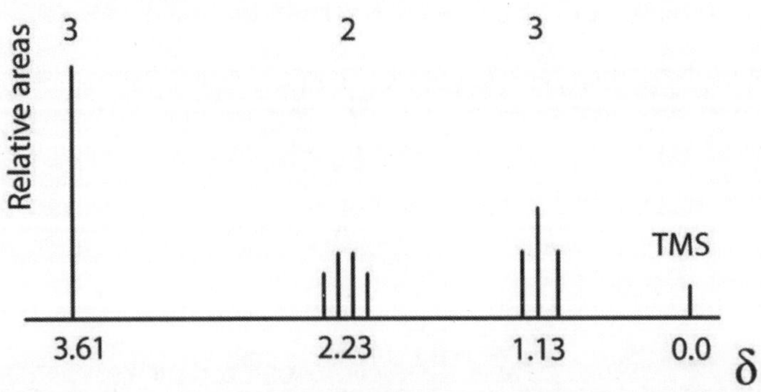

Which of the following compounds is most consistent with the ^{1}HNMR above?

- O **A.** $CH_3CH_2COOCH_3$
- O **B.** $CH_3COCH_2OCH_3$
- O **C.** $CH_3CH_2OCH_2CH_2CH_3$
- O **D.** C_4H_6O

Question 30

Ethylene glycol, a component of antifreeze, is poisonous to humans. Its sweet taste can lead to accidental ingestion or allow its deliberate use as a murder weapon. Ethylene glycol becomes toxic after undergoing oxidation reactions catalyzed by alcohol dehydrogenase. The antidote is high doses of ethanol, which inhibits oxidation of ethylene glycol by competing for the alcohol dehydrogenase active site. Which of the following best describes the role of ethanol in the treatment of ethylene glycol poisoning?

- O **A.** A reducing agent
- O **B.** A depressant
- O **C.** A competitive inhibitor
- O **D.** A non-competitive inhibitor

Question 31

Nearsightedness (myopia) is a condition where an image is formed in front of the retina. Corrective lenses can help to focus light on the retina. If the radius of curvature of corrective lenses for myopia is 80 cm, what is the refractive power in diopters?

- O **A.** +80
- O **B.** -80
- O **C.** +2.5
- O **D.** -2.5

Question 32

Nitrites are used for the curing of meat to prevent bacterial growth. Nitrites in meat can react with degradation products of amino acids, forming nitrosamines, which are known carcinogens. Which of the following is consistent with the structure of nitrite?

○ A. 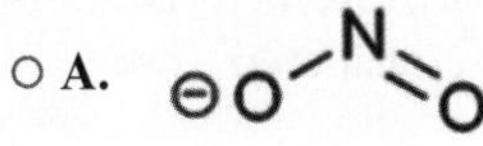

○ B. 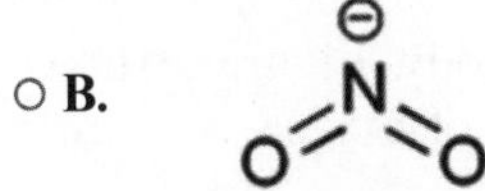

○ C. 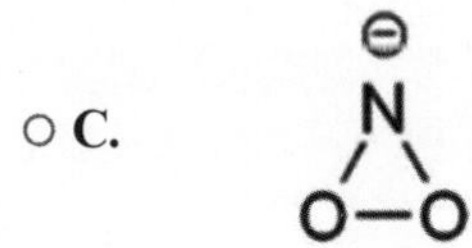

○ D. $^{\ominus}O-\overset{\oplus}{N}=O$

Passage 6 (Questions 33–36)

At 29,029 feet, Mount Everest is the world's highest mountain and one of the most dangerous. As of 2016, about 6.5% of the roughly 4,000 climbers who have attempted a summit died, most in an area called the Death Zone where the percentage of oxygen in the air is too low and tissues receive an insufficient amount of oxygen. Figure 1 shows the percentage of hemoglobin in the blood that is saturated with oxygen to form oxyhemoglobin as a function of the partial pressure of oxygen in the air. A saturation percentage below 90 is considered low.

As the oxygen partial pressure decreases, climbers become susceptible to hypoxia, a condition that occurs when the body is deprived of an adequate supply of oxygen. Hypoxia can lead to fatigue, nausea and potentially unconsciousness. Past a certain point there is not enough oxygen to sustain the body. Figure 2 shows the relationship between the total pressure for different altitudes and the volume percentage of oxygen.

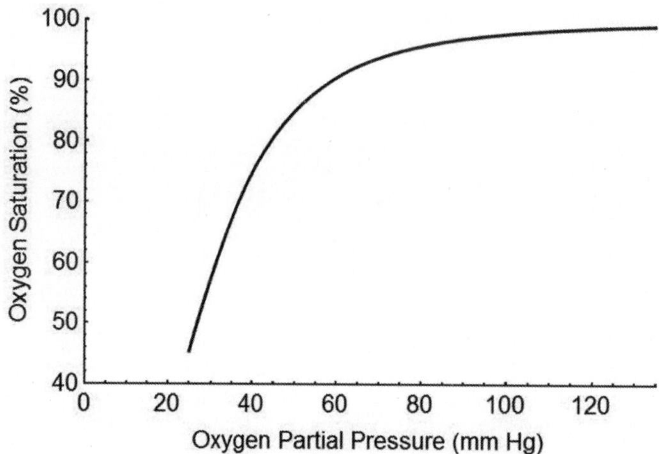

Figure 1 Percentage of oxygen saturation in hemoglobin versus the oxygen partial pressure

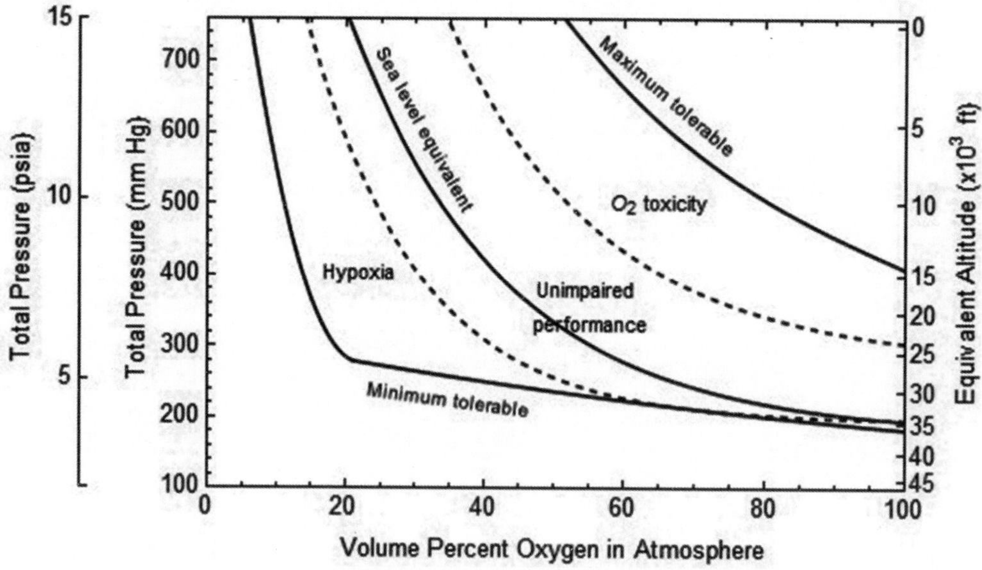

Figure 2 Pressure and oxygen percentage as a function of altitude

Figure 1 adapted from Julie-Ann Collins, Aram Rudenski, John Gibson, Luke Howard and Ronan O'Driscoll, Breathe, 2015. Figure 2 adapted from Man-System Integration Standards Volume 1, National Aeronautics and Space Administration, 1995.

Question 33

Climbers have a higher chance of surviving the Death Zone if they take supplemental oxygen delivered through a face mask. How does the supplemental oxygen affect the body?

- O **A.** Increases oxygen flow rate
- O **B.** Increases percent oxygen saturation
- O **C.** Decreases oxygen partial pressure
- O **D.** Decreases chance of oxygen toxicity

Question 34

At sea level, what is the optimal oxygen partial pressure?

- O **A.** 1-3 psia
- O **B.** 3-6 psia
- O **C.** 6-8 psia
- O **D.** 8-10 psia

Question 35

At 5 psia of total pressure, what is the minimum percentage of oxygen-saturated hemoglobin a climber needs?

- O **A.** 20%
- O **B.** 45%
- O **C.** 60%
- O **D.** 85%

Question 36

At 20,000 feet, at what volume percent oxygen does hypoxia set in?

- O **A.** 20%
- O **B.** 35%
- O **C.** 45%
- O **D.** 60%

Passage 7 (Questions 37–40)

An organic chemist was attempting to prepare alkyl halides from alcohols. Three experiments were performed.

Experiment 1

Sodium chloride was reacted with 1-butanol using sulfuric acid as a catalyst. Two alkyl halides were produced.

$$CH_3CH_2CH_2CH_2OH + NaCl \xrightarrow{H_2SO_4} \underset{\textit{Product 1}}{CH_3CH_2CH(Cl)CH_3} + \underset{\textit{Product 2}}{CH_3CH_2CH_2CH_2Cl} + H_2O$$

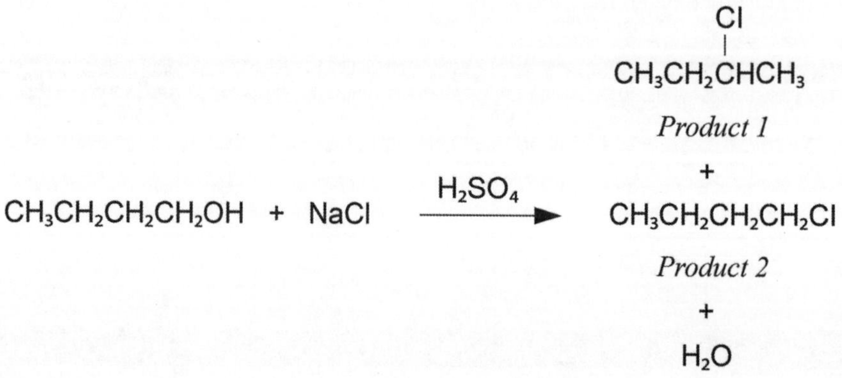

Experiment 2

Chlorine gas was reacted with 1-butanol. Four different products were produced in varying amounts. The two most abundant products are listed.

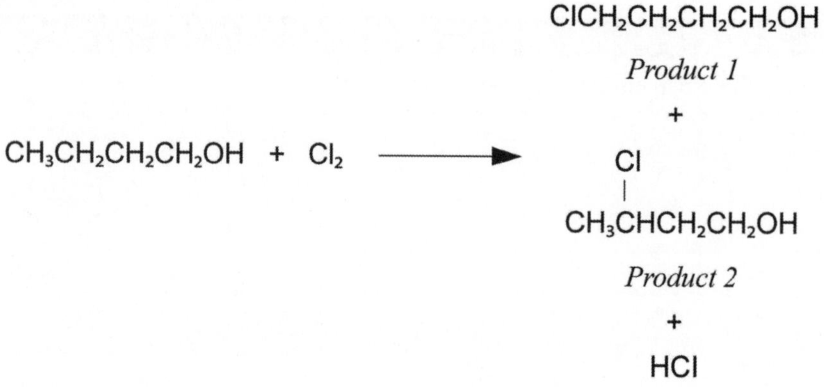

$$CH_3CH_2CH_2CH_2OH + Cl_2 \longrightarrow \underset{\textit{Product 1}}{ClCH_2CH_2CH_2CH_2OH} + \underset{\textit{Product 2}}{CH_3CH(Cl)CH_2CH_2OH} + HCl$$

Experiment 3

Hydrogen chloride was reacted with 1-butanol. Two alkyl halides were produced.

$$CH_3CH_2CH_2CH_2OH + HCl \longrightarrow \underset{\textit{Product 1}}{CH_3CH_2CH(Cl)CH_3} + \underset{\textit{Product 2}}{CH_3CH_2CH_2CH_2Cl} + H_2O$$

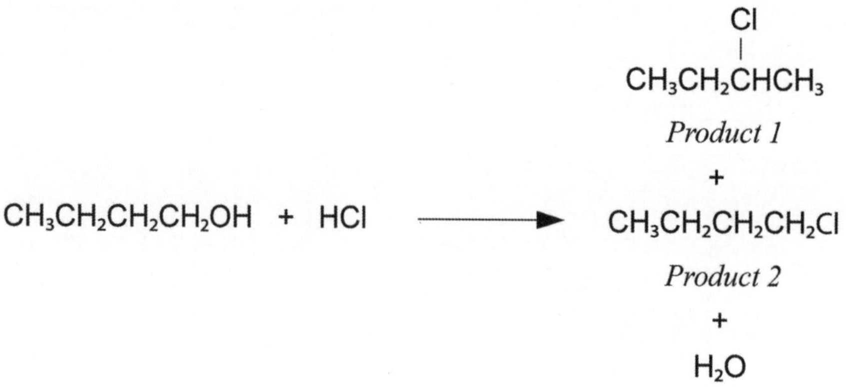

Question 37

Which of the following accounts for there being two products in Experiment 1?

- ○ **A.** The heat of formation for the reaction in Experiment 1 does not favor one product over the other.
- ○ **B.** A proton shifts from the 2 carbon position to the 1 carbon position in some molecules.
- ○ **C.** Product 1 and product 2 are formed by the same mechanism.
- ○ **D.** Product 1 and product 2 are equally stable.

Question 38

The catalyst in Experiment 1 has the function of:

- ○ **A.** protonating the chloride ion after it dissociates from the sodium to form the strong acid HCl.
- ○ **B.** increasing the temperature of the reaction so that its rate of reaction increases.
- ○ **C.** protonating the oxygen of 1-butanol in order to form a good leaving group
- ○ **D.** providing protons so that a hydride shift can occur to form a stable carbocation.

Question 39

When HCl was replaced with HF in Experiment 3 only a small amount of product formed. Which of the following explains this phenomenon?

- ○ **A.** HF is a weak acid.
- ○ **B.** Fluoride ions do not react well with carbon due to there being a large difference in electronegativity between the two species.
- ○ **C.** Upon dissociating, the proton from the HF molecule will not protonate the oxygen atom of 1-butanol.
- ○ **D.** Fluoride ions form F_2 gas at a quicker rate than fluoride bonds with carbon.

Question 40

If product 1 in Experiment 3 were the only desired product, which of the following should be reacted with HCl?

○ **A.**

```
               OH
               |
CH3CH2CH2CH2
```

○ **B.**

```
    OH
    |
CH3CHCH2CH3
```

○ **C.** $CH_3CH_2OCH_2CH_3$

○ **D.**

```
    OHOH
    |  |
CH3CHCHCH3
```

Passage 8 (Questions 41–44)

Polyprotic acids are those capable of dissociating more than one ionizable hydrogen. Carbonic acid, H_2CO_3, is an example of a polyprotic acid. It is formed when carbon dioxide dissolves in water. The solubility of CO_2 in water is quite sensitive to pH.

Reaction I

$CO_2 + H_2O \leftrightarrow H_2CO_3$

Carbonic acid has two ionization equilibria with each having a distinct acid dissociation constant (K_a):

Reaction II

$H_2CO_3 + H_2O \leftrightarrow H_3O^+ + HCO_3^-$

Reaction III

$HCO_3^- + H_2O \leftrightarrow H_3O^+ + CO_3^{2-}$

Carbon dioxide diffuses out of cells and is transported in blood in a few different ways: less than 10% dissolves in the blood plasma, about 20% binds to hemoglobin, while about 70% is converted to carbonic acid to be carried to the lungs.

Carbonic anhydrase is an enzyme present in red blood cells (RBCs) containing zinc coordinated with histidine at the active site that catalyzes the reversible hydration of carbon dioxide. Binding of the substrate carbon dioxide occurs at a hydrophobic pocket. The mechanism at the active site can be summarized below.

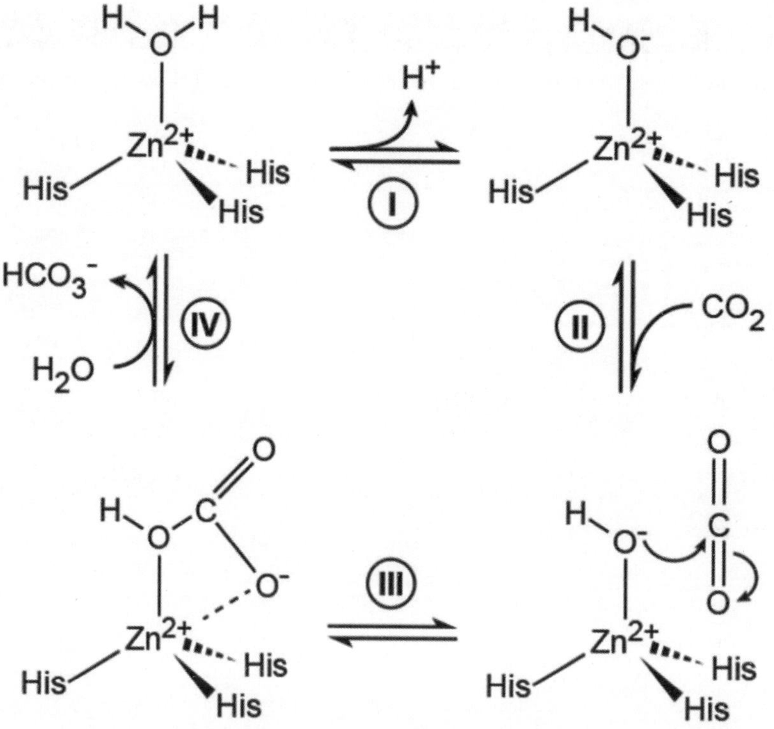

Question 41

According to the Bronsted-Lowry acid-base theory, which of the following species is the conjugate base of carbonic acid?

- ○ **A.** OH^-
- ○ **B.** HCO_3^-
- ○ **C.** CO_3^{2-}
- ○ **D.** H_3O^+

Question 42

It can be assumed that Reaction III is the rate-limiting step of the net reaction of Reactions II and III. What best accounts for this assumption?

- ○ **A.** H_2CO_3 is a stronger acid than HCO_3^-
- ○ **B.** Reaction II has a slower rate of reaction than Reaction III
- ○ **C.** Reaction II has a smaller equilibrium constant
- ○ **D.** HCO_3^- is a weaker base than CO_3^{2-}

Question 43

As shown in Reaction II and Reaction III, carbonic acid ionizes in a stepwise manner. Consequently, two equilibrium expressions (K_{a1} and K_{a2}) can be written for each ionization step. The first ionization K_{a1} is much larger than the second ionization constant K_{a2}. Which of the following statements would correctly explain why the value of K_{a1} is much larger than that of K_{a2} for carbonic acid?

- ○ **A.** Carbonic acid is a weak acid and so is completely ionized resulting in a large K_{a1}.
- ○ **B.** It is much easier to remove H^+ from the first ionization step of carbonic acid as it is uncharged.
- ○ **C.** There really should not be a great difference between the two ionization constants (K_{a1} and K_{a2}) as both released H^+ ions are from carbonic acid.
- ○ **D.** As the concentration of H^+ released from the first ionization is much larger than the second ionization, this will increase the possibility of the second ionization concentration to be large

Question 44

Which of the following is likely true about the activity of carbonic anhydrase in RBCs?

I. Carbonic anhydrase increases the rate of Reaction I by bringing the reactants into close proximity.
II. The higher the pH, the greater the activity of carbonic anhydrase in the hydration of carbon dioxide.
III. The activity of carbonic anhydrase leads to increased carbon dioxide in RBCs in the lungs.

- ○ **A.** I only
- ○ **B.** II only
- ○ **C.** I and III only
- ○ **D.** I, II and III

The following questions are NOT based on a descriptive passage (Questions 45–48).

Question 45

A Doppler study of a patient's aorta was used to determine the speed of blood flow at 0.40 m/s in the thoracic aorta and then at a point 0.4 m away, 0.20 m/s in the abdominal aorta. Assuming that the blood flow slowed at a constant rate, what is the rate that the blood slowed between the 2 points measured along the aorta?

- ○ **A.** 0.15 m/s^2
- ○ **B.** 0.30 m/s^2
- ○ **C.** 1.50 m/s^2
- ○ **D.** 3.00 m/s^2

Question 46

From the following, choose the potential energy profile for an S_N2 reaction:

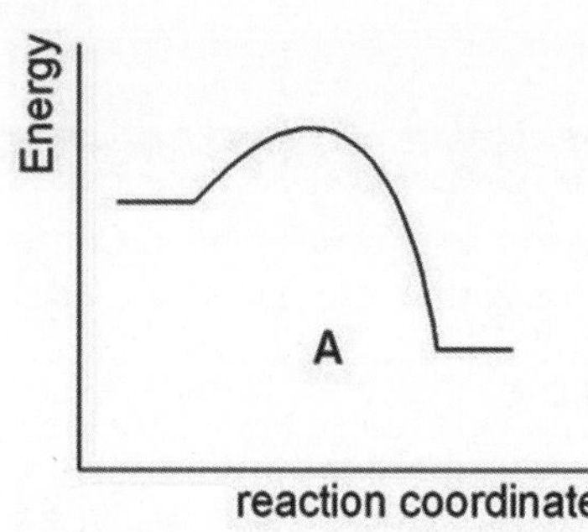

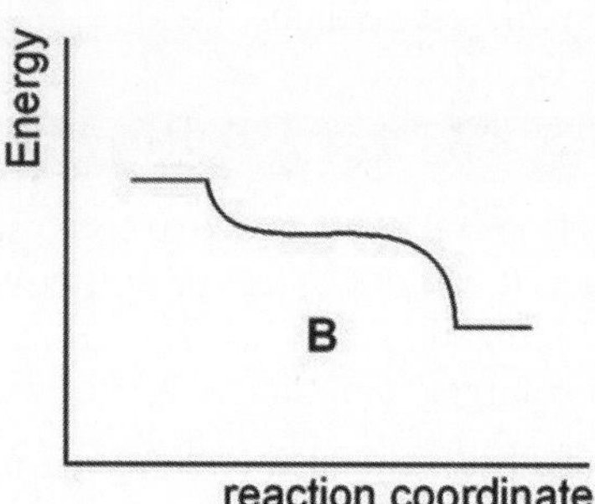

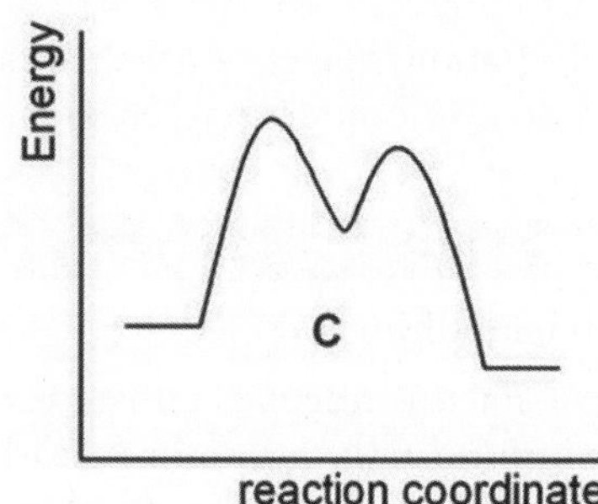

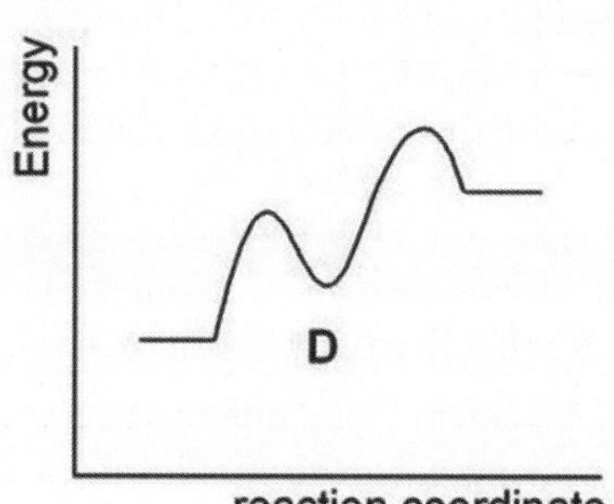

- ○ **A.** A
- ○ **B.** B
- ○ **C.** C
- ○ **D.** D

Question 47

Which of the following is NOT characteristic of hydrogen bonding?

- ○ **A.** The hydrogen atom involved must be covalently bonded to a very electronegative atom.
- ○ **B.** The hydrogen bonds are typically weaker than ionic or covalent bonds.
- ○ **C.** The other atom involved in the hydrogen bond (not the hydrogen atom) must be covalently bonded to a hydrogen atom.
- ○ **D.** The other atom involved in the hydrogen bond (not the hydrogen atom) must possess at least one lone pair of electrons.

Question 48

Identify the correct order of the following molecules with respect to their ability to form hydrates, from highest to lowest (Me = methyl).

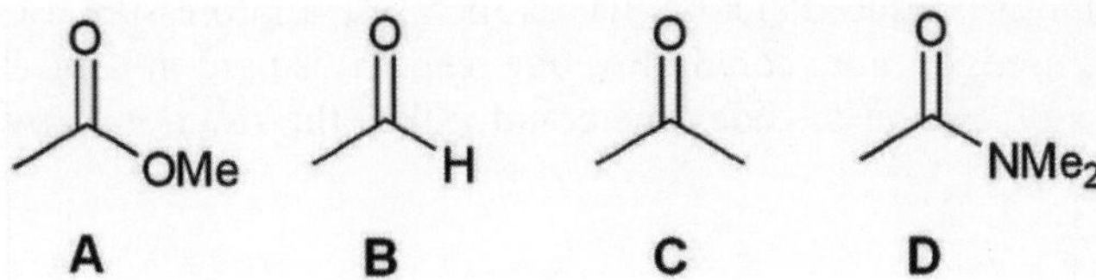

- ○ **A.** A > B > C > D
- ○ **B.** B > C > A > D
- ○ **C.** C > B > D > A
- ○ **D.** D > A > C > B

Passage 9 (Questions 49–52)

From the ideal gas equation PV = nRT, it is possible to determine the molar mass of a gas once the other physical variables are known. One technique for doing this involves the production of a known volume of the gas from one of the reactions in which it is produced at a known temperature and pressure. In the reaction, stoichiometric amounts of the reactants are used, or more commonly, one reactant is used in large excess. For example, in order to determine the molar mass of carbon dioxide, one could utilize the reaction between carbonates and acid as shown in Reaction I.

Reaction I

$MgCO_3 + 2HCl \rightarrow MgCl_2 + CO_2(g) + H_2O$

The reaction is carried out in a closed vessel attached to a water manometer (a thin U-tube filled with water) where the difference in the height of the two levels in the two arms can be used to determine the pressure inside the vessel. This is due to the fact that the relative levels in the two arms gives the **difference** in pressure between the atmosphere and the vessel.

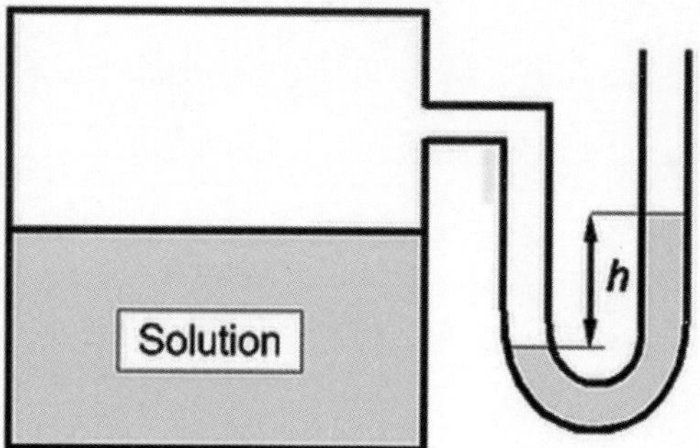

35.00 grams of $MgCO_3$ were placed into the reaction vessel and 150 mL of 5 M HCl were subsequently added. After all the $MgCO_3$ had reacted, the difference in height of the water in the two arms of the manometer was read.

Question 49

Given the density of water is 1000 kg m^{-3} and that gravitational acceleration g = 9.8 m s^{-2}, calculate the pressure inside the reaction vessel if the level of water in the right arm of the manometer was 50 cm higher than in the left arm.

- ○ **A.** 4900 N m^{-2} + atmospheric pressure
- ○ **B.** 490 N m^{-2} + atmospheric pressure
- ○ **C.** 9800 N m^{-2} + atmospheric pressure
- ○ **D.** 980 N m^{-2} + atmospheric pressure

Question 50

How should the ideal gas equation be rearranged to allow for the determination of the molecular mass of the gas? (The mass of the gas is designated by "w" and the molar mass of the gas is designated by "M" for this question and the following two questions)

- o **A.** M = wPT/(RV)
- o **B.** M = RV/(wPT)
- o **C.** M = wRT/(PV)
- o **D.** M = PV/(wRT)

Question 51

If Reaction I was exothermic and the temperature of the reaction vessel ended up being higher than expected, if the initial temperature was used in the equation how would the recorded value of M compare to its predicted value?

- o **A.** It would be higher than expected.
- o **B.** It would be lower than expected.
- o **C.** It would be the same.
- o **D.** The direction of change of the value of M cannot be predicted from the data given.

Question 52

CO_2 happens to be quite soluble in water. How would this affect the value of M obtained in the experiment?

- o **A.** It would be higher than expected.
- o **B.** It would be lower than expected.
- o **C.** It would be the same.
- o **D.** The direction of change of the value of M cannot be determined from the data given.

Passage 10 (Questions 53–56)

Flexible endoscopes have revolutionized many areas of diagnostic medicine by helping to visualize internal structures such as the respiratory tract, stomach, and colon. Unlike a rigid endoscope, a flexible endoscope can bend and thus go around "corners." The consequence is less discomfort for the patient and the endoscope can be advanced farther into the cavity under examination.

A typical endoscope has various channels, such as for irrigation, suction, surgical manipulation, illumination, and imaging. The image from the patient is transmitted along bundles of optical fibers containing separate layers of glass, or more specifically, silica. Each optical fiber consists of a cylindrical *core* surrounded by a *cladding*. Light enters one end of a fiber and is total internally reflected repeatedly until it exits the fiber at the opposite end. Because of the difference in the index of refraction of the two layers, total internal reflection confines the light waves within the core of the fiber.

A model for a segment of an optical fiber in longitudinal section is shown in Figure 1. A beam of light enters one end of the fiber at an angle with respect to the axis of the fiber. Assume that the interface between the air and the optical fiber is a flat plane.

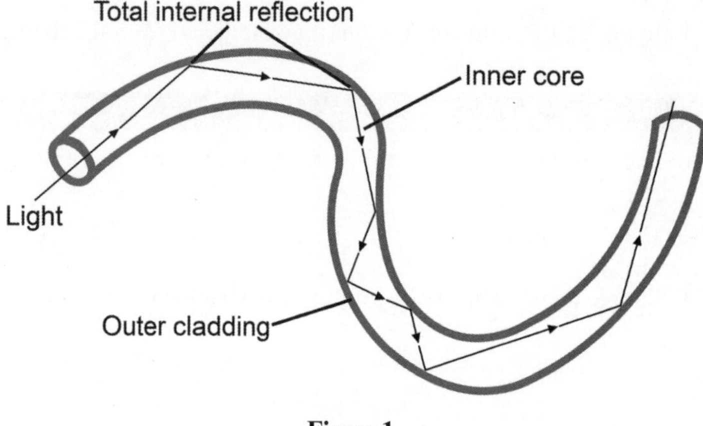

Figure 1

The optical density of a material is given by the index of refraction n. Snell's law states that the ratio of the sines of the angles of incidence and refraction is equivalent to the reciprocal of the ratio of the indices of refraction.

Question 53

For the best image quality, which of the following conditions should be met?

I. The cladding must have a higher optical density than the core.
II. Light rays must be incident to the core-cladding interface at angles of incidence greater than the critical angle.
III. The core must not absorb a significant amount of light.

- ○ **A.** II only
- ○ **B.** I and II only
- ○ **C.** II and III only
- ○ **D.** I, II and III

Question 54

The critical angle of the core-cladding interface is given by:

- ○ **A.** critical angle = $\sin^{-1}(n_{cladding}/n_{core})$
- ○ **B.** critical angle = $\sin^{-1}(n_{core}/n_{cladding})$
- ○ **C.** critical angle = $\sin^{-1}(1/n_{core})$
- ○ **D.** critical angle = $\sin^{-1}(1/n_{cladding})$

Question 55

Consider the following graphs of the sine of the angle of refraction (y axis) vs. the sine of the angle of incidence (x axis). Which of the following is consistent with Snell's law?

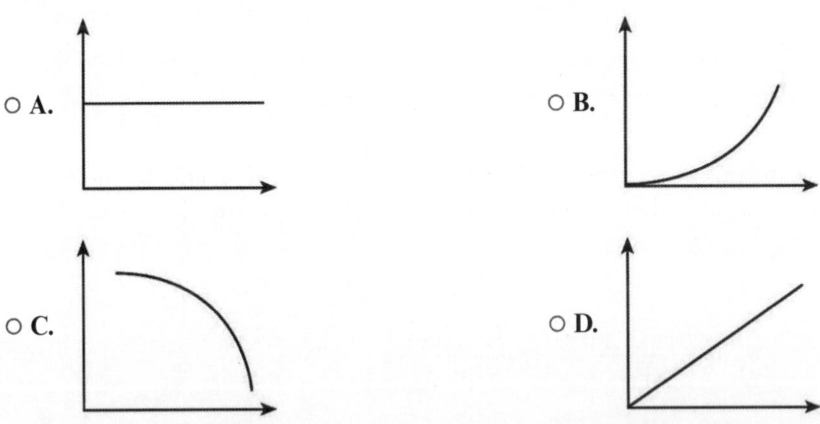

Question 56

A spherical air bubble is rising in a small pool of clear gastrointestinal fluid and is illuminated from one side by an endoscope. What happens to a ray of light incident on the air bubble at A?

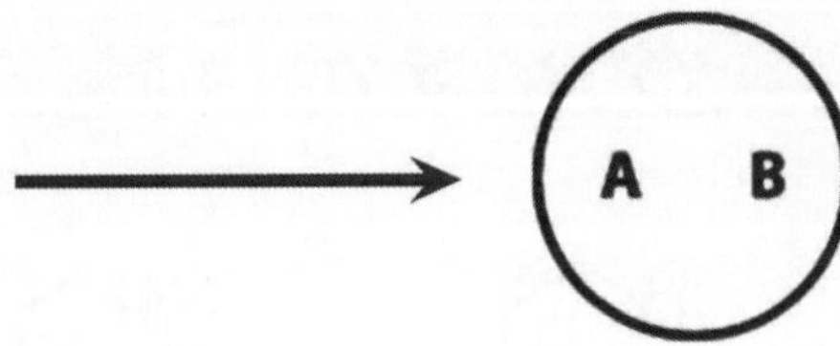

- ○ **A.** Reflection at both surfaces
- ○ **B.** Reflection at A; no reflection at B
- ○ **C.** Reflection at B; no reflection at A
- ○ **D.** no reflection at either surface

The following questions are NOT based on a descriptive passage (Questions 57–59).

Question 57

Consider Figure 1 and the Michaelis-Menten equation.

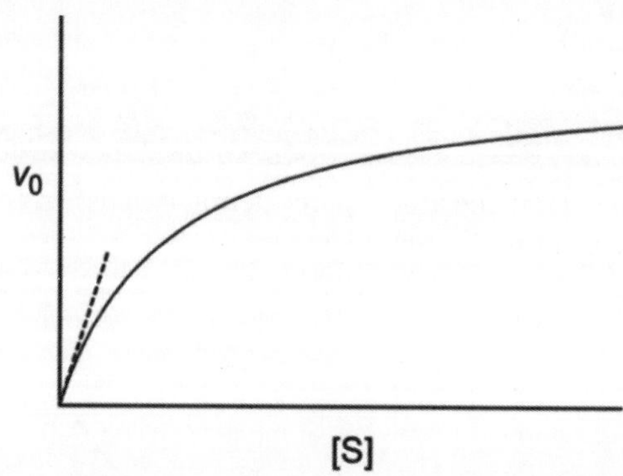

Figure 1 Initial velocity v_0 versus substrate concentration [S] in an enzyme-catalyzed reaction demonstrating Michaelis-Menten kinetics. The dashed line indicates the slope of the curve when [S] << K_m.

The Michaelis-Menten equation:

$$v_0 = \frac{k_{cat}[E_t][S]}{[S] + K_m} = \frac{V_{max}[S]}{[S] + K_m}$$

Which of the following corresponds to the slope of the dashed line in Figure 1?

- O **A.** (1/2)[S]
- O **B.** V_{max}/K_m
- O **C.** k_{cat}/K_m
- O **D.** $1/V_{max}$

Question 58

Which of the following molecules are chiral?

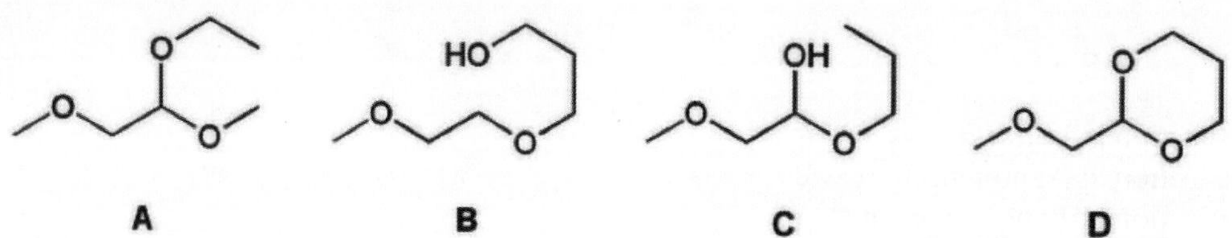

- O **A.** A and B
- O **B.** B and C
- O **C.** C and D
- O **D.** A and C

Question 59

Estimate the number of times that your heart beats in one year.

- O **A.** 4.2 x 10^7
- O **B.** 4.2 x 10^9
- O **C.** 4.2 x 10^{11}
- O **D.** 4.2 x 10^{13}

CANDIDATE'S NAME ____________________________

RAW SCORE AND SCALED SCORE ____________________________

GS-4
Mock Exam 4 of 7
Solutions at MCAT-prep.com

GS-4 Section II: Critical Analysis and Reasoning Skills (CARS)

Questions: 1-53
Time: 90 minutes

INSTRUCTIONS: This test contains nine passages, each of which is followed by several questions. After reading the passage, select the best answer to each question. If you are unsure of the answer, eliminate the alternatives you know to be false then select an answer from the remaining alternatives. To indicate your selection, use a pencil to blacken the corresponding circle next to the answer choice and/or you can use the answer document at the back of this book. No marks are deducted for wrong answers.

The computer-based real MCAT has an on-screen highlighter function and ~~STRIKEOUT~~ function. These tools help to spotlight text or assist in the process of elimination. You may use a yellow highlighter for this paper-based exam and/or a pen (or preferably a pencil to make it easier should you change your mind) to mark text. At the time of publishing, both highlighting and strikeout functions can be used for passages, questions and answer choices. You can also flag a question to review later should time remain.

For the real exam, you will be provided with a dry erase board which is a white laminated noteboard booklet accompanied by a fine point marker. The noteboard includes 9 graph-lined pages for you to write though you cannot erase. You can simulate the experience with a fine point marker on a noteboard or with 8” x 14” plain graph paper.

Please note: For the real MCAT, a small number of field-tested questions will remain unscored.

This practice test has been designed exclusively to test knowledge and thinking skills. This exam may contain hypothetical statements and/or express controversial ideas. Statements contained herein do not necessarily reflect the policy, position, or view of RuveneCo Inc. or MCAT-prep.com.

START EXAM ONLY WHEN TIMER IS READY.

Passage 1 (Questions 1–6)

The "Theatre of the Absurd" is a term coined by Hungarian-born critic Martin Esslin, who made it the title of his 1962 book on the subject. The term refers to a particular type of play which first became popular during the 1950s and 1960s and which presented on stage the philosophy articulated by French philosopher Albert Camus in his 1942 essay, "The Myth of Sisyphus," in which he defines the human condition as basically meaningless. Camus argued that humanity had to resign itself to recognizing that a fully satisfying rational explanation of the universe was beyond its reach; in that sense, the world must ultimately be seen as absurd.

Esslin regarded the term "Theatre of the Absurd" merely as a "device" through which he meant to bring attention to certain fundamental traits discernible in the works of a range of playwrights. The playwrights loosely grouped under the label of the "absurd" attempt to convey their sense of bewilderment, anxiety, and wonder in the face of an inexplicable universe. According to Esslin, the five defining playwrights of the movement are Eugène Ionesco, Samuel Beckett, Jean Genet, Arthur Adamov, and Harold Pinter, although these writers were not always comfortable with the label and sometimes preferred to use terms such as "Anti-Theater" or "New Theater." Other playwrights associated with this type of theatre include Tom Stoppard, Arthur Kopit, Friedrich Dürrenmatt, Fernando Arrabal, Edward Albee, N.F. Simpson, Boris Vian, Peter Weiss, Vaclav Havel, and Jean Tardieu.

The most famous, and most controversial, absurdist play is probably Samuel Beckett's *Waiting for Godot*. The characters of the play are strange caricatures who have difficulty communicating the simplest of concepts to one another as they bide their time awaiting the arrival of Godot. The language they use is often ludicrous, following a cyclical pattern, seeming to end in precisely the same condition it began, with no real change having occurred. In fact, it is sometimes referred to as "the play where nothing happens." Its detractors count this a fatal flaw and often turn red in the face fomenting on its inadequacies. It is mere gibberish, they cry, eyes nearly bulging out of their head—a prank on the audience disguised as a play. The play's supporters, on the other hand, describe it is an accurate portrayal of the human condition in which "the more things change, the more they are the same." Change, they argue, is only an illusion.

In 1955, the famous character actor Robert Morley predicted that the success of *Waiting for Godot* meant "the end of theatre as we know it." His generation may have gloomily accepted this prediction, but the younger generation embraced it. They were ready for something new—something that would move beyond the old stereotypes and reflect their increasingly complex understanding of existence.

Whereas traditional theatre attempts to create a photographic representation of life as we see it, the Theatre of the Absurd aims to create a ritual-like, mythological, archetypal, allegorical vision, closely related to the world of dreams. The focal point of these dreams is often man's fundamental bewilderment and confusion, stemming from the fact that he has no answers to the basic existential questions: why we are alive, why we have to die, why there is injustice and suffering. Ionesco defined the absurdist everyman as "Cut off from his religious, metaphysical, and transcendental roots ... lost; all his actions become senseless, absurd, useless." The Theatre of the Absurd, in a sense, attempts to reestablish man's communion with the universe. Dr. Jan Culik writes, "Absurd Theatre can be seen as an attempt to restore the importance of myth and ritual to our age, by making man aware of the ultimate realities of his condition, by instilling in him again the lost sense of cosmic wonder and primeval anguish. The Absurd Theatre hopes to achieve this by shocking man out of an existence that has become trite, mechanical and complacent. It is felt that there is mystical experience in confronting the limits of human condition."

Crabb, J. P. (2006, Sept 02). Theatre of the Absurd. *Theatre Database*. Retrieved from www.theatredatabase.com/20th_century/theatre_of_the_absurd.html.

Question 1

Based on passage information, the playwrights under discussion in this passage used absurdity in order to:

- ○ **A.** provide a respite from the humdrum ordinariness of normal life.
- ○ **B.** shock viewers who believed all theater should reflect life realistically.
- ○ **C.** make viewers newly aware of the absurdity of human life.
- ○ **D.** express their real selves and the uniquely strange way they experienced life.

Question 2

One can infer from the passage information that "Theatre of the Absurd" plays:

I. contain naturalistic dialogue based on the rhythms of speech.
II. involve plots based on those of classical myths.
III. alter viewers' perceptions of reality after they leave the theater.

- ○ **A.** I and III
- ○ **B.** I, II, and III
- ○ **C.** III only
- ○ **D.** I only

Question 3

Based on passage information, it can be inferred that in Samuell Beckett's play *Waiting for Godot*:

- ○ **A.** the characters are mouthpieces for the author in accurately describing the absurdity of existence.
- ○ **B.** the concept of waiting is given cosmic significance as both characters and audience wait for something that will never occur.
- ○ **C.** the author provides an ambivalent statement on human existence because while the characters' lives do not improve, they also do not get any worse.
- ○ **D.** Beckett caricatures the ridiculous and shallow people of his time through the stilted words and actions of the characters.

Question 4

The author implies that the "Theatre of the Absurd" could be considered a:

- ○ **A.** branch of realism.
- ○ **B.** step in the evolution toward today's artistic forms.
- ○ **C.** template for producing artistic works.
- ○ **D.** genre of literature.

Question 5

An author who wished to critique Theatre of the Absurd might make all of the following claims EXCEPT:

- ○ **A.** Plays in which nothing happens are undramatic, and lose their value once the initial novelty wears off.
- ○ **B.** Ancient forms of storytelling like myth have just as much to tell us about the human condition as avant-garde forms like Theatre of the Absurd.
- ○ **C.** Life is not inherently absurd; instead its meaning comes from the struggle for justice.
- ○ **D.** The most effective way to highlight life's absurdity is to reveal it through strict realism.

Question 6

The author's tone in paragraph 3 discussing critics of *Waiting for Godot* can be described as:

- ○ **A.** analytical.
- ○ **B.** persuasive.
- ○ **C.** mocking.
- ○ **D.** definitional.

Passage 2 (Questions 7–11)

In order to use archaeological methods to gain a better understanding of the consumption and waste in packaged food products in contemporary Australian society, it is first essential to understand why archaeological methods could be useful in this scenario. Wylie explains that archaeology "could teach us about the conditions of life, the reasons for cultural change and persistence, affinity and diversity, that manifested themselves in the gritty particulars of the archaeological record."

It is thus not unreasonable to think that archaeological methods could also be applied to research questions set in a contemporary environment. According to the Contemporary and Historical Archaeology in Theory (CHAT) Group, Contemporary Archaeology is an area of archaeological research that is most interested in the more recent past. The hallmark of contemporary archaeology is that it involves the application of archaeological thinking to the contemporary or modern world. It is often informed by anthropological material culture studies and is characterised by applying traditional archaeological methods and practices to new uses.

The reason for developing this branch of archaeology is to allow traditional archaeological methods to make a contribution to broader social scientific studies of the contemporary world. Methods can include the study of material things such as objects, landscapes, buildings and material heritage through to sociological, geographical and political studies of the modern world.

Schofield and Harrison outline the main archaeological methods that can be used in a contemporary archaeology study. They suggest that while it is largely a matter of transferring traditional archaeological methods and skills, our cultural backgrounds and life experiences will potentially influence the way the material, which is often very familiar, is interpreted. There will also be differences in the natural decay, which because of the close temporal proximity, does not occur as readily in a contemporary setting. In the area of garbage, traditionally a rich source of material in archaeology studies, the fact that garbage is now regularly collected and transported to a specific location instead of being found in close proximity to the home or place of origin, changes the way that material can be interpreted.

The principle archaeological method that has been used in this study was artifact analysis. In the analysis of food packaging categories, the principle features were material and branding. There were also other complicating factors around the increasingly elaborate system of domestic recycling that means that similar items can end up in up to three completely separate waste streams. The type of information that was garnered from the material included the origin of the packaged food, how much was actually used, use by and best by dates, overall dietary habits and the amount and level of processed food in the total food waste stream.

Traditional research methods to address these types of research questions include consumer surveys, interviews and focus groups. While these methods have some value, it is also true that most people tend to underestimate the amount of food waste that occurs in their household. However, using contemporary archaeological methods over a period of time can provide actual data on what and how much people waste.

Starting in 1973, Dr. William Rathje and his students at the University of Arizona initiated the Garbage Project [4–6]. Quantitative data from garbage bins was compared with information known about the residents who owned them. The results indicated that information people freely volunteered about their consumption habits did not always tally with the contents of their garbage bins. For example, alcohol consumption was proven to be significantly higher in reality than in the questionnaires completed by the people studied. Such findings have highlighted the difference between people's self-reported and actual behaviours.

Lehmann, La. (2015, Feb). The Garbage Project Revisited: From a 20th Century Archaeology of Food Waste to a Contemporary Study of Food Packaging Waste. *Sustainability*, 7(6), 6994–7010. doi:10.3390/su7066994.

Question 7

This passage introduces a study on food waste. In doing so, it provides an explanation of which of the following?

- ○ **A.** Why it is relevant to study modern sites and items
- ○ **B.** Why and how traditional archaeological methods were adapted for the modern sites
- ○ **C.** What is uniquely difficult about the study of food waste
- ○ **D.** Where food waste can be found and the forms it takes

Question 8

The discussion of location in paragraphs 4 and 5 implies that:

- ○ **A.** traditional archaeology does not deal with waste products because its primary focus is on useful items that have been preserved.
- ○ **B.** traditional archaeology incorrectly assumed that garbage is always discarded near the place where it was created.
- ○ **C.** it is easier to provide an archaeological analysis of garbage if different types of garbage are pre-sorted into different sites.
- ○ **D.** traditional archaeology deals with sites where all the garbage has been discarded in a location near where it was created.

Question 9

Based on passage information, the BEST alternate example of Contemporary Archaeology would be:

- ○ **A.** a study of contemporary speech patterns at home versus at work, captured via digital recording.
- ○ **B.** a study on grocery purchases and eating habits done via supermarket sales records.
- ○ **C.** a study of how space is used in an office based on patterns of wear and tear.
- ○ **D.** a study of erosion on a mountain range over the last 10 years based on patterns of erosion.

Question 10

Based on the passage, we can assume that archaeological methods are not the most adequate in a situation where:

- ○ **A.** people are likely to accurately remember and honestly report their use of an item.
- ○ **B.** it is important to know the reasons behind individual item choices.
- ○ **C.** artifacts from multiple people or households have been discarded in one spot with no way to tell which item belonged to whom.
- ○ **D.** the primary topic of study is the discrepancy between the actual facts of people's lifestyles and their self-perceived lifestyle.

Question 11

Based on the final paragraph, other good uses for archaeological methods would be all of the following EXCEPT:

- ○ **A.** a study on the smoking patterns of drinkers conducted using trash inside bars.
- ○ **B.** a study on energy use in homes investigating how much power is wasted by leaving doors open and lights on.
- ○ **C.** a study of trash at a senior living facility investigating whether residents take their medications as often as prescribed.
- ○ **D.** a survey of recycling bins in busy and deserted areas indicating whether people recycle more regularly when others are watching.

Passage 3 (Questions 12–18)

For many instructors, the opportunity to teach Jane Austen is an occasion to share with students their love for a favorite author. One might imagine that students in these classes are excited about reading Austen's novels. Many of them have seen film adaptations of the novels; some have even read an actual novel or two before taking the class. I have encountered a very different kind of teaching situation, however: reading Austen with students who bring little or no excitement about Austen's novels to their college literature classroom.

John Jay, the institution where I teach, is one of about two dozen colleges that make up City University of New York (CUNY), the only public university in New York City, attended by approximately 200,000 students. Unique within CUNY as a federally registered "Hispanic-Serving Institution," John Jay enrolls about 15,000 students drawn primarily from working-class populations that arrive in New York City from every corner of the world.

Most of these students come to college having heard of very few writers in English, and some with no familiarity with literature at all. Their academic careers are tales of tremendously risky personal transformation. These students discover college literature classrooms (as well as other disciplines in the humanities) as spaces in which to become more competent thinkers about society and culture. Their experience studying the humanities goes against the expectations cultivated by parents and teachers who warn them about the dangers of failing to follow cultural norms, acquire academic credentials, and pursue the economic and social benefits of higher education.

Often for the first time, students find that a college literature classroom legitimizes doubts and conversations about the threats and warnings that brought them to college in the first place. At the cost of disrupting the safe, pragmatic plan they had presented to their parents and to themselves, they question committing to an occupation that would give them job security and social status. They choose instead to use the little time they have in college to look directly at the ideologies, social norms, and historical patterns that shape the lives of individuals: to question how they think, why they like what they like, why they do what they do.

From this constituency come the English majors who learn about the stature of Austen in various corners of U.S. popular culture, watch the films, read the novels, and still commonly refuse to develop a taste for them. In a situation where students abandon the values and priorities that brought them to college in the name of the new pleasures they discover in literature, their unwillingness to appreciate a popular canonical writer such as Austen is instructive. When they say they cannot enjoy Austen, students insist that Austen's work is not a good instrument for the kind of corrosive examination they have learned to desire.

Rectifying "one of the great anomalies of literary history" (Johnson xiii), feminist scholarship has re-configured Austen's canonical position and given her texts new historical and biographical interpretive frameworks. The novelist now enjoys the distinctive status of a female canonical figure deeply and deliberately immersed in the political matter of her day. Female characters in novels such as *Persuasion* could be read as ideological experiments testing the shape and currency of desirable masculinity and femininity in the setting Austen delineates. The novel seems to ask, Can there be "true love" outside the social norm that sanctions acceptable emotion and ties it to marriage, property, and the family?

I assign *Persuasion* because I share much of the enthusiasm of other professional critics about the novel as an important critical treatment of the politics of the modern family, gender norms, and affect. I like to believe that I use Austen's texts as instruments of social and cultural critique. This is the kind of pedagogy that brings my students to the literature classroom because they are excited to treat reading literary texts as a way to engage with their own burning ideological concerns.

Neither my excitement about *Persuasion*, nor the critics' sense of the novel's edginess, however, transfers to my students. They remain reluctant and unsympathetic readers of the novel. They disagree with the many professional critical readers who argue that Austen's novels critique societal norms and hierarchies. Anticipating readers' dissatisfaction with the politics of Austen's novels, Gary Kelly insists that present-day readers cannot expect to find their ideological and political concerns adequately represented in a nineteenth-century text. He proposes that "if Austen were considered a feminist, it would be by her participating in a feminism of her time, and not of ours."

Rather than aiming to turn students into "good" readers by positing authoritative readings as interpretive points of arrival, our class discussion has examined the grounds and implications of students' defiance. Their resistance is worth examining because it makes explicit and questionable the teacher's expectation that students would become better critics of society and culture by appreciating Austen's work in the way critics do. Precisely because they believe in the goals of the "heroic pedagogy," however, students disagree with the critics' claim that *Persuasion* is a novel subversive of the gender or class order.

Jokic, O. (2014). Teaching to the Resistance: What to Do When Students Dislike Austen. *Persuasions On-Line, a Publication of the Jane Austen Society of North America.* Retrieved from jasna.org.

Question 12

An assumption of the author in paragraphs 2 through 4 is that:

- A. students from underprivileged backgrounds are more unwilling than others to pursue the humanities as a route to questioning their assumptions.
- B. students from Hispanic backgrounds have more difficulty than US-born white students in finding cultural common ground with authors like Austen.
- C. students from underprivileged backgrounds are more likely than others to be encouraged to use college as a pragmatic route to a high-status career.
- D. traditional college English classes fail to provide for the needs of students from underprivileged backgrounds.

Question 13

Based on passage information, the type of students the teacher did NOT encounter in Jane Austen classrooms were:

- A. from educated backgrounds looking for socially critical literature.
- B. from underprivileged backgrounds questioning the need to be pragmatic.
- C. who reproach Austen for her extreme feminist gender-biased views.
- D. who reproach Austen for lack of relevant social criticism.

Question 14

According to the author, why is it ironic that her students reject Austen?

- A. The same subversive mode of reading that college English professors encourage leads students to reject her work as too conservative.
- B. The students who could most benefit from the lessons of Austen are those least likely to understand them.
- C. While Austen expresses concerns similar to those of these students, the style in which she expresses them makes them hard to understand.
- D. Middle-class white students are more likely to enjoy Austen even though her works critique the mentality of people like them.

Question 15

What does paragraph 6 most likely mean by "one of the greatest anomalies of literary history"?

- A. The unique willingness of Austen to question hierarchies of gender and class.
- B. The uniquely ambivalent position of Austen as an author who is both conservative and subversive.
- C. The inability of chauvinist critics throughout history to understand Austen's critique of gender ideology.
- D. The uniquely misguided omission of Austen from the canon of great feminist authors.

Question 16

Based on passage information, the author primarily sees college humanities classes as an opportunity to:

- ○ **A.** learn to appreciate the great authors of the Western tradition.
- ○ **B.** learn how to think critically about beliefs one has taken for granted.
- ○ **C.** learn how to read and appreciate literature in the way professional critics do.
- ○ **D.** acquire the cultural advantages of more privileged students.

Question 17

Which of the following would NOT constitute an example of the type of reading the author encourages?

- ○ **A.** Analyzing an unconventional female character as an example of rebellion against standards for ladylike behavior.
- ○ **B.** Analyzing the pressures that are placed on a main character to reject the man she has chosen to marry.
- ○ **C.** Analyzing a male character for the way his investment in conventional "chivalry" determines his behavior.
- ○ **D.** Analyzing a scene in which a character commits a faux pas to better understand the social etiquette of the time.

Question 18

Which of the following would the passage author deem an important criterion in evaluating literary works?

- ○ **A.** Ability to break free of the standards and beliefs of the society in which they were created
- ○ **B.** Sophistication with which they portray and analyze the ideological system of their time
- ○ **C.** Relevance to politically literate current-day readers
- ○ **D.** Standing in critical hierarchies

Note: This page is left blank so that the passage would be visible without turning pages while assessing the passage-based questions.

Passage 4 (Questions 19–25)

> "I believe that the use of noise to make music will continue and increase until we reach a music produced through the aid of electrical instruments which will make available for musical purposes any and all sounds that can be heard."
>
> —John Cage, The Future of Music: Credo

Noise music has a complex history and takes on many different forms and elements. It is a term used to describe varieties of avant-garde music and sound art that may use elements such as cacophony, dissonance, atonality, noise, indeterminacy, distortion, repetition, randomness, and acoustic, electronic, traditional, and non-traditional sounds in their realization. Noise music may also incorporate manipulated recordings, static, hiss and hum, feedback, live machine sounds, custom noise software, circuit bent instruments, and non-musical vocal elements that push noise towards the ecstatic.

The Futurist art movement was important for the development of the noise aesthetic, as was the Dada art movement (a prime example being the Antisymphony concert performed on April 30, 1919 in Berlin), and later the Surrealist and Fluxusart movements, specifically the Fluxus artists of the 60's and 70's, which included noise experimenters such as Joe Jones and Yoko Ono.

Contemporary noise music is often associated with extreme volume and distortion, particularly in the popular music domain, with examples such as Jimi Hendrix's use of feedback, Sonic Youth and Lou Reed's Metal Machine Music. However, many noise musicians are keenly aware of dynamics and build them into their pieces. Genres such as industrial, industrial techno, lo-fi music, black metal, and glitch music employ noise-based materials.

Definitions of noise music shift over time. Ben Watson, in his article "Noise as Permanent Revolution," points out that Ludwig van Beethoven's "Grosse Fuge" (1825) "sounded like noise" to his audience at the time. Indeed, Beethoven's publishers persuaded him to remove it from its original setting as the last movement of a string quartet. He did so, replacing it with a sparkling Allegro. They subsequently published "Grosse Fuge" separately under the title "Op. 133."

Though the works of the noted cultural critics Jean Baudrillard, Georges Bataille and Theodor Adorno, Paul Hegarty (2007) traces the history of "noise" back to 18th century concert hall music. He defines noise at different times as "intrusive, unwanted," "lacking skill, not being appropriate" and "a threatening emptiness." Hegarty contends that it is John Cage's composition "4'33", in which an audience sits through four and a half minutes of "silence" (Cage 1973), that represents the beginning of noise music proper. For Hegarty, "noise music", as with "4'33", is made up of incidental sounds that represent perfectly the tension between "desirable" sound (properly played musical notes) and undesirable "noise" that make up all noise music from Erik Satie to NON to Glenn Branca. In *Noise: The Political Economy of Music* (1985), Jacques Attali explores the relationship between noise music and the future of society. He indicates that noise in music is a predictor of social change and demonstrates how noise acts as the subconscious of society—validating and testing new social and political realities.

In common use, the word noise means unwanted sound or noise pollution. In electronics, noise can refer to the electronic signal corresponding to acoustic noise (in an audio system) or the electronic signal corresponding to the (visual) noise commonly seen as "snow" on a degraded television or video image. In signal processing or computing, it can be considered data without meaning; that is, data that is not being used to transmit a signal, but is simply produced as an unwanted by-product of other activities. Noise can block, distort, or change the meaning of a message in both human and electronic communication. White noise is a random signal (or process) with a flat power spectral density. In other words, the signal contains equal power within a fixed bandwidth at any center frequency. White noise is considered analogous to white light which contains all frequencies. Oddly enough, for Michel Serres (1982) in *The Parasite*, noise factors are the beginning of order or novelty. One can certainly view aesthetic movements as introductions of dissonance within established orders, from this perspective. Such as the introduction of noise and dissonance in rock and roll music, with the use of various gadgetry, such as stomp boxes, echoes, distortion pedals, and other variations of the noise motif.

Cage, J. (1938). The Future of Music: Credo. Seattle, Washington.

Nechvatal, J. (2011). Immersion into Noise: Noise Music. *Michigan Publishing, Open Humanities Press*. Retrieved from http://dx.doi.org/10.3998/ohp.9618970.0001.001. University of Michigan Library.

Question 19

What is the passage's definition of noise music?

- ○ **A.** Music that features unconventional elements like electronic sound and nontraditional instruments
- ○ **B.** Music that intentionally combines sounds in a manner that is generally deemed musically undesirable
- ○ **C.** Music that incorporates ambient sound and incidental noise
- ○ **D.** Music that includes abrasive or unpleasant sounds and is thus disliked by most people

Question 20

The anecdote about Beethoven in paragraph 5 implies that:

- ○ **A.** the Grosse Fuge now sounds musical to audiences because expectations for possible musical sounds have changed.
- ○ **B.** many sounds that seem like noise to us could have seemed musical to audiences of Beethoven's time.
- ○ **C.** people in Beethoven's time were less tolerant of music that sounded like "noise" than people in our time.
- ○ **D.** the Grosse Fuge was influential and helped pave the way for later noise music.

Question 21

One possible reason for the author's choice of epigraph is to show that:

- ○ **A.** listeners have embraced electronic music but do not understand its roots in the noise genre.
- ○ **B.** Cage represents the misleading view that noise music must be based on electronic sound.
- ○ **C.** Cage's prediction came true, suggesting that the role of noise in music has become greater.
- ○ **D.** now that music is dominated by electronic instruments, the divide between music and pure noise has disappeared.

Question 22

Based on passage information, the main role of social conventions about music genres is to:

- ○ **A.** make clear to listeners what to expect as a legitimate part of the musical experience.
- ○ **B.** dictate what elements go into a piece of music.
- ○ **C.** provide a set of criteria that helps listeners to judge the quality of the piece.
- ○ **D.** provide a set of criteria that helps listeners decide if they like a work of music or not.

Question 23

What would NOT necessarily count as an example of analogous to noise in a different medium other than sound?

- ○ **A.** A perfume that employs undesirable smells like sweat and dirt.
- ○ **B.** Non-representative painting in which the canvas is covered in abstract shapes.
- ○ **C.** A deliberately unflattering line of fashions that makes the figure look shapeless.
- ○ **D.** A film that deliberately leaves in mistakes, such as line misreadings and continuity errors.

Question 24

Many critics are discussed within the passage, each with a particular view of noise. Which of the following views is NOT represented in the passage?

- ○ **A.** Noise in music is connected to large-scale changes in society.
- ○ **B.** Noise as a genre had its true beginning before the 20th century.
- ○ **C.** Noise is a common element in the birth of new genres.
- ○ **D.** Noise reflects the ugliness of the mechanized society that produced it.

Question 25

Which of the following assertions is LEAST supported in the text?

- ○ **A.** Definitions of noise music modify over time.
- ○ **B.** Noise musicians sought to break music-related conventions.
- ○ **C.** The history of noise music is intricate and it manifests itself in many different ways.
- ○ **D.** Jacques Attali argued that noise music reflects social changes.

Passage 5 (Questions 26–31)

Critical thinking has been described as "the correct assessing of statements"; "thinking about thinking"; "knowing how to think"; "the intellectually disciplined process of actively and skillfully conceptualizing, applying, analyzing, synthesizing, and/or evaluating information gathered from, or generated by, observation, experience, reflection, reasoning, or communication, as a guide to belief and action"; and "the process of purposeful, self-regulatory judgment, which uses reasoned consideration to evidence, context, conceptualizations, methods, and criteria."

These understandings of what critical thinking is can be grouped into two groups: Narrow, and Broad. Broad definitions equate critical thinking with the cognitive processes and strategies involved in decision making, problem solving, or inquiry – as with Robert H. Ennis' claim that it is "reflective and reasonable thinking that is focused on deciding what to believe or do." Limited definitions focus on the evaluation or appraisal processes behind the formulation of judgments – that is, as one of the essential elements involved in problem solving, decision making, and alike cognitive tasks.

Critical thinking, whether conceived broadly or narrowly, implies curiosity, skepticism, reflection, and rationality. Philosophers further link it to the commitment to the social and political practice of participatory democracy, willingness to imagine or remain open to considering alternative perspectives, willingness to integrate new or revised perspectives into our ways of thinking and acting, and willingness to foster criticality in others.

There is a reasonable level of consensus among experts that individuals or groups engaged in strong critical thinking take into consideration:

- Observed evidence;
- Context (e.g., setting or environment, historical background);
- Evaluation criteria (e.g., logic, clarity, credibility, accuracy, precision, relevance, depth, breadth, significance, and fairness); and
- Theoretical constructs framing the problem or question at hand.

In an article for The Center of Skeptical Inquiry, James Lett listed six rules, or tests, that a critical thinker may utilize. These can be conceived as evaluation criteria that are commonly associated with the scientific method and are:

- Falsifiability (i.e., has limited scope, is specific, not overgeneralized)
- Logic (i.e., proceeds from a deduction)
- Comprehensiveness (i.e., adequately covers what it purports to cover)
- Honesty (i.e., is ethically and morally sound)
- Replicability (i.e., can be repeated in a study, or observation)
- Sufficiency (i.e., is quantitatively sound, there is "enough" data

Many proponents of critical thinking stop short of evaluating the most basic criteria, or values, by which they make judgments. They understand the concept of critical thinking only within conventional frames of reference of a society. A more profound view encourages appraisal of frameworks or sets of criteria by which judgments are made. This deeper level of critical thinking counteracts egocentric, ethnocentric, or doctrinaire judgments, which result when thinkers fail to appraise fundamental assumptions or standards.

Ennis, R. H. (1985 Oct). A logical basis for measuring critical thinking skills. *Educational Leadership, 43*(2), 44-48. Retrieved from https://eric.ed.gov/?id=EJ327936

Lett, J. (1990, Winter). A Field Guide to Critical Thinking. *Skeptical Inquirer*, *14*(2).

Question 26

According to the passage, which of the following is the LEAST representative example of critical thinking?

○ **A.** Determining whether conclusions are valid
○ **B.** Deciding what course of action to take
○ **C.** Selecting the most relevant standards for prioritizing options
○ **D.** Listing what is known about something

Question 27

One weakness of the passage could be inferred to be:

- ○ **A.** lack of examples of critical thinking, as applied to different contexts.
- ○ **B.** lack of discussion of alternate understandings of critical thinking.
- ○ **C.** lack of discussion of practical applications of critical thinking.
- ○ **D.** lack of discussion of the role of bias and preconception in hindering critical thinking.

Question 28

Which of the following would constitute an example of the "deeper level of critical thinking" discussed in the last paragraph of the passage?

- ○ **A.** Basing one's decided course of action on a forecast of how it will affect one over a period of months or years.
- ○ **B.** Engaging in critical thinking for its own sake, such as solving a mathematical equation once thought to be impossible.
- ○ **C.** Questioning whether ideas based on scientific studies are more valid than ideas based on people's self-reported experiences.
- ○ **D.** Questioning whether it is more fair to appoint panelists in a 50/50 male-female ratio, or based purely on one's perception of merit.

Question 29

The most comprehensive title for the passage would be:

- ○ **A.** Metacognition: Thinking About Thinking
- ○ **B.** The Narrow and Broad Definitions of Critical Thinking
- ○ **C.** Critical Thinking and Its Applications
- ○ **D.** Critical Thinking: An Overview

Question 30

The "evaluation criteria" in paragraph four and Lett's rules in paragraph five differ in which of the following ways?

I. The first focuses on general characteristics, while the second provides guidelines for ruling something in or out as an example of critical thinking.
II. The first refers to evidence upon which a conclusion is based, while Lett's rules focus on premises, logic and theoretical frameworks.
III. Only Lett's rules can be inferred to have quantitative applications.

- ○ **A.** I, II, and III
- ○ **B.** II and III
- ○ **C.** I and III
- ○ **D.** I only

Question 31

Based on passage information, for which of the following is critical thinking the LEAST relevant?

- ○ **A.** Thinking about the best public policies and ways to carry them out.
- ○ **B.** Thinking about and addressing citizens' needs when such actions are found to be fruitful.
- ○ **C.** Describing systems of government such as democracy, theocracy, autocracy, and oligarchy.
- ○ **D.** Ability to evaluate politicians' statements and decide whether they make sense.

Passage 6 (Questions 32–37)

The concept of a 'tourist bubble' – which is similar to what Cohen (1972, 166) has called the environmental bubble – was coined by Smith (1978, 6) to denote the tendency of tourists to stay among themselves and to be 'physically "in" a foreign place but socially "outside" its culture'. It was later used for the segregation of tourism areas from local residential spaces as a way to create familiar cultural environments where tourists could feel safe. Judd (1999, 36) employed the tourist bubble concept in this sense with respect to the refurbishment of downtown areas in American cities to form tourism and leisure areas that were meant to provide the traveller with a 'secured, protected and normalized environment'. Minca (2000) employed the term 'Bali syndrome' to denote a similar process of spatial segregation ('re-territorialization') of tourist spaces in Bali.

At first sight, the tourist bubble concept seems to be relevant primarily to enclave-like forms of mass tourism such as theme parks, all-inclusive resorts, international-style hotels or cruise ships and less so for small-scale destinations like the one studied in this paper. Several authors have shown, however, that the tourist bubble may equally apply to alternative forms of tourism such as backpacking (Jacobsen 2003, 74; Noy and Cohen 2005) or ecotourism (Carrier and Macleod 2005). Based on their study of ecotourism destinations in Jamaica and the Dominican Republic, Carrier and Macleod (2005) have shown that the interactions between ecotourists and their attention to the local nature and culture are often abstracted from historical and social contexts. They coined the notion of 'ecotourist bubble' to refer to the ignorance of context in ecotourism.

Abstraction from cultural contexts also occurs in the 'commoditization of culture process' (Greenwood 1978, 137) that occurs in response to tourists' desire for 'authentic' experiences (MacCannell 1973, 597). In this process, often a 'staged authenticity' emerges (MacCannell 1973, 595-596) with 'invented traditions' which are disconnected from the population's historical context. In Alter do Chão the changes in a local cultural event, the Sairé festival, can be interpreted as such a 'commoditization of culture' process. As we will illustrate below, this festival evolved from a local cultural festivity into a big commercial event in which reference is made to the disputed notion of 'Borari Indians', and new elements were introduced in order to attract a larger number of tourists. A similar process is described by Grünewald (2002) in his study of tourism and cultural revival among the 'Pataxó Indians' in southern Bahia, Brazil. Stimulated by the agents in the tourist industry, the Pataxó – in reality consisting of five ethnicities with no common language or background – were turned into 'performing primitives' who sell 'invented objects' and 'produced traditions'. Rather than losing authenticity, the Pataxó experience this change as 'cultural revival' that gives them a special status in the region.

The easy adoption of a 'new' indigenous identity and 'invented traditions' and the interpretation of these as a 'cultural revival' suggests a relationship with what Perz et al. (2008) call the racial-ethnical reclassification process that occurred in Brazil during the 1990s. Following the new constitutional rights that indigenous people acquired in 1988, self-identification as being 'indigenous' emerged as a way to reassert political and territorial claims. This process created a new 'post-traditional Indian' (Warren 2001) who Perz et al. (2008, 13) describe as follows:

> These are people of indigenous descent who live in the fragmented remnants of their traditional cultures but for whom those remnants constitute a central reference for their identity. Post-traditional Indians actively seek to rediscover, recuperate, and reinvigorate cultures that conquest and colonization disrupted. It is this orientation that distinguishes post-traditional Indians from non-Indians and often proves infectious, especially given the legal avenue that indigenous identity offers for land acquisition.

The authors (Perz et al. 2008, 27) estimate that reclassified indigenous people constituted almost half of Brazil's indigenous population in 2008 and that the process accounted for 79 per cent of indigenous population growth in Brazil during the 1990s.

Reproduced in part from Ros-Tonen, M. A., & Werneck, A. F. (2009). Small-scale Tourism Development in Brazilian Amazonia: The Creation of a 'Tourist Bubble'. *European Review of Latin American and Caribbean Studies | Revista Europea De Estudios Latinoamericanos Y Del Caribe,0*(86), 59. doi:10.18352/erlacs.9610

Question 32

What is the main topic of this passage?

- ○ **A.** Ecotourism as a form of tourism bubble
- ○ **B.** People's motives for choosing to self-identify as indigenous
- ○ **C.** Tourism bubbles and their effects on indigenous identity in places like Brazil
- ○ **D.** Tourism and cultural identity

Question 33

The author's statement in paragraph 3 that "Rather than losing authenticity, the Pataxó experience this change as 'cultural revival' that gives them a special status in the region." suggests that:

- ○ **A.** contrary to what some have claimed, there is nothing "inauthentic" about the popular concept of the Pataxó, since it has been adopted by these people themselves.
- ○ **B.** tourism may have paradoxical effects, since it is through the interactions with tourist culture that many Pataxó learn about their own culture.
- ○ **C.** tourism may have paradoxical effects, since it can give people a sense of identity, even if this identity is based on inaccurate information.
- ○ **D.** the Pataxó disagree with anthropologists and historians on the history of their people and the existence of a Pataxó identity.

Question 34

Based on passage information, other examples of a tourist bubble could include all of the following EXCEPT:

- ○ **A.** a visitor to Greece who visits ancient temples but does not explore modern sites or activities.
- ○ **B.** a visitor to a Sandals resort who chooses a destination primarily for the weather and beaches.
- ○ **C.** a foreign exchange student who stays with a host family but continues to enjoy an upper-middle-class lifestyle.
- ○ **D.** a hiker in Thailand who explores nature but stays in hostels populated by other Western visitors.

Question 35

According to the passage, indigenous people sometimes become "performing primitives" for tourists. Based on passage information, this is probably because:

- ○ **A.** visitors desire to see real culture of minority groups but lack knowledge about their lives and history.
- ○ **B.** visitors desire to meet members of minority groups but do not want to know about the cultural differences that set them apart.
- ○ **C.** visitors desire to see performances by members of indigenous groups but do not want to interact with them one-on-one.
- ○ **D.** visitors want to see indigenous people act out ancient rituals but do not want to learn about their current culture.

Question 36

What might the author recommend someone do if they want to learn about the real traditions of a region like Alter do Chão?

- ○ **A.** Take a low-budget hiking or backpacking trip to see the region up close
- ○ **B.** Attend small local festivals that are specific to a subculture.
- ○ **C.** Experience the culture of oppressed groups instead of just the dominant group.
- ○ **D.** Immerse themselves in the country for a longer period of time.

Question 37

The quote from Perz et al. is introduced in the second-to-last in order to:

- ○ **A.** critique post-traditional Indians for their shallow understanding of their own culture.
- ○ **B.** critique western colonizers for robbing indigenous people of their culture.
- ○ **C.** describe an orientation to culture that has a arisen in part thanks to tourism.
- ○ **D.** distinguish between two types of indigenous people, traditional and post-traditional.

Passage 7 (Questions 38–43)

Evolutionary Psychology (EP) can be seen as developing from the work of Symons, John Tooby and Leda Cosmides at the University of California, Santa Barbara. EP proposes that "much, if not all, of our behavior can be explained by appeal to internal psychological mechanisms" that "are adaptations—products of natural selection—that helped our ancestors get around the world, survive and reproduce" (Downes 2008).

Put simply, humans evolved to survive in the Pleistocene era ("environment of evolutionary adaptation"; EEA) (1.8 million to 10,000 years ago) and we are carrying that "equipment" in the modern world. "Human behaviors are not a direct product of natural selection but rather the product of psychological mechanisms that we were selected for" (Downes 2008). This "argument-for-design" approach assumes that humans are evolutionarily adapted for the EEA, not necessarily for today (Byrne 2000).

Tooby and Cosmides (2005) summarized the principles of EP as:

- The brain is a "computer" designed by natural selection;
- Human behavior comes from this "evolved computer";
- The cognitive programs within the "computer" allowed the first humans to survive and reproduce effectively;
- These cognitive programs may, thus, not be adaptive now as the environment has changed from the EEA;
- The brain is made up of many different programs ("massive modularitys"; Samuels 1998)

This last notion prompted Buller (2009) to coin the phrase "pop EP" to describe aspects of EP that offer "grand and encompassing claims about human nature for popular consumption." Buller listed three fallacies of "pop EP":

1. Analysis of Pleistocene problems tells us about the evolution of the mind.

It is argued that we can understand human psychology by knowing how it evolved in the first humans. But there is little direct information from fossils about many aspects of early human life, particularly social, and the fossils may relate to a species of early hominid that have become extinct. Many speculations have to be made: "our ancestors' motivational and cognitive processes would have been selectively responsive to certain features of the physical and social environments, and this selective responsiveness would have determined which environmental factors affected human evolution. So to identify the adaptive problems that shaped the human mind, we need to know something about ancestral human psychology. But we don't." (Buller 2009)

2. It is possible to discover why certain human traits evolved.

In biology, the comparative method allows researchers to understand the evolution of differences between closely related species with a common ancestor. For example, two species of bird from a common ancestor, one with a long beak and the other with a short beak. "Correlating trait differences with specific environmental variations can indicate the environmental demands to which a trait is adapted." (Buller 2009)

This is not possible with human traits because closely related species to humans, like chimpanzees, do not share certain behaviors like language, or other hominids of the genus Homo (eg: Homo erectus) are not here to compare.

Language, for example, may have "emerged" not due to specific adaptive pressure, but because of the availability of extra "computational space" in the expanding cortex (Clark 1997) . On the other hand, language may have come from "the re-molding of pre-existing adaptations" (known as "exaptations").

3. The modern human has a "Stone Age mind."

Though some human psychological mechanisms evolved in the Pleistocene era, some are older than that in evolutionary terms. Panksepp and Panksepp (2000) described emotions as one such example. Emotions such as Care, Panic, and Play have evolutionary origins in early primates, and Fear, Rage, Seeking, and Lust as pre-mammalia.

On the other hand, human evolution has continued since early humans, so we are not stuck in the Stone Age completely. Not to mention the changes in the environment, namely technology and industrial developments, since then. Evolutionary changes in the human genome have been found as recently as 5000 years ago, and it is estimated that humans have evolved faster in the past 10,000 years than since the split from a common ancestor with chimpanzees.

Tooby, J., & Cosmides, L. (2015). Conceptual Foundations of Evolutionary Psychology. *The Handbook of Evolutionary Psychology,* 5-67. doi:10.1002/9780470939376.ch1

Question 38

What is the author's purpose in introducing the claim that "language may have come from "the re-molding of pre-existing adaptations" (known as "exaptations").

- ○ **A.** It is impossible to know how language evolved unless we know what traits it emerged from.
- ○ **B.** The claim that language emerged simply because of extra computational space is implausible because there are so many other possible explanations.
- ○ **C.** It is impossible to know the exact course human evolution took because there are many possible ways a trait could have emerged.
- ○ **D.** The concept of exaptations is more plausible than that of specific selection pressure for language.

Question 39

If one was to accept the notion that the brain is a computer that can be programmed, it would most reasonably follow that:

- ○ **A.** we can always ascertain the response if we know the stimulus.
- ○ **B.** knowledge comes after the program (a posteriori).
- ○ **C.** knowledge is already there before the program (a priori).
- ○ **D.** knowledge consists of combinations of some minimal unit of information.

Question 40

What is the main thesis of Evolutionary Psychology?

- ○ **A.** Behavior is a result of determined responses to stimuli.
- ○ **B.** Behavior is the result of adapted internal psychological mechanisms.
- ○ **C.** Behavior is the result of evolutionary mutated random psychological mechanisms.
- ○ **D.** Behavior is an evolutionary feature that is determined by which behaviors were selected for.

Question 41

We can infer that the three fallacies identified by the passage are the product of "pop EP"'s:

- ○ **A.** inaccurate understanding of how evolution works.
- ○ **B.** overly limited view of which traits can be selected for.
- ○ **C.** desire to make the differences between modern humans and our stone age ancestors seem greater than they really are.
- ○ **D.** desire to find simple explanations by connecting modern behavior to stone age conditions.

Question 42

According to passage information, how does evolutionary psychology relate to natural selection?

- ○ **A.** Psychological mechanisms are selected for, and in turn cause behavior.
- ○ **B.** Natural selection determines the form of humansocial groups, which determines what psychological skills we need.
- ○ **C.** Evolutionary adaptive psychological mechanisms are the result of chance and mutation while natural selection views these as biological apparatus geared for survival.
- ○ **D.** Behaviors are selected for, and over time, the needed behavioral repertoire determines the psych skills we develop.

Question 43

The author might agree with a work arguing that humans could become evolutionarily adapted to modern circumstances if:

- ○ **A.** people were more often subjected to the pressures of natural selection by dying.
- ○ **B.** the same conditions persisted for sufficiently long.
- ○ **C.** modern civilization required traits that could be selected for.
- ○ **D.** society changed more rapidly, producing pressure to adapt.

Passage 8 (Questions 44–48)

In his 1907 lecture, "Anthropology," the "father of American Anthropology" Franz Boas identified two basic questions for anthropologists: "Why are the tribes and nations of the world different, and how have the present differences developed?" These questions were clarified with the explanation that the object of anthropological study was unrelated to anatomical, physiological, and mental individual traits. Instead, it related to the diversity of cultural characteristics, as found in groups of men from every social class, and residing in varied geographical areas. Anthropologists should look into the causes and the temporal sequence of events behind such diversity.

These questions represent a break from then generalized assumption that people who lacked written records lacked history; only those with written records had a history or past. Some authors suggested that the difference between these two kinds of societies (with and without written records) were behind the reason why history, sociology, economics and other alike writing-based disciplines were important for understanding societies with written records, and anthropology was critical for understanding societies without writing.

Boas rejected this argument. He understood all societies to have a history, and all societies to be proper objects of anthropological study. For him, the history of whatever type of society could be investigated through the analysis of aspects besides written texts. Thus, in his 1904 article, "The History of Anthropology," Boas discussed how anthropology dedicated itself to "a domain of knowledge" that thus far had not been the concern of any other research field - namely, "the biological history of mankind in all its varieties; linguistics applied to people without written languages; the ethnology of people without historic records; and prehistoric archaeology."

Boas also dismissed the social and cultural evolution theories of historians and social theorists of the 18th and 19th centuries, especially those most dominant, as nothing but speculative. He endeavored to establish an evidence-based discipline that would base its claims on rigorous empirical study.

One of Boas' most important books, *The Mind of Primitive Man* (published in 1911), integrated his theories and established a program that was expected to dominate American anthropology for the next fifteen years. There, he claimed that, in any given population, biology, language, and culture are autonomous domains; each is an equally important dimension of human nature that cannot be reduced, overlapped, or merged with any other. He further emphasized that these aspects, in any considered group of people, are the product of historical developments and subjected to evolution mechanisms. Specific cultural environments that had evolved over time would shape individual behavior as much as longitudinally-evolved biological or linguistic environments. And, with such assumption, cultural plurality becomes a fundamental feature of humankind, in the same way that a plurality of phenotypes is.

In the very same book, Boas appealed to the scientific community, reminding scientists that all knowledge has moral consequences that should be taken into account even when searching for the truth. This humanistic concern also embedded his final book remarks, where he pointed out that anthropological investigations opened way for "greater tolerance of forms of civilization different from our own." People should "look on foreign races with greater sympathy and with a conviction that, as all races have contributed in the past to cultural progress in one way or another", they will continue to do so given "a fair opportunity."

Boas, F. (1904). The History of Anthropology. *Science,20*, 513-524. Boas, F. (1908). *Anthropology*. Lecture presented at Columbia University Press, 1908 in Columbia University, New York.
Boas, F. (2015). *The Mind of Primitive Man*. London: Forgotten Books.

Question 44

The thrust of Boas' studies in anthropology could be said to be marked by arguing for the similarity between:

- ○ **A.** anthropology and sociology.
- ○ **B.** scientific and philosophical approaches to tracing cultural history.
- ○ **C.** written texts and physical evidence.
- ○ **D.** literate and non-literate cultures.

Question 45

In the light of what is stated about the variables that Boas isolated as critical for the study of mankind (paragraph 5), it can be inferred that culture:

I. evolves only when biology and language also evolve.
II. develops over time through its own mechanisms.
III. is linguistically or symbolically determined.

- ○ **A.** I and II
- ○ **B.** II and III
- ○ **C.** I only
- ○ **D.** II only

Question 46

The author quotes Boas in the passage's conclusion to:

- ○ **A.** show that Boas' belief in cultural relativism trumped his belief in science.
- ○ **B.** stress that Boas was a voice for multiculturalism.
- ○ **C.** show that Boas was more progressive than other anthropologists of his time.
- ○ **D.** show that anthropology cannot progress without respect for other cultures.

Question 47

Which of the following would undermine Boas' claims the most?

- ○ **A.** The discovery that Boas described inaccurately the history of a tribe of people in an essay
- ○ **B.** The discovery that literate civilizations had a culture beyond what was conveyed in written texts
- ○ **C.** The discovery that culture developed exclusively due to dissemination rather than parallel development
- ○ **D.** The discovery that all civilizations have certain features in common such as dance, body decoration, and rituals for eating

Question 48

Based on passage information, Boas' role in anthropology is similar to that of:

- ○ **A.** a biologist discovering that there are essential features that help to distinguish between different types of organisms.
- ○ **B.** a psychologist arguing that all diagnostic tests should be carefully calibrated to ensure they measure what they purport to.
- ○ **C.** a nutritionist arguing that all healthy diets contain the same essential nutrients.
- ○ **D.** a linguist arguing that all languages are equally sophisticated at conveying thought, no matter what specific features they have.

Passage 9 (Questions 49–53)

A play is a story devised to be presented by actors on a stage before an audience.

It is, of course, true that the very greatest plays have always been great literature as well as great drama. The purely literary element—the final touch of style in dialogue—is the only sure antidote against the opium of time. Now that Aeschylus is no longer performed as a playwright, we read him as a poet. But, on the other hand, we should remember that the main reason why he is no longer played is that his dramas do not fit the modern theatre,—an edifice totally different in size and shape and physical appointments from that in which his pieces were devised to be presented. In his own day he was not so much read as a poet as applauded in the theatre as a playwright; and properly to appreciate his dramatic, rather than his literary, appeal, we must reconstruct in our imagination the conditions of the theatre in his day. The point is that his plays, though planned primarily as drama, have since been shifted over, by many generations of critics and literary students, into the adjacent province of poetry; and this shift of the critical point of view, which has insured the immortality of Aeschylus, has been made possible only by the literary merit of his dialogue. When a play, owing to altered physical conditions, is tossed out of the theatre, it will find a haven in the closet only if it be greatly written. From this fact we may derive the practical maxim that though a skilful playwright need not write greatly in order to secure the plaudits of his own generation, he must cultivate a literary excellence if he wishes to be remembered by posterity.

This much must be admitted concerning the ultimate importance of the literary element in the drama. But on the other hand it must be granted that many plays that stand very high as drama do not fall within the range of literature. A typical example is the famous melodrama by Dennery entitled *The Two Orphans*. This play has deservedly held the stage for nearly a century, and bids fair still to be applauded after the youngest critic has died. It is undeniably a very good play. It tells a thrilling story in a series of carefully graded theatric situations. It presents nearly a dozen acting parts which, though scarcely real as characters, are yet drawn with sufficient fidelity to fact to allow the performers to produce a striking illusion of reality during the two hours' traffic of the stage. It is, to be sure—especially in the standard English translation—abominably written. One of the two orphans launches wide-eyed upon a soliloquy beginning, "Am I mad?... Do I dream?"; and such sentences as the following obtrude themselves upon the astounded ear,—"If you persist in persecuting me in this heartless manner, I shall inform the police." Nothing, surely, could be further from literature. Yet thrill after thrill is conveyed, by visual means, through situations artfully contrived; and in the sheer excitement of the moment, the audience is made incapable of noticing the pompous mediocrity of the lines.

In general, it should be frankly understood by students of the theatre that an audience is not capable of hearing whether the dialogue of a play is well or badly written. Such a critical discrimination would require an extraordinary nicety of ear, and might easily be led astray, in one direction or the other, by the reading of the actors. The rhetoric of Massinger must have sounded like poetry to an Elizabethan audience that had heard the same performers, the afternoon before, speaking lines of Shakespeare's. If Mr. Forbes-Robertson is reading a poorly-written part, it is hard to hear that the lines are, in themselves, not musical. Literary style is, even for accomplished critics, very difficult to judge in the theatre. Some years ago, Mrs. Fiske presented in New York an English adaptation of Paul Heyse's *Mary of Magdala*. After the first performance—at which I did not happen to be present—I asked several cultivated people who had heard the play whether the English version was written in verse or in prose; and though these people were themselves actors and men of letters, not one of them could tell me. Yet, as appeared later, when the play was published, the English dialogue was written in blank verse by no less a poet than Mr. William Winter. If such an elementary distinction as that between verse and prose was in this case inaudible to cultivated ears, how much harder must it be for the average audience to distinguish between a good phrase and a bad!

The fact is that literary style is, for the most part, wasted on an audience. The average auditor is moved mainly by the emotional content of a sentence spoken on the stage, and pays very little attention to the form of words in which the meaning is set forth. At Hamlet's line, "Absent thee from felicity a while"—which Matthew Arnold, with impeccable taste, selected as one of his touchstones of literary style—the thing that really moves the audience in the theatre is not the perfectness of the phrase but the pathos of Hamlet's plea for his best friend to outlive him and explain his motives to a world grown harsh.

Hamilton, C. M. (2016). *Theory of the Theatre, and Other Principles of Dramatic Criticism*. CreateSpace Independent Publishing Platform.

Question 49

The passage characterizes the relationship between literature and drama in which of the following ways?

- O **A.** The two are completely different art forms because what is good as drama is bad judged as literature.
- O **B.** They are closely related because a work must have literary qualities to be truly satisfactory as drama.
- O **C.** The relationship is a matter of perspective because a viewer may choose to experience a work as drama or as literature.
- O **D.** The two are related yet different because great drama is sometimes great literature, but not always.

Question 50

The author's argument would be most strongly contradicted by evidence showing that:

- O **A.** most plays that succeed as dramatic works of theater are well written as literature.
- O **B.** audiences can intuitively grasp whether a line of dialogue sounds well written, and this affects their enjoyment of a play.
- O **C.** many people who are otherwise skilled writers cannot create dramatic dialogue that sounds naturalistic.
- O **D.** many plays that are greatly admired as literature are rarely performed, and lack suspense.

Question 51

The passage implies that the drama includes elements that literature does not, including all of the following EXCEPT:

- O **A.** visual impressions.
- O **B.** the skill of the actors.
- O **C.** the pacing of a well-directed performance.
- O **D.** the suspense of series of well-planned scenes.

Question 52

An example analogous to the relationship between drama and literature the author describes would be:

- O **A.** rock music, in which successful lyrics cannot always stand alone as poetry.
- O **B.** opera, in which there is no spoken dialogue and sung music must advance the plot.
- O **C.** TV sitcoms, in which viewers prefer a show that has both humor and a well-developed plot.
- O **D.** ballet, in which excellent musicianship is essential for dancing to be effective.

Question 53

One possible critique of the author's logic is that:

- O **A.** he is not consistent regarding whether a play without literary qualities can remain successful for long periods of time.
- O **B.** he is inconsistent as to whether audiences enjoy plays like The Two Orphans with poor writing style.
- O **C.** he fails to provide evidence for his thesis that a good drama need not be good as literature.
- O **D.** he fails to provide evidence for his claim that audiences cannot tell the difference between good and bad dialogue.

CANDIDATE'S NAME ______________________________

RAW SCORE AND SCALED SCORE ______________________

GS-4 Section III: Biological and Biochemical Foundations of Living Systems

Questions: 1-59
Time: 95 minutes

INSTRUCTIONS: Of all the questions on this test, most are organized into groups preceded by a passage. After evaluating the passage, select the best answer to each question in the group. Fifteen questions are independent of any descriptive passage or each other. Similarly, select the best answer to these questions. If you are unsure of an answer, eliminate the alternatives that you know to be incorrect and select an answer from the remaining alternatives. To indicate your selection, use a pencil to blacken the corresponding circle next to the answer choice and/or you can use the answer document at the back of this book. No marks are deducted for wrong answers.

The computer-based real MCAT has an on-screen highlighter function and ~~STRIKEOUT~~ function. These tools help to spotlight text or assist in the process of elimination. You may use a yellow highlighter for this paper-based exam and/or a pen (or preferably a pencil to make it easier should you change your mind) to mark text. At the time of publishing, both highlighting and strikeout functions can be used for passages, questions and answer choices. You can also flag a question to review later should time remain.

For the real exam, you will be provided with a dry erase board which is a white laminated noteboard booklet accompanied by a fine point marker. The noteboard includes 9 graph-lined pages for you to write though you cannot erase. You can simulate the experience with a fine point marker on a noteboard or with 8” x 14” plain graph paper.

You may consult the periodic table at any point during the science subtests.

Please note: For the real MCAT, a small number of field-tested questions will remain unscored.

This practice test has been designed exclusively to test knowledge and thinking skills. This exam may contain hypothetical statements and/or express controversial ideas. Statements contained herein do not necessarily reflect the policy, position, or view of RuveneCo Inc. or MCAT-prep.com.

START EXAM ONLY WHEN TIMER IS READY.

Passage 1 (Questions 1–5)

Neisseria meningitidis (meningococcus) is a Gram-negative bacterium that is found commonly in the upper respiratory tract of humans but is often asymptomatic. However, infections sometimes cause meningitis and septicemia, which can have serious consequences and even lead to the death of infected patients. *N. meningitidis* colonizes the upper respiratory tract using a variety of strategies, including immune evasion and adhesion to epithelial cells.

Type four pili (Tfp) mediate DNA uptake, bacterial aggregation, and adhesion. Tfp are filamentous fibers that are composed of thousands of subunits of PilE (the major pilin) together with accessory pilins that are arranged in a helical configuration. These structures play an important role in host cell interactions via CD-147. Previous studies demonstrated that *N. meningitidis* strains that lack *pilE* have a reduced ability to adhere to human airway cultures or epithelial cells *in vitro*. Tfp are also required for colonization of the vascular endothelium. After colonization they promote bacterial survival and pathogenesis by facilitating the resistance to blood flow and microcolony formation, inflammation, migration across the blood-brain barrier, and transformation.

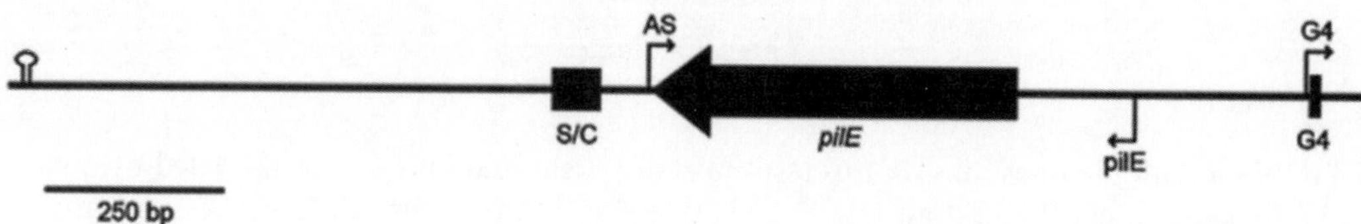

Figure 1 The location of the promoter sequence of the *pilE* locus in *N. meningitidis*.

The organization of the *pilE* locus is shown in Figure 1. In some strains it undergoes phase and antigenic variation in response to changes in the environment, which provides a mechanism for immune evasion and could alter the properties of Tfp. A study was performed to clone the *cis* AS promoter (downstream) and a 752-bp adjacent fragment (upstream). The antisense (AS) RNA encompasses sequences complementary to *pilE* and its 5′ untranslated region (UTR), but it does not possess a Shine-Dalgarno sequence. The PCR product was cloned flanking an erythromycin resistance cassette. The resulting bacterial strains were grown in a variety of stresses to assess their growth under different conditions, including 0.5 M NaCl, 0.5 M KCl, 6% sucrose, or 0.15% H_2O_2 (Figure 2). The expression of AS RNA did not affect *pilE* expression significantly, and *pilE* is expressed at all stages of growth in strains that both express and do not express AS RNA.

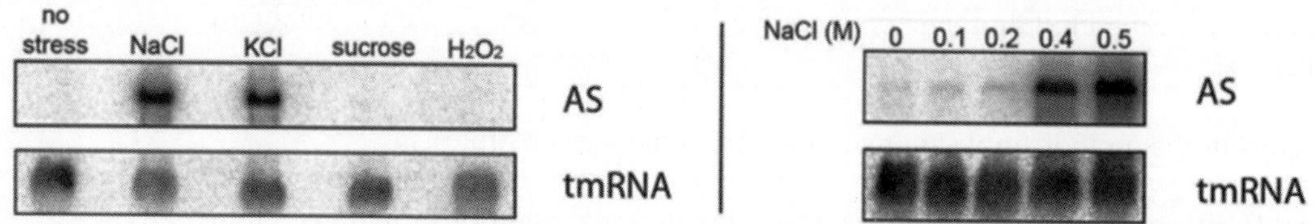

Figure 2 Northern blot of total RNA from wild-type *N. meningitidis* grown in the presence of different stresses (left panel) and different salt concentrations (right panel). A 50-nt probe [(AS)pilE-1] that hybridizes specifically to the AS RNA 533 nt downstream of the AS promoter was used.

Transcription of the AS RNA can affect the levels of the corresponding sense transcript via a variety of mechanisms, such as altering the RNA stability or binding to the 5′ UTR regions (UTRs) to modulate ribosome binding and subsequent protein expression. The AS RNA was mapped using a single forward primer and several reverse primers to assess whether it encompasses the entire *pilE* coding region with or without the 5′ UTR. The results are shown in Figure 3 and Figure 4.

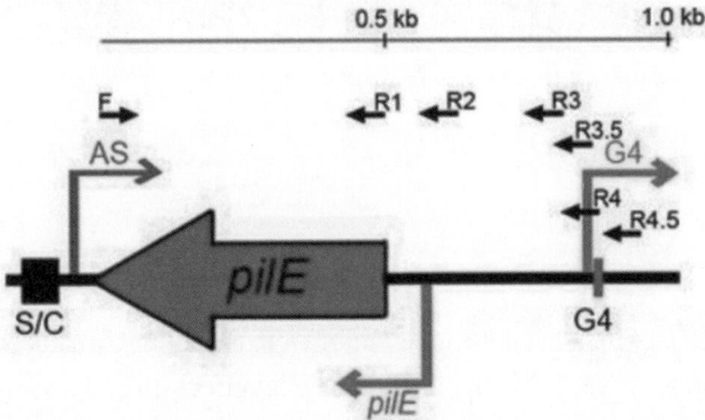

Figure 3 Characterization of the 5′ and 3′ ends of the AS transcript using RT-PCR. The short black arrows show the hybridization positions of the PCR primers (F and R1–R4.5). The scale bar at the top shows the distance from the AS transcriptional start site.

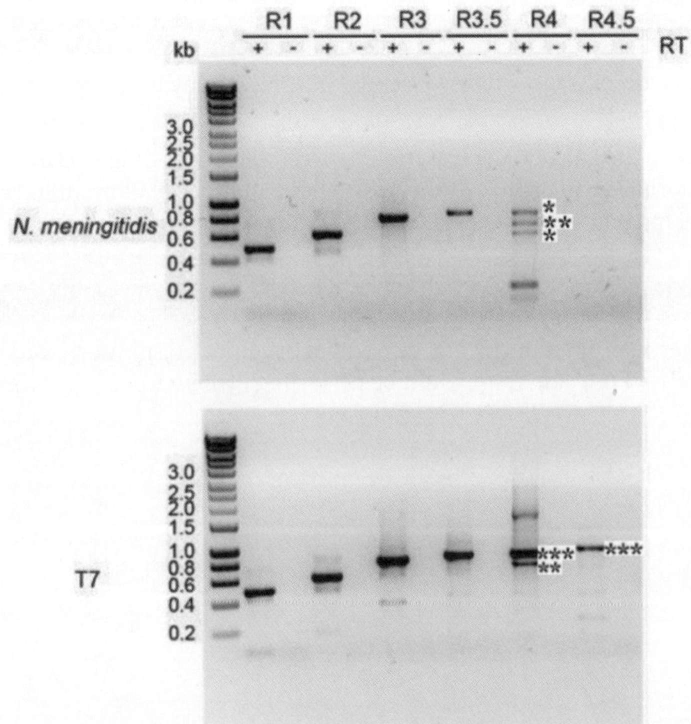

Figure 4 Agarose gels of the PCR products amplified using cDNAs from *N. meningitidis* total RNA (upper panel) or AS RNA synthesized using T7 bacteriophage RNA polymerase (lower panel). The presence (+) or absence (−) of reverse transcriptase (RT) in the reaction is shown. One asterisk (*) indicates nonspecific products amplified from rRNA. Two asterisks (**) indicate truncated PCR products (as determined using sequencing). Three asterisks (***) indicate the full-sized product.

Adapted from Journal of Bacteriology (jb.asm.org); 1757.

Question 1

Based on the information presented in the passage, which of the following statements is most true about the AS RNA?

- ○ **A.** It is exactly complementary to the corresponding sense RNA.
- ○ **B.** Its expression is regulated by osmotic stress.
- ○ **C.** It is translated into a protein that protects against salt stress.
- ○ **D.** It is expressed ubiquitously.

Question 2

Within or before which primer sequence does the AS transcript terminate?

- O **A.** 2
- O **B.** 3
- O **C.** 4
- O **D.** 4.5

Question 3

Based on the passage, the expression of AS RNA likely has what effect on *pilE* expression?

- O **A.** Stabilizes
- O **B.** Destabilizes
- O **C.** Induces its degradation
- O **D.** Unknown

Question 4

Based on the information in the passage, which role could *pilE* NOT play in the adherence to host cells?

- O **A.** Binding to CD-147
- O **B.** Steric hindrance to modulate the interaction between the host cell and Tfp
- O **C.** Inducing a conformational change at the host cell membrane to allow an interaction with CD-147
- O **D.** Stabilizing the Tfp complex at the host cell membrane

Question 5

An aspirate (sample) of mucous containing evidence of an active upper respiratory tract infection due to *N. meningitidis* was acquired. If a DNA analysis would be performed, where would the *pilE* gene most likely be found?

- O **A.** Kinetochore
- O **B.** Centromere
- O **C.** Euchromatin
- O **D.** Heterochromatin

Note: This page is left blank so that the passage would be visible without turning pages while assessing the passage-based questions.

Passage 2 (Questions 6–9)

Aside from diabetes, thyroid disease is the most common glandular disorder. Over 10 million North Americans are treated for thyroid conditions, often an underactive or overactive gland. Overwhelmingly, women between the ages of 20 and 60 are much more likely than men to succumb to these conditions. The etiology lies in the failure of the immune system to recognize the thyroid gland as part of the body and thus antibodies are sent to attack the gland.

The plasma proteins that bind thyroid hormones are albumin, a prealbumin called thyroxine-binding prealbumin (TBPA), and a globulin with an electrophoretic mobility, thyroxine-binding globulin (TBG). The free thyroid hormones in plasma are in equilibrium with the protein-bound thyroid hormones in the tissues. Free thyroid hormones are added to the circulating pool by the thyroid. It is the free thyroid hormones in plasma that are physiologically active and imbalances in these hormones result in thyroid disease.

In addition, in humans there are four small parathyroid glands that produce the hormone, parathormone, which is a peptide composed of 84 amino acids. Parathormone and the thyroid hormone calcitonin work antagonistically to regulate the plasma calcium and phosphate levels. Overactive parathyroid glands, hyperparathyroidism, can lead to an increase in the level of calcium in plasma and tissues.

Table 1 Different plasma proteins and their binding capacity and affinity for thyroxine.

Protein	Plasma Level (mg/dl)	Thyroxine Binding Capacity (micro g/dl)	Affinity for thyroxine	Amount of thyroxine bound in normal plasma (micro g/dl)
Thyroxine binding globulin (TBG)	1.0	20	High	7
Thyroxine binding prealbumin (TBPA)	30.0	250	Moderate	1
Albumin	...	1000	Low	None
Total protein-bound thyroxine in plasma	...	...	...	8

Question 6

According to Table 1, it would be expected that:

- O **A.** TBG has the highest binding capacity for thyroxine while TBPA has the highest affinity.
- O **B.** TBG has the highest binding capacity for thyroxine while albumin has the lowest affinity.
- O **C.** albumin has the highest binding capacity for thyroxine while TBPA has the highest affinity.
- O **D.** albumin has the highest binding capacity for thyroxine while TBG has the highest affinity.

Question 7

This question refers to Figure 1.

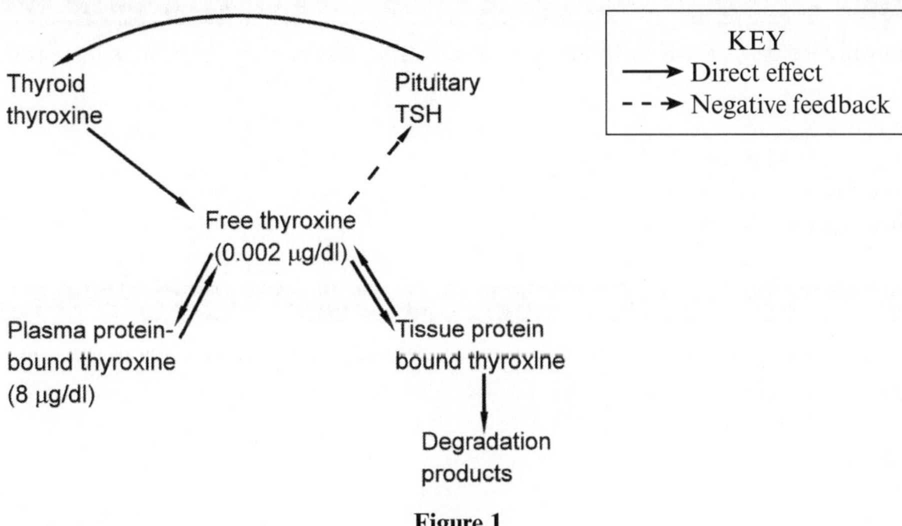

Figure 1

According to the equilibrium shown in Figure 1, an elevation in the concentration of free thyroid hormone in the plasma is followed by:

- O **A.** an increase in tissue protein-bound thyroxine.
- O **B.** an increase in tissue protein-bound thyroxine and plasma protein-bound thyroxine.
- O **C.** an increase in the amount of TSH secreted from the pituitary gland.
- O **D.** an increase in both the amount of TSH secreted from the pituitary gland and the release of thyroxine from the thyroid gland.

Question 8

Symptoms of hypothyroidism and hyperthyroidism, respectively, likely include:

- O **A.** a fine tremor and diminished concentration.
- O **B.** brittle nails and kidney stones.
- O **C.** rapid heart beat and increased irritability.
- O **D.** lethargy and nervous agitation.

Question 9

Which of the following cell types would be expected to be maximally stimulated in a patient with hyperparathyroidism?

- O **A.** Osteoclasts
- O **B.** Osteoblasts
- O **C.** Fibroblasts
- O **D.** Chondrocytes

The following questions are NOT based on a descriptive passage (Questions 10–13).

Question 10

A compound that only increases the Km for an enzyme-substrate reaction would be most consistent with which of the following?

- O **A.** An activator
- O **B.** A competitive inhibitor
- O **C.** An uncompetitive inhibitor
- O **D.** A noncompetitive inhibitor

Question 11

The difference between the bacterium Lactobacillus and the eukaryote *Trichomonas* is that *Lactobacillus* has no:

- O **A.** ribosomes.
- O **B.** cell wall.
- O **C.** plasma membrane.
- O **D.** lysosomes.

Question 12

After fertilization, the zygote will develop into a female if:

- O **A.** the egg possesses an X chromosome.
- O **B.** the secondary oocyte possesses an X chromosome.
- O **C.** the zygote possesses an X chromosome.
- O **D.** the sperm possesses an X chromosome.

Question 13

A combination of which of the following amino acids is most likely to be found in the transmembrane domains of integral membrane proteins?

- O **A.** Tyrosine, Glutamate, Lysine and Methionine
- O **B.** Valine, Alanine, Leucine, and Isoleucine
- O **C.** Threonine, Glycine, Arginine and Histidine
- O **D.** Alanine, Histidine, Glutamine and Arginine

Note: This page is left blank so that the passage would be visible without turning pages while assessing the passage-based questions.

Passage 3 (Questions 14–18)

The last step in translation involves the cleavage of the ester bond that joins the complete peptide chain to the tRNA corresponding to its C-terminal amino acid. This process of *termination*, in addition to the termination codon, requires release factors (RFs). The freeing of the ribosome from mRNA during this step requires the participation of a protein called ribosome releasing factor (RRF).

Cells usually do not contain tRNAs that can recognize the three termination codons. In *E. coli*, when these codons arrive on the ribosome they are recognized by one of three release factors. RF-1 recognizes UAA and UAG, while RF-2 recognizes UAA and UGA. The third release factor, RF-3, does not itself recognize termination codons but stimulates the activity of the other two factors.

The consequence of release factor recognition of a termination codon is to alter the peptidyl transferase center on the large ribosomal subunit so that it can accept water as the attacking nucleophile rather than requiring the normal substrate, aminoacyl-tRNA.

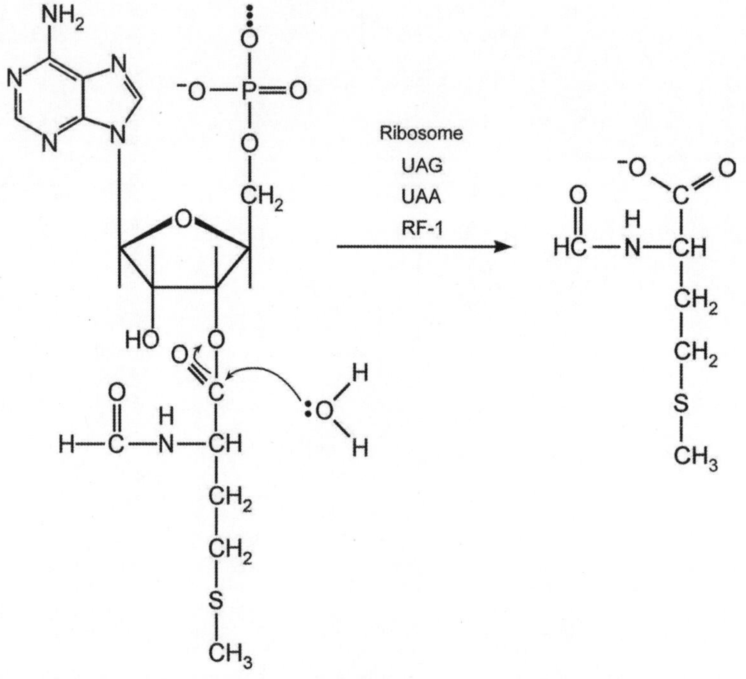

Ribosome
UAG
UAA
RF-1

Figure 1

Question 14

Where would the RFs be expected to be found in the cell?

- O **A.** Within the nuclear membrane
- O **B.** Floating in the cytosol
- O **C.** In the matrix of the mitochondria
- O **D.** Within the lumen of the smooth endoplasmic reticulum

Question 15

The alteration to the peptidyl transferase center during the termination reaction serves to convert peptidyl transferase into a(n):

- O **A.** exonuclease
- O **B.** lyase.
- O **C.** esterase.
- O **D.** ligase.

Question 16

Sparsomycin is an antibiotic that inhibits peptidyl transferase activity. The effect of adding this compound to an *in vitro* reaction in which *E. coli* ribosomes are combined with methionine aminoacyl-tRNA complex, RF-1 and the nucleotide triplets, UAG and UAA, would be to:

- O **A.** inhibit hydrolysis of the amino acid, allowing polypeptide chain extension.
- O **B.** inhibit peptide bond formation causing the amino acid to be released.
- O **C.** induce hydrolysis of the aminoacyl-tRNA complex.
- O **D.** inhibit both hydrolysis of the aminoacyl-tRNA complex and peptide bond formation.

Question 17

If the water in the reaction in Figure 1 was labeled with ^{18}O, which of the following molecules would contain ^{18}O at the end of the reaction?

- O **A.** The free amino acid
- O **B.** The phosphate group of the tRNA molecule
- O **C.** Oxygen-containing molecules in the cytoplasm
- O **D.** The ribose moiety of the tRNA molecule

Question 18

In the genetic code, many codons that code for the same amino acid differ by only one nitrogenous base. The main advantage of this is that:

- O **A.** the code is universal.
- O **B.** DNA replication is simplified.
- O **C.** point mutations are less effective.
- O **D.** the code is non-overlapping.

Passage 4 (Questions 19–22)

In spite of their structural and physiological resemblance, hemoglobin and myoglobin molecules differ in many respects. While hemoglobin transports H^+, O_2, and CO_2, in the blood, myoglobin is the main oxygen carrier of the muscle. The binding of oxygen by hemoglobin is regulated by H^+, CO_2, and organic phosphate. These molecules, when attached to the protein part of the hemoglobin, affects the oxygen binding properties of hemoglobin. This effect is termed *allosteric interaction.*

One of the main differences of hemoglobin and myoglobin is that the latter is not an allosteric molecule. Furthermore, the oxygen dissociation curves of both molecules are different. That is, when fractional occupancy of the oxygen-binding sites arc plotted against partial pressures of oxygen for either molecules, the myoglobin curves tend to be hyperbolic, while hemoglobin curves tend to be sigmoidal.

Finally, myoglobin shows no change in oxygen binding over a broad range of pH, nor does CO_2 have a noticeable effect on it. While with hemoglobin, the acidity enhances the release of oxygen.

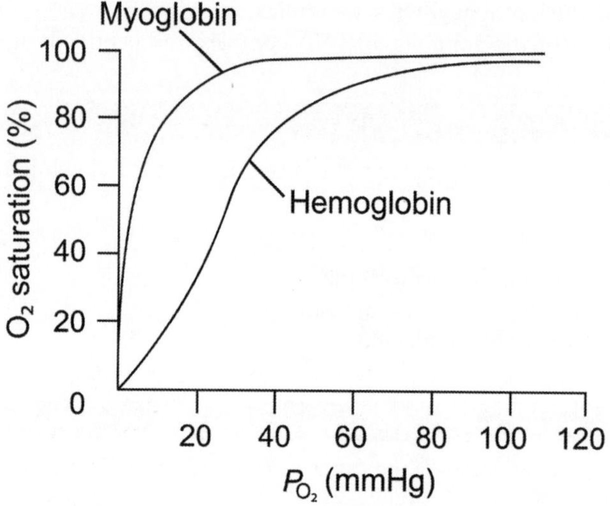

Figure 1 O_2 Dissociation Curves of Hemoglobin and Myoglobin

Question 19

Which of the following can be concluded from the information provided?

I. The binding of O_2 to hemoglobin enhances the binding of additional O_2 to the same hemoglobin molecule.
II. Hemoglobin has a lower affinity for oxygen compared to myoglobin.
III. The affinity of myoglobin and hemoglobin for oxygen is dependent on the pH of the environment.

- **A.** I and II only
- **B.** I and III only
- **C.** II and III only
- **D.** I, II, and III

Question 20

The saturation level of hemoglobin is expected to be about 100% in the:

- O **A.** capillaries of active muscles.
- O **B.** ventricle of the heart.
- O **C.** pulmonary vein.
- O **D.** pulmonary artery.

Question 21

Fetal hemoglobin is slightly different from adult hemoglobin in its structure and function. For the developing fetus to obtain oxygen, there must be a transfer of oxygen from the mother's blood to the fetal blood of the placenta. Fetal blood must be able to load oxygen at the same time that the mother's hemoglobin is unloading oxygen. This difference is best represented by which of the following hemoglobin dissociation curve relationships?

- O **A.** The fetal dissociation curve must be to the right of the adult curve.
- O **B.** The fetal dissociation curve must be to the left of the adult curve.
- O **C.** The fetal dissociation curve must be the same as the adult dissociation curve.
- O **D.** The fetal hemoglobin dissociation curve must be the same as the fetal myoglobin dissociation curve.

Question 22

Hemoglobin found in humans is composed of four chains that can each bind one oxygen molecule. Given a fully saturated hemoglobin molecule, the sigmoidal shape of the oxygen saturation curve in humans is an indication of which of the following?

- O **A.** The first oxygen molecule dissociates from the heme component, while the next three dissociate from the globin component.
- O **B.** It becomes easier to lose the second and third oxygen molecules.
- O **C.** It becomes more difficult to lose the second and third oxygen molecules.
- O **D.** The fourth oxygen molecule dissociates from the heme component, while the previous three dissociate from the globin component.

Passage 5 (Questions 23–26)

Helper T cells play a vital function in the immune system, and aid in a variety of roles depending on the subset they belong to. The development of Th1 and Th2 cells are influenced by the activities of several cytokines, all of which are carefully modulated by a complex system of signal transduction pathways.

Figure 1 illustrates a simplified overview of the molecules and proteins involved in helper T cell differentiation, and how they interact.

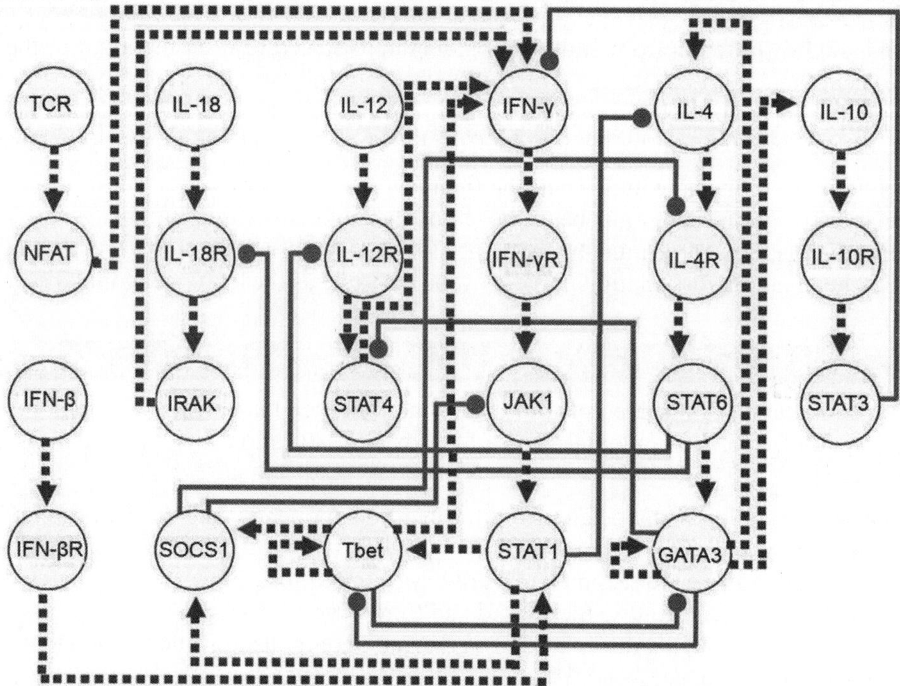

Figure 1 Regulatory pathway of proteins involved in T helper cell differentiation. Positive interactions are shown with dashed lines, while negative interactions are shown as solid lines.

Adapted from Mendoza L, Xenarios I, "A method for the generation of standardized qualitative dynamical systems of regulatory networks," Theor Biol Med Model (2006).

Question 23

Based on the information provided, an overexpression of GATA3 would most likely lead to:

- ○ **A.** an increase in Tbet activity.
- ○ **B.** degradation of STAT4.
- ○ **C.** a decrease in IL-4R activity.
- ○ **D.** a decrease in IFN-γ activity.

Question 24

Mouse experiments have shown that SOCS1 knockouts, where SOCS1 is not active, are lethal, with 100% mortality rates by the third week. The mutation causes a number of effects, the most significant of the following is likely to include:

- ○ **A.** decreased IL-4R activity.
- ○ **B.** overexpression of T-bet.
- ○ **C.** overexpression of IL-12.
- ○ **D.** deactivation of STAT6.

Question 25

Interleukin-4 (IL-4) induces the differentiation of naive helper T cells into Th2 cells. Once activated, Th2 cells produce additional IL-4. This is an example of:

- O **A.** antigen presentation.
- O **B.** a positive feedback loop.
- O **C.** isotype switching.
- O **D.** gene modification.

Question 26

Identify the organ (or organ system) where precursor T cells develop into fully competent but not yet activated T cells.

- O **A.** The lymph nodes
- O **B.** The bone marrow
- O **C.** The thymus
- O **D.** The white pulp of the spleen

The following questions are NOT based on a descriptive passage (Questions 27–30).

Question 27

After radioactive iodine ^{131}I is injected into the vein of a patient, where would ^{131}I concentration be expected to be highest?

- O **A.** Liver
- O **B.** Small intestines
- O **C.** Thyroid
- O **D.** Cardiac muscle cells

Question 28

Which of the following body systems in humans is implicated in thermoregulation and transportation of components of the immune and endocrine systems?

- O **A.** The lymphatic system
- O **B.** Skin
- O **C.** The excretory system
- O **D.** The circulatory system

Question 29

A new protein is designed which requires a phosphorylation reaction in order to be functional. Which of the following will lower the activation energy for the required reaction?

- O **A.** Kinase
- O **B.** Isomerase
- O **C.** Amylase
- O **D.** Phosphatase

Question 30

The isoelectric point (pI) is the pH at which a particular molecule carries no net electrical charge in the statistical mean. Consider Figure 1.

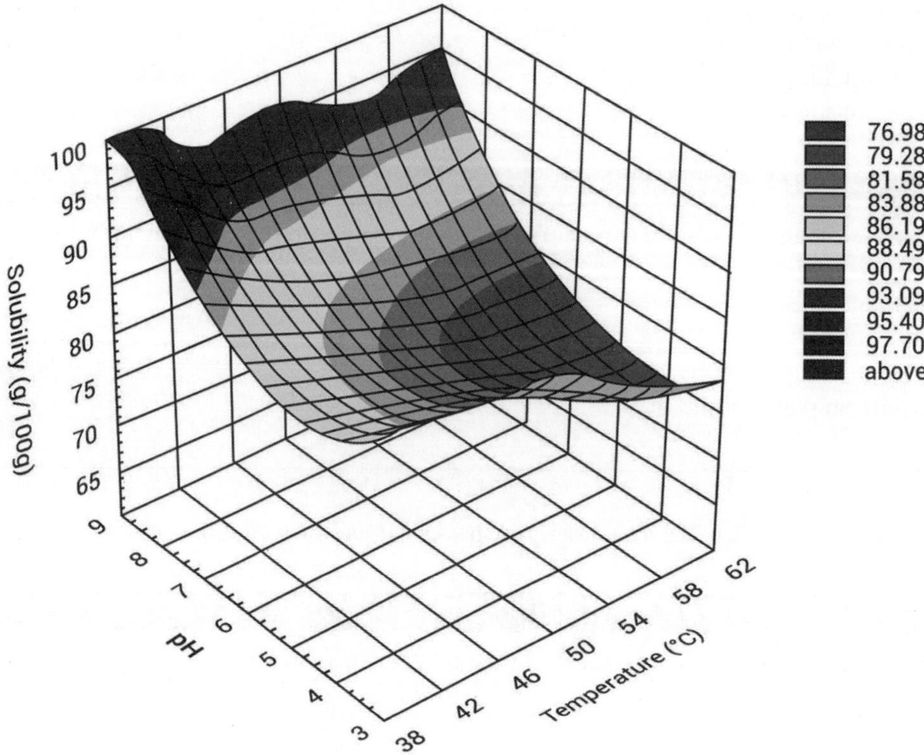

Figure 1 Three-dimensional surface plot generated for whey protein solubility in water as a function of temperature and pH (Ref. Food Science and Technology 38(1):77-80 · February 2005)

Which of the following can be inferred from Figure 1?

- O **A.** Whey proteins have a net positive charge at a pH of 9.
- O **B.** Whey proteins have their lowest solubility below 70 g/100 g.
- O **C.** Whey proteins demonstrate increased solubility with increasing temperature.
- O **D.** Whey proteins have a pI below a pH of 7.

Passage 6 (Questions 31–34)

A *monoclonal antibody* is a single pure antibody produced in quantity by a cultured clone of an immune cell called a B lymphocyte. Prior to the development of the monoclonal antibody, the only means of producing large quantities of specific antibodies was immunization of animals with as purified an antigen as possible. But such an antigen still contained many epitopes. Consequently, the antibodies produced by the animals were polyclonal antibodies, with a different antibody produced for each epitope. Now monoclonal antibodies are produced by a single clone of genetically identical cells derived from a single stimulated antibody-producing cell. They can be prepared in large quantities by using special cells called *hybridomas.*

B-lymphocytes that produce antibodies can become cancerous. A myeloma is a cancer, or unchecked proliferation, of an antibody-producing cell. Because a myeloma begins as a single cell, all of its progeny constitute a clone of identical lymphocytes. In 1975, a technique was developed for combining the growth characteristics of myeloma cells and the special characteristics of normal immune spleen cells. In doing so, they developed a "hybrid" cell called a hybridoma, which is a specific antibody-producing factory. In such cells the myeloma portion provides immortality and thus large quantities of monoclonal antibody; the immune lymphocyte portion provides the information for the specificity of the antibody. The technique for making hybridoma cells is as follows:

1. The selected antigen is injected into the spleen of a mouse.

2. The spleen is removed and the antibody-synthesizing cells from the spleen are fused with myeloma cells to make hybridoma cells.

3. Hybridoma cells are grown in a selective culture medium.

4. Individual hybridoma cells are separated into wells and clones are grown.

5. Each clone produced is tested for the desired antibody.

Question 31

What property of spleen cells makes them appropriate for creating hybridomas?

- ○ **A.** Their ability to produce ATP in large quantities
- ○ **B.** Their predetermined antibody specificity
- ○ **C.** Their immortal nature
- ○ **D.** The rate at which they divide

Question 32

Which of the following biological processes would be inhibited by the removal of an adult human spleen?

- ○ **A.** The production of red blood cells
- ○ **B.** The production of T cells
- ○ **C.** The production of monocytes
- ○ **D.** The destruction of red blood cells

Question 33

Based on the passage, does the antigen need to be purified before being injected into the mouse?

- ○ **A.** No, the separation of the hybridoma cells into wells makes purification unnecessary.
- ○ **B.** No, only one type of antibody is produced in spleen cells in response to the antigen.
- ○ **C.** Yes, the injected antigen contains many epitopes.
- ○ **D.** Yes, an unpurified antigen would kill the mouse.

Question 34

One would expect that the culture medium chosen:

- ○ **A.** permitted the growth of unfused myeloma and spleen cells as well as hybridoma cells.
- ○ **B.** permitted the growth of hybridomas, but inhibited the growth of unfused myeloma and spleen cells.
- ○ **C.** permitted the growth of unfused myeloma and spleen cells, but inhibited the growth of hybridoma cells.
- ○ **D.** permitted the growth of spleen and hybridoma cells, but inhibited the growth of unfused myeloma cells.

Passage 7 (Questions 35–38)

Glycine (gly or G) is the simplest of the 20 amino acids commonly found in proteins. Since it only has hydrogen for a side chain, it is the only achiral amino acid. In fact, due to its minimal side chain, glycine can fit into hydrophilic or hydrophobic environments.

Glycine

Although most glycine is found in proteins, free glycine is also found in body fluids. Glycine and gamma-aminobutyric acid (GABA) are the major inhibitory neurotransmitters in the central nervous system.

Table 1 Properties of Glycine

Molecular formula	$C_2H_5NO_2$
Molecular mass	75.07 g mol^{-1}
Density	1.607 g/cm^3
Solubility in water	24.99 g/100 mL (25 °C)
Acidity (pK_a)	2.3 (carboxyl), 9.6 (amino)
Isoelectric point	pH 6.0

Experiment: Glycine's Flexibility at the Active Site

Glycine's small size means that it can occupy parts of protein structures that are forbidden to other amino acids (e.g. tight turns in structures). This means that there is much more conformational flexibility in glycine. In a revealing experiment, X-ray crystallographic data of 23 enzymes was analyzed to determine the properties of amino acids involved in active site cavity (pocket) regions. These regions were found to be rich in G-X-Y or Y-X-G oligopeptides, where X and Y are various amino acids (see Figure 1). Other regions of the enzyme molecules have significantly fewer of these sequences. These features suggest that glycine residues may provide flexibility necessary for enzyme active sites to change conformation, and the G-X-Y or Y-X-G oligopeptides may be a motif for the formation of enzyme active sites.

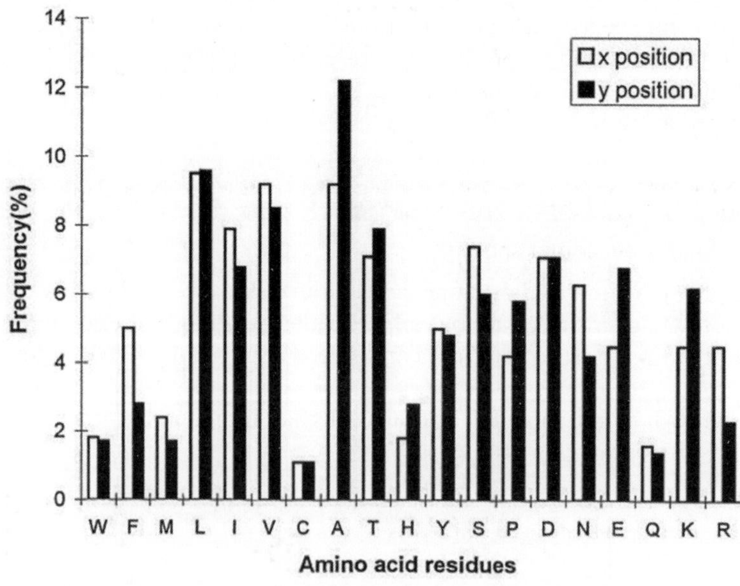

Figure 1 Frequency of amino acid residues observed in x and y positions in the G-X-Y or Y-X-G oligopeptides. Taken from the data set of 381 G-X-Y or Y-X-G oligopeptides in 23 enzymes examined.

Adapted from Yan BX, Sun YQ (1997) Glycine residues provide flexibility for enzyme active sites. J Biol Chem 272(6):3190–3194.

Question 35

Glycine is predominantly deprotonated at:

- O **A.** pH > 2.3
- O **B.** pH > 6.0
- O **C.** pH > 7.0
- O **D.** pH > 9.6

Question 36

The pH of cytoplasm typically ranges from 7.0 to 7.4. Which form of glycine predominates in cytoplasm?

- O **A.** H_3N^+-CH_2-COO^-
- O **B.** H_3N^+-CH_2-COOH
- O **C.** H_2N-CH_2-COOH
- O **D.** H_2N-CH_2-COO^-

Question 37

A small quantity of glycine is placed in a buffer solution of pH 2.0 and an electric field is applied. What will happen to the glycine sample?

- O **A.** It will migrate to the anode.
- O **B.** It will migrate to the cathode.
- O **C.** It will not migrate.
- O **D.** It will migrate, but in an unpredictable direction.

Question 38

Consider Figure 1 and examples of the most common amino acids found at the active site of the enzymes in the experiment. In general, what are the most likely features of the oligopeptide residues at sites on the substrates that bind to the enzymes in the experiment?

- O **A.** Small, hydrophilic
- O **B.** Large, ionic
- O **C.** Small, polar
- O **D.** Large, hydrophobic

Passage 8 (Questions 39–44)

The *lac* operon includes three genes that are required for lactose metabolism in some bacteria including *E. coli*. The operon contains *lacZ*, *lacY*, and *lacA*, which encode β-galactosidase, lactose permease, and galactoside O-acetyltransferase, respectively. It also contains three operator sequences (O1, O2, and O3). During lactose metabolism, lactose permease transports lactose into the cell, where β-galactosidase cleaves it into glucose and galactose. β-galactosidase also converts lactose to its isomer allolactose. The operon is under the strict control of a variety of proteins that regulate the expression of the *lacZ*, *lacY*, and *lacA* genes in the absence of lactose, or when an alternative and more efficient energy source is available. For example, IPTG, which mimics the function of allolactose, serves as an inducer of the *lac* operon although it is not a β-galactosidase substrate.

Table 1 Transcription from the *lac* operon in the presence of a variety of sugars and proteins.

Sugars present			Proteins present		*lacZ* transcription
Lactose	Allolactose	Glucose	LacI	CAP	
+	-	-	-	+	+++
+	-	+	-	-	-
-	-	-	+	+	-
-	-	+	+	-	-
+	+	-	+	+	++
+	+	-	+	-	-

The ability of activator and repressor proteins to regulate transcription from the *lac* operon involves a series of mechanisms including DNA looping, which can alter the proximity and/or alignment of enhancer DNA sequences. The activity of the protein that inhibits transcription from the *lac* operon (named LX for the purpose of this passage) is regulated by a process known as trans-translation, whereby the *ssrA* RNA causes ribosomes to pause at the 3′ end of the mRNA and add a short peptide tag to the C-terminus of the protein. The effect of *ssrA* on β-galactosidase activity was assessed in wild-type and *ssrA* mutant cells after *lac* transcription had been activated using IPTG, a molecule that mimics allolactose and triggers the transcription of the *lac* operon (Figure 1). The *ssrA* mutant contains a protease-resistant tag at its C-terminus, in which two Ala residues have been replaced with Asp. These mutations render *ssrA* inactive.

The tagging of LX requires its binding to operator sequences in the *lac* operon. To assess which operator is important, a study performed mutagenesis experiments, and the tagging of LX was assessed (Figure 2).

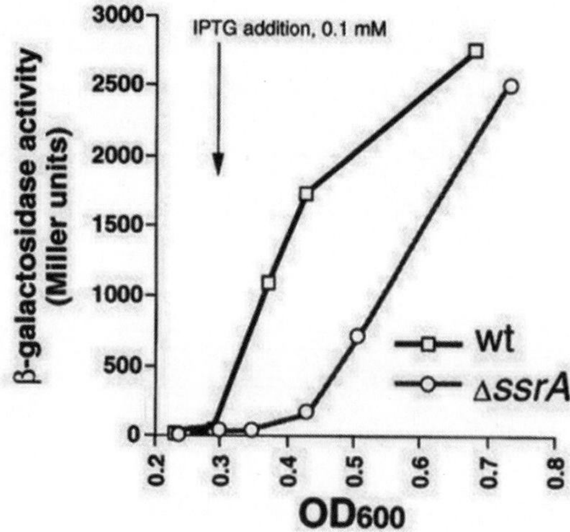

Figure 1 β-galactosidase activity in cells containing wild-type (wt) and mutant *ssrA* after the addition of IPTG.

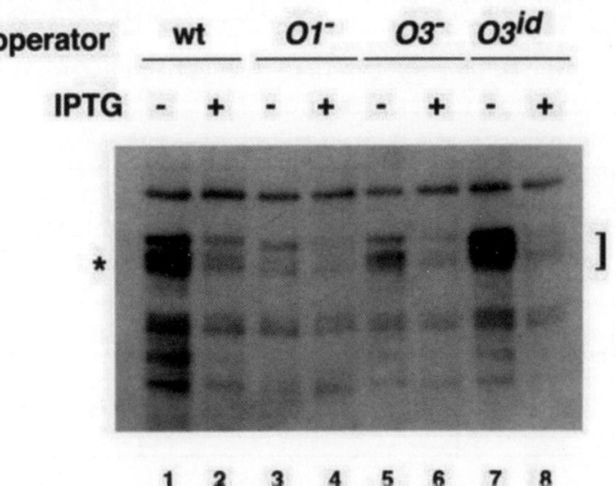

Figure 2 Cells containing wild-type operator sequences, mutated O1 ($O1^-$), mutated O3 ($O3^-$), and the ideal O3 operator ($O3^{id}$) were transfected with LX, grown in the presence or absence of IPTG, and LX was immunoprecipitated using specific antibodies. LX tagging was then assessed using immunoblotting.

Data partly based on nih.gov, PMC313975.

Question 39

Based on the information in Table 1, what are the roles of LacI and CAP?

- A. LacI is a transcriptional activator and CAP is a transcriptional repressor.
- B. LacI is a transcriptional activator and CAP is a transcriptional activator.
- C. LacI is a transcriptional repressor and CAP is a transcriptional activator.
- D. LacI is a transcriptional repressor and CAP is a transcriptional repressor.

Question 40

Based on the data in Table 1, what is the likely role of CAP in regulating transcription from the *lac* operon?

- A. It prevents the activity in the absence of sugar.
- B. It potentiates the activity in the absence of sugar.
- C. It prevents the activity of LacI.
- D. It potentiates the activity of LacI.

Question 41

Based on the data in Figure 1 and the passage, which of the following statements describes the activities that *ssrA* might have on LX?

- A. Inhibit its activity and increase DNA binding
- B. Inhibit its activity and decrease DNA binding
- C. Enhance its activity and increase DNA binding
- D. Enhance its activity and decrease DNA binding

Question 42

In an experiment, *E. coli* cells with the full *lac* operon (lac) or inactive *lacZ* (ΔlacZ) were grown with lactose or IPTG and the induction of lactose permease was measured.

	Lactose	IPTG	Lactose permease
lac	+	-	+
	-	+	+
ΔlacZ	+	-	-
	-	+	+

The results indicate that:

- O **A.** *lacZ* is inactivated by lactose.
- O **B.** *lacY* is regulated by *lacZ*.
- O **C.** β-galactosidase is necessary for the expression of lactose permease.
- O **D.** allolactose is necessary to induce the *lac* operon.

Question 43

While there are multiple mechanisms that can regulate transcription of the *lac* operon, the *lac* repressor protein, which is not encoded by the *lac* operon, likely works by:

- O **A.** preventing RNA polymerase from binding to the promoter.
- O **B.** deactivating *lacZ*.
- O **C.** downregulating β-galactosidase expression.
- O **D.** preventing glucose from being transported into the cell.

Question 44

Researchers wishing to express a recombinant protein in *E. coli* cloned the target gene into an expression vector controlled by the *lac* promoter. However, the *E. coli* strain chosen for the cell culture has a mutation that renders *lacI* dysfunctional, resulting in:

- O **A.** twice the necessary IPTG for target protein expression.
- O **B.** downregulation of target protein expression.
- O **C.** the inactivation of the *lac* operon.
- O **D.** constitutive expression of the target protein.

The following questions are NOT based on a descriptive passage (Questions 45–48).

Question 45

A library of DNA fragments results from the use of which of the following?

- O **A.** DNA ligase
- O **B.** Restriction endonucleases
- O **C.** Recombinant DNA
- O **D.** Single-stranded plasmids

Question 46

Superoxide dismutase 1 is an enzyme implicated in amyotrophic lateral sclerosis (Lou Gehrig's disease) which has a copper ion bound to the active site. In this enzyme, copper most likely functions as a(n):

- ○ **A.** coenzyme.
- ○ **B.** cofactor.
- ○ **C.** allosteric activator.
- ○ **D.** allosteric inhibitor.

Question 47

Consider the following diagram.

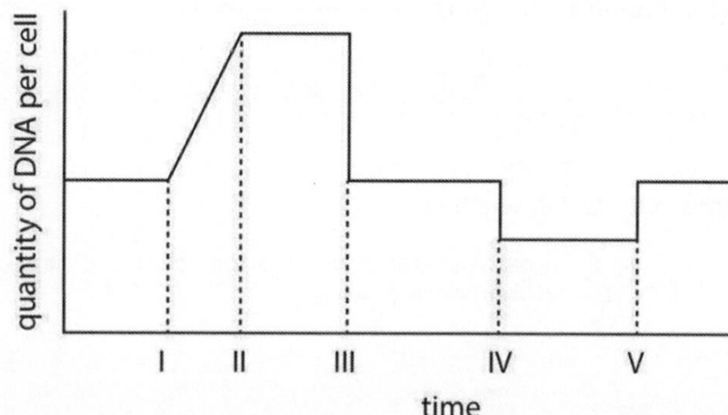

Which of the following is most consistent with the quantity of DNA per cell at the end of the first meiotic division?

- ○ **A.** I
- ○ **B.** II
- ○ **C.** III
- ○ **D.** IV

Question 48

Consider the following reaction.

$2e^- + H^+$

What is the product of the reaction above?

- ○ **A.** NAD^+
- ○ **B.** NADH
- ○ **C.** NADH + H
- ○ **D.** NADH + H^+

Passage 9 (Questions 49–52)

The polymerase chain reaction (PCR) is a powerful biological tool that allows the rapid amplification of any fragment of DNA without purification. In PCR, DNA primers are made to flank the specific DNA sequence to be amplified. These primers are then extended to the end of the DNA molecule with the use of a heat-resistant DNA polymerase. The newly synthesized DNA strand is then used as the template to undergo another round of replication.

The 1st step in PCR is the melting of the target DNA into 2 single strands by heating the reaction mixture to approximately 94 °C, and then rapidly cooling the mixture to allow annealing of the DNA primers to their specific locations. Once the primer has annealed, the temperature is elevated to 72 °C to allow optimal activity of the DNA polymerase. The polymerase will continue to add nucleotides until the entire complimentary strand of the template is completed at which point the cycle is repeated (Figure 1).

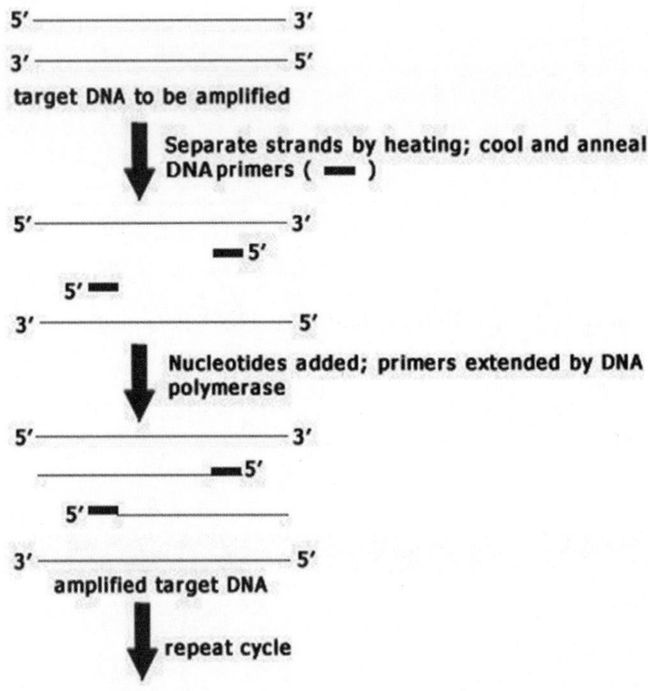

Figure 1

One of the uses of PCR is sex determination, which requires amplification of intron 1 of the amelogenin gene. This gene found on the X-Y homologous chromosomes has a 184 base pair deletion on the Y homologue. Therefore, by amplifying intron 1 females can be distinguished from males by the fact that males will have 2 different sizes of the amplified DNA while females will only have 1 unique fragment size.

Question 49

The polymerase chain reaction most likely resembles which of the following cellular process?

- O **A.** Transcription of DNA
- O **B.** Protein synthesis
- O **C.** DNA replication
- O **D.** Translation

Question 50

Which of the following statements could be used to correctly describe the overall polymerase chain reaction?

- O **A.** It is an anabolic reaction that breaks down new DNA strands.
- O **B.** It is an anabolic reaction that synthesizes new DNA strands.
- O **C.** It is a catabolic reaction that breaks down new DNA strands.
- O **D.** It is a catabolic reaction that synthesizes new DNA strands.

Question 51

What would PCR amplification of an individual's intron 1 of the amelogenin gene reveal if the individual were male?

- O **A.** One type of intron 1 since the individual has one X chromosome and one Y chromosome.
- O **B.** Two types of intron 1 since the individual has only one X chromosome.
- O **C.** One type of intron 1 since the individual has only one X chromosome.
- O **D.** Two types of intron 1 since the individual has one X chromosome and one Y chromosome.

Question 52

Both copies of intron 1 of the amelogenin gene on the 2 sex chromosomes can be referred to as:

- O **A.** homologous chromosomes.
- O **B.** recessive traits.
- O **C.** alleles.
- O **D.** spliced RNA.

Passage 10 (Questions 53–56)

Several models have been developed for relating changes in dissociation constants to changes in the tertiary and quaternary structures of oligomeric proteins. One model suggests that the protein's subunits can exist in either of two distinct conformations, R and T. At equilibrium, there are few R conformation molecules: 10 000 T to 1 R and it is an important feature of the enzyme that this ratio does not change. The substrate is assumed to bind more tightly to the R form than to the T form, which means that binding of the substrate favors the transition from the T conformation to R.

The conformational transitions of the individual subunits are assumed to be tightly linked, so that if one subunit flips from T to R the others must do the same. The binding of the first molecule of substrate thus promotes the binding of the second and if substrate is added continuously, all of the enzyme will be in the R form and act on the substrate. Because the concerted transition of all of the subunits from T to R or back, preserves the overall symmetry of the protein, this model is called the *symmetry model*. The model further predicts that allosteric activating enzymes make the R conformation even more reactive with the substrate while allosteric inhibitors react with the T conformation so that most of the enzyme is held back in the T shape.

Experiment Evaluating Non-Symmetry Model Enzymes

Experiments were performed with enzyme conformers that did not obey the symmetry model. The data is summarized in Figure 1.

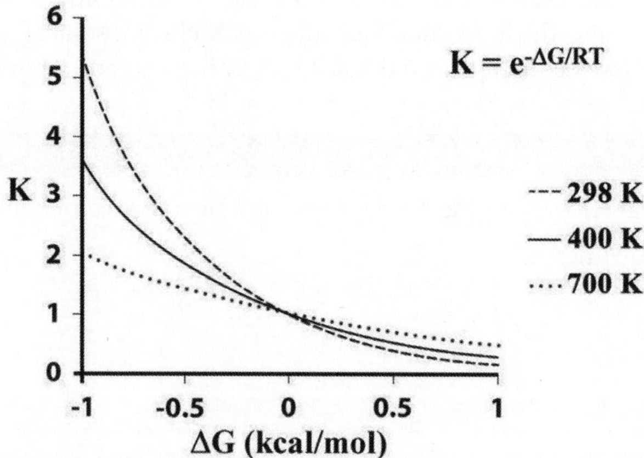

Figure 1 Equilibrium distribution of two conformers at different temperatures given the free energy of their interconversion. (modified from Mr.Holmium)

Question 53

What assumption is made about the T and R conformations and the substrate?

- O **A.** In the absence of any substrate, the T conformation predominates.
- O **B.** In the absence of any substrate, the R conformation predominates.
- O **C.** In the absence of any substrate, the T and R conformations are in equilibrium.
- O **D.** In the absence of any substrate, the enzyme exists in another conformation, S.

Question 54

The symmetry model describes a form of cooperative binding. Most enzymes do not engage in cooperative binding. The predicted shape of a graph representing reaction rate versus the addition of substrate to most enzymes would be expected to be:

- O **A.** a hyperbola.
- O **B.** a straight line with a positive slope.
- O **C.** a straight line with a negative slope.
- O **D.** sigmoidal.

Question 55

Allosteric enzymes differ from other enzymes in that they:

- O **A.** are not denatured at high temperatures.
- O **B.** are regulated by compounds which are not their substrates and which do not bind to their active sites.
- O **C.** they operate at an optimum pH of about 2.0.
- O **D.** they are not specific to just one substrate.

Question 56

All of the following statements are consistent with Figure 1 EXCEPT:

- O **A.** the products must have less free energy than the reactants in the exergonic reactions at the various temperatures.
- O **B.** the equation for the equilibrium constant K used to construct the graph is derived from $\Delta G = -RT \ln K$
- O **C.** the 3 different temperature curves intersect at a point where the reaction is at equilibrium.
- O **D.** higher temperatures favor relatively more of the more stable conformer.

The following questions are NOT based on a descriptive passage (Questions 57–59).

Question 57

Human mRNA with a length of 210 nucleotides likely codes for a protein of:

- O **A.** approximately 210 amino acids.
- O **B.** between 70 – 210 amino acids.
- O **C.** exactly 70 amino acids.
- O **D.** less than 70 amino acids.

Question 58

Which of the following is NOT consistent with the β anomer of D-glucose?

- O **A.** 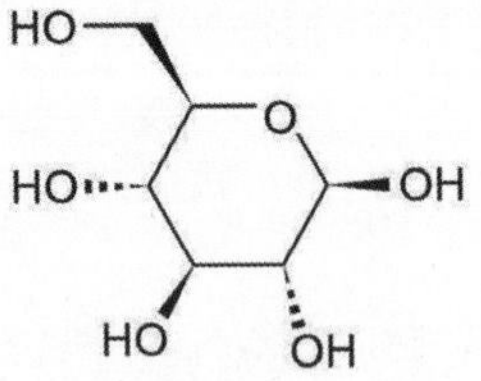
- O **B.** 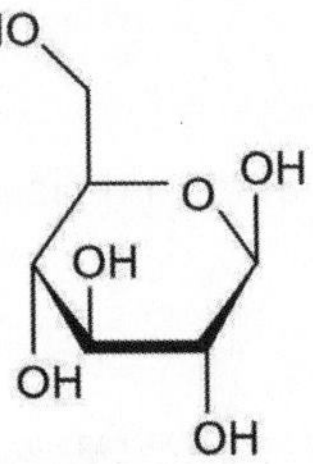
- O **C.** 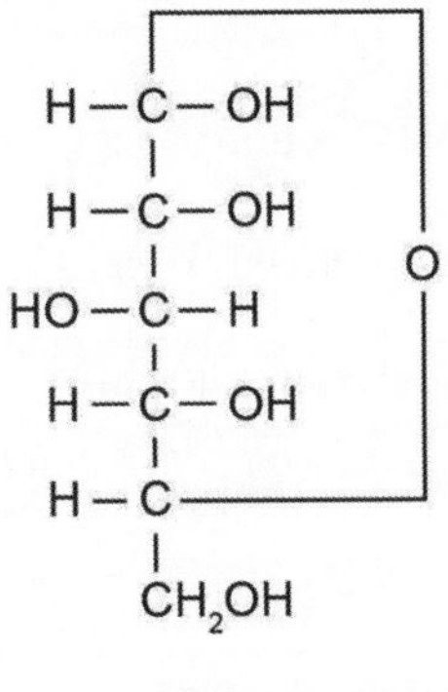
- O **D.**

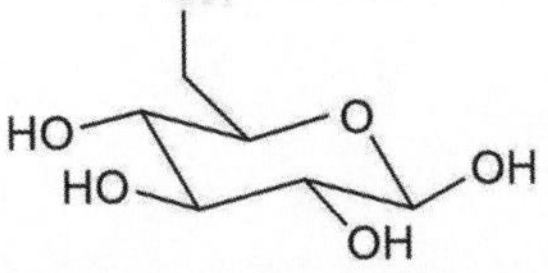

Question 59

Which of the following contains an incorrect statement about a metabolic process?

- O **A.** Glycolysis is catabolic, because a large molecule is broken into smaller ones, with a net production of high-energy molecules.
- O **B.** Glycogenolysis is catabolic because it involves breaking larger molecules into smaller ones.
- O **C.** Glycogenesis is anabolic because it consumes energy in the form of ATP in order to build a larger molecule from smaller ones.
- O **D.** Gluconeogenesis is anabolic because it is a synthesis reaction, consuming energy as ATP and GTP.

CANDIDATE'S NAME ____________________

RAW SCORE AND SCALED SCORE ____________________

GS-4
Mock Exam 4 of 7
Solutions at MCAT-prep.com

GS-4 Section IV: Psychological, Social, and Biological Foundations of Behavior

Questions: 1-59
Time: 95 minutes

INSTRUCTIONS: Of all the questions on this test, most are organized into groups preceded by a passage. After evaluating the passage, select the best answer to each question in the group. Fifteen questions are independent of any descriptive passage or each other. Similarly, select the best answer to these questions. If you are unsure of an answer, eliminate the alternatives that you know to be incorrect and select an answer from the remaining alternatives. To indicate your selection, use a pencil to blacken the corresponding circle next to the answer choice and/or you can use the answer document at the back of this book. No marks are deducted for wrong answers.

The computer-based real MCAT has an on-screen highlighter function and ~~STRIKEOUT~~ function. These tools help to spotlight text or assist in the process of elimination. You may use a yellow highlighter for this paper-based exam and/or a pen (or preferably a pencil to make it easier should you change your mind) to mark text. At the time of publishing, both highlighting and strikeout functions can be used for passages, questions and answer choices. You can also flag a question to review later should time remain.

For the real exam, you will be provided with a dry erase board which is a white laminated noteboard booklet accompanied by a fine point marker. The noteboard includes 9 graph-lined pages for you to write though you cannot erase. You can simulate the experience with a fine point marker on a noteboard or with 8" x 14" plain graph paper.

Please note: For the real MCAT, a small number of field-tested questions will remain unscored.

This practice test has been designed exclusively to test knowledge and thinking skills. This exam may contain hypothetical statements and/or express controversial ideas. Statements contained herein do not necessarily reflect the policy, position, or view of RuveneCo Inc. or MCAT-prep.com.

START EXAM ONLY WHEN TIMER IS READY.

Passage 1 (Questions 1–4)

Several studies have been conducted to better understand the effect keeping a journal can have on patients. Through the practice of journaling, patients can learn about identification, regulation, and expression of emotions either in private or in therapeutic contexts. It can be cathartic and work as a reflective and life-changing practice. Some scholars have attempted to explain the effects of keeping a journal with theories around cognitive change, habituation, or changes in working memory.

In 2003, James W. Pennebaker, one of the key scholars to write about journaling therapy, and Sherlock Campbell conducted a study that used latent semantic analysis in order to categorize journal entries of three different purposive samples, composed of individuals who had been previously subjected to an individual psychotherapeutic intervention. They were interested in whether similarities in the writing content predicted health changes. The study looked at three different samples, which consisted of (1) 74 first-year students, (2) 50 upper division students, and (3) 59 maximum-security prisoners. Table 1 displays the demographic distribution of the samples.

Table 1 Demographic Distribution of Samples 1, 2, and 3

	(1)	(2)	(3)
Total n	74	50	59
Male n	35	14	59
Female n	39	36	0
Mean age	17.9	19.8	35.4
SD	0.4	2.6	9.5

The participants were randomly assigned to two conditions. They either had to write about superficial topics or about emotional topics. They all were asked to write 15–20 minutes per day for 3–5 consecutive days. Considered for analysis were the content of their journals (wording similarity), the type of pronouns used (use similarity), and the number of illness-related physician visits in the university/prison health center two months before and four months after the psychotherapeutic intervention (that is, changes in frequency of illness-related physician visits).

Table 2 Correlation between Essay Similarity and Change in Frequency of Illness-related Physician Visits for Experimental Participants

	Sample		
Semantic space	First-year students (n = 35)	Upper-division students (n = 25)	Psychiatric inmates (n = 33)
Content	−.05	.08	.25
Style	.34*	.51**	.43*
Particle	.38*	.51**	.41*
Preposition	.20	.32	.14
Conjunction, article	.18	.38	.08
Auxiliary verb	−.22	.10	.22
Pronoun	.35*	.50**	.43**

$*p \le .05$. $**p \le .01$.

Source: Adapted from S.R. Campbell & J.W. Pennebaker, "The Secret Life of Pronouns: Flexibility in Writing Style and Physical Health." Copyright 2003 Psychological Science.

The results showed that the factor most clearly associated with recovery was the use of personal pronouns. Patients whose writing changed perspective from day to day were less likely to seek medical treatment during the follow-up period. Table 2 displays how similarity of writing content and style correlates with frequency of physician visits for the experimental group. Content and style were each operationalized as semantic spaces—that is, as frequencies of words occurring together. Those scores were noted as content and style coefficients. Those coefficients were then compared between sequential essays and computed into similarity ratings. Those were averaged in order to get the overall similarity ratings. A higher rating signified more similarity.

Question 1

Which statement corresponds best to the results displayed in Table 2?

- O **A.** Statistically significant health improvements were found only for the group of upper-division students.
- O **B.** The more consistent the participants' writing styles were, the more likely they were to see a physician after the intervention.
- O **C.** The more dissimilar the participants' writing style, the more likely they were to visit a physician after the intervention.
- O **D.** Only the experimental group experienced a significant change in the frequency of physician visits, which could be explained by the content of their writing style.

Question 2

Which of the following procedures would most likely NOT help to enhance the reliability and validity of the study described in the passage?

- O **A.** Creating a new sample that includes participants from different sociodemographic backgrounds
- O **B.** Asking participants to continue writing in the journal for a period of six months, and perform a longitudinal comparison of the style, content, and physician visit–related data in different moments in time
- O **C.** Assisting less literate participants with the diary writing by brainstorming with them before summing up the results for them in the diary
- O **D.** Only counting illness-related visits to the physician, not injury- or routine checkup–related visits

Question 3

A journaling exercise consisting of describing decision-making preferences would most likely aim at assessing:

- O **A.** the four temperaments of Hippocrates' medical theory of personality.
- O **B.** the extravert and introvert attitudes used in analytical psychology.
- O **C.** Carl Jung's thinking and feeling personality types.
- O **D.** type A and type B personality categories.

Question 4

Which of the following theories would most likely argue that people's linguistic skills are determined by the environment, such as the praises received when employing rich vocabulary?

- O **A.** Behaviorism
- O **B.** Nativism
- O **C.** Social interactionism
- O **D.** Structuralism

Passage 2 (Questions 5–9)

The terms "puberty" and "adolescence" are sometimes used interchangeably. Yet puberty is often reserved to refer exclusively to the human developmental stage during which endocrine changes indicate children's transition into adulthood. These changes are mostly related to the awakening of the biological clock that commands neurons to start releasing gonadotropin-releasing hormone (GnRH). On the other hand, the term adolescence is often reserved by specialists for concomitant psychological and social changes. In both cases, however, changes hold a reproductive purpose.

Authors like Erik Erikson, Sigmund Freud, James Marcia, Jean Piaget, Lawrence Kohlberg, and G. Stanley Hall have all tried to explain the psychosocial changes that occur during adolescence from different perspectives and approaches. In brief, adolescents go through a sometimes strenuous process of individuation brought about partly by the burgeoning of sexual traits and the acquisition of adult-like thinking styles, roles, and statuses. Individuals' self-concept and identity, whether ethnic, cultural, social, or sexual, are generally clarified, restructured, or redefined. Although puberty marks its beginning, the end of the adolescence, by being dependent on the achievement and/or development of a certain psychosocial position and identity, is more difficult to pin down.

In accordance with the biopsychosocial model, it is, like childhood, a critical period in which experienced adversities of different orders can create long-term if not permanent vulnerabilities or deficits that seriously affect the person. For example, sometimes adolescents make less healthy, positive, or constructive behavioral choices (e.g., risk-taking, boundary testing, drug use, deviance, or crime) which can impact their identity and maturation process in the long run.

Pregnancy during this stage often results from a combination of teenagers' desire to establish intimate relationships and their risk-taking tendency. This behavior and its outcome have been subjected to preventive measures in many Western countries. As found by the U.S. National Center for Health Statistics, the teen birth rate has declined over the past 20 years. In 1991, the U.S. teen birth rate was 61.8 births per 1,000 adolescent females, compared with 26.5 births per 1,000 adolescent females in 2013. Figure 1 below details these findings.

These results seem to suggest that adopted preventive measures and social changes have successfully reduced what is currently regarded in these countries as an undesirable outcome of adolescent risk-taking behavior.

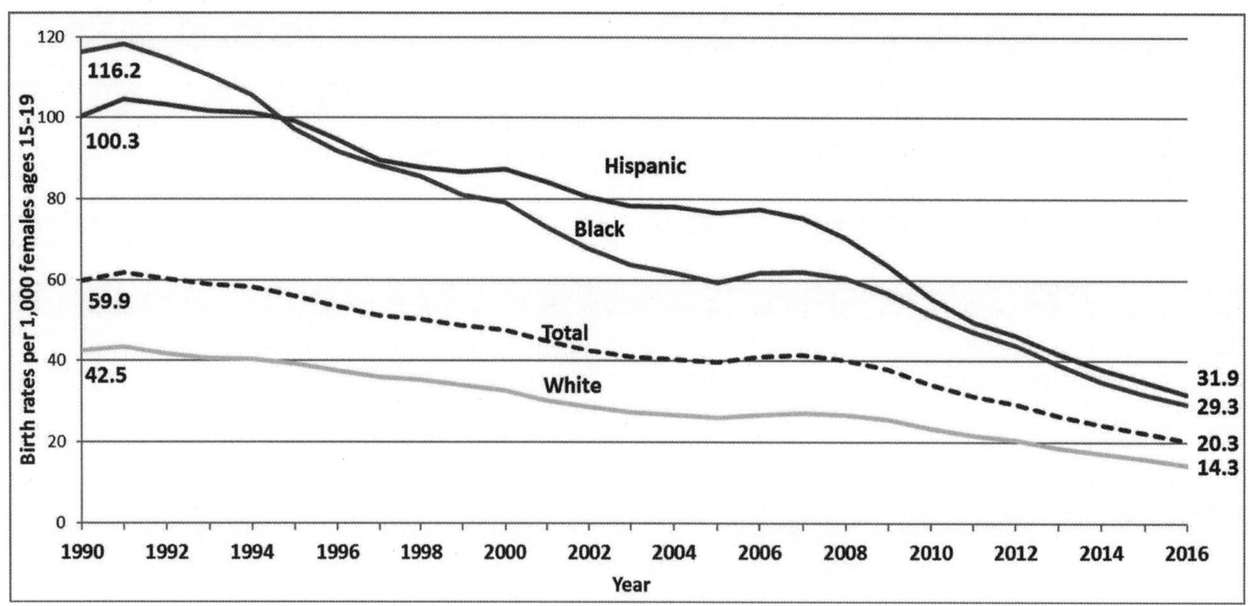

Figure 1 Birth rates per 1,000 females aged 15–19, by race/ethnicity, 1990–2018

Sources: J. Marcia, "Identity in Adolescence," in Handbook of Adolescent Psychology. *Copyright 1980 John Wiley & Sons; J.A. Martin, B.E. Hamilton, & S.J. Ventura, "Births: Final Data for 2018." Copyright 2018 U.S. National Center for Health Statistics.*

Question 5

Which of the following options does NOT correctly describe pubertal endocrine changes?

- O **A.** Steroid hormones start influencing the formation of secondary sex traits in peripheral tissues, regulating GnRH neurons via a neuroendocrine feedback loop, and facilitating social behaviors by central nervous system actuation.
- O **B.** Luteinizing hormone and follicle-stimulating hormone act on the testes and ovaries to initiate the production of sperm, eggs, and steroid hormones.
- O **C.** GnRH is produced by specialized neurons located in the pituitary and is responsible for initiating the production of gonadotropins, namely luteinizing hormone and follicle-stimulating hormone.
- O **D.** Acquired gender specific secondary traits are for women, the enlargement of breasts and erection of nipples, the growth of body hair, and the widening of hips. For men, these include the growth of body and facial hair, the squaring of the face, and the increase of muscle mass.

Question 6

The term "latency" is sometimes used to situate the onset of adolescence. Which author adopts this term to describe a stage of human development; what is his/her approach to human development; and how could that stage be succinctly described (author; approach; description, respectively)?

- O **A.** G. Stanley Hall; biopsychosocial approach; quietness before the storm
- O **B.** Sigmund Freud; psychoanalytic approach; interiorization of social norms
- O **C.** B.F. Skinner; behaviorist approach; reward and punishment learning
- O **D.** Erik Erikson; psychoanalytic approach; identity and role confusion

Question 7

According to Lawrence Kohlberg's theory referenced in the passage, which of the following tasks could reveal whether an adolescent from the United States had developed normally and gone beyond the children's developmental stage?

- O **A.** Balancing weights of different dimensions on an old-fashioned two-plate balance scale
- O **B.** Describing what someone with a difficult life story was likely feeling and thinking, and might likely do
- O **C.** Identifying the most likely emotions, intentions, actions, and thoughts of people in photographs
- O **D.** Providing arguments in favor and against killing a dictator who has killed millions of people

Question 8

The passage referred to how the adolescent undergoes a sometimes strenuous individuation process that involves identity formation. According to James Marcia, which of the following identity statuses implies an identity crisis?

- O **A.** Identity diffusion
- O **B.** Moratorium
- O **C.** Foreclosure
- O **D.** Identity achievement

Question 9

If the total annual birth rates per 1,000 females aged 15–19 identified in Figure 1 were transformed into a bar chart, which of the following options would most closely represent the conclusions drawn from Figure 1?

○ **A.**

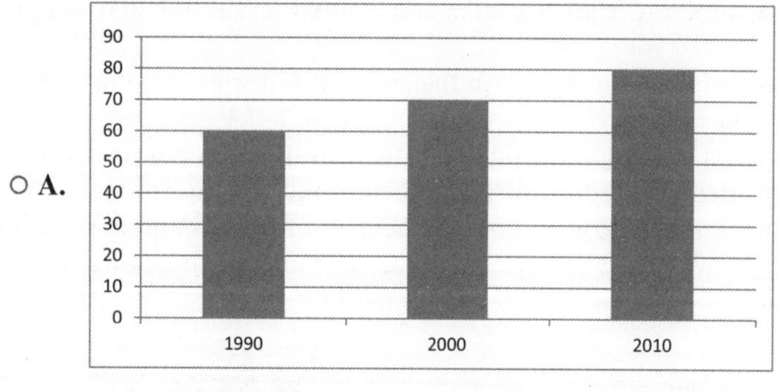

○ **B.**

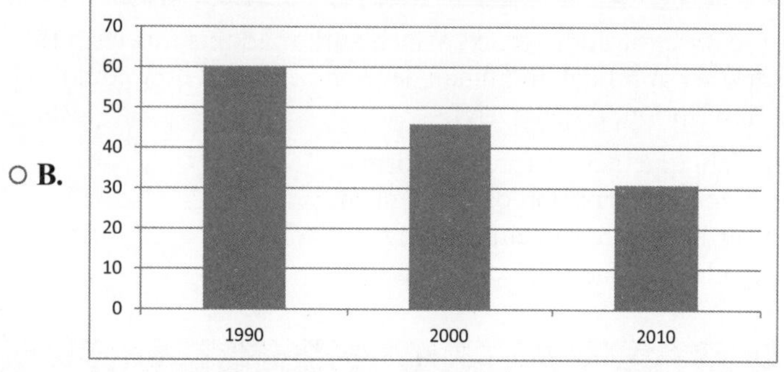

○ **C.**

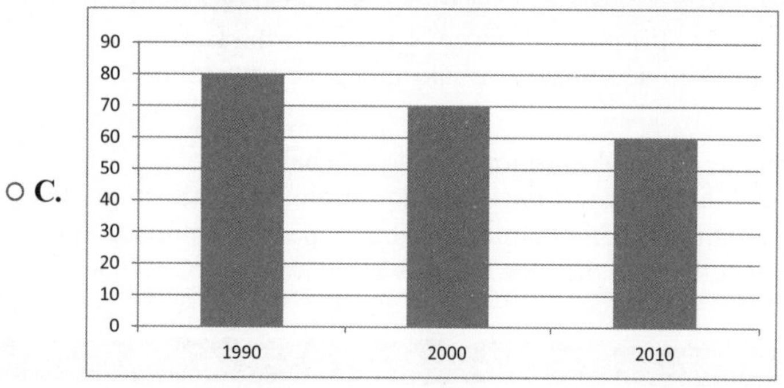

○ **D.**

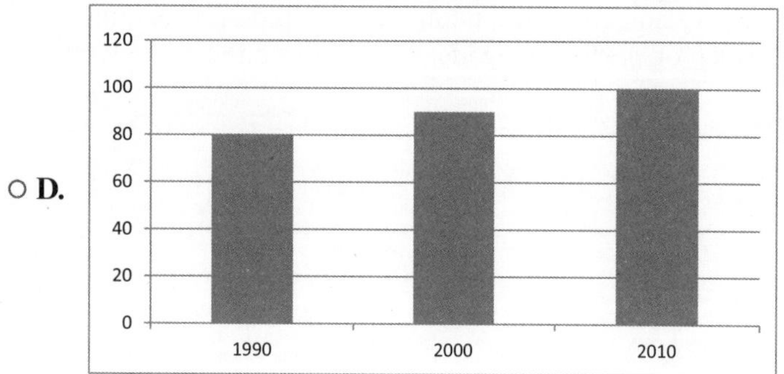

The following questions are NOT based on a descriptive passage (Questions 10–13).

Question 10

Paul Broca's research showed that certain functions of the brain are lateralized, i.e., centralized in a single hemisphere of the brain. What particular function was Broca studying?

- O **A.** Problem solving
- O **B.** Language production
- O **C.** Facial recognition
- O **D.** Language comprehension

Question 11

Which of the laws below is NOT one of the principles of Gestalt psychology?

- O **A.** Law of similarity
- O **B.** Law of discontinuation
- O **C.** Law of proximity
- O **D.** Law of Prägnanz

Question 12

A recognition test consists of presenting one photo at a time in random order from three ten-photo sets (famous actors; family and oldest friends; and strangers). Which of the following diagnoses would better apply to results evidencing that someone was unable to recognize equally photos from every set?

- O **A.** Astereognosis
- O **B.** Visual agnosia
- O **C.** Apperceptive agnosia
- O **D.** Prosopagnosia

Question 13

Which category of Robert K. Merton's model of deviance would best explain why some people engage in criminal acts or other deviant activities in order to become wealthy?

- O **A.** Conformity
- O **B.** Innovation
- O **C.** Ritualism
- O **D.** Rebellion

Passage 3 (Questions 14–17)

Society has become very sensitive to any type of information that may be interpreted as stereotypical (involving beliefs), as well as prejudiced (involving evaluations) or discriminatory (involving behaviors). Open expressions of stereotyping, prejudice, discrimination, racism, and any other type of "ism" are socially censured, sometimes sanctioned, and thereby avoided by anyone who wishes to be socially approved. The way advertisement has changed over the years clearly illustrates how these issues are culturally regulated. In the light of social and cultural North American norms, the ad reproduced in Figure 1 could have been published 70 years ago—yet it was published in 2011. For this reason, it might be regarded as discriminatory.

Nevertheless, as Susan Fiske remarked in 2000, "everyone must categorize in order to function"—a process that is a stepping stone toward (if not synonymous with) stereotyping. It is naïve to think otherwise. Even people's memory of others has been shown to be biased. Outgroup members tend to be confused with one another in memory, being mainly remembered for their stereotyped attributes. In contrast, the ingroup members tend to preserve in memory their distinctive and idiopathic traits.

Implicit prejudice experiments further revealed that people's exposure to stereotype-congruent stimuli, concerning (at least) ethnicity, race, age, and gender, increased the odds of biased social judgments. That is, simply knowing a stereotype existed and having stereotype-relevant information cognitively made available to people seemed to suffice for prejudiced responses to come about. Importantly, these prejudiced responses sometimes occurred against people's will, intention, awareness, and/or manifested views about the topic. Neuropsychologically, these responses activated the subcortical network for quick information processing, which is linked to autonomic and behavioral systems. Particularly, the amygdala was active during covert (vs. overt) prejudiced attitude manifestation. This neuropsychological results seem to suggest that prejudices are the fruit of difficult-to-change neurological processes and as natural as categorization processes.

However, criticism was raised about the implicit prejudice paradigm. Specifically, testing procedures seemed to be unable to conceal their aim of testing prejudice. Given the current censuring of such attitudes, amygdala activation could partly result from participants' fear of being judged as prejudiced. In addition, attitude change research using classic conditioning and diversity education has had promising results. Such interventions seem to hold the potential to bring societies closer the ideal pursued by many Western countries of unprejudiced societies.

This Mother's Day,
Get Back To
The Job
That Really
Matters.
Mr.
Clean.

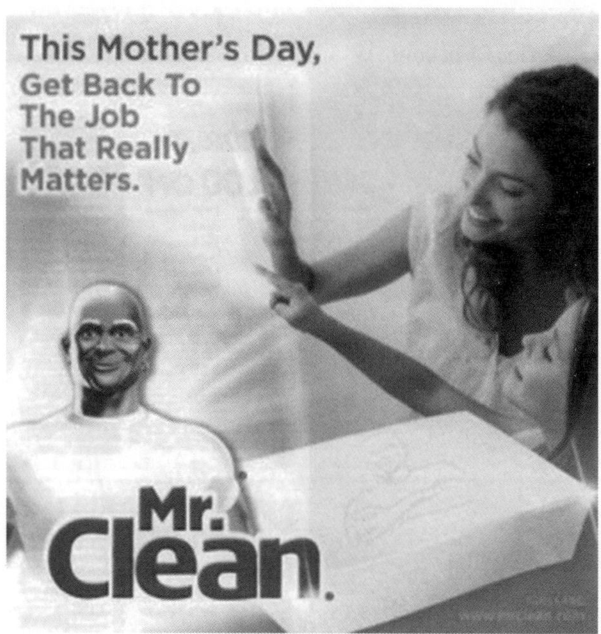

Figure 1 Mr. Clean advertisement

Sources: Adapted from S. Fiske, "Stereotyping, Prejudice, and Discrimination at the Seam between the Centuries: Evolution, Culture, Mind, and Brain." Copyright 1999 John Wiley & Sons; Mr. Clean, "Mother's Day" [advertisement]. Copyright 2011 P&G.

Question 14

Which of the following reactions would likely involve the activation of systems other than the autonomic nervous system?

- O **A.** Waking up in the middle of the night to urinate
- O **B.** Meeting a person one fancies and feeling one's heart start to race along with sweating profusely
- O **C.** Hitting someone in the face after seeing that person get physically violent with a child
- O **D.** Unwillingly throwing up one's dinner after being scared to death by a movie

Question 15

Which of the following interpretations of the ad in Figure 1 would be the LEAST discriminatory for a third-wave feminist?

- O **A.** It suggests that women should feel happy when cleaning the house, by portraying them smiling while cleaning the house alongside their young daughters.
- O **B.** It suggests that women are above both men and children by placing them at the top of the ad, and men and children at the bottom.
- O **C.** It suggests that women lack the muscular strength needed for performing their most important job, which is house cleaning alongside their daughters.
- O **D.** It suggests that women should celebrate mothers' special day by house cleaning alongside their daughters.

Question 16

Taking into account the information described in the passage and available knowledge about stereotypes, which of the following conclusions regarding Muzafer Sherif's classical intergroup relationship experiment entitled Robbers Cave would most likely consist of a statistical type I error?

- O **A.** Discriminatory behavior toward outgroups depends on contextual factors.
- O **B.** Groups are perceived as homogeneous entities lacking in interindividual diversity, even when they are constituted at random.
- O **C.** Familiarization and behavior-mimicking allows outgroup members to become ingroup members.
- O **D.** People advantage outgroup (vs. ingroup) members, seeing negative traits as situational and positive traits as dispositional.

Question 17

An implicit prejudice research paradigm would necessarily involve:

- O **A.** the presentation of stimuli below the threshold of perception.
- O **B.** the testing of people's automatic information processing of stereotype-relevant attributes.
- O **C.** the selection of two groups that act as outgroup and ingroup.
- O **D.** a brief explanation of the aims of the experiment prior to the testing of individuals.

Passage 4 (Questions 18–22)

When studying the prevalence of crime and deviance, a researcher may rely upon statistics. These tell us a number of things, including that Black men are overrepresented at all levels of the criminal justice system, from stop-and-search to imprisonment, leading some to believe that they have higher levels of criminal involvement. These statistics helped to form the stereotype of the "criminal black man," an image of a dangerous outlaw who should be feared by the population. This stereotype spread through media channels and reached society.

According to Jeffrey Reiman, the "criminal black man" stereotype is further mirrored in the treatment of ethnic minorities by the criminal justice system. Through the reactions of those who represent the justice system while interacting with those who apparently fit the disseminated stereotype the label is reinforced further. This is especially true for individual officers. According to Brinkerhoff and colleagues, officers have a unique power in the criminal justice system. They have autonomy and can make arrests without anyone having made a complaint against an individual. Research implies that police officers also have high levels of community alienation and high group identification. This is often on ethnic lines, and given the high proportion of white officers, some research suggests that many lay the blame of crime at the door of Black populations, even in some instances believing that there is something inferior in Black culture that leads to crime.

There are alternative interpretations of the very same data. Specifically, feminists would emphasize the "man" in the "criminal Black man" stereotype and would see the higher percentage of male criminality as the most obvious trend in crime statistics. For them, the most startling aspect is that men commit more crimes of most types than women. Many would further assume that this is a structural problem in society. Other interpretations would suggest that the "problem" is not one of gender at all and that the real problem is capitalism, which is "criminogenic"—inherently crime producing.

There are various theories on the causes of crime, methods of crime prevention, and of effective crime punishment. One causal theory simply relates to the idea that interacting with certain people will lead to criminal behavior. This theory is often used to explain the overrepresentation of Black men in crime statistics. A fascinating example of this is rioting. During a riot, many people get involved in criminal activity through being swept up by the group. This happens regardless of race, and in the absence of both personal history of such acts and persuasive actions from the other members. Thus the group is argued to lead to a loss of accountability and identity for the individual, which at times may mean committing crimes alongside other group members.

Prejudice and stereotypes are prevalent at every level of society, and beliefs about crime may not respond to the actual reality of criminality. Imagine a scenario in which the police receives numerous calls from citizens claiming they have been accosted in a mall parking lot, the assailant hitting them on the head with the butt of a gun before demanding money. The victims cannot identify the criminal. However, they may have an image of what the criminal may look like. How will the media report it? How will the general population view the crime? Criminological research in general shows that a primary identifier will be the criminal's race. And if the stereotype is used to fill in a memory gap, the "criminal Black man" may be perhaps unfairly implicated.

Sources: Adapted from John Hagan, "Many Colors of Crime: Inequalities of Race, Ethnicity, and Crime in America." Copyright 2006 New York University Press; D.B. Brinkerhoff, L.K. White, S.T. Ortega, R. Weitz, Essentials of Sociology. *Copyright 2010 Wadsworth Publishing Co.*

Question 18

According to the passage, capitalism is "criminogenic." With which of the theories below would this statement most likely fit?

- O **A.** Feminism
- O **B.** Marxism
- O **C.** Functionalism
- O **D.** Postmodernism

Question 19

If, in the scenario given in the passage, the criminal had been ordered to commit the crime by the leader of his/her gang, though the person would not have behaved that way without the order and it was not a "copycat" crime, which concept could most effectively explain what triggered this behavior?

- O **A.** Obedience
- O **B.** Conformity
- O **C.** Internalization
- O **D.** Informational influence

Question 20

What construct would explain why someone from an African race might fear being judged more severely by society, as a 'criminal Black man', even though they were committing a first offense to help a friend to pay medical bills?

- O **A.** Differential association
- O **B.** Diffusion of responsibility
- O **C.** Cognitive dissonance
- O **D.** Stereotype threat

Question 21

According to the information provided in the passage, which of the concepts below would best explain the behavior of people in riots?

- O **A.** Peer pressure
- O **B.** Deindividuation
- O **C.** Social facilitation
- O **D.** Social loafing

Question 22

Which concept could explain most effectively the views of the police officers expressed in the passage?

- O **A.** Ethnocentrism
- O **B.** Institutional discrimination
- O **C.** Racialization
- O **D.** Orientalism

Passage 5 (Questions 23–27)

Everyone dreams. If not of better futures, then at least during the night, whether or not one intends to. Biologists' interest in dreams began with the observation that the eyelids of sleeping adults did not move for approximately 20 minutes of each sleep hour. This was coined the "no eye movement" (NEM) period. This discovery, published around 1950, led to extensive sleep research involving observational studies and the registry of the brain activity of sleeping adults via electroencephalogram (EEG) and electrooculography (EOG) techniques. Through these procedures, the most well-known sleep stage, the rapid eye movement (REM) period, was discovered.

The quick saccadic eye movements of REM, along with jerkiness, are found to be good discriminators between waking and sleeping periods. During REM, great cortical activity is registered, suggesting, in contrast with popular biologists' views at the time, that sleep is not a "completely passive phenomenon." Although dreaming is not limited to REM periods, dreams that occur during this period tend to be more vivid, complex, emotional, and easier to remember. As for NEM (No Eye Movement), this period was subsequently divided into several sleep stages, all generally currently named after REM as NREM (Non–rapid Eye Movement) stages), thereby reinforcing the pivotal importance of REM.

For biologists, these discoveries were surprising, principally because evidence showed that the brain was not at rest during sleep. However, those who had been studying dreams as well as psychiatric disorders had already given credit to the importance of sleeping and dreaming for people's psychological lives. An example is Sigmund Freud and his book *The Interpretation of Dreams*, an approach that was taken a step further by Carl Jung. Both psychoanalytic thinkers thoroughly studied the content of their own and their patients' dreams, believing them to be the most direct way to access the mysterious and hard-to-reveal unconscious. They argued that they could better understand people's psychological disorders, conflicts, and desires by interpreting their dreams, and thereby better help them on the pathway to mental health.

The psychiatric approach to psychological disorders often involves the prescription of drugs. These may quantitatively and qualitatively affect sleep, such as by suppressing REM, causing lucid or morbid dreaming; or unanticipated sleep, a symptom of narcolepsy. For example, as experimentally found, compared with baseline, fluoxetine (the serotonin-increasing active substance in an antidepressant widely prescribed in the 1990s and early 2000s) statistically and significantly diminished people's ability to recall their dreams. Moreover, the dreams that were remembered were less vivid and detailed. Thus the drug was considered to act as an REM sleep suppressor. Although REM's functions are partly unknown, they are likely important. Therefore efforts were and are being made to avoid this side effect. Apparently dreams still keep their secrets, from dreamers and scientists alike.

Sources: Adapted from E. Aserinsky, The Discovery of REM Sleep. *Copyright 1996 Taylor & Francis Group.*

Question 23

In the passage it is remarked that EEGs were used in the first sleep studies. What is this technique, how could it have helped in concluding that sleep was not a "passive phenomenon," and which of the figures below would most likely illustrate the results obtained by this technique during REM sleep?

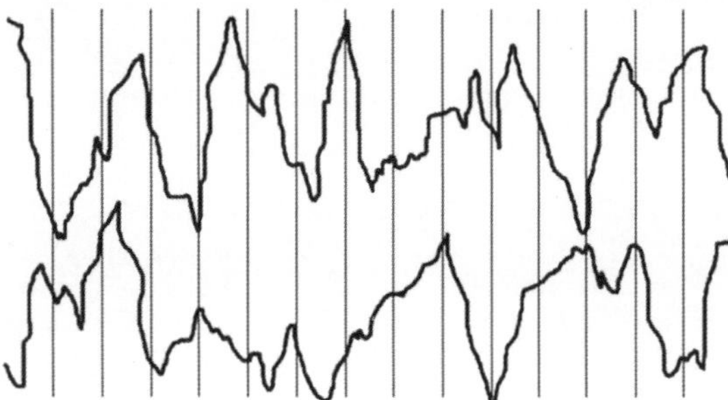

Figure 1 Example of sleep activity measurements

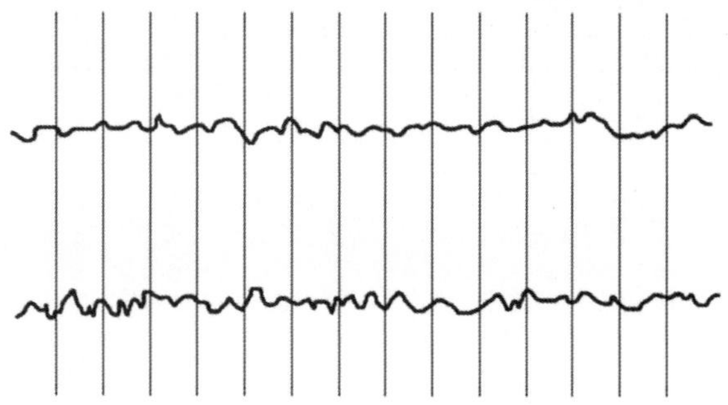

Figure 2 Example of sleep activity measurements

- ○ **A.** The EEG registers electromagnetic brain activity, hence indicating whether the brain is passive or active during the assessment period. Figure 1 most probably illustrates measurements obtained during REM.
- ○ **B.** The EEG registers electrical brain activity, hence indicating whether the brain is passive or active during the assessment period. Figure 1 most probably illustrates measurements obtained during REM.
- ○ **C.** The EEG registers electromagnetic brain activity, hence indicating whether the brain is passive or active during the assessment period. Figure 2 most probably illustrates measurements obtained during REM.
- ○ **D.** The EEG registers electrical brain activity, hence indicating whether the brain is passive or active during the assessment period. Figure 2 most probably illustrates measurements obtained during REM.

Question 24

Which of the following techniques or events were regarded as useful for the study of the id at the time when biologists made the discovery of NEM?

- ○ **A.** Diary writing, agenda setting, and pro–con analysis
- ○ **B.** Meditation, sense of humor, and fantasies
- ○ **C.** Hypnosis, slips of the tongue, and free association
- ○ **D.** fMRIs, EEGs, and MEGs

Question 25

Although the main functions of each sleep stage in humans are not precisely known, evidence is being gathered in support of several hypotheses. Which of the following does NOT accurately describe one of these hypotheses?

- ○ **A.** REM consolidates, at a synaptic level, memories created during that day's awake period. NREM stage 2 consolidates memories at a system level.
- ○ **B.** NREM stages 1, 2, 3, and 4 represent a continuum of increasing depth. Their specific duration varies during the course of sleep, throughout the lifespan, and across genders.
- ○ **C.** Wakefulness (process C) is regulated by circadian rhythms. It progressively alternates with sleep (process S), which is a homeostatic drive.
- ○ **D.** Metabolic stress triggers degenerative processes. Sleep counteracts such effects.

Question 26

Which of the following statistical procedures would best test whether experimental and control group differences were statistically significant, in a week-long study that involved studying before sleep and recalling material the next morning in a point-graded survey, and which subjected the experimental group to week-long REM sleep deprivation?

- ○ **A.** Descriptive statistics
- ○ **B.** Spearman correlations
- ○ **C.** Linear regression
- ○ **D.** Mixed ANOVA

Question 27

Which of the following phenomena best describes a possible drug side-effect that consists of starting to become aware that one is dreaming while the dreaming is taking place?

- ○ **A.** Lucid dreaming
- ○ **B.** Latent content dreaming
- ○ **C.** Paradoxical sleep
- ○ **D.** Prodromal dreaming

The following questions are NOT based on a descriptive passage (Questions 28–31).

Question 28

In which of Jean Piaget's cognitive development stages would children be, if, given two pieces of clay of equal mass, a block and a flattened disk, they said that the flattened disk had more clay and was heavier because it looked bigger?

- ○ **A.** The concrete operational stage
- ○ **B.** The sensorimotor stage
- ○ **C.** The formal operational stage
- ○ **D.** The preoperational stage

Question 29

Which parts of the brain are the LEAST critically important when people engage in the process of writing something by hand on a piece of paper?

- ○ **A.** The visual cortex and the left angular gyrus
- ○ **B.** The cingulate cortex
- ○ **C.** Broca's and Wernicke's areas
- ○ **D.** The parietal lobe

Question 30

The sensory system in charge of spatial orientation, and formed by the utricle, saccule, and three semicircular canals, is called the:

- ○ **A.** vestibular system.
- ○ **B.** auditory system.
- ○ **C.** otolithic system.
- ○ **D.** cochlear system.

Question 31

Emile Durkheim, a sociologist of the functionalist school, employed the term "anomie" to explain, among other things, the levels of suicide and crime in a society. In which of the examples below will a state of anomie NOT likely be felt?

- ○ **A.** After a revolution in which a new government seizes power
- ○ **B.** During an economic depression, such as after the Wall Street crash of 1929
- ○ **C.** In North Korea, a country whose citizens' thoughts and actions are greatly controlled by the government
- ○ **D.** In modern-day New York, a place that is a "melting pot" of thousands of contrasting cultures and lifestyles

Note: This page is left blank so that the passage would be visible without turning pages while assessing the passage-based questions.

Passage 6 (Questions 32–35)

Attention-deficit/hyperactivity disorder (ADHD) is a psychiatric diagnosis more frequently attributed to children than to adults, with prevalence set between 3% and 7% for the younger population. It is characterized by impulsivity, hyperactivity, and sustained attention deficits. Children seem unable to concentrate for moderately long periods of time on the same task. Consequently they have difficulties in traditional learning settings where they are asked to sit still and remain quiet, and are often regarded as having social and conduct problems. These traits are endophenotypes, that is, diagnostically important phenotypes thought to be caused by specific genes.

In recent years, based on Alan Baddeley and Graham Hitch's working memory model, some studies have proposed working memory deficits as a potential endophenotype of the disorder. Evidence has been gathered to support this proposition. For example, Lisa Kasper and colleagues' 2012 meta-analysis assessed studies that included 8- to 16-year-olds, a control and an ADHD group, reported phonological and/or visuospatial scores separately, and provided sufficient data for adequately calculating between-group effect sizes of working memory performance. They also inspected the effects of the following potential moderators: age, gender, trials per set (low vs. high number of testing trials and thus the amount of strain placed on working memory), performance metric (total correct trials vs. stimuli correct), response modality (recognition vs. recall), and central executive demand (low vs. high).

For 29 visuospatial studies, there was a significantly large between-group effect size of 0.74 (95% confidence interval = 0.53 to 0.95). That is, children with ADHD, in comparison with controls, performed worse on tasks involving visual and/or spatial information. As for phonological tasks, as assessed by 34 studies, the significantly large between-group effect size was 0.69 (95% confidence interval = 0.53 to 0.84). In other words, children diagnosed with ADHD also performed worse than controls on tasks involving auditory verbal information. The results regarding the investigated moderators' effects, calculated via meta-regression analysis, are specified in Table 1. It illustrates which variables more significantly interfered with each group performance. Overall this study, along with several others that yielded similar conclusions, supports the inclusion of working memory deficits among ADHD behavioral symptoms—though not necessarily among the traits constitutive of an endophenotype of this diagnosis.

Table 1 Weighted Regression Model for Phonological (PH) and Visuospatial (VS) Working Memory Component Moderators

	PH			VS		
	χ^2	df	p	χ^2	df	P
Regression	24.99	6	0.001	27.11	6	0.001
Residual	25.76	24	0.366	22.32	22	0.441
R	0.49			0.55		
Moderators	β	Z	P	β	Z	P
Constant	0.71			0.95		
Percent female	−0.3	−1.99	0.046*	−0.558	−3.72	0.001***
Age	−0.233	−1.52	0.127	−0.191	−1.20	0.229
Trials per set size	0.477	2.27	0.023*	0.390	2.26	0.024*
Response modality	0.581	2.71	0.007**	0.689	3.63	0.001***
Performance metric	0.245	1.62	0.105	−0.055	−0.361	0.719
Central executive demand	0.320	2.09	0.037*	0.377	2.29	0.022*

Notes:
χ^2: chi-square value; df: degrees of freedom; p: significance levels, or likelihood of randomly obtaining a result at least as extreme as that observed, even when the null hypothesis is true, and * $p<0.5$; ** $p<0.1$; *** $p<0.01$;
R^2: variance accounted for by the model; β: standardized beta weight, or the standard deviation change in the dependent variable per each standard deviation change in the independent variable; Z: regression coefficient divided by its standard error.

Source: Adapted from L.J. Kasper, R.M. Alderson, & K.L. Hudec, "Moderators of Working Memory Deficits in Children with Attention-deficit/Hyperactivity Disorder (ADHD): A Meta-analytic Review." Copyright 2012 Elsevier Ltd.

Question 32

The central executive, from Alan Baddeley and Graham Hitch's working memory model, included in the study described in the passage, is thought to operate by:

- ○ **A.** determining which memory is relevant for storing incoming information: phonological memory for auditory, visuospatial memory for visual and spatial, episodic memory for events, and semantic memory for meanings.
- ○ **B.** retrieving needed information from long-term memory and directing it, along with incoming sensory input, to the appropriate subcomponent under its control (phonological loop and visuospatial sketchpad).
- ○ **C.** controlling the flow of information between its subsidiary memories: the phonological, visuospatial, episodic, semantic, and procedural.
- ○ **D.** managing attentional resources, dividing and focusing attention when needed, and replacing irrelevant with relevant information in its subsidiary temporary storage systems.

Question 33

Which of the following conclusions is supported by the findings presented in Table 1?

- ○ **A.** Younger children diagnosed with ADHD performed significantly worse than older children with the same diagnosis on phonological and visuospatial tasks.
- ○ **B.** Children from the feminine gender diagnosed with ADHD performed significantly worse than children with the same diagnosis from the masculine gender on phonological tasks, and extremely significantly worse on visuospatial tasks.
- ○ **C.** Children with ADHD performed significantly or extremely significantly worse on phonological and visuospatial tasks involving greater cognitive demand, as assessed via trials per set and response modality.
- ○ **D.** Performance metric was the most relevant moderator for both phonological and visuospatial tasks.

Question 34

Which of the following psychological functions would be the LEAST necessary for a one minute long task involving counting out loud the number of people going up (vs. going down) a flight of stairs in jeans, amidst people going up and down the stairs in a variety of outfits?

- ○ **A.** Episodic memory
- ○ **B.** Selective attention
- ○ **C.** Working memory
- ○ **D.** Arithmetic

Question 35

Which of the following sentences concerning memory-related biological processes is INCORRECT?

- ○ **A.** The hippocampus and the medial temporal lobe are thought to be more important to the formation of declarative (vs. procedural) memories.
- ○ **B.** The cerebellum and the striatum are more important for the formation of procedural (vs. declarative) memories.
- ○ **C.** Short-term memory formation involves the synthesis of new protein via the intervention of cytoplasmic and nuclear molecules, whereas long-term memory does not.
- ○ **D.** Although it does not apply to every type of long-term potentiation, the maxim is that "cells that fire together wire together."

Passage 7 (Questions 36–40)

The shiny carrot and the lazy donkey are often used as symbols of motivation. There is hope in this metaphor, as the one who at first seems unwilling manages to carry on with his duties with a little incentive. Nevertheless, motivation is not always or necessarily a fruit of laziness or generated extrinsically. As often happens with symbols, the truth of motivation is not literally represented by this image..

Avolition, or lack of motivation, is a symptom of several psychiatric diagnoses, such as depression and schizophrenia (though absent from the *Diagnostic and Statistical Manual of Mental Disorders, 5th Edition, DSM-5*, for depression). In these cases, therapists often seek to find what is blocking individuals from wanting to act and live fully and how such desire might be gained—in other words, what their "carrot" may be.

There are several theories as to what motivates individuals, each including motivators of all sorts, along with consequences, and implications. This research diversity and interest partly results from the general consensual acknowledgment that motivation is critical for many different research areas and interferes with a multitude of biopsychosocial aspects, from job performance to well-being.

For instance, David McClelland's acquired needs theory applies to goal accomplishment and distinguishes three main types of motivation: achievement, authority or power (personal or institutional), and affiliation. Each individual is usually mainly driven by a single type of motivation, although the other two types may also influence him or her at times. This approach emphasizes interindividual variability. Yet for some scholars, this set of motivations is incomplete and/or fails to highlight universal motivations, such as thirst and death. Indeed, not everyone is motivated by achievement, power, and affiliation—for example, the clinically depressed.

Even so, this approach has generated extensive research about goal achievement. A recent study followed up evidence suggesting that goal commitment and goal progress affected motivation. The designed task involved charitable fundraising. The sample included both regular donors, added to the "hot list" due to their past record of high commitment to charitable causes, and participants whose commitment to charitable causes was uncertain because they merely manifested their interest in compassion and had never contributed to a fundraiser. These were included in the "cold list." Both these groups received one of two types of letters about the campaign, one emphasizing how much had been already accomplished in terms of fundraising (To-Date, or information about the present), and another emphasizing how much was still required to accomplish the campaign's aim (To-Go, or information about the future). These operationalized goal achievement progress. Thus, the research had a 2x2 between-subjects design, and its results are illustrated in Figure 1. The analysis of variance (ANOVA) results were $F(1, 242)=10.47$, $p \leq 0.01$.

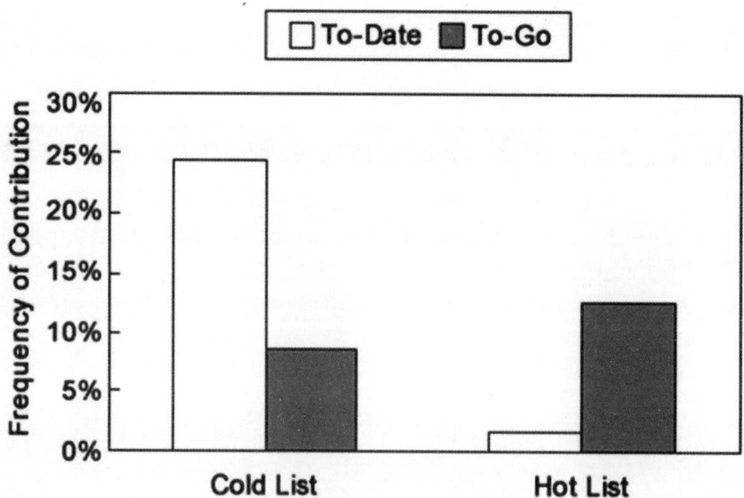

Figure 1 Charity contributions per commitment certainty (cold vs. hot list) and type of information (To-Go vs. To-Date)

Source: Adapted from M. Koo & A. Fishbach, "Dynamics of Self-Regulation: How (Un)accomplished Goal Actions Affect Motivation." Copyright 2008 Journal of Personality and Social Psychology.

Question 36

Which of the following statistical conclusions is supported by Figure 1 and the ANOVA results described in the passage?

- ○ **A.** Both goal commitment and goal achievement progress independently helped to predict with high statistical significance the participants' contributions.
- ○ **B.** There was a highly significant statistical interaction between goal commitment and goal achievement progress, both factors affecting participants' contributions.
- ○ **C.** Both goal commitment and goal achievement progress were statistically highly significant and negatively correlated with participants' contributions.
- ○ **D.** There was a highly significant statistical difference between the effects of the two types of goal achievement progress.

Question 37

In the passage, the carrot was described as an extrinsic motivator. Which of the following type of motivator is usually paired with it as its opposite, and how could it be best defined?

- ○ **A.** Internal motivators are those that are determined by internal processes and instinctive needs, such as one's emotional state and hunger.
- ○ **B.** Innate motivators are those that are determined by genetic predispositions, such as one's extraversion or introversion.
- ○ **C.** Intrinsic motivators are those that are determined by one's own sense of accomplishment and pleasure, such as enjoying playing a game.
- ○ **D.** Biopsychosocial motivators are those that are determined by biological, psychological, or social factors, such as the impact of relationships with peers on one's well-being and mental health.

Question 38

In the passage, avolition is said to be a symptom of depression. Yet it was not adopted by the DSM-5 for differential diagnostic purposes. Which of the following core symptoms were actually included in the DSM-5 for the diagnosis of a typical major depressive episode?

- ○ **A.** Depressed humor, hallucinations, insomnia, occasional panic attacks, and loss of interest
- ○ **B.** Anhedonia, feelings of worthlessness, feelings of sadness, weight loss, and insomnia
- ○ **C.** Psychomotor agitation, paranoia, isolation, aggressiveness, and incoherent speech
- ○ **D.** Motor retardation, hypersomnia, weight gain, lethargy, and refusal to speak

Question 39

A single, long-term unemployed man in his 30s seeks work daily so as to pay for lodging and food but could not care less about his singleness. How would Abraham Maslow's hierarchy of needs theory of motivation explain his unwillingness to find a partner?

- ○ **A.** Such willingness cannot develop until his more basic physiological needs have been satisfied.
- ○ **B.** His sexual drive has a lower intensity than other more pressing primary drives, such as hunger.
- ○ **C.** The relational and sexual drive has been sublimated into the more culturally and socially elevated willingness to work.
- ○ **D.** Such unwillingness is the result of attributional processes that deem his professional situation to be the only factor responsible for his discontentment.

Question 40

The passage remarks that "goal commitment and goal progress" affect motivation. Which of the following sentences best describes how motivation was operationalized in the research design of the study in the passage?

- ○ **A.** Motivation was the dependent variable.
- ○ **B.** Motivation was the moderator.
- ○ **C.** Motivation was a sample selection requisite.
- ○ **D.** Motivation was not operationalized.

Passage 8 (Questions 41–44)

The way one expresses emotions and the way one expresses organizationally desired emotions (emotional labor) are two core aspects of emotional expression in organizational environments. These concepts are not necessarily always concordant with each other and are known to affect satisfaction, performance, and professional relationships.

For example, in the medical profession, emotions are often supposed to remain tacit and invisible. Medical staff members are encouraged to modulate their emotions in front of patients and other staff even when confronted with emotionally intense and challenging situations such as the diagnosis of a fatal disease. Tension can arise when the emotions that the professional feels are in constant conflict with the organizationally desired emotions that must be displayed. This tension is called emotional dissonance. Ways of coping with this dissonance include surface acting and deep acting. Emotional contagion (or the spreading of emotions between people and groups) further complicates this task. Emotions are highly dependent on surroundings and relationships and therefore difficult to control.

Contagion has been shown to occur in different experimental settings that involve face-to-face and even audio and visual exposure to emotional stimuli. To better understand what happened in an online social network with regard to emotional reactions such as emotional contagion, a controversial study manipulated the newsfeed of different Facebook users without their knowledge. One group received a newsfeed that had been filtered to reduce between 10% and 90% of the positive emotional content posted by others. Another group received a newsfeed that had been filtered to reduce 10% and 90% of the negative content of others' posts. The influence of those experimental conditions was measured with a count of the negative or positive posts by the users following the stimulus. The sample of the study consisted of 155000 participants per condition, chosen via a random selection of all users who accessed Facebook's functions in English. The experiment found statistically significant results, although a very small effect size.

Sources: Adapted from A. Kramer, J. Guillory, & J. Hancock, "Experimental Evidence of Massive-scale Emotional Contagion through Social Networks." Copyright 2014 Proceedings of the National Academy of Sciences.

Question 41

The Facebook study was expanded via the recruitment of users residing in Asian countries and choosing Asian language settings, and users residing in Western countries and choosing English language settings. According to current empirical evidence related to cultural differences in emotional expression, what should researchers expect to observe in this new study?

- ○ **A.** The Asian sample would be less likely to express personal emotions explicitly.
- ○ **B.** The high-context sample and the low-context sample would be equally likely to express personal emotions explicitly.
- ○ **C.** The Asian sample would be more likely to express two specific personal emotions: pride and anger.
- ○ **D.** The individualist culture would be more likely to express two specific personal emotions: friendliness and shame.

Question 42

Which of following concepts associated with the dramaturgical approach could be a form of emotional labor as defined in the passage?

- ○ **A.** Surface acting
- ○ **B.** Backstage work
- ○ **C.** Self-handicapping
- ○ **D.** Self-verification

Question 43

A waiter in a restaurant wants to greet his customers in a way that is perceived as socially accommodating. In order to convincingly display this and leave a positive, welcoming first impression on people of different cultures, the waiter would likely have to pay the LEAST attention to his:

- ○ **A.** Kinesics
- ○ **B.** Paralinguistics
- ○ **C.** Verbalizations
- ○ **D.** Proxemics

Question 44

Which of the items below could be included in an instrument seeking to measure, in an ordinal scale, which and how organizational factors influenced employees' emotional labor experiences (question: answer option, respectively)?

- ○ **A.** Do you receive sufficient support through your supervisors in your workplace?: Yes/no
- ○ **B.** Please describe how well you feel supported in your hospital: Field for open answers provided
- ○ **C.** The person who supports me most in my daily work is: Head of department/supervisor/manager/administrator/technician
- ○ **D.** I receive the support that I need in order to perform well in my workplace: Strongly agree/agree/neutral/disagree/strongly disagree

---

The following questions are NOT based on a descriptive passage (Questions 45–48).

Question 45

Researchers want to conduct a study to predict who is going to be the next president among seven candidates for a country with the same rules for voting than the United States. Which of the following methods would be the most suitable, reliable, and commonly used for this purpose?

- ○ **A.** Focus groups
- ○ **B.** Qualitative research design
- ○ **C.** Systematic literature review
- ○ **D.** Opinion poll

Question 46

Stanley Milgram's controversial, famous, standardized and replicated lab experiment was introduced to participants as a study of learning. However, it was actually studying whether people would obey authority even if it meant harming others. Participants were informed of this deception at the end of the experiment. According to this study's description, which of the following criticisms could be made?

- ○ **A.** Lack of a debrief
- ○ **B.** Lack of ecological validity
- ○ **C.** Lack of an operational definition of obedience
- ○ **D.** Lack of reliability

Question 47

Which of the theories below best describes the feeling of unease someone of the Muslim religion may feel if they were to fail to follow the dietary restrictions imposed by Islam at a restaurant during a social outing with friends who do not adhere to the same beliefs?

- ○ **A.** Groupthink
- ○ **B.** Protest consumption
- ○ **C.** Peer pressure
- ○ **D.** Cognitive dissonance

Question 48

Pierre Bourdieu suggests that middle-class children have "cultural capital," which refers to a set of symbolic assets that can convey privilege in society, such as tastes, knowledge, and skills. With this comes a "set of ingrained dispositions that dictate cultural behavior." Which of the concepts below is the name that Bourdieu gives to this?

- O **A.** Anomie
- O **B.** Praxis
- O **C.** Habitus
- O **D.** Ascribed status

Passage 9 (Questions 49–52)

Social inequality has long existed. The destruction of Europe after World War II served as a platform for many colonies to develop liberation movements. As years progressed, social liberation movements became more active, principally in the so-called developing and Third World countries. The idea of revolution began to grow mainly among the people of Latin America.

With the triumph of the Cuban Revolution in 1959, the idea of social revolts to change the status quo was extrapolated to other countries, and guerrilla movements saw their biggest expansion ever, principally in colonies in Africa and Southeast Asia. The aim was to redistribute the means of production to the communities. These ideas were in radical contrast to capitalist processes, which usually allowed only specific members of society to accumulate wealth. Simultaneously, a distinct way of thinking sociologically was born with the 1959 book entitled *The Sociological Imagination*. It established a radical new method of investigating societies that reconciled the study of individuals with that of society.

With some exceptions, such as Vietnam, the radical movements failed across the world and were then subject to the international credit institutions' instructions that introduced the rule of privately owned companies in the state. It has been argued that the reform package promoted for developing countries by the International Monetary Fund (IMF) and World Bank led to greater global inequality in the long run.

In health, a change was also brought about in 1948, when the World Health Organization (WHO) broadened the definition of health from exclusively absence of disease to a vaster area of issues involving physical, emotional, and psychic aspects. This change in perspective prevailed. For example, in 2015, WHO sent out a fact sheet stating that more than 50% of children's deaths under the age of 5 worldwide occurred from preventable or easily treated causes associated with social inequality in access to public health, such as lower income, which is highly correlated with higher rates of preventable deaths.

Source: Adapted from World Health Organization, "Children: Reducing Mortality." Copyright 2016 http://www.who.int.

Question 49

The author of the book cited in the passage, and one of the main founders of an influent macrosociology school, was:

- O **A.** C. Wright Mills
- O **B.** Robert Nisbet
- O **C.** Max Weber
- O **D.** Erving Goffman

Question 50

Stanley Milgram illustrated how individuals perform the most harmful acts when coerced or simply solicited by an authority figure, even when they originally hold pacifist values. What was the name given to this phenomenon?

- ○ **A.** Peer pressure
- ○ **B.** Deindividuation
- ○ **C.** Conformity
- ○ **D.** Obedience

Question 51

Evelyn Kitagawa and Philip Hauser conducted a study in 1973 and used findings to illustrate how life expectancy of 25-year-old US women linearly and positively correlated with education level. Which of the following Figures most likely illustrates the found relationship pattern?

○ **A.**

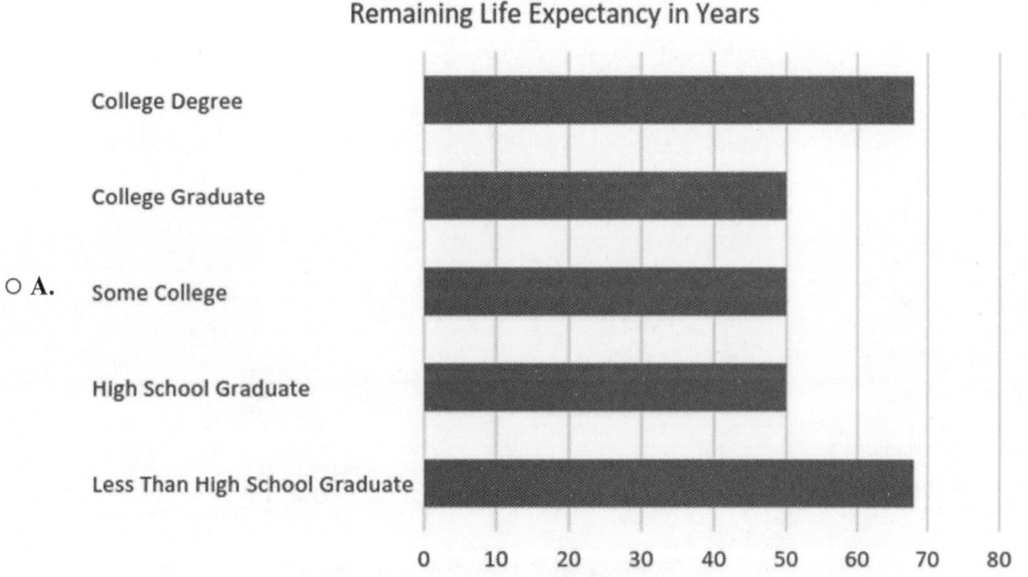

Figure 1 Remaining life expectancy per education level in 25-year-old women, USA, 2005

○ **B.**

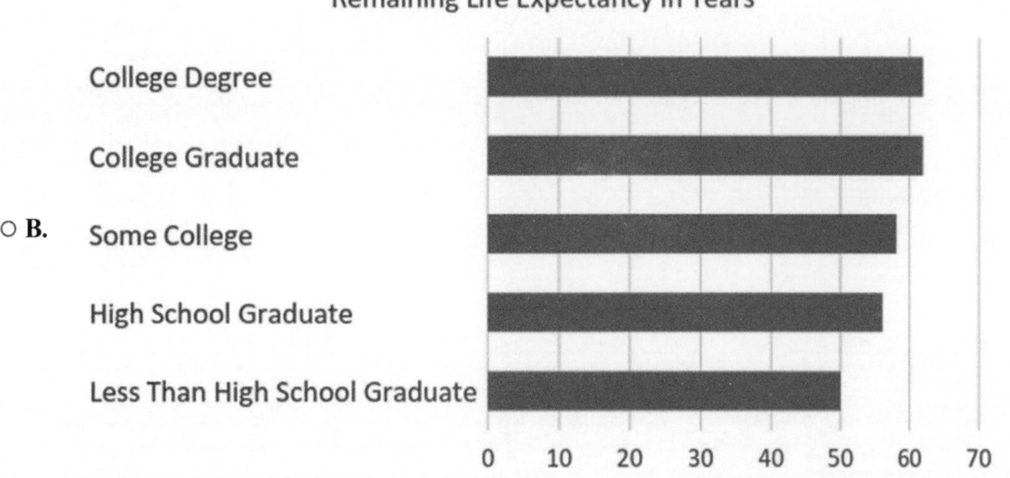

Figure 2 Remaining life expectancy per education level in 25-year-old women, USA, 2005

○ C.

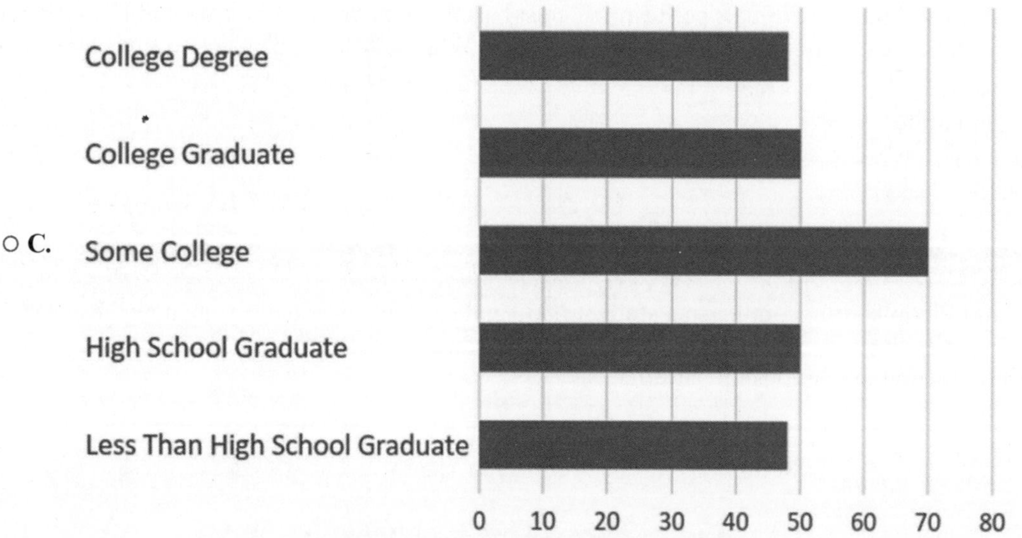

Figure 3 Remaining life expectancy per education level in 25-year-old women, USA, 2005

○ D.

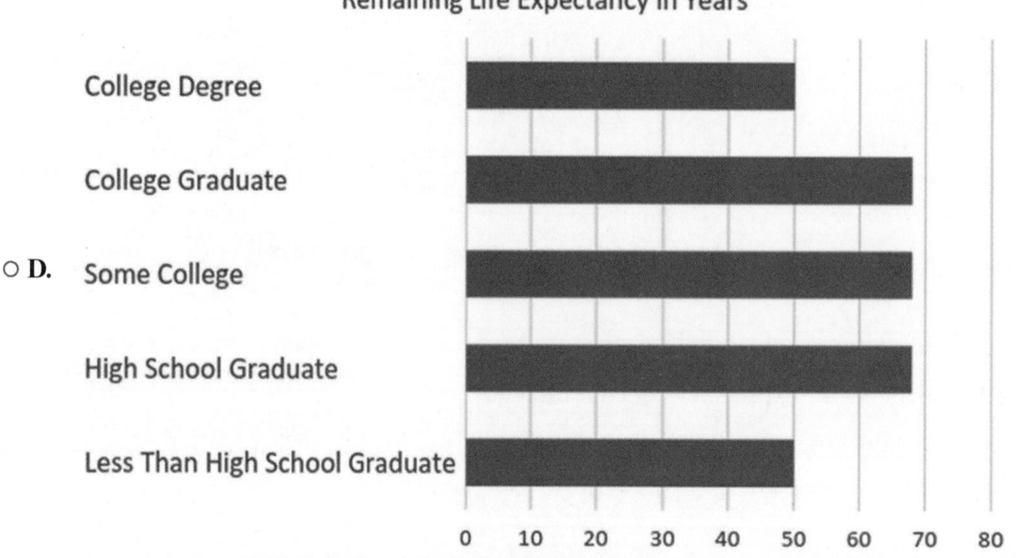

Figure 4 Remaining life expectancy per education level in 25-year-old women, USA, 2005

Question 52

Figure 1 below represents the global distribution of wealth per quintile of population, where the first quintile includes the 20% of the population with the lowest-income and the fifth quintile includes the richest 20% of the population. Which of the following observations most accurately describes the illustrated data?

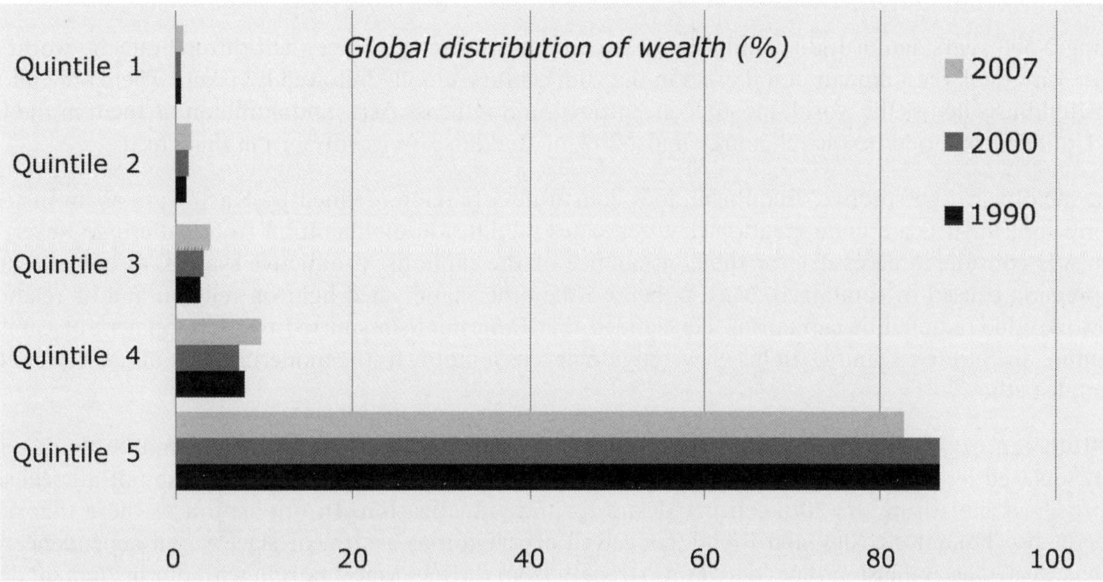

Figure 1 Percentage of world's wealth per quintile; 1–5 are the poorest to richest quintiles

Source: Adapted from I. Ortiz & M. Cummins, "Global Inequality: Beyond the Bottom Billion." Copyright 2014 www.unicef.org.

○ **A.** The graph reveals no data about distribution of wealth.
○ **B.** The richest 20% of the world's population concentrates more than 80% of the wealth.
○ **C.** The richest quintile concentrates less than 5% of the world's wealth.
○ **D.** Wealth is similarly distributed across quintiles.

Passage 10 (Questions 53–56)

Buddhism is most commonly referred to as a philosophy rather than a religion due to the lack of a celestial god to look up to at its center. Instead, it is based upon the teachings of Siddhartha Gautama, also known as Buddha, the Enlightened. According to the definition given by practicums, it is an ascesis, understood as the building of a path leading toward perfection.

Emerging 2,500 years ago in India, Buddhism has continuously spread since then throughout the world, being the creed with the largest growth in followers in the 20th century, closely followed by Islam. There are almost 400 million Buddhists across the world, mostly concentrated in Southeast Asia, and a million of them in the United States. Unlike most monotheistic religions, almost 30% of Buddhists were not born in that creed.

From a sociological perspective, Buddhism does constitute a religion, defined by Karl Marx as an instrument of oppression, for it is a human creation that generates the illusion of liberation from suffering. Nevertheless, religion was considered necessary for the continuance of the capitalist productive system, as compensates for the oppression caused by capitalism. Max Weber, on the other hand, shed light on religion and its relationship to the work ethic required by capitalism. He claimed that Protestantism spurred the development of capitalism, constituting an "elective affinity." In his view, religion acts as a motor to the modernization of society built upon the capitalist ethos.

In the 19th century, Émile Durkheim believed that the social influence of religion would be weakened and possibly replaced by organic solidarity, while in 1908 Georg Simmel looked upon the creation of a laical society. Both processes constitute the 20th-century desire for individualization. In opposition to these theories, the founder of psychoanalysis, Sigmund Freud, conceived of religion as a form of slavery and dependence. In his work, it is treated as an illusion that "derives its strength from the fact that it falls in with our instinctual desires." In this sense, it is a natural "attempt to get control of our sensory world" similar to childhood neurosis.

Source: Adapted from S. Freud, New Introductory Lectures on Psychoanalysis. *Copyright 1933 W.W. Norton & Co.*

Question 53

What does Émile Durkheim mean by "organic solidarity"?

- ○ **A.** Social revolution
- ○ **B.** A complementary form of social bond
- ○ **C.** Alienation
- ○ **D.** An ideal type of capitalist society

Question 54

Which of the following is NOT one of the three ideal types of religious activity recognized by Max Weber in *Economy and Society* (1922)?

- ○ **A.** World-flying mysticism
- ○ **B.** World-rejecting asceticism
- ○ **C.** Inner-world asceticism
- ○ **D.** Calvinist Protestantism

Question 55

The famous differentiation between religion and religiosity is most often attributed to:

- ○ **A.** Karl Marx.
- ○ **B.** Georg Simmel.
- ○ **C.** Auguste Comte.
- ○ **D.** Herbert Spencer.

Question 56

Which are the parts of the psychic apparatus according to Freudian psychoanalysis?

- O **A.** Neurosis and psychosis
- O **B.** Schizophrenia and normality
- O **C.** Id, ego, and superego
- O **D.** Ego and alter ego

The following questions are NOT based on a descriptive passage (Questions 57–59).

Question 57

From the attachment theory perspective, which of the concepts below best describes the case of an abused woman, who spent most of her childhood in isolation, mostly tied to a chair, and was never allowed to form an attachment to anyone?

- O **A.** Deprivation
- O **B.** Privation
- O **C.** Isolation
- O **D.** Affectionless psychopathy

Question 58

What social norm is supported by experimental findings showing that the more participants liked their "partners" (whom they believed to be a participant but actually was a researcher), the more likely they were to accept to buy them cake, and principally when they had previously been offered free juice from them?

- O **A.** Reciprocity
- O **B.** Door-in-the-face
- O **C.** Compliance
- O **D.** Altruism

Question 59

The three elements of social identity theory are:

- O **A.** identification, comparison, and group focus.
- O **B.** categorization, identification, and comparison.
- O **C.** categorization, comparison, and group focus.
- O **D.** identification, categorization, and group focus.

Full-length MCAT Practice Test GS-5

Periodic Table of the Elements

You may consult this page anytime you wish during the following exam sections:

- Section I: Chemical and Physical Foundations of Biological Systems
- Section III: Biological and Biochemical Foundations of Living Systems

On the real exam, the computer-based shortcut to see the periodic table is Alt + T.

1 **H** 1.0																	2 **He** 4.0
3 **Li** 6.9	4 **Be** 9.0											5 **B** 10.8	6 **C** 12.0	7 **N** 14.0	8 **O** 16.0	9 **F** 19.0	10 **Ne** 20.2
11 **Na** 23.0	12 **Mg** 24.3											13 **Al** 27.0	14 **Si** 28.1	15 **P** 31.0	16 **S** 32.1	17 **Cl** 35.5	18 **Ar** 39.9
19 **K** 39.1	20 **Ca** 40.1	21 **Sc** 45.0	22 **Ti** 47.9	23 **V** 50.9	24 **Cr** 52.0	25 **Mn** 54.9	26 **Fe** 55.8	27 **Co** 58.9	28 **Ni** 58.7	29 **Cu** 63.5	30 **Zn** 65.4	31 **Ga** 69.7	32 **Ge** 72.6	33 **As** 74.9	34 **Se** 79.0	35 **Br** 79.9	36 **Kr** 83.8
37 **Rb** 85.5	38 **Sr** 87.6	39 **Y** 88.9	40 **Zr** 91.2	41 **Nb** 92.9	42 **Mo** 95.9	43 **Tc** (98)	44 **Ru** 101.1	45 **Rh** 102.9	46 **Pd** 106.4	47 **Ag** 107.9	48 **Cd** 112.4	49 **In** 114.8	50 **Sn** 118.7	51 **Sb** 121.8	52 **Te** 127.6	53 **I** 126.9	54 **Xe** 131.3
55 **Cs** 132.9	56 **Ba** 137.3	57 **La*** 138.9	72 **Hf** 178.5	73 **Ta** 180.9	74 **W** 183.9	75 **Re** 186.2	76 **Os** 190.2	77 **Ir** 192.2	78 **Pt** 195.1	79 **Au** 197.0	80 **Hg** 200.6	81 **Tl** 204.4	82 **Pb** 207.2	83 **Bi** 209.0	84 **Po** (209)	85 **At** (210)	86 **Rn** (222)
87 **Fr** (223)	88 **Ra** (226)	89 **Ac**** (227)	104 **Unq**** (261)	105 **Unp** (262)	106 **Unh** (263)	107 **Uns** (262)	108 **Uno** (265)	109 **Une** (267)									
			*	58 **Ce** 140.1	59 **Pr** 140.9	60 **Nd** 144.2	61 **Pm** (145)	62 **Sm** 150.4	63 **Eu** 152.0	64 **Gd** 157.3	65 **Tb** 158.9	66 **Dy** 162.5	67 **Ho** 164.9	68 **Er** 167.3	69 **Tm** 168.9	70 **Yb** 173.0	71 **Lu** 175.0
			**	90 **Th** 232.0	91 **Pa** (231)	92 **U** 238.0	93 **Np** (237)	94 **Pu** (244)	95 **Am** (243)	96 **Cm** (247)	97 **Bk** (247)	98 **Cf** (251)	99 **Es** (252)	100 **Fm** (257)	101 **Md** (258)	102 **No** (259)	103 **Lr** (260)

CANDIDATE'S NAME ______________________________

RAW SCORE AND SCALED SCORE ______________________

GS-5
Mock Exam 5 of 7
Solutions at MCAT-prep.com

GS-5 Section I: Chemical and Physical Foundations of Biological Systems

Questions: 1-59
Time: 95 minutes

INSTRUCTIONS: Of all the questions on this test, most are organized into groups preceded by a passage. After evaluating the passage, select the best answer to each question in the group. Fifteen questions are independent of any descriptive passage or each other. Similarly, select the best answer to these questions. If you are unsure of an answer, eliminate the alternatives that you know to be incorrect and select an answer from the remaining alternatives. To indicate your selection, use a pencil to blacken the corresponding circle next to the answer choice and/or you can use the answer document at the back of this book. No marks are deducted for wrong answers.

The computer-based real MCAT has an on-screen highlighter function and ~~STRIKEOUT~~ function. These tools help to spotlight text or assist in the process of elimination. You may use a yellow highlighter for this paper-based exam and/or a pen (or preferably a pencil to make it easier should you change your mind) to mark text. At the time of publishing, both highlighting and strikeout functions can be used for passages, questions and answer choices. You can also flag a question to review later should time remain.

For the real exam, you will be provided with a dry erase board which is a white laminated noteboard booklet accompanied by a fine point marker. The noteboard includes 9 graph-lined pages for you to write though you cannot erase. You can simulate the experience with a fine point marker on a noteboard or with 8” x 14” plain graph paper.

You may consult the periodic table at any point during the science subtests.

Please note: For the real MCAT, a small number of field-tested questions will remain unscored.

This practice test has been designed exclusively to test knowledge and thinking skills. This exam may contain hypothetical statements and/or express controversial ideas. Statements contained herein do not necessarily reflect the policy, position, or view of RuveneCo Inc. or MCAT-prep.com.

START EXAM ONLY WHEN TIMER IS READY.

Passage 1 (Questions 1–6)

Terpenes are major biosynthetic building blocks that are multiple units of the 5-carbon hydrocarbon isoprene (IUPAC name: 2-methyl-1,3-butadiene). Two isoprene units in a structure make a monoterpene, and four isoprene units make a diterpene. Sesqui- and sester- are prefixes indicating one and a half and two and a half, respectively. In other words, a sesterterpene contains 25 carbon atoms.

β-Carotene ('provitamin A') is an important natural terpene. It is a strongly colored red-orange pigment abundant in plants and fruits. Carotene is the substance in carrots, pumpkins and sweet potatoes that colors them orange and is the most common form of carotene in plants.

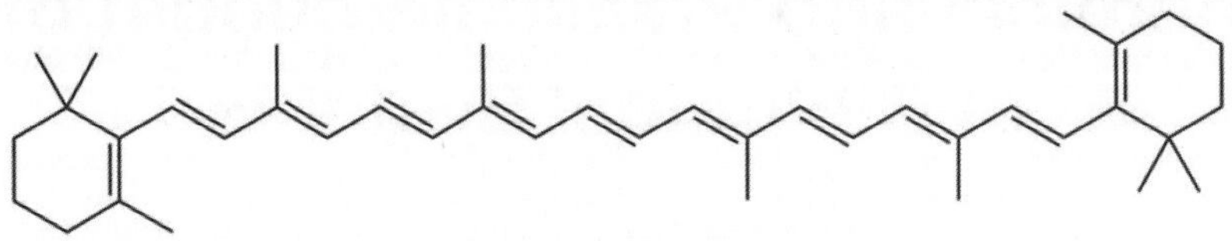

β-Carotene ($C_{40}H_{56}$)

In nature, β-carotene is a precursor (inactive form) to vitamin A, which unlike β-carotene, is yellow-colored. Vitamin A (retinol) has multiple functions: it is important for growth and development, for the maintenance of the immune system and good vision.

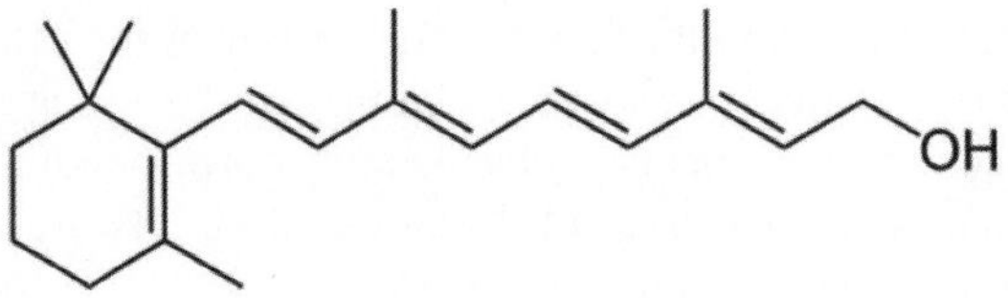

OH

Vitamin A (retinol; $C_{20}H_{30}O$)

Limonene is a cyclic terpene found in relatively high concentrations in citrus fruits.

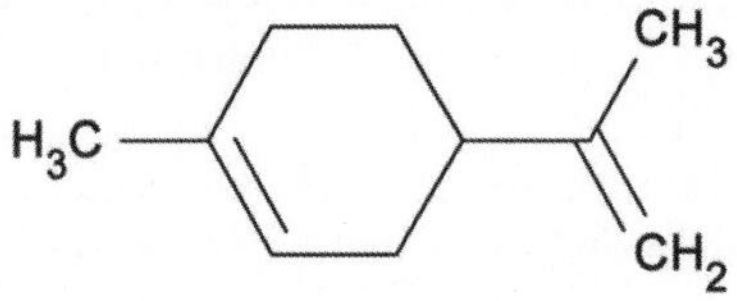

CH_3

H_3C

CH_2

Limonene ($C_{10}H_{16}$)

Question 1

β-Carotene can be best classified as which of the following?

- A. Sesquiterpene
- B. Sesterterpene
- C. Diterpene
- D. Tetraterpene

Question 2

Both β-carotene (provitamin A) and limonene can be metabolized to form vitamin A. Given as a ratio of β-carotene to limonene, what is the ratio of vitamin A obtainable?

- A. 1:1
- B. 2:1
- C. 4:1
- D. 16:1

Question 3

Vitamin A is considered to be a terpenoid. The essential difference between terpenoids and terpenes is that the former has one or more additional functional groups. How many bonds must be made between separate isoprene units, which are easily isomerized in polymers, to construct one vitamin A molecule?

- O **A.** 2
- O **B.** 3
- O **C.** 4
- O **D.** More than 4

Question 4

There are four main retinol binding proteins, they are: RBP, CRBP, IRBP, and CRALBP. RBP and CRBP are cup shape proteins with a single domain. The active site where the ligand is bound is a cavity which is likely which of the following?

- O **A.** Polar
- O **B.** Lipophilic
- O **C.** Anionic
- O **D.** Cationic

Question 5

Compounds such as dimethylsulfoxide (DMSO) have been used historically to deliver pharmaceuticals topically, as its unique structure makes it not only able to dissolve a variety of drugs, but also to penetrate the skin and other cellular membranes without damaging them.

$$H_3C-S(=O)-CH_3$$

DMSO

Recently, scientists have isolated a family of carboxylate-group-containing cyclic monoterpenes (i.e. terpenoids) from the plant *Perilla frutescens* that are also capable of freely penetrating cellular membranes. The scientists concluded that these terpenenoids were able to do so:

- O **A.** because of structural similarities to DMSO.
- O **B.** because of their low molecular mass.
- O **C.** by increasing membrane gaps by repulsion with bilayer lipid heads.
- O **D.** through osmosis.

Question 6

Plant pigments can be separated using a technique called thin layer chromatography (TLC), which separates mixtures into distinct compounds. The mixture is applied on a thin layer of adsorbent material on a plate, and then dipped in a solvent, which is drawn up the plate via capillary action. Different compounds are drawn up the plate at different rates, resulting in separation, analogous to black ink being separated into its various color compounds.

An experiment was set up using the crushed leaves of two different spinach plants, whose green color is mostly provided by chlorophyll, but also contains a significant amount of β-carotene. Of the two plants, one was infected with a virus that forces some of the cells to express dioxygenase, an enzyme that cleaves β-carotene into retinol. On the plate applied with the infected spinach, assuming that chlorophyll only appears as one band, one would expect to see:

- O **A.** only green and orange bands.
- O **B.** a distinct yellow band, in addition to green and orange bands.
- O **C.** only a yellow band.
- O **D.** one green band and two orange bands.

Passage 2 (Questions 7–10)

Despite its age, one of the vital tools required to monitor and maintain awareness of potential soft tissue injury after a nuclear accident (i.e. Fukushima, Chernobyl, Three Mile Island) is the relatively simple Geiger counter.

The Geiger counter is an innovative method used to detect radioactive emissions and many other types of particles and energy and was devised by Geiger, in conjunction with Muller in the early 1900's. The apparatus works on the principle that many types of small particles and energy (in particular radioactive emissions) convert a gas into a conductor of electricity. The instrument itself consists of a glass tube into which two metal electrodes are sealed: a central cathode and the cylindrical anode lining the glass tube as shown in Figure 1.

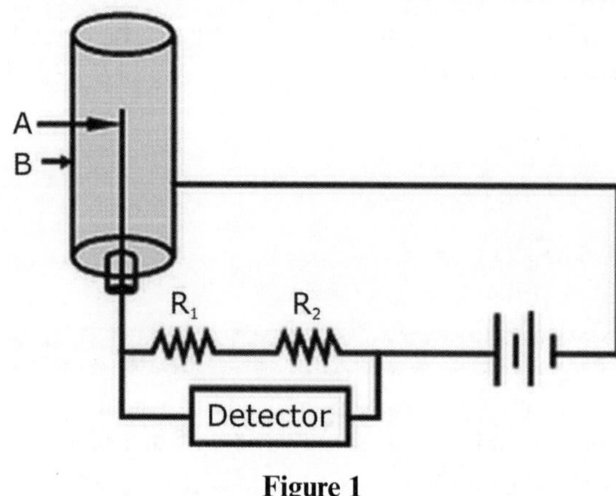

Figure 1

The anode A is a tungsten wire running along the axis of the tube while the cathode B is a thin aluminium cylinder around the circumference of the tube. A potential difference of about 500 V is maintained between the electrodes. The ionizing radiation/particles enters through a mica window and when it interacts with the argon gas present inside the tube (at a pressure of 1300-1600 Pa along with 6% ethanol), the argon atoms are ionized giving rise to cations and free electrons. As the charged particles thus generated are attracted to the electrodes of opposite sign, they are accelerated and ionize other previously neutral argon atoms.

The force exerted on a charged particle in an electric field of strength E is given by F = q E where q = charge on the particle in coulombs. The energy of a particle under a potential difference of V volts is given by E = q V where E = energy of particle.

Mass of an electron = 9.1×10^{-31} kg

Mass of a proton = 1.7×10^{-27} kg

Mass of a neutron = 1.7×10^{-27} kg

Charge on electron = 1.6×10^{-19} C

Question 7

As both the argon cation and electron are accelerated to electrodes of opposite sign, they both have the same initial velocity. Ionization of the gaseous atoms present is dependent only on the velocity of collision. Assuming that they both have the same initial velocity, which of the following statements is true?

- O **A.** Both electron and cation will yield the same number of charged particles.
- O **B.** The electron will yield more charged particles.
- O **C.** The argon cation will yield more charged particles.
- O **D.** The answer cannot be determined without knowing the exact value of the initial velocity.

Question 8

What is the energy of an alpha particle (a helium nucleus) under a potential difference of 20 V?

- O **A.** 3.5×10^{-18} J
- O **B.** 3.2×10^{-18} J
- O **C.** 1.3×10^{-18} J
- O **D.** 6.4×10^{-18} J

Question 9

A sudden voltage drop across the resistors in Figure 1 appears as a pulse to the detector. If $R_2 = 2R_1$ and R_2 is removed from the circuit, what will the new voltage drop be if the current remains unchanged?

- O **A.** 1/2 the original value
- O **B.** 1/3 the original value
- O **C.** 1/6 the original value
- O **D.** The same as the original value

Question 10

Three types of electromagnetic radiation, P, Q and R, were allowed to enter the Geiger counter. Assuming that the current flow is due only to electron motion and that the ionizing power of radiation is directly proportional to its energy, what is the sequence of P, Q and R in order of increasing wavelength (λ)?

Current obtained from P = 1.50 A

Current obtained from Q = 0.75 A

Current obtained from R = 1.00 A

- O **A.** $\lambda_P < \lambda_R < \lambda_Q$
- O **B.** $\lambda_P < \lambda_Q < \lambda_R$
- O **C.** $\lambda_Q < \lambda_R < \lambda_P$
- O **D.** $\lambda_Q < \lambda_P < \lambda_R$

The following questions are NOT based on a descriptive passage (Questions 11–14).

Question 11

Consider the following ray diagrams, where the object point $\boldsymbol{O}$, the image point $\boldsymbol{I}$ and the focal points $\boldsymbol{F_1}$ and $\boldsymbol{F_2}$ of a concave lens are indicated. Which diagram is accurate?

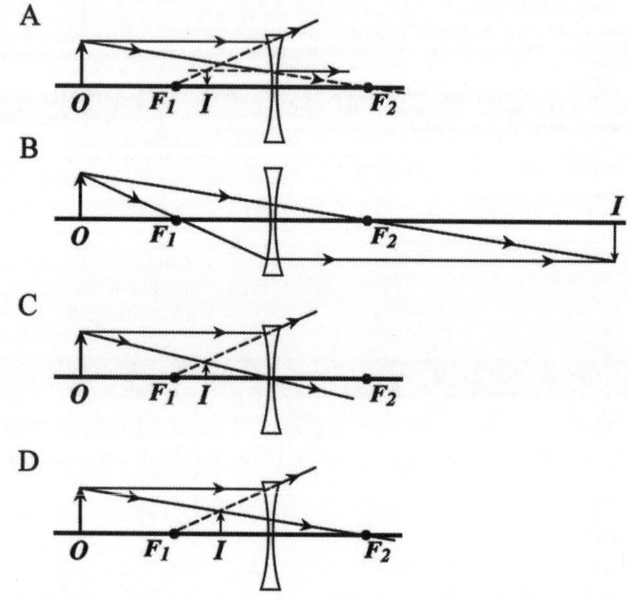

- ○ **A.** A
- ○ **B.** B
- ○ **C.** C
- ○ **D.** D

Question 12

Consider the following reaction.

COOCH3
NaBH4
MeOH
O
Br
H
COOCH3
HO
Br
H

The infrared spectrum of the product can be distinguished from that of the starting material by the:

- ○ **A.** disappearance of IR absorption at 3360 cm^{-1}.
- ○ **B.** disappearance of IR absorption at 2820 cm^{-1}.
- ○ **C.** appearance of IR absorption at 3360 cm^{-1}.
- ○ **D.** appearance of IR absorption at 1740 cm^{-1}.

Question 13

How many different linear tetrapeptides of leu_2val_2 are possible?

- ○ **A.** 4
- ○ **B.** 6
- ○ **C.** 8
- ○ **D.** 16

Question 14

The data in Table 1 were collected for Reaction I:

Reaction I

$2X + Y \rightarrow Z$

Table I

Exp.	[X] in M	[Y] in M	Initial rate of reaction
1	0.050	0.100	2×10^{-4}
2	0.050	0.200	8×10^{-4}
3	0.200	0.100	8×10^{-4}

Identify the rate law for Reaction I.

- ○ **A.** Rate = $k[X]^2[Y]$
- ○ **B.** Rate = $k[X]^2[Y]^2$
- ○ **C.** Rate = $k[X][Y]^2$
- ○ **D.** Rate = $k[X][Y]$

Passage 3 (Questions 15–18)

Figure 1 illustrates a solubility based characterization procedure, often used by organic chemists, for the qualitative analysis of monofunctional organic compounds. Table 1 lists the organic compounds comprising the various solubility classes of compounds from Figure 1.

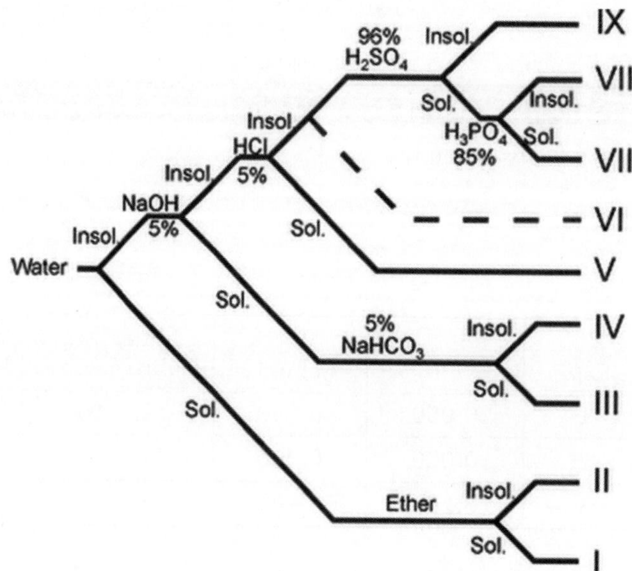

Figure 1 Solubility (Sol.) and insolubility (Insol.) of various compounds in different solvents.

Table 1

Group	Compounds
I	Salts of organic acids, amino acids, amine chlorides Sugars (carbohydrates) and other polyfunctional compounds with hydrophilic substituents
II	Arenesulfonic acids Monofunctional carboxylic acids, alcohols, ketones, aldehydes, esters, amides and nitriles with 5 or less carbon atoms Monofunctional amines with 6 or less carbon atoms
III	Phenols with ortho- and/or para- electron withdrawing groups, beta-diketones Carboxylic acids with 6 or more carbon atoms
IV	Sulfonamides, nitro-compounds with alpha-hydrogens Phenols, oximes, enols, imides and thiophenols with 6 or more carbon atoms
V	Some oxy-ethers, anilines, aliphatic amines with 8 or more carbon atoms
VI	Neutral compounds containing sulfur or nitrogen with 6 or more carbon atoms
VII	Ethers with 7 or less carbon atoms Monofunctional esters, aldehydes, ketones, cyclic ketones, methyl ketones with between 6 and 8 carbon atoms; epoxides
VIII	Ethers, most other ketones Unsaturated hydrocarbons, aromatic compounds, particularly those which possess activating groups
IX	Alkanes, alkyl and aryl halides Aromatic compounds with electron withdrawing substituents, diaryl ethers

Question 15

The result from combining phenols and water can be explained by the fact that phenols:

- O **A.** can hydrogen bond.
- O **B.** cannot hydrogen bond.
- O **C.** are large compounds.
- O **D.** have an aromatic ring.

Question 16

Benzoic acid should be soluble in which of the following solvent pairs?

- O **A.** Water and 5% HCl
- O **B.** 5% NaOH and 5% $NaHCO_3$
- O **C.** 5% HCl and 5% NaOH
- O **D.** 85% H_3PO_4 and 5% NaOH

Question 17

The significance of the number of carbons present in compounds from Group VI is most consistent with which of the following statements?

- O **A.** Increasing the number of carbons increases the hydrophobic moiety.
- O **B.** Six carbon compounds are cyclical.
- O **C.** The number of carbons relates to the group number.
- O **D.** Compounds with six or more carbons are always amphoteric.

Question 18

According to the information provided, all of the following compounds would be included in the water soluble group EXCEPT:

- O **A.** O O H H
- O **B.** O O
- O **C.** OH O
- O **D.** H HO OH H

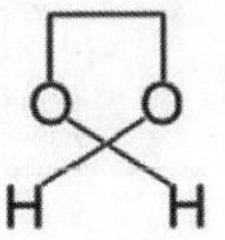

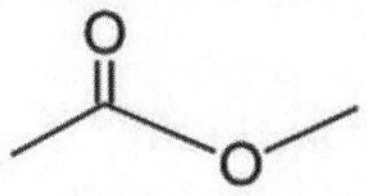

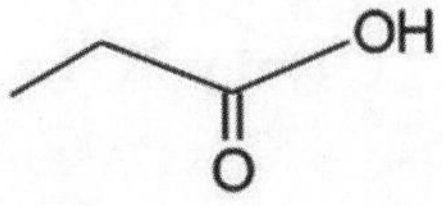

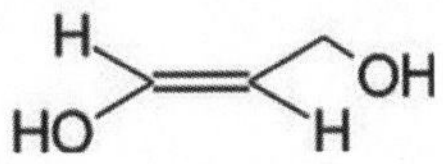

Passage 4 (Questions 19–22)

Testosterone, a steroid androgen, or male sex hormone, is synthesized according to the following pathway.

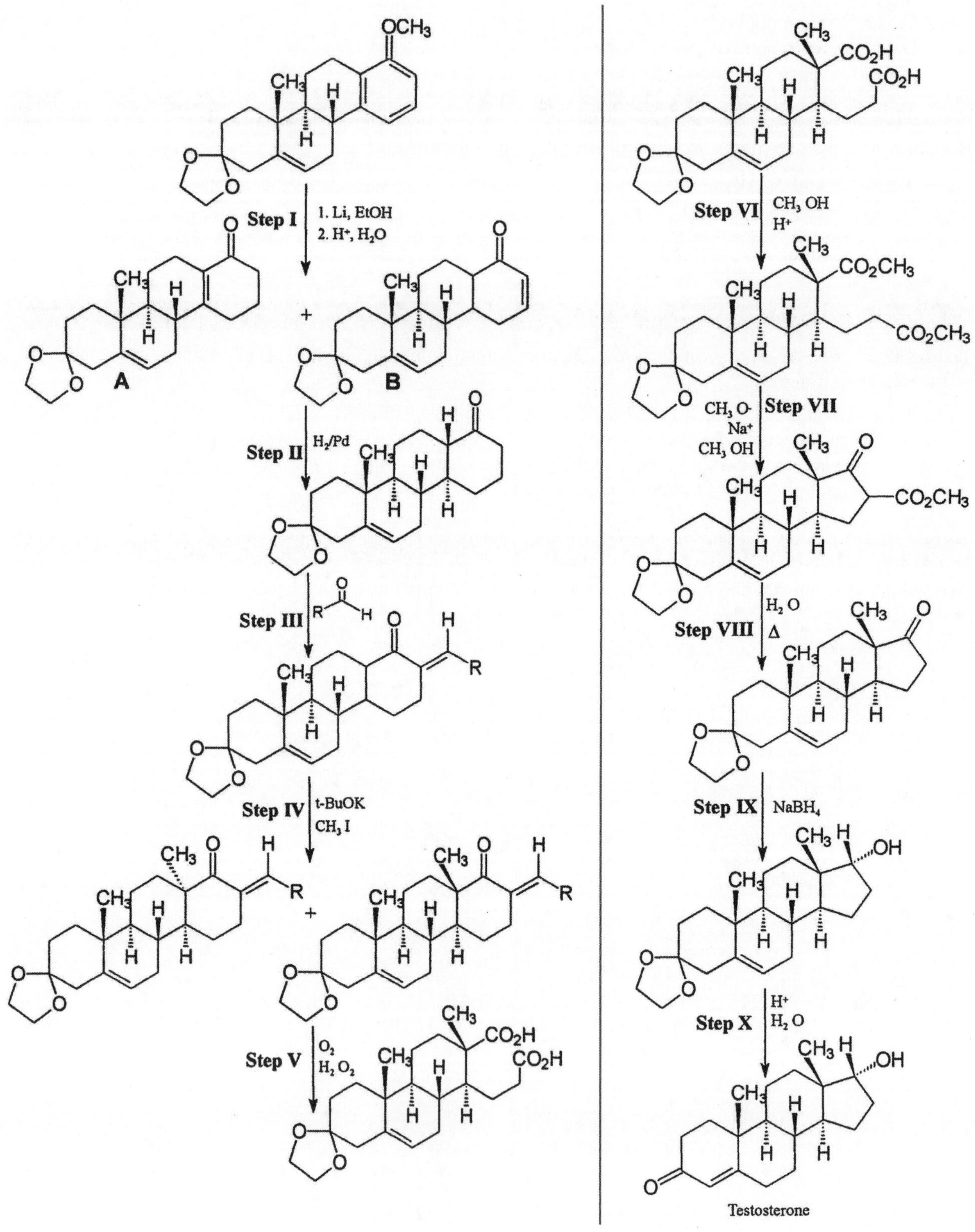

Step I: 1. Li, EtOH 2. H^+, H_2O → A + B

Step II: H_2/Pd

Step III: RCHO

Step IV: t-BuOK, CH_3I

Step V: O_2, H_2O_2

Step VI: CH_3OH, H^+

Step VII: CH_3O^- Na^+, CH_3OH

Step VIII: H_2O, Δ

Step IX: $NaBH_4$

Step X: H^+, H_2O

Testosterone

Question 19

What is the product of the following acid-catalyzed reaction?

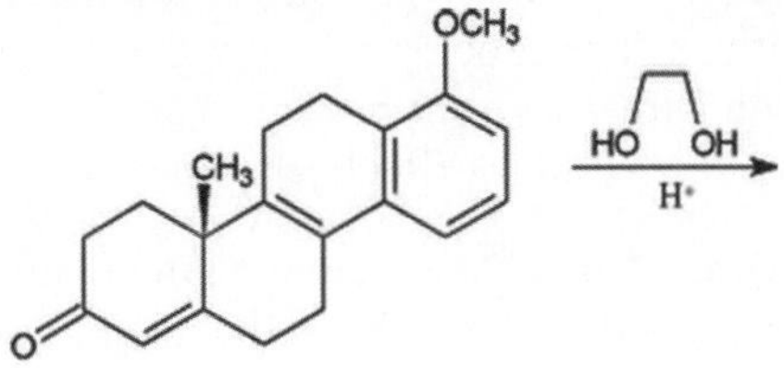

OCH3 CH3 HO OH H+

○ A. OCH3 CH3 HO OH

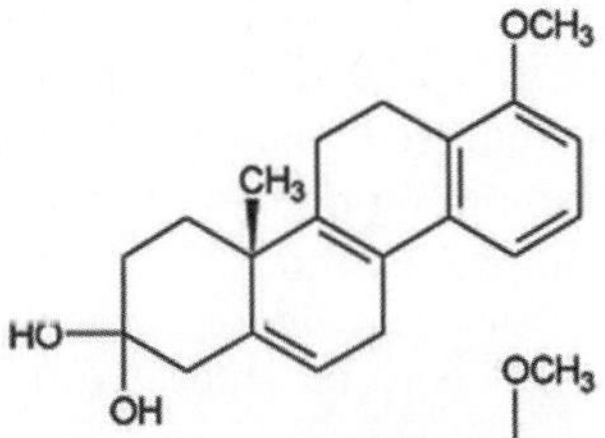

○ B. OCH3 CH3 HO H

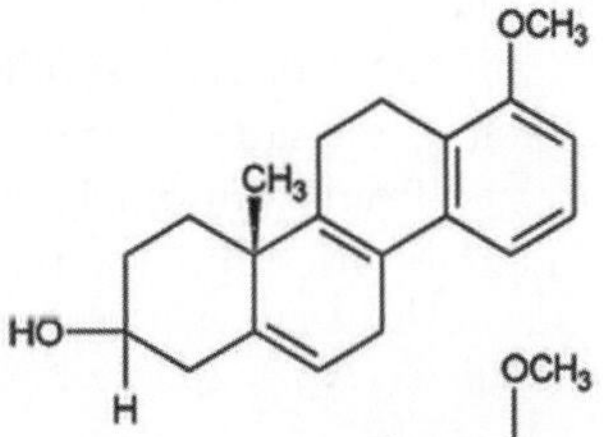

○ C. OCH3 CH3 O O

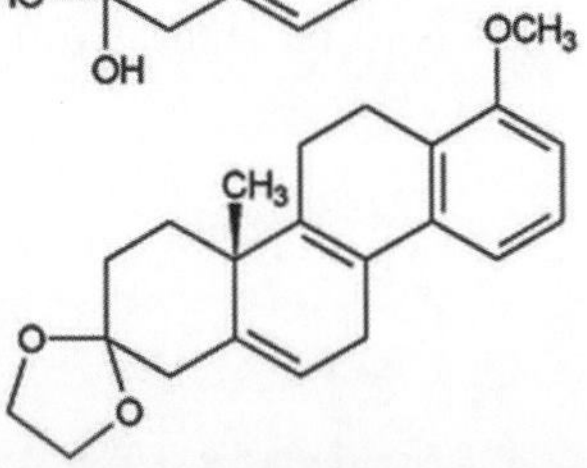

○ D. OCH3 CH3 HO

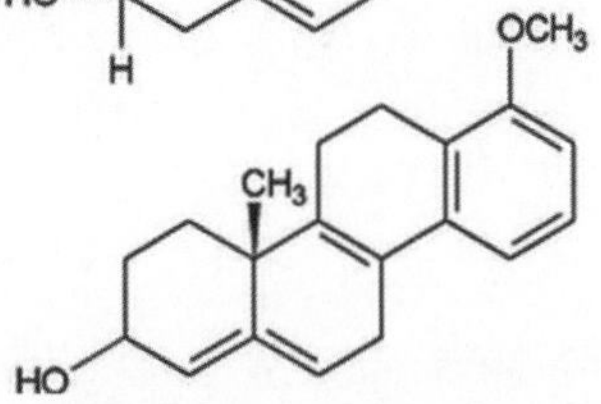

Question 20

The synthesis of testosterone from the following precursor has been reported.

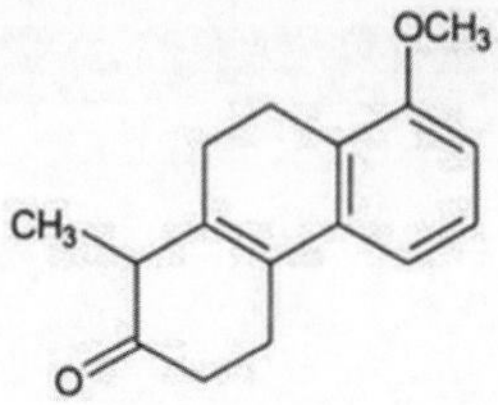

OCH3 CH3 O

Which of the following is formed when a solution of the above compound is treated with lithium diisopropylamide (LDA), given that LDA is a hindered molecule whose conjugate acid has a pK_a of approximately 40?

- ○ **A.** A hemi-acetal
- ○ **B.** An enolate ion
- ○ **C.** A radical anion
- ○ **D.** A ketal

Question 21

Step 1 generated a mixture of cyclohexene derivatives A and B. Products A and B can most easily be distinguished from each other by ^{1}HNMR because:

- ○ **A.** Product A has fewer vinylic protons than Product B.
- ○ **B.** Product A has more vinylic protons than Product B.
- ○ **C.** Product A has more protons than Product B.
- ○ **D.** Product A has more sigma bonds than Product B.

Question 22

In the synthesis of testosterone, Step IX is what type of reaction?

- ○ **A.** A catalytic hydrogenation reaction
- ○ **B.** A reduction reaction
- ○ **C.** A saponification reaction
- ○ **D.** A dehydration reaction

Passage 5 (Questions 23–27)

Due to the fact that many cations form sparingly soluble salts, a method known as *selective precipitation* can be used to separate a mixture of cations. The process involves the addition of a soluble salt containing an anion which forms a sparingly soluble salt with one or more of the cations. If it forms a sparingly soluble salt with only one of the cations in solution, then that cation is effectively separated out of solution.

However, this is not usually the case. More often than not a number of cations in solution will form sparingly soluble salts with the anion. Separation then depends on the magnitude of the K_{sp} value of the sparingly soluble salts that could be formed. The smaller the K_{sp} value for a salt, the earlier it will precipitate out of solution relative to the other salts. Thus the process is similar to a titration: the anion is added gradually in increasing amounts and precipitating each of the salts separately, then the precipitate is removed when all of that particular cation species has been extracted from solution. This is used extensively in the mining industry in the purification of various metal ores and in laboratories in the separation of ions from various bodily fluids.

A mixture of bismuth (Bi^{3+}), silver (Ag^+), zinc (Zn^{2+}) and copper (Cu^{2+}) cations is to be separated using sodium sulfide (Na_2S).

$K_{sp}(Bi_2S_3) = 1.0 \times 10^{-97}$

$K_{sp}(Ag_2S) = 2.0 \times 10^{-49}$

$K_{sp}(ZnS) = 1.0 \times 10^{-21}$

$K_{sp}(CuS) = 9.0 \times 10^{-36}$

Question 23

The K_{sp} expression for Bi_2S_3 is:

- ○ **A.** $[Bi_2^{3+}][S_3^{2-}]$
- ○ **B.** $[Bi^{3+}][S^{2-}]$
- ○ **C.** $[Bi^{3+}]^2[S^{2-}]^3$
- ○ **D.** $[Bi^{3+}]^3[S^{2-}]^2$

Question 24

Cyanide ions (CN^-) could also have been used to precipitate the cations. If after all the cations have been precipitated, the concentration of CN^- is 0.02 M, calculate the pH of the solution given that:

$CN^- + H_2O \rightarrow HCN + OH^-$

$K_b = 1.39 \times 10^{-5}$

- ○ **A.** 8.6
- ○ **B.** 9.8
- ○ **C.** 7.7
- ○ **D.** 10.7

Question 25

If in a solution containing only Zn^{2+}, the concentration of zinc ions is 5.0×10^{-3} M, what concentration of S^{2-} is required to just begin the precipitation of zinc sulfide?

- ○ **A.** 5.0×10^{-24} M
- ○ **B.** 2.0×10^{-19} M
- ○ **C.** 3.2×10^{-11} M
- ○ **D.** 5.0×10^{-3} M

Question 26

An unknown cation X^+ was added to the original solution of cations and was found to precipitate before Ag_2S but after Bi_2S_3. Which of the following gives a plausible value for the solubility product of X_2S?

- O **A.** 3.4×10^{-99}
- O **B.** 1.4×10^{-15}
- O **C.** 8.0×10^{-28}
- O **D.** 4.0×10^{-53}

Question 27

The CuS from the selective precipitation was collected, purified and equal weights of it placed into each of two beakers. Beaker 1 contained distilled water and beaker 2 contained a 0.01 M $Cu(NO_3)_2$ solution. Which of the following statements is true?

- O **A.** More of the CuS will dissolve in beaker 1.
- O **B.** More of the CuS will dissolve in beaker 2.
- O **C.** Equal amounts of CuS will dissolve in both beakers.
- O **D.** No CuS will dissolve in either beaker.

The following questions are NOT based on a descriptive passage (Questions 28–31).

Question 28

What is the order of increasing acidity for the following compounds?

I. 4-methylpentanoic acid
II. 3-chloropentanoic acid
III. 2-bromopentanoic acid
IV. 2,2-dichloropentanoic acid

- **A.** I < II < III < IV
- **B.** IV < III < II < I
- **C.** I < III < II < IV
- **D.** II < III < I < IV

Question 29

Coniine, a poisonous neurotoxin, is illustrated below. What is the hybridization of C2 in coniine?

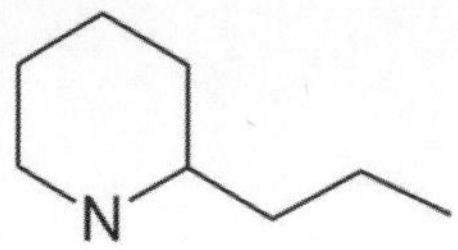

N

- **A.** sp
- **B.** sp^2
- **C.** sp^3
- **D.** sd^4

Question 30

What would be the expected change in the solubility of a gas when a solution containing the gas is heated and when a solution containing the gas has the pressure over the solution decreased, respectively?

- **A.** Increase, increase
- **B.** Increase, decrease
- **C.** Decrease, increase
- **D.** Decrease, decrease

Question 31

The structure of 1,1-dichloroethane, which used to be used as a surgical inhalational anesthetic, is shown below.

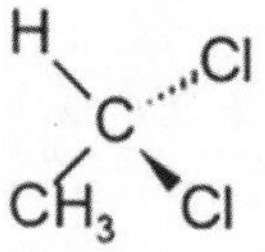

H
Cl
C
CH_3 Cl

If a beam of plane polarized light is passed through a large collection of 1,1-dichloroethane molecules, would emerge with the plane of polarization having rotated:

- **A.** 0°
- **B.** 90°
- **C.** 60°
- **D.** 180°

Note: This page is left blank so that the passage would be visible without turning pages while assessing the passage-based questions.

Passage 6 (Questions 32–35)

The cardiac action potential differs significantly in different portions of the heart. The specialized pacemaker cells have the ability to spontaneously depolarize, and it is the pacemaker potential that drives the self-generated rhythmic firing, known as 'cardiac muscle automaticity'.

The action potential (AP) in cardiac cells depends upon the activity of several types of ion channels, and the voltage-gated potassium channel is vital for normal cardiac electrical activity.

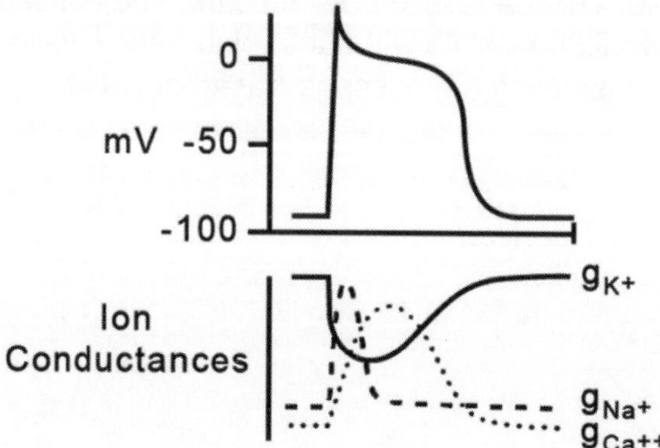

Figure 1 Action potential and ion flow in cardiac myocytes

The primary role of potassium channels in cardiac action potentials is cell repolarization. The *human ether à-gogo related gene* (hERG1) channel is responsible for a major component of the potassium current flow and is a voltage-activated, outward rectifying K^+ channel.

hERG1 is a gene that codes for a protein known as $K_v11.1$, the alpha subunit of a potassium ion channel. When this channel's ability to conduct electrical current across the cell membrane is inhibited it can result in a potentially fatal disorder termed 'Long QT syndrome'.

Stereoselectivity in pharmacodynamics and pharmacokinetics has shown the *chiral toxicity* of some molecules in the hERG1 channel, leading to a reduction in K^+ flow. A growing number of drugs have been shown to have similar effects on the AP, leading to life-threatening ventricular arrhythmias known as *Torsades de Pointes*.

Chirality is a very common feature of marketed drugs, which have distinct three-dimensional structures and potentially different biological activities. Both the pharmacodynamic and pharmacokinetic properties can differ between enantiomers, as well as between individuals taking the drug due to metabolic polymorphisms. A number of clinically successful drugs in the market have had the tendency to inhibit hERG1, and create a risk of sudden death as a side effect, which has made hERG1 inhibition an important characteristic that must be avoided during drug development.

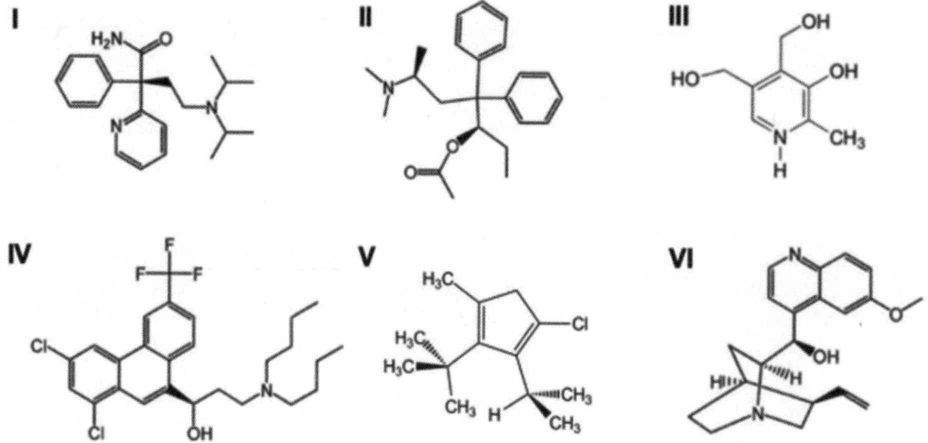

Figure 2 Medications under evaluation for potential hERG1 effects

Question 32

Given the same scale as the one in Figure 1, which of the following action potential traces in cardiac myocytes is most consistent with the effects of a hERG1 channel inhibitor?

○ **A.**

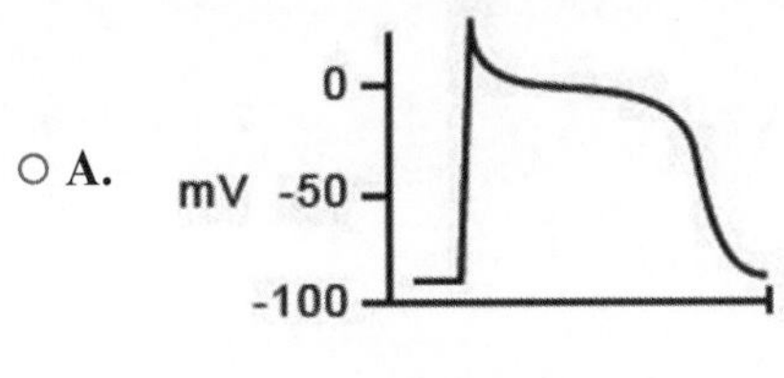

○ **B.**

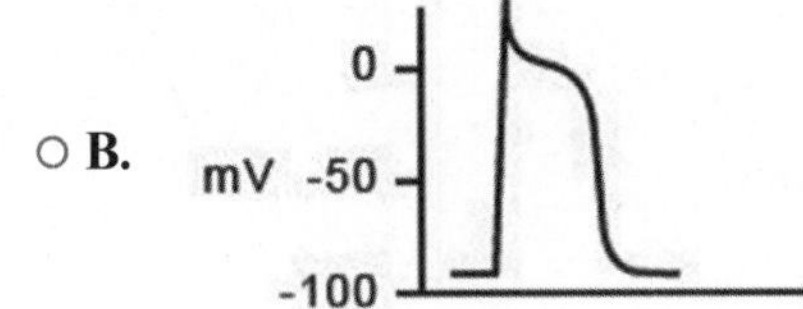

○ **C.**

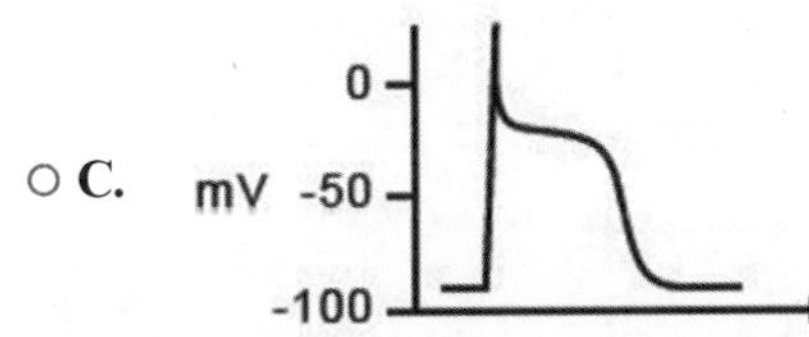

○ **D.**

0
mV -50
-100

Question 33

Consider two cardiac myocytes joined together by intercalated disks. The cell on the left has repolarized and the cell on the right is experiencing a wave of depolarization. Which of the following is most consistent with the electric field lines for the two cardiac myocytes?

○ **A.**

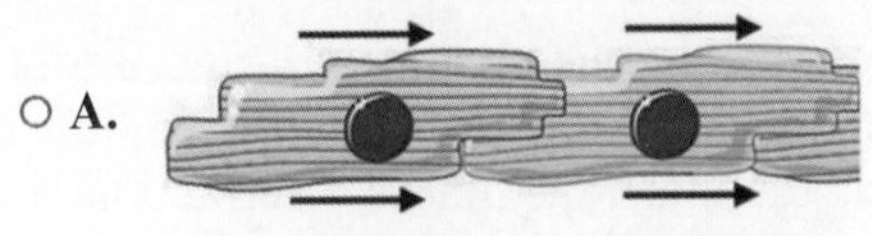

○ **B.**

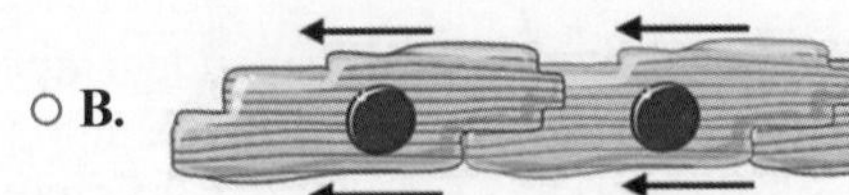

○ **C.**

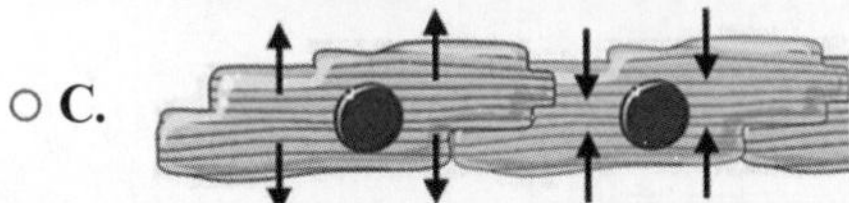

○ **D.**

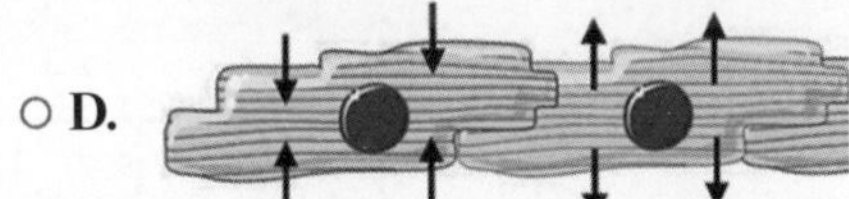

Question 34

How many of the six medications in Figure 2 are NOT chiral?

○ **A.** 0
○ **B.** 1
○ **C.** 2
○ **D.** More than 2

Question 35

A study was performed in which Compound V from Figure 2 was radiolabeled, injected into a patient and its metabolite was evaluated and found to rotate plane-polarized light to the right. Based on the experiment, which of the following is the correct conclusion?

○ **A.** The substrate rotates plane-polarized light to the left.
○ **B.** The substrate rotates plane-polarized light to the right.
○ **C.** The enzyme must be achiral.
○ **D.** The enzyme must be chiral.

Passage 7 (Questions 36–39)

Consider the diagram of the human eye.

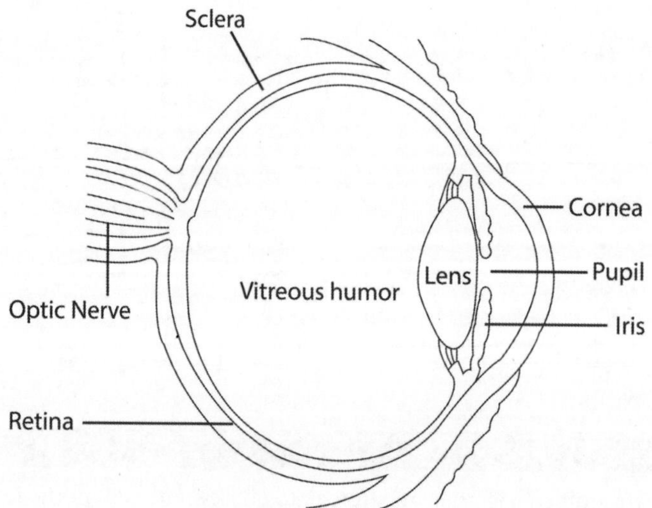

Figure 1 Basic anatomy of the human eye

Like any wave, the speed of a light wave is dependent upon the properties of the medium. In the case of an electromagnetic wave, the speed of the wave depends upon the optical density of that material. One indicator of the optical density of a material is the index of refraction value of the material. Index of refraction values (represented by the symbol n) are numerical index values that are expressed relative to the speed of light in a vaccum.

Component	Index of Refraction
Air	1
Cornea	1.38
Vitreous humor	1.34
Lens	1.40

Myopia (also known as near-sightedness and short-sightedness) and hyperopia (also known as far-sightedness or long-sightedness) are among the most common anomalies of vision. Someone with myopia can see near objects clearly, but cannot focus properly on distant objects. This is caused by the eyeball being elongated, so that the distance between the lens and the retina is too great. Someone with hyperopia can see distant objects clearly, but cannot focus properly on near objects. This is because the lens focuses the sharpest image behind the retina, instead of on it.

Artificial (glass or plastic) lenses are sometimes used to correct visual anomalies. The thin lens equation relates the objective distance to the lens o, the image distance to the lens i, and the focal length f of a lens as indicated below.

$$1/o + 1/i = 1/f$$

Question 36

To focus an image on the retina, the components of the eye which are primarily implicated are which of the following?

- O **A.** Pupil and vitreous humor
- O **B.** Iris and Cornea
- O **C.** Cornea and Lens
- O **D.** Lens and Iris

Question 37

The greatest deviation (refraction) of light would be expected at which of the following interfaces?

- O **A.** Lens – vitreous humor
- O **B.** Cornea - air
- O **C.** Pupil - lens
- O **D.** Cornea - lens

Question 38

Which of the following lenses would most reasonably be used to correct myopia and hyperopia, respectively?

- O **A.** convex, convex
- O **B.** convex, concave
- O **C.** concave, convex
- O **D.** concave, concave

Question 39

The power of a lens is its ability to bend light – the greater the power, the greater the refraction of light. The power of a lens is measured in diopters (D) which is equal to the inverse of the focal length calculated in meters. If a thin convex lens has real image at 18 cm from the lens when an object is placed at 36 cm in front of the lens, what is the power of the lens?

- O **A.** + 8.3 D
- O **B.** - 8.3 D
- O **C.** + 8.3×10^{-2} D
- O **D.** - 8.3×10^{-2} D

Passage 8 (Questions 40–43)

Sucrose is metabolized in the human body through a complicated series of chemical reactions whose net result is the same as the complete combustion of sucrose.

Reaction 1

$C_{12}H_{22}O_{11(s)} + 12\ O_{2(g)} \Leftrightarrow 12\ CO_{2(g)} + 11\ H_2O_{(l)}$

A bomb calorimeter (see Figure 1) is useful for measuring the heat evolved in the combustion of sucrose. The reactants are held in a water-tight steal bomb which is surrounded by water. A thermometer measures the change in water temperature after the reaction. A stirrer ensures that equal heating occurs. The reaction is initiated by momentary electric heating of a length of iron wire covered with the reactants. The heat of reaction is determined by measuring the total quantity of heat absorbed by the water, taking into account the heat capacity of the calorimeter. The heat capacity of the calorimeter used in the experiment was 4.9 kJ/°C.

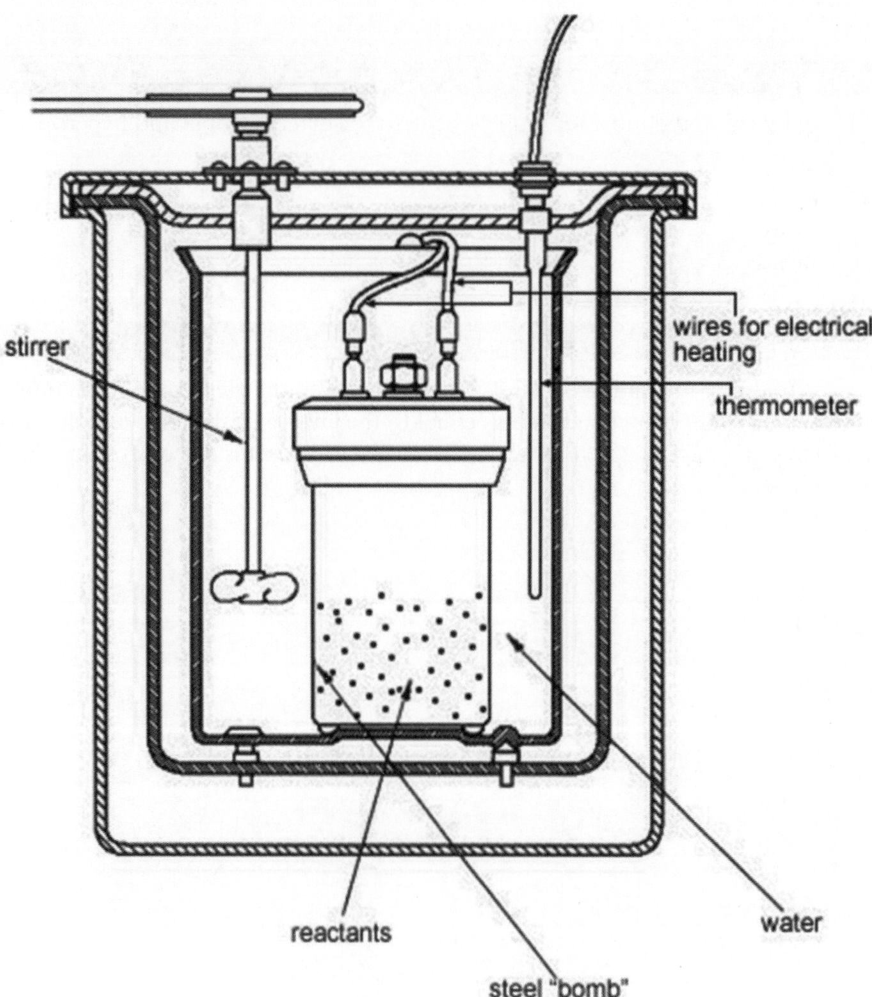

Figure 1 Standard configuration of a bomb calorimeter

Question 40

All of the following are necessary for Reaction 1 to occur, EXCEPT:

- ○ **A.** oxygen gas.
- ○ **B.** ignition source.
- ○ **C.** sucrose.
- ○ **D.** water.

Question 41

If the water temperature rose 20 °C what quantity of heat would be generated by the combustion reaction?

- ○ **A.** 0 kJ
- ○ **B.** 9.8 kJ
- ○ **C.** 98 kJ
- ○ **D.** 980 kJ

Question 42

When the water in the calorimeter rises in temperature, the mercury in the thermometer initially drops before it rises to correspond to the temperature of the water, what explains this phenomenon?

- ○ **A.** Mercury has a higher boiling point than water.
- ○ **B.** The specific heat of mercury is greater than water.
- ○ **C.** The glass of the thermometer expands upon being heated.
- ○ **D.** The temperature of the mercury is less than that of the glass.

Question 43

Approximately how many grams of oxygen gas are consumed upon the combustion of 5 g of sucrose?

- ○ **A.** 0.21 g
- ○ **B.** 2.0 g
- ○ **C.** 5.6 g
- ○ **D.** 12 g

The following questions are NOT based on a descriptive passage (Questions 44–47).

Question 44

Consider the following diagram illustrating hydrophobic bonding between X and Y in an aqueous medium where each bent line symbolizes a water molecule.

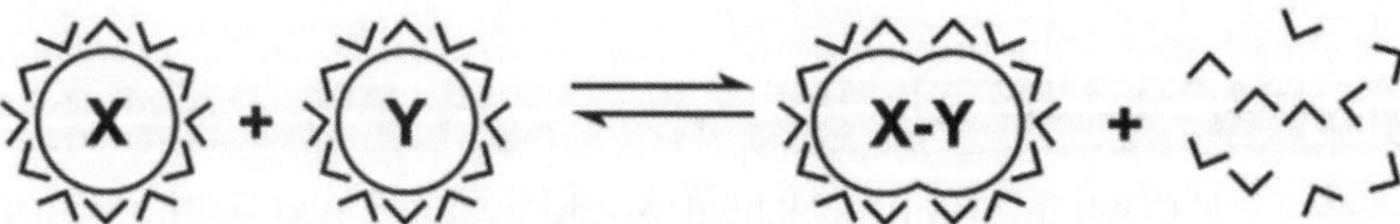

Which of the following most accurately describes the cause of the hydrophobic bond X-Y?

- O **A.** An electrostatic attraction between X and Y
- O **B.** The nonpolar force of attraction between X and Y
- O **C.** Net gain in entropy
- O **D.** Overall positive Gibbs free energy

Question 45

Fas/APO-1 is a transmembrane receptor which, when stimulated, may activate intracellular mechanisms leading to cell death. **Fas/APO-1** is likely:

- O **A.** a phospholipid.
- O **B.** a complex carbohydrate.
- O **C.** synthesized in the nucleus.
- O **D.** synthesized by rough endoplasmic reticulum.

Question 46

The cruising altitude of most planes is about 10,000 meters above sea level where there is less air above the plane pushing down, so the air pressure is lower (about 20 kPa outside compared to about 100 kPa atmospheric pressure at sea level). To keep everyone comfortable inside the plane, the cabin is pressurized to about 75 kPa. The passenger doors on a 747 are about 1 meter wide by 2 meters tall.

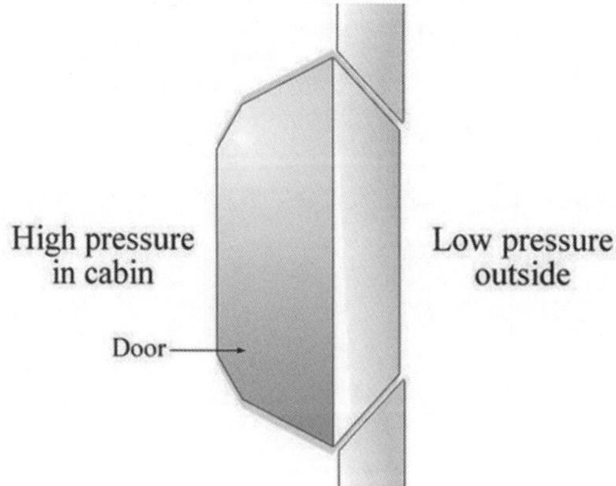

If a metric ton is 1000 kg, to pull the door open at 10,000 meters is equivalent to moving how many metric tons? (the acceleration due to gravity can be approximated as 10 m/s^2)

- O **A.** 5×10^{-2} tons
- O **B.** 0.8 tons
- O **C.** 2 tons
- O **D.** 11 tons

Question 47

In the presence of a competitive inhibitor, an enzyme-catalyzed reaction consistent with Michaelis–Menten kinetics would be expected to have:

- ○ **A.** the Km for the reaction unchanged.
- ○ **B.** the Vmax for the reaction unchanged.
- ○ **C.** the Vmax and Km for the reaction changed.
- ○ **D.** the Vmax and Km for the reaction unchanged.

Passage 9 (Questions 48–52)

Aurora kinase is an important cell cycle regulator in animal cells. One of the substrates of aurora kinase is a nuclear protein called histone. Aurora kinase phosphorylates histone to produce histone-P. The reaction catalyzed by aurora kinase obeys Michaelis-Menten kinetics. According to the Michaelis-Menten model, the rate of product formation, V_0, can be described by the following equation:

$$V_0 = \frac{V_{max} * [S]}{K_m + [S]}$$

in which V_0 is the initial reaction rate, V_{max} is the maximum reaction rate, K_m refers to the Michaelis constant, and $[S]$ is the substrate concentration.

The turnover rate for an enzyme refers to the number of substrate molecules converted into product molecules by an enzyme molecule per unit of time when the enzyme is saturated with substrate. Under these conditions, the reaction proceeds at the maximum rate and the turnover rate, k_{cat}, can be calculated according to the following formula:

$$k_{cat} = V_{max} / [E]$$

where $[E]$ is the enzyme concentration.

Experiment: Kinetic Properties of Aurora Kinase

To study the properties of aurora kinase, the rate of histone phosphorylation by aurora kinase was measured and the results are shown in the graph below (Figure 1).

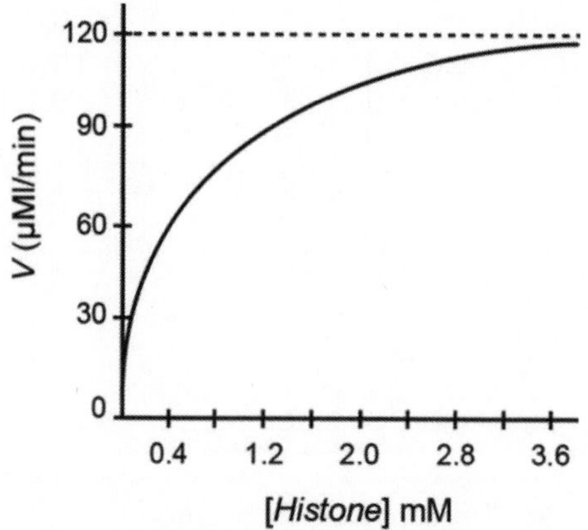

Figure 1 The rate of histone phosphorylation by aurora kinase as a function of substrate concentration. The velocity is given per mg of enzyme.

To investigate the mechanisms of aurora kinase inhibition, two different drugs, A and B, were used. The enzyme activity was recorded in the presence of each drug and plotted as a Lineweaver-Burk plot (Figure 2).

I.

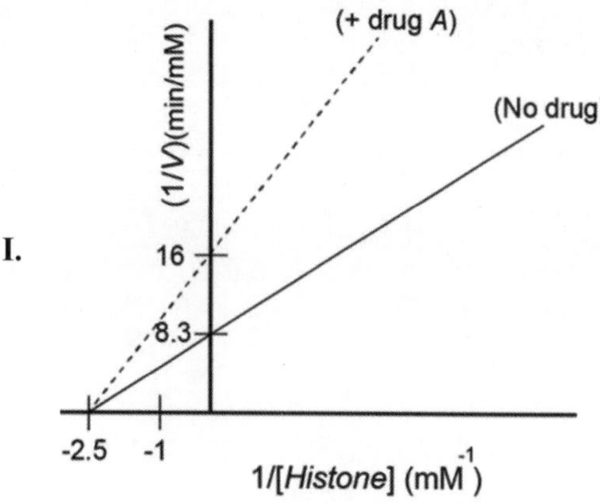

II.

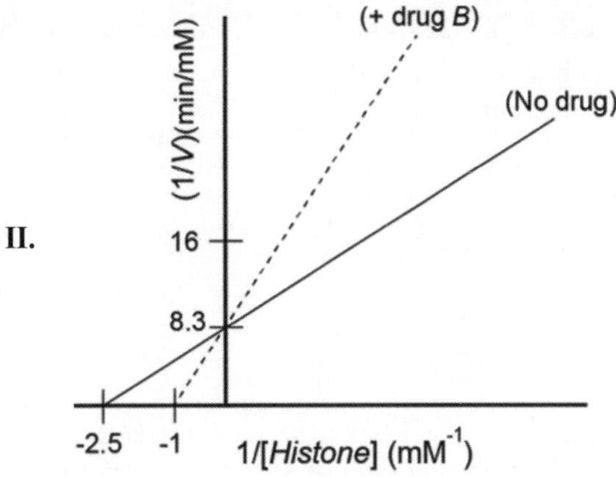

Figure 2 The Lineweaver-Burk plot of Aurora kinase activity in the presence or absence of two drugs. **I.** The effect of drug A on Aurora kinase activity. **II.** The effect of drug B on Aurora kinase activity. The velocity is given per mg of enzyme.

Question 48

From the data presented in Figure 1, which of the following would be the best approximation of the initial reaction rate when histone concentration is 2 mM?

- O **A.** 90 μM of histone-P per minute per mg of aurora kinase
- O **B.** 95 μM of histone-P per minute per mg of aurora kinase
- O **C.** 100 μM of histone-P per minute per mg of aurora kinase
- O **D.** 120 μM of histone-P per minute per mg of aurora kinase

Question 49

Based on the data shown in Figure 2, which of the following is consistent with the effect of drug A and B on aurora kinase activity?

- O **A.** Drug A: K_m changed to 1 mM; and Drug B: V_{max} changed to 62.5 μmol/min
- O **B.** Drug A: K_m changed to 100 mM; and Drug B: V_{max} changed to 60 μmol/min
- O **C.** Drug A: V_{max} changed to 62.5 μmol/min; and Drug B: K_m changed to 1 mM
- O **D.** Drug A: V_{max} changed to 60 μmol/min; and Drug B: K_m changed to 100 mM

Question 50

Consider the graphs of aurora kinase activity presented in Figure 2. What type of inhibition is likely exerted by drugs A and B?

- O **A.** Drug A is competitive, drug B is non-competitive
- O **B.** Drug A is non-competitive, drug B is competitive
- O **C.** Drug A is competitive, drug B is mixed
- O **D.** Drug A is mixed, drug B is competitive

Question 51

The dissociation constant for aurora kinase bound in a complex with histone was measured as 25 μM. What is the affinity constant between aurora kinase and histone?

- O **A.** 0.04 μM^{-1}
- O **B.** 40 μM^{-1}
- O **C.** 2.5 μM^{-1}
- O **D.** 4 μM^{-1}

Question 52

The active site of kinase aurora inhibitors contain a gatekeeper residue at a hinge region that can hydrogen bond (·····) to a substrate as shown in the diagram below.

Hinge Region

Gatekeeper residue

Hydrophobic pocket

Solvent exposed area

What is the substrate shown?

- O **A.** NAD
- O **B.** NADH + H^+
- O **C.** GTP
- O **D.** ATP

Passage 10 (Questions 53–56)

The electronic structure of the atom has always been of interest to scientists. From the model of atomic organization by Rutherford to Bohr's revolutionary application of Planck's quantum theory, the world of science has marvelled at how electrons are arranged around a central nucleus. One of the first instruments used to study this phenomenon made use of ionization via electron bombardment. The ease with which the successive ionizations of the atom could be achieved gave an indication of the magnitude of the attractive forces between the nucleus and the electrons and the type of organization present. The apparatus used is represented in Figure 1.

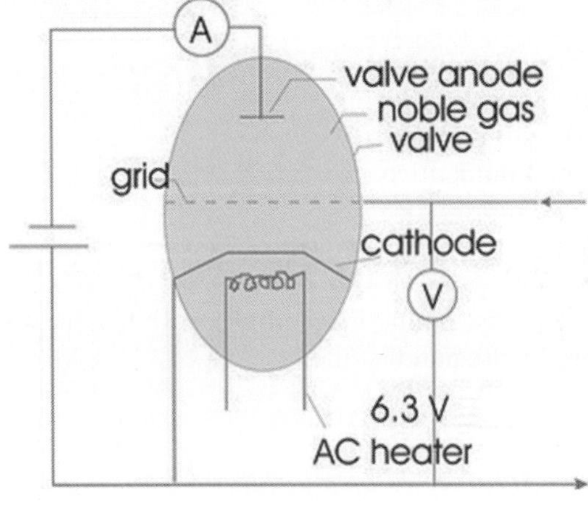

Figure 1

When the cathode is heated from the 6.3 V AC supply, electrons are emitted from its surface. These electrons fall on the grid (which is positive) and a current flows in the cathode/grid circuit. As electrons stream from the cathode toward the grid, they bombard atoms of the gas under study (in this case a noble gas) inside the valve. As the potential difference between the cathode and the grid is increased, electrons are accelerated through the valve at greater and greater speeds. As the kinetic energy of the electrons continues to increase, it eventually becomes great enough such that on collision with an atom, the most loosely bound electron is removed from the atom to yield a cation. The cations are attracted to the negative terminal and the electrons to the positive terminal and this leads to a sudden increase in the reading from the ammeter. The kinetic energy of the bombarding electrons can be calculated from the voltage of the system via the following formula:

$E = e \times V$

e = charge on an electron (1.6×10^{-19} C)

V = voltage

E = kinetic energy of one bombarding electron in joules (J) = energy required to ionize one atom or ion

Mass of electron = 9.1×10^{-31} kg

1 eV = 1.6×10^{-19} J

Question 53

What is the approximate force on an electron, emitted from the cathode, which experiences an acceleration of 2.5×10^{12} m s^{-2}?

- O **A.** 2.8×10^{-6} N
- O **B.** 1.4×10^{-6} N
- O **C.** 2.3×10^{-18} N
- O **D.** 1.2×10^{-18} N

Question 54

How does the force exerted on the cations relate to the force exerted on the electrons given that the mass of the cation involved is 6.7×10^{-27} kg?

- O **A.** The force acting on the cation is equal to the force acting on the electron.
- O **B.** The force acting on the electron is approximately 3,700 times that of the force acting on the cation.
- O **C.** The force acting on the electron is 7,400 times the force acting on the cation.
- O **D.** The force acting on the electron is 14,800 times the force acting on the cation.

Question 55

A sharp increase in the ammeter reading was observed when the voltage was 22 V. What is the ionization energy in terms of eV mol^{-1} ?

- O **A.** 1.15×10^{6}
- O **B.** 2.10×10^{6}
- O **C.** 1.32×10^{25}
- O **D.** 1.15×10^{25}

Question 56

What is the velocity of an electron which has a kinetic energy of 1.82×10^{-19} J?

- O **A.** 4.0×10^{12} m s^{-1}
- O **B.** 2.0×10^{6} m s^{-1}
- O **C.** 8.0×10^{12} m s^{-1}
- O **D.** 6.4×10^{5} m s^{-1}

The following questions are NOT based on a descriptive passage (Questions 57–59).

Question 57

Consider the following potential energy diagram for a reversible reaction. Which of the following best describes the reaction illustrated in the diagram?

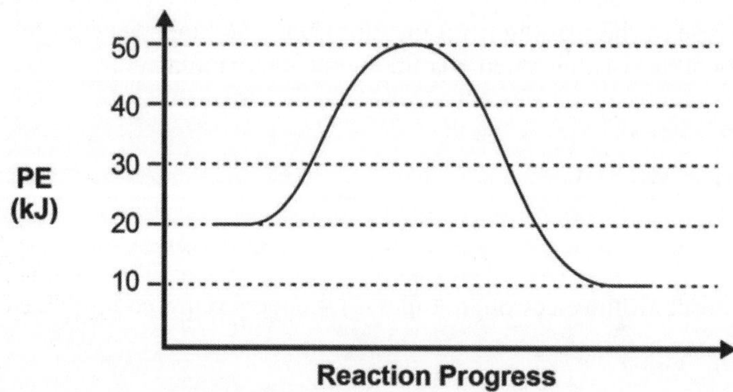

- O **A.** For the forward reaction: activation energy: 30 kJ; ΔH: +10 kJ
- O **B.** For the reverse reaction: activation energy: 30 kJ :ΔH: -10 kJ
- O **C.** For the reverse reaction: activation energy: 40 kJ; ΔH: +10 kJ
- O **D.** For the forward reaction: activation energy: 40 kJ; ΔH: -10 kJ

Question 58

Consider the following form of van der Waal's equation that corrects for the pressure and volume of real gases (*a*, *b* and R are constants, P is pressure, V is volume and T is temperature).

$$\left(P + \frac{a}{V^2}\right)(V - b) = RT$$

In the fundamental quantities of mass (M), length (L) and time (T), the dimensions of the constant *a* would be consistent with which of the following?

- O **A.** $M L^5 T^{-2}$
- O **B.** $M L^{-1} T^{-2}$
- O **C.** $M L^2 T$
- O **D.** L^6

Question 59

In order to become active, a Map kinase has to undergo phosphorylation of its catalytic domain on amino acids 183 and 185 according to the primary structure. To create a catalytically inactive Map kinase - a kinase dead mutant - the most likely substitution within its active domain would be:

- O **A.** A183T185.
- O **B.** Y183A185.
- O **C.** G183A185.
- O **D.** S183Y185.

CANDIDATE'S NAME ____________________________________

RAW SCORE AND SCALED SCORE ___________________________

GS-5
Mock Exam 5 of 7
Solutions at MCAT-prep.com

GS-5 Section II: Critical Analysis and Reasoning Skills (CARS)

Questions: 1-53
Time: 90 minutes

INSTRUCTIONS: This test contains nine passages, each of which is followed by several questions. After reading the passage, select the best answer to each question. If you are unsure of the answer, eliminate the alternatives you know to be false then select an answer from the remaining alternatives. To indicate your selection, use a pencil to blacken the corresponding circle next to the answer choice and/or you can use the answer document at the back of this book. No marks are deducted for wrong answers.

The computer-based real MCAT has an on-screen highlighter function and ~~STRIKEOUT~~ function. These tools help to spotlight text or assist in the process of elimination. You may use a yellow highlighter for this paper-based exam and/or a pen (or preferably a pencil to make it easier should you change your mind) to mark text. At the time of publishing, both highlighting and strikeout functions can be used for passages, questions and answer choices. You can also flag a question to review later should time remain.

For the real exam, you will be provided with a dry erase board which is a white laminated noteboard booklet accompanied by a fine point marker. The noteboard includes 9 graph-lined pages for you to write though you cannot erase. You can simulate the experience with a fine point marker on a noteboard or with 8" x 14" plain graph paper.

Please note: For the real MCAT, a small number of field-tested questions will remain unscored.

This practice test has been designed exclusively to test knowledge and thinking skills. This exam may contain hypothetical statements and/or express controversial ideas. Statements contained herein do not necessarily reflect the policy, position, or view of RuveneCo Inc. or MCAT-prep.com.

START EXAM ONLY WHEN TIMER IS READY.

Passage 1 (Questions 1–6)

Writers have long drawn on the experiences of war to examine themes such as race, power, democracy, and human behavior under conditions of stress. Partly through addressing these and similar issues with unprecedented candor and realism, U.S. war literature matured during and after World War II. Hundreds of war novels eventually appeared, some of outstanding craftsmanship. Many American poets did impressive work, and wartime journalism and postwar memoirs often exhibited a new subtlety and clarity.

World War II novels comprise the most varied category in U.S. war literature. Harry Brown tells of small-unit combat in *A Walk in the Sun* (1944). John Hersey's *A Bell for Adano* (1944) suggests that the integrity of most Americans abroad will ultimately outweigh the arrogance and cruelty of a few. Hersey also wrote *Into the Valley* (1943) and *Hiroshima* (1946), both reportorial classics, as well as the novels *The Wall* (1950), about the Warsaw Ghetto, and *The War Lover* (1959), a Freudian tale of bomber pilots in England.

Saul Bellow's *Dangling Man* (1944) ends disturbingly before its draftee protagonist goes overseas. Life in North Africa and Italy beguiles the GIs in John Horne Burns's *The Gallery* (1947). Like many novels, *The Gallery* features self-seeking officers, decent enlisted men, and kind-hearted foreign women, but a chapter about gay Allied soldiers was controversial. John Hawkes' surrealistic *The Cannibal* (1949) portrays occupied Germany as a landscape of gothic horrors, and Jerzy Kozinski takes a macabre view of Nazi-occupied Poland in *The Painted Bird* (1965). William Gardner Smith's *Last of the Conquerors* (1948) shows black soldiers in occupied Germany as better treated by German civilians than by fellow Americans. John Oliver Killens' *And Then We Heard the Thunder* (1962) dramatically portrays a comparable social contradiction in wartime Austria.

In his deeply pessimistic *The Naked and the Dead*, Norman Mailer mixes realistic details of the Pacific war with profound fears about the future of democracy. In this novel, war has given frightening power to autocrats like General Cummings and sadists like Sergeant Croft. Only chance and heroic endurance, embodied in Private Ridges and Private Goldstein, offer a glimmer of hope in a dark human and natural landscape.

James Jones published the best-selling *From Here to Eternity* in 1951, describing the life of the rebellious Private Prewitt in Hawaii before Pearl Harbor. Considered shocking in language and detail at the time it was published, its brutal depiction of army life angered some skeptical critics. But Jones's ability to write powerfully and insightfully about soldiers was confirmed in *The Thin Red Line* (1962), an outstanding combat-oriented novel.

Almost immediately following World War II was the Korean War (1950–1953). Richard Hooker's novel *MASH: A Novel About Three Army Doctors* was a black comedy set in Korea during the war; it was later made into a movie and a successful television series.

The U.S. Army Air Force in Joseph Heller's *Catch-22* (1961) is a world of caricatures and tortured logic. But beneath the slapstick, *Catch-22* satirizes greed, gullibility, ambition, corruption, and complacency. Captain Yossarian is at the mercy of corrupt and inept bosses and colleagues. He finally rejects a system that demands infinite loyalty despite its cruelty to the individual. Heller's theme is that of the individual in an irrational, impersonal society, but during the Vietnam War many readers eagerly endorsed military idiocy as the book's actual message.

In Slaughterhouse Five (1969), Kurt Vonnegut shuttles Private Billy Pilgrim between 1945 Dresden, a future America, and a zoo on the planet Tralfamidor. Hardly a straightforward "antiwar" novel, *Slaughterhouse Five* seems to counsel resignation in the face of the world's horrors. Also influenced by science fiction, Thomas Pynchon's avant-garde *Gravity's Rainbow* (1973) focuses on Nazi development of "vengeance weapons" near the end of the war.

War literature has a deep tradition dating back to the Greek and Roman culture, and its representations are as varied as the responses to war in life, solidifying the study as a genre in itself within the rubric of literary history and the contextual analysis of texts. Many universities now offer this genre of study within the corpus of English studies.

Reproduced in part from: The Gale Group, Inc. (2005). Literature, World War II. Retrieved from https://www.encyclopedia.com/defense/energy-government-and-defense-magazines/literature-world-war-ii

Question 1

Based on passage information, we can infer that one key goal of war literature is to:

- O **A.** critique the army leadership structure for inefficiency and ineffective tactics.
- O **B.** promote a pacifistic agenda that suggests violence is never justified.
- O **C.** satirize both antiwar pacifists and pro-war hawks as unrealistic and out of touch.
- O **D.** reveal the negative aspects of war through realistic depictions of army life.

Question 2

Based on the discussion of Catch-22, we can infer that readers' interpretations were affected by a bias against:

- O **A.** U.S. involvement in World War II.
- O **B.** the U.S. military.
- O **C.** violence in any form.
- O **D.** realistic depictions of war.

Question 3

The passage's discussion of war novels suggests that overall, they:

- O **A.** reinforced the individual heroism of the soldier in times of war.
- O **B.** presented a balanced view contrasting the flaws of the army with the good done by U.S. military action.
- O **C.** depicted the harm caused by jingoism.
- O **D.** focused on the horrors of war with little hope of justifying such actions.

Question 4

In *Catch-22*, the famous "catch" is that a soldier can avoid flying dangerous combat missions by being diagnosed as insane, but requesting a psychiatric evaluation is taken as proof of sanity, ensuring that a soldier will be declared fit to fly. From this we can conclude that according to the novel:

- O **A.** the Army is more irrational and cruel than other large institutions.
- O **B.** the Army's "logic" is irrational and frustrates individual desires.
- O **C.** the Army's policies are designed to outsmart the simplistic and naïve thinking of ordinary soldiers.
- O **D.** the Army is more concerned with making policies than with actually conducting the war.

Question 5

Generically, this passage takes the form of:

- O **A.** literary criticism.
- O **B.** historicist criticism.
- O **C.** literary history.
- O **D.** literary theory.

Question 6

Based on the passage, the literary tactics used for creating well-crafted war novels could also be used on all of the following EXCEPT:

- O **A.** a pseudo-memoir about the Hollywood filmmaking process from a crew member's perspective.
- O **B.** a light comedy infusing the life of a lowly trash collector with a sense of romance and heroism.
- O **C.** a satirical novel about a U.S. presidential election.
- O **D.** a mock-heroic tale of trying to get a simple expense report approved in a Byzantine corporate bureaucracy.

Passage 2 (Questions 7–12)

When thinking about the suitability of the 'critical period' concept to the particular case of the acquisition of languages, there exist two preliminary questions that cannot be avoided: (i) What is (and what is not) a critical period for the development of any given organic capacity? (ii) Does language actually belong to the kind of phenomena to which the concept may be aptly applied? Surprisingly enough, an ample majority of the sources on the topic of the critical period for language seem to sidestep both questions. As for the second question, while language is customarily referred to as the target of critical period effects in the relevant literature, what one ultimately discovers is that what is suggested there to be subject to such effects are the putative organic bases underlying the acquisition, storing or use of languages; so on reflection, the corresponding approaches seem to implicitly adhere to the view that languages are not qua languages the locus of critical period effects.

As for the first question, most views seem to conceptualize the critical period for language as a scheduling of sorts, which inadvertently introduces an unacceptable teleological bias into a developmental matter. In this paper, after reviewing the current consensus about why and how language is specifically thought to be a capacity subject to maturational control or critical period effects, we argue that by means of a clarification of the developmental character of languages and, in parallel, of critical period effects in developmental phenomena at large, one may avoid the cumulative odd implications of connecting these two issues.

It has been known for a long time that children are more apt than adults to learn non-native linguistic systems. To wit, Juan Huarte de San Juan, one of the founding figures of the field of Cognitive Psychology, expressed with the following words in 1575 what for many continues to sound as a paradox:

The extent to which imagination and understanding seem to be improper skills in order to learn languages is clearly demonstrated by childhood, for while being the age at which men are the less gifted in them both, yet children, as already observed by Aristotle, learn any single language better than older men, in spite of the latter being more rational. And no one needs to remember us this, for common experience amply shows it, as when a thirty or forty years old native from Biscay [Basque Country] comes to Castile, and he never learns the Romance language, but if he is a child, within two or three years he looks as if born in Toledo. (Huarte de San Juan 1575/1991: 151; authors' translation)

If one wants to learn Latin or any other language, she better does it while still a child, for if she waits until the body becomes rigid and gains its proper perfection, she will never succeed. (Huarte de San Juan 1575/1991: 60; authors' translation)

Efforts at scientifically clarifying this paradox, however, had to wait some four hundred years, after the focus was again put on the question by Wilder Penfield and Lamar Roberts, paving the way to the groundbreaking work of Eric Lenneberg, to whom present conceptions and factual knowledge on the issue are profoundly in debt. As a matter of fact, Lenneberg's landmark postulation of a critical period for language acquisition, as an associated aspect to its maturationally controlled character, was a generalization based on his first-hand observations on the recovery patterns from traumatic aphasias at different age ranges, starting from very young children.

Specifically, he discovered that children before 3 years (re)acquired their mother tongue almost as if they had not suffered any trauma, but that from that point on the following pattern was attested: From 4 to 10 years, gradual (re)acquisition without residual signs of impairment; around 15 years, gradual (re)acquisition with residual signs of impairment; and from 15 years on, unpredictable pattern of recovery, as it is typical of adult aphasias associated to strokes and so on.

From these observations, Lenneberg concluded that a window of opportunity existed for first language acquisition that extended from age 2 until the onset of puberty, out of which normal levels of grammatical competence were not guaranteed at all. The indirectness of Lenneberg's method, far from problematic, was the perfect strategy to remedy the (fortunate) scarcity of related natural experiments—as children almost unexceptionally receive sufficient linguistic stimulation from the very onset of the relevant period, and there are (obvious) ethical impediments to performing them in artificial conditions. Nevertheless, some new cases of feral children were known and studied with care after Lenneberg's untimely death, yet only to confirm his predictions.

Balari, S., & Lorenzo, G. (2015). Should It Stay or Should It Go? A Critical Reflection on the Critical Period for Language. *Biolinguistics*. 9, 8-42.

Question 7

What is the author's view on a critical period for language?

- ○ **A.** The evidence for a critical period is weak because supporting research is indirect and lacking conceptual rigor.
- ○ **B.** Language is subject to critical period effects because if there were not, post-adolescents could reliably learn language.
- ○ **C.** Observational research confirms that there is a window of opportunity for learning languaes, although the research is conceptually weak.
- ○ **D.** Determining whether there is a critical period is not as important as understanding the psychological basis of development.

Question 8

Based on passage information, what are the author's reasons for arguing that "the indirectness of Lenneberg's method [was] far from problematic"?

- ○ **A.** The cases Lennenberg studied mimicked the effects of childhood language deprivation, which occurs very rarely.
- ○ **B.** Direct research is not well suited to linguistics studies.
- ○ **C.** His research was more ethical than those of researchers who experimented on human subjects by depriving them of language.
- ○ **D.** Although indirect research cannot prove anything, it is clinically useful for the treatment of aphasic people.

Question 9

The author refers in paragraph 2 to a "teleological bias." "Telos" refers to an ultimate end or purpose. This critique would be most consistent with which of the following statements?

- ○ **A.** By introducing the concept of scheduling, scholars assume all pre-adolescent language learning results in the goal of perfect fluency.
- ○ **B.** By introducing the concept of scheduling, scholars assume language learning to be a goal of the brain, rather than simply a part of development.
- ○ **C.** Scholars assume language learning will occur if people are exposed to a normal amount of speech during the time window.
- ○ **D.** Scholars are basing their views on their opinion that learning language well is desirable, instead of remaining neutral.

Question 10

Based on passage content, we might expect the later portions of this article to:

- ○ **A.** call into question the notion that language learning is subject to a developmental window.
- ○ **B.** provide a more specific definition of exactly which cognitive abilities are involved in developing the ability to learn a language.
- ○ **C.** argue that people most reliably learn language when they are exposed to it before puberty.
- ○ **D.** question the concept of developmental windows as it relates to all forms of human development.

Question 11

Which of the following hypothetical facts would count as a "paradox" like the one the author mentions in paragraph 3?

- ○ **A.** Children have worse memories than adults, but their preferences in food and flavors are mostly set in childhood.
- ○ **B.** Children heal more quickly from injuries than adults, but have a higher mortality rate.
- ○ **C.** Children have a less perfect command of language than adults, but speak more often.
- ○ **D.** Children are smaller than adults, but eat more compared to their body weight.

Question 12

We might guess that the author cites Juan Huarte de San Juan as "one of the founding figures of the field of Cognitive Psychology" because he:

- O **A.** devised plausible explanation for phenomena that had previously been unexplained.
- O **B.** observed aspects of psychology accurately and minutely.
- O **C.** conducted experiments to study aspects of thought.
- O **D.** devised theories and explanations similar to those we now know to be true.

Note: This page is left blank so that the passage would be visible without turning pages while assessing the passage-based questions.

Passage 3 (Questions 13–17)

I forget what veteran public speaker it was who gave this advice to a beginner: "Write out your speech; and be especially careful about writing the parts in which you give way to your feelings." Though I believe the counsel to be excellent, and, on all important occasions, have acted upon it, I have never committed the written matter to memory. That is for several reasons, though one – that I could not if I tried – is sufficient. Even if I could learn a speech by heart, I agree with Mr. Bright that the burden of going through the process would be intolerable. However, this is a question of idiosyncrasy. I know of at least one admirable speaker who is said to learn every word by heart, and whose charming delivery omits no comma of the original.

The use, to me, of writing, sometimes of rewriting half a dozen times over, that which I threw aside when I had finished it, was to make sure that the framework of what I had to say–its logical skeleton, so to speak–was, so far as I could see, sound and competent to bear all the strain put upon it. I very early discovered that an argument in my head was one thing, and the same argument written out in dry bare propositions quite another in point of trustworthiness. In the latter case, assumptions supposed to be certain while they lay snug in one's brain had a trick of turning out doubtful; consequences which seemed inevitable proved to be less tightly connected with the premises than was desirable; and telling metaphors showed a curious capacity for being turned to account by the other side. I have often written the greater part of an address half a dozen times over, sometimes upsetting the whole arrangement and beginning on new lines, before I felt I had got the right grip on my subject.

A subordinate, but still very important use of writing, when one has to speak, is that the process brings before the mind all the collateral suggestions which are likely to arise out of the line of argument adopted. Psychologically considered, public speaking is a very singular process. One half of the speaker's mind is occupied with what he is saying; the other half with what he is going to say. And if the field of vision of the prospective half is suddenly crossed by some tempting idea which has not already been considered, the speaker is not at all unlikely to follow it. But if he does, Heaven knows where he may turn up; or what bitter reflections may be in store for him, when the report of his speech stares him in the face next morning. Cynical as the latter part of the advice which I have quoted may sound, it is just when the strange intoxication which is begotten by the breathless stillness of a host of absorbed listeners weakens the reason and opens the floodgates of feeling that the check of the calmly considered written judgment tells, even if its exact words are forgotten.

As to notes, my experience may be of interest to that unfortunate mortal the average Englishman, who, as you say, finds it the hardest thing in the world to stand up and speak for ten minutes without looking, or at least feeling, either a fool or a coward. Of that form of suffering I do not believe that the average Englishman knows half as much as I do. For twenty years I never got up to speak without my tongue cleaving to the roof of the mouth; and if the performance was a lecture, without an idée fixe that I should have finished all I had to say long before the expiration of the obligatory hour; and, at first, I clung to my copious MS. as a shipwrecked mariner to a hencoop. My next stage was to use brief but still elaborate notes–not unfrequently, however, having the big MS. in my pocket to fall back upon in case of an emergency, which, by the way, never arose. Then the notes got briefer and briefer, until I have known occasions on which they came down to a paragraph. But the aid and comfort afforded by that not too legible scrawl upon a short sheet of paper was inexpressible.

Twice in my life I have been compelled to swim without floats altogether–to renounce even a sheet of note-paper. On one of these occasions, I had to address an audience to some extent hostile, upon a topic which required very careful handling, and I had taken unusual pains in writing my discourse with the intention of practically reading many parts of it. But the assemblage was a very large one; and when I came face to face with it I saw, at a glance, that, if I meant to be heard, looking at notes was out of the question. So I took my courage in my two hands, put my papers down, and left them untouched; while the discourse, in a way quite unaccountable to me, rolled itself off as if I had been a phonograph, in order and matter, though not in words, as it was written.

In spite of this tolerably plain evidence that if I were put to it I could very well do without notes, I have never willingly been without them–at any rate in my pocket. At public dinners and ordinary public meetings they have long ceased to come out; but, on more serious occasions, I have always had them before me, though I very often forgot to look at them. I think they acted as a charm against that physical nervousness, which I have never quite got over, and the origin of which has always been a puzzle to me. With every respect for the public, I cannot say I ever felt afraid of an audience; and my cold hands and dry mouth used to annoy me when my hearers were only students of my class, as much as at other times. The late Lord Cardwell once told me that Sir Robert Peel never got up to speak in the House of Commons without being in what schoolboys call a "funk;" and I fancy from what I have heard of great speakers that this trouble of their weaker brethren is much better known to them than people commonly suppose.

Huxley, T. (1988, October 24). How to Become an Orator. *Pall Mall Gazette*, 1-2.

Question 13

What is the main topic of this passage?

- O **A.** The importance of relying on written notes when speaking in public
- O **B.** The irrationality of stage fright when speaking in public
- O **C.** The role of written notes as opposed to memorization in public speaking
- O **D.** The difference between novice and experienced public speakers

Question 14

Huxley argues that the writer should think about "collateral suggestions which are likely to arise" because:

- O **A.** if one brings up points one just has just thought of while speaking, they may undermine the point.
- O **B.** this will make the finished speech more comprehensive because it covers related questions.
- O **C.** thinking about possible counter-arguments will allow one to rebut them more effectively.
- O **D.** this will help the writer determine if they point they are trying to make is really accurate.

Question 15

The author overall argues that if one writes out a speech, as opposed to not involving the writing process in speech preparation:

- O **A.** the quality of the speech will be the same, but one will have a paper copy as reassuring backup.
- O **B.** some spontaneity will be lost and it will be more difficult for listeners to hear.
- O **C.** one will be able to deliver a speech with few errors because wording will be pre-determined.
- O **D.** the logic will be more rigorous, even if the actual words change in the delivery.

Question 16

One can infer that potential dangers to the public speaker include which of the following?

I. Giving a speech that is much shorter than the allotted time
II. Ad-libbing pointless or illogical material
III. Making analogies that actually benefit the opposing side

- O **A.** I and II
- O **B.** I, II, III
- O **C.** II only
- O **D.** II and III

Question 17

An analogy that expresses the function of written notes to a speaker like Huxley might be:

- O **A.** a recipe to a first-time cook.
- O **B.** blueprints to an architect.
- O **C.** an inspiration board to a fashion designer.
- O **D.** sheet music to a concert pianist.

Passage 4 (Questions 18–24)

According to a widely accepted view, to be opposed in this book, the empirical sciences can be characterized by the fact that they use "inductive methods," as they are called. According to this view, the logic of scientific discovery would be identical with inductive logic, i.e. with the logical analysis of these inductive methods.

It is usual to call an inference "inductive" if it passes from singular statements (sometimes also called "particular" statements), such as accounts of the results of observations or experiments, to universal statements, such as hypotheses or theories. Now it is far from obvious, from a logical point of view, that we are justified in inferring universal statements from singular ones, no matter how numerous; for any conclusion drawn in this way may always turn out to be false; no matter how many instances of white swans we may have observed, this does not justify the conclusion that all swans are white.

The question whether inductive inferences are justified, or under what conditions, is known as the problem of induction. The problem of induction may also be formulated as the question of the validity or the truth of universal statements which are based on experience, such as the hypotheses and theoretical systems of the empirical sciences. For many people believe that the truth of these universal statements is "known by experience"; yet it is clear that an account of an experience, an observation or the result of an experiment can in the first place be only a singular statement and not a universal one. Accordingly, people who say of a universal statement that we know its truth from experience usually mean that the truth of this universal statement can somehow be reduced to the truth of singular ones, and that these singular ones are known by experience to be true; which amounts to saying that the universal statement is based on inductive inference. Thus to ask whether there are natural laws known to be true appears to be only another way of asking whether inductive inferences are logically justified.

Yet if we want to find a way of justifying inductive inferences, we must first of all try to establish a principle of induction. A principle of induction would be a statement with the help of which we could put inductive inferences into a logically acceptable form. In the eyes of the upholders of inductive logic, a principle of induction is of supreme importance for scientific method: "This principle," says Reichenbach, "determines the truth of scientific theories. To eliminate it from science would mean nothing less than to deprive science of the power to decide the truth or falsity of its theories. Without it, clearly, science would no longer have the right to distinguish its theories from the fanciful and arbitrary creations of the poet's mind."

Now this principle of induction cannot be a purely logical truth like a tautology or an analytic statement. Indeed, if there were such a thing as a purely logical principle of induction, there would be no problem of induction; for in this case, all inductive inferences would have to be regarded as purely logical or tautological transformations, just like inferences in deductive logic. Thus the principle of induction must be a synthetic statement; that is, a statement whose negation is not self-contradictory but logically possible. So the question arises why such a principle should be accepted at all, and how we can justify its acceptance on rational grounds. Some who believe in inductive logic are anxious to point out, with Reichenbach, that "the principle of induction is unreservedly accepted by the whole of science and that no man can seriously doubt this principle in everyday life either." Yet even supposing this were the case, for after all, "the whole of science" might err, I should still contend that a principle of induction is superfluous, and that it must lead to logical inconsistencies.

That inconsistencies may easily arise in connection with the principle of induction should have been clear from the work of Hume; also, that they can be avoided, if at all, only with difficulty. For the principle of induction must be a universal statement in its turn. Thus if we try to regard its truth as known from experience, then the very same problems which occasioned its introduction will arise all over again. To justify it, we should have to employ inductive inferences; and to justify these we should have to assume an inductive principle of a higher order; and so on. Thus the attempt to base the principle of induction on experience breaks down, since it must lead to an infinite regress.

Popper, K. R. (2010). *The logic of scientific discovery*. London: Routledge.

Question 18

Popper's main idea in this passage can be reasonably expressed through which of the following statements?

- O **A.** Deductive logic is preferable to inductive logic.
- O **B.** The methods of empirical science are marked by circular reasoning.
- O **C.** Inductive reasoning is subject to unavoidable logical difficulties.
- O **D.** Only tautological statements can be unreservedly accepted as true.

Question 19

Based on passage information, the problem of induction is best represented by which of the following hypothetical conclusions?

- O **A.** Thunder and lightning were observed to occur consecutively 100 times, so they are not always concurrent (occurring at the same time).
- O **B.** Rain has followed thunder 100 times, so rain always follows thunder
- O **C.** Thunder and lightning were observed to occur within seconds of each other 100 times, so we can hypothesize they are related.
- O **D.** Lightning has struck 100 times in county A but 0 times in the neighboring county B, so it is likely county B will be struck next.

Question 20

Based on passage information, which of the following is tested against experience with observation and experiment?

- O **A.** Inductive logic
- O **B.** Deductive logic
- O **C.** Empirical sciences
- O **D.** Hypotheses and theories

Question 21

According to passage information, the inductive statement would be:

- O **A.** a principle that demonstrates why inductive reasoning is valid.
- O **B.** an example that shows why the conclusion being argued for is true.
- O **C.** the theoretical reasoning behind the claim that inductive reasoning is not valid.
- O **D.** a rule allowing one to distinguish between a good and bad example of inductive reasoning.

Question 22

Which of the following would NOT count as an example of the inductive problem?

- O **A.** A scientist notes that all known species need water to live and determines that if life exists on other planets, they will have water.
- O **B.** A scientist observes a species that reproduces asexually and determines that it is possible for life to exist without sexual reproduction.
- O **C.** A scientist observes that there are no known organisms that live longer than a redwood tree and conclude that the redwood is the longest-lived species.
- O **D.** A person has been taking the bus observes that it never comes on time, and concludes that she does not need to be on time to the bus stop the next day.

Question 23

According to the author, Reichenbach organizes a principle of induction around:

- O **A.** the establishment of logical inferences.
- O **B.** consensus of the scientific community.
- O **C.** logically derived theoretical formulations.
- O **D.** other inductive tautologies.

Question 24

The author's point in arguing that the principle of induction must be a synthetic statement is that:

- O **A.** there is no such thing as a statement that MUST be true.
- O **B.** verifying inductive reasoning through deductive reasoning does not work.
- O **C.** a self-evidently true statement cannot be used to prove the accuracy of a statement that is not self-evidently true.
- O **D.** a statement is true only if its negation is self-contradictory.

Note: This page is left blank so that the passage would be visible without turning pages while assessing the passage-based questions.

Passage 5 (Questions 25–31)

That modern human have language and speech, and that our remote ancestors did not, are two incontrovertible facts. But there is no consensus on when the transition from non-language to language took place, nor any consensus on the species of the first language users. Some authors regard language as the exclusive province of anatomically modern humans [AMH], whereas others argue that at least proto-language in some form, if not full modern language, can be found in some earlier species.

Neanderthals have a key position in this debate, being a late major side branch in human evolution with human-like capacities in many other respects, notably a brain at least as large as ours. Their capacity for language or speech has been discussed in numerous papers over the years, stretching from Lieberman & Crelin (1971) over Schepartz (1993) to Benítez-Burraco et al. (2008) and Barceló-Coblijn (2011). The latter offers what is presented as a "biolinguistic approach" to the issue, but unfortunately the approach is neither comprehensive nor stringent.

Ever since Neanderthals were discovered in the 19th century, there has been a lively debate over whether they are a separate species from us or not — Homo neanderthalensis or Homo sapiens neanderthalensis? I am not going into the naming debate here, as the name per se is irrelevant to the topic of this article; instead I will call Neanderthals 'Neanderthals', and call the people indistinguishable from ourselves 'anatomically modern humans' [AMH].

In this paper, I will explore what fossil, archeological, genetic, and other evidence can, and cannot, say about Neanderthal language. All modern human populations have language, obviously, and there is no evidence of any difference in language capacity between living human populations. Given that language has at least some biological substrate, parsimony (see Section 2.1) implies that the most recent common ancestor of all modern humans had language, and had all the biological prerequisites for language.

The fossil record of AMH goes back to nearly 200,000 years ago in Africa. The molecular data likewise strongly support a common origin for all extant humans somewhere around 100–200,000 years ago. The relation between population divergence times and genetic coalescence times is non-trivial (Hurford & Dediu 2009), but it is hard to reconcile the genetic data with a common ancestor of all modern humans living much less than 100,000 years ago. This is consistent also with fossil and archeological evidence indicating that modern humans had spread across much of the Old World more than 50,000 years ago. It follows that the origin of the human language faculty is very unlikely to be more recent than 100,000 years ago (Johansson 2011). This 100,000-year limit brings us back to a time when Neanderthals and AMH were living side by side, with similar material culture, and quite possibly encountering each other in the Middle East. Did only one of them have language, or both?

As noted in just about every paper ever published on language in prehistory, language does not fossilize. Thus the evidence bearing on Neanderthal language is necessarily indirect, and bridging theories (Botha 2008) are required in order to make inferences about the presence or absence of language in an extinct species. A few general methodological issues are discussed in this section.

Parsimony as a general concept is basically the same as Occam's razor — do not multiply entities needlessly, keep theories as simple as possible, and in the choice between two alternative explanations that both explain the data prefer the simpler one. In the context of inferring the evolutionary history of a group of organisms, parsimony has the more specialized meaning that the simplest history should be preferred, simplest in the sense of requiring the smallest amount of evolutionary change. The main use of parsimony is in choosing between several alternative hypotheses about the branching pattern of the family tree — the pattern minimizing the total amount of evolutionary change is to be preferred.

The general idea is quite old, but it was formalized and elaborated by Hennig (1966) under the label cladistics. A byproduct of the use of parsimony in the choice of family tree hypothesis is that it also supplies inferences about the features of the common ancestor at each branching point of the tree. Parsimony is based on the assumption that evolution is unlikely to repeat itself. In the case of complex features, dependent on multiple co-evolved genes, this is a highly reliable assumption. The evolution of a complex feature is a rare occurrence, so it is very unusual for the same complex feature to evolve twice in different organisms.

The corollary of this is that if we do observe the same complex feature in two related organisms, we can safely assume that it evolved only once, and that their common ancestor possessed it already. In the case of language, this means that any language-related features displayed by for example chimpanzees today, were most likely present already in the common ancestor of us and chimpanzees, and did not evolve for human-level linguistic purposes. This has the corollary that if chimps and modern humans share a feature, then all other species that are also descended from the common ancestor of chimps and modern humans, notably all extinct hominins (including Neanderthals), most likely also possessed that feature. In the absence of positive evidence to the contrary, we can thus safely assume that all features shared by chimps and modern humans were also present in Neanderthals.

Johansson, S. (2013). The Talking Neanderthals: What Do Fossils, Genetics, and Archeology Say? *Biolinguistics,7*, 35-74. Retrieved from https://www.biolinguistics.eu/index.php/biolinguistics/article/view/283/295.

Question 25

The author suggests making inferences on Neanderthal language use based on:

- O **A.** features of anatomically modern humans, since the two are very similar.
- O **B.** features of common ancestor shared by humans and Neanderthals, since Neanderthals evolved from them.
- O **C.** shared features of humans and chimps, according to the parsimony principle.
- O **D.** features of chimps, since Neanderthals evolved from a similar species.

Question 26

Which of the following is NOT a main topic of the passage?

- O **A.** Why other scholars have failed to adequately explore the subject of Neanderthal language
- O **B.** What can be known about possible language capacity of Neanderthals
- O **C.** The most valid sources of information about Neanderthal language abilities
- O **D.** The relationship between humans and Neanderthals

Question 27

The author's main reason for introducing information about the possible time frame for the emergence of anatomically modern humans is to:

- O **A.** point out the difficulty of finding fossil-based evidence for events so remote in time.
- O **B.** point out the uncertainty that exists even in answering relatively simple questions like when the human species first appears.
- O **C.** point out that it is difficult to speculate about the relationship between humans and Neanderthals when we do not know which appeared first.
- O **D.** point out that the language faculty most likely evolved at or before the time that Neanderthals came into existence.

Question 28

The author's point would be most strongly refuted by evidence that:

- O **A.** Neanderthals were hostile to anatomically modern humans, and the two subspecies rarely interacted.
- O **B.** Neanderthals practiced human-like activities such as adorning the body and burying the dead.
- O **C.** it is common in evolution for a trait to disappear and reappear multiple times in the same lineage based on fluctuations in the environment.
- O **D.** the common ancestor of humans, Neanderthals and chimps, was much more similar to chimps than to either of the other two species.

Question 29

Which of the following traits can we infer, based on passage information, would best be studied by making inferences through Occam's Razor?

- ○ **A.** Mating practices and monogamy vs. polygamy
- ○ **B.** Burial practices and treatment of the dead
- ○ **C.** Diet and plant/animal species most commonly eaten
- ○ **D.** Tooth shape and what diet the species was most adapted to

Question 30

Based on passage information, we could be fairly certain that Neanderthals had some speech ability if we knew that:

- ○ **A.** Neanderthals and humans were descended from a common ancestor.
- ○ **B.** language would have been as beneficial to Neanderthals as it was to anatomically modern humans.
- ○ **C.** language abilities can evolve in a relatively short period of time.
- ○ **D.** the ancestors of modern humans could already speak before the species split off from Neanderthals.

Question 31

The author suggests that the principle of parsimony is relevant to family trees because:

- ○ **A.** it suggests that if two species with a common ancestor share a feature, the ancestor did too.
- ○ **B.** it suggests that family trees are generally very simple.
- ○ **C.** it suggests that the amount of evolutionary change between each branching point in the ladder is minimal.
- ○ **D.** it suggests that if a species and its ancestor share a feature, other descendants of the ancestor species will too.

Note: This page is left blank so that the passage would be visible without turning pages while assessing the passage-based questions.

Passage 6 (Questions 32–36)

Kitsch can be defined as the reduction of aesthetic objects or ideas into easily marketable forms. Some theorists of postmodernism see the "kitschification" of culture as one symptom of the postmodern condition. The term can be as difficult to define as its companion term, "camp," since there are so many disparate examples that can be cited as kitsch. Jean Baudrillard provides us with a useful definition: "The kitsch object is commonly understood as one of that great army of 'trashy' objects, made of plaster of Paris [stucco] or some such imitation material: that gallery of cheap junk—accessories, folksy knickknacks, 'souvenirs,' lampshades or fake African masks—which proliferate everywhere, with a preference for holiday resorts and places of leisure." As Baudrillard goes on, "To the aesthetics of beauty and originality, kitsch opposes its aesthetics of simulation: it everywhere reproduces objects smaller or larger than life; it imitates materials (in plaster, plastic, etc.); it apes, forms or combines them discordantly; it repeats fashion without having been part of the experience of fashion."

Kitsch tends to simplify and trivialize complex ideas by reducing them to black-and-white stereotypes. It is oriented to the masses and thus tends towards a lowest-common denominator so that anyone can relate; it tends to be tied to mass consumption and thus to profit-making entertainment. As Baudrillard puts it, "This proliferation of kitsch, which is produced by industrial reproduction and the vulgarization at the level of objects of distinctive signs taken from all registers (the bygone, the 'neo,' the exotic, the folksy, the futuristic) and from a disordered excess of 'ready-made' signs, has its basis, like 'mass culture,' in the sociological reality of the consumer society." Kitsch remains, on the whole, completely unselfconscious and without any political or critical edge. When kitsch becomes especially self-conscious, it begins to tip over into camp.

"Camp" is derived from the French slang term camper, which means "to pose in an exaggerated fashion." Susan Sontag argued in her 1964 notes on "camp" that camp was an attraction to the human qualities which expressed themselves in "failed attempts at seriousness," the qualities of having a particular and unique style, and of reflecting the sensibilities of the era. It involved an aesthetic of artifice rather than of nature. Indeed, hard-line supporters of camp culture have long insisted that "camp is a lie that dares to tell the truth."

With the emergence of postmodernism in the 1980s, the borders between kitsch and high art again became blurred. One development was the approval of what is called "camp taste"—which may be related to, but is not the same as camp when used as a "gay sensibility." Camp, in some circles, refers to an ironic appreciation of that which might otherwise be considered corny, such as singer and dancer Carmen Miranda with her tutti-frutti hats, or otherwise kitsch, such as popular culture events that are particularly dated or inappropriately serious, such as the low-budget science fiction movies of the 1950s and 1960s.

A hypothetical example from the world of painting would be a kitsch image of a deer by a lake. In order to make this camp, one could paint a sign beside it, saying "No Swimming." The majestic or romantic impression of a stately animal would be punctured by humor; the notion of an animal receiving a punishment for the breach of the rule is patently ludicrous. The original, serious sentimentality of the motif is neutralized, and thus it becomes camp.

Much of pop art attempted to incorporate images from popular culture and kitsch. These artists strove to maintain legitimacy by saying they were "quoting" imagery to make conceptual points, usually with the appropriation being ironic. In Italy, a movement arose called the Nuovi-nuovi ("new new"), which took a different route: instead of "quoting" kitsch in an ironic stance, it founded itself in a primitivism, which embraced ugliness and garishness, emulating kitsch as a sort of anti-aesthetic.

Felluga, D. (2011, January 31). Terms used by Postmodernists. *Introductory Guide to Critical Theory*. Purdue U. Retrieved from https://www.cla.purdue.edu/english/theory/postmodernism/terms/termsmainframe.html
Kitsch. (2015, January 18). *Shim-pua marriage - The Art and Popular Culture Encyclopedia*. Retrieved from http://www.artandpopularculture.com/Kitsch
Kitsch. (2007). Retrieved from https://www.cs.mcgill.ca/~rwest/wikispeedia/wpcd/wp/k/Kitsch.htm

Question 32

According to the passage, high-culture artists' use of kitsch elements is defined by:

- O **A.** assimilating low culture and high culture, unrefined art and elitist art.
- O **B.** occupying the nexus between camp and kitsch.
- O **C.** quoting imagery to convey ideas.
- O **D.** co-opting stereotypes and cultural norms.

Question 33

What is the passage's overall purpose?

- O **A.** To critique kitsch
- O **B.** To defend kitsch as a source of artistic inspiration
- O **C.** To distinguish kitsch from camp
- O **D.** To provide a definition of kitsch

Question 34

When kitsch is transformed into camp, it can be reasonably inferred that the resulting work would display:

- O **A.** sarcasm.
- O **B.** parody.
- O **C.** horrifying or frightening elements.
- O **D.** surrealism.

Question 35

According to passage information, kitsch can be identified because it:

I. copies sophisticated ideas without finesse.
II. always has a political or critical aspect.
III. is oriented toward people who are not knowledgeable about a technique or style.

- O **A.** I and II
- O **B.** II only
- O **C.** II and III
- O **D.** I and III

Question 36

Which of the following would NOT constitute an example of kitsch becoming camp similar to the example in paragraph 5?

- O **A.** Remaking a sentimental family sitcom to include self-aware jokes about genre conventions.
- O **B.** A melodramatic female movie role being reprised by a male drag performer.
- O **C.** A comedy television show poking fun at the stylistic features of infomercials and reality television.
- O **D.** A popular humorous slogan from postcards and t-shirts being converted into a meme and shared widely on social media.

Passage 7 (Questions 37–42)

In most modern instances, interpretation amounts to the philistine refusal to leave the work of art alone. Real art has the capacity to make us nervous. By reducing the work of art to its content and then interpreting that, one tames the work of art. Interpretation makes art manageable, conformable.

This philistinism of interpretation is more rife in literature than in any other art. For decades now, literary critics have understood it to be their task to translate the elements of the poem or play or novel or story into something else. Sometimes a writer will be so uneasy before the naked power of his art that he will install within the work itself - albeit with a little shyness, a touch of the good taste of irony - the clear and explicit interpretation of it. Thomas Mann is an example of such an overcooperative author. In the case of more stubborn authors, the critic is only too happy to perform the job.

The work of Kafka, for example, has been subjected to a mass ravishment by no less than three armies of interpreters. Those who read Kafka as a social allegory see case studies of the frustrations and insanity of modern bureaucracy and its ultimate issuance in the totalitarian state. Those who read Kafka as a psychoanalytic allegory see desperate revelations of Kafka's fear of his father, his castration anxieties, his sense of his own impotence, his thralldom to his dreams. Those who read Kafka as a religious allegory explain that K. in *The Castle* is trying to gain access to heaven, that Joseph K. in *The Trial* is being judged by the inexorable and mysterious justice of God. Another oeuvre that has attracted interpreters like leeches is that of Samuel Beckett. Beckett's delicate dramas of the withdrawn consciousness - pared down to essentials, cut off, often represented as physically immobilized - are read as a statement about modern man's alienation from meaning or from God, or as an allegory of psychopathology.

Proust, Joyce, Faulkner, Rilke, Lawrence, Gide... one could go on citing author after author; the list is endless of those around whom thick encrustations of interpretation have taken hold. But it should be noted that interpretation is not simply the compliment that mediocrity pays to genius. It is, indeed, the modern way of understanding something, and is applied to works of every quality. Thus, in the notes that Elia Kazan published on his production of *A Streetcar Named Desire*, it becomes clear that, in order to direct the play, Kazan had to discover that Stanley Kowalski represented the sensual and vengeful barbarism that was engulfing our culture, while Blanche Du Bois was Western civilization, poetry, delicate apparel, dim lighting, refined feelings and all, though a little the worse for wear to be sure. Tennessee Williams' forceful psychological melodrama now became intelligible: it was about something, about the decline of Western civilization. Apparently, were it to go on being a play about a handsome brute named Stanley Kowalski and a faded mangy belle named Blanche Du Bois, it would not be manageable.

It doesn't matter whether artists intend, or don't intend, for their works to be interpreted. Perhaps Tennessee Williams thinks Streetcar is about what Kazan thinks it to be about. It may be that Cocteau in *The Blood of a Poet* and in *Orpheus* wanted the elaborate readings which have been given these films, in terms of Freudian symbolism and social critique. But the merit of these works certainly lies elsewhere than in their "meanings." Indeed, it is precisely to the extent that Williams' plays and Cocteau's films do suggest these portentous meanings that they are defective, false, contrived, lacking in conviction.

It is always the case that interpretation of this type indicates a dissatisfaction (conscious or unconscious) with the work, a wish to replace it by something else.

Interpretation, based on the highly dubious theory that a work of art is composed of items of content, violates art. It makes art into an article for use, for arrangement into a mental scheme of categories.

Sontag, S. (1966). *Against Interpretation*. Farrar, Straus and Giroux.

Question 37

Which of the following is a possible implied weakness of the play A Streetcar Named Desire?

- O **A.** It lacks a meaning.
- O **B.** It is overly melodramatic.
- O **C.** It suggests an overblown meaning for the events it portrays.
- O **D.** The events and story of the play seem unrealistic and lack conviction.

Question 38

What can BEST be inferred about the artist's "intention" based on passage information?

- O **A.** It is not necessarily important since authors can be wrong about the meaning of their work.
- O **B.** It is important because authors' desire for their work to be read straightforwardly should not be ignored.
- O **C.** Critics assume their contrived interpretations reflect what authors really intended, but they are wrong.
- O **D.** Critics should respect author's desire for their works not to be interpreted.

Question 39

Which of the following is a possible weakness of Sontag's argument?

- O **A.** She fails to provide examples for her general statements.
- O **B.** She equates forms of criticism that are in opposition to each other and have many incompatible assumptions.
- O **C.** She fails to provide alternative accounts for the meaning of the texts she discusses.
- O **D.** She fails to consider forms of interpretations that describe the meaning of the events of a text.

Question 40

From passage information, how are literary analysts characterized?

- O **A.** Parasitic
- O **B.** Unimaginative
- O **C.** Relativistic
- O **D.** Objective

Question 41

The author's use of the term "philistine" ("a person who is hostile or indifferent to culture and the arts") implies that critics are:

- O **A.** under-appreciative or under-valuing of a work of art.
- O **B.** ignorant of the traditions of criticism surrounding a work.
- O **C.** insensitive to the nuances and stylistic features of a work.
- O **D.** remote and critically detached from the work of art.

Question 42

Based on her comments about "the highly dubious theory that a work of art is composed of items of content," Sontag would likely approve of:

- O **A.** a work exploring how a work reflects the author's biography.
- O **B.** a work discussing the strengths and weaknesses of other critics' interpretations.
- O **C.** a work that explores how a work's formal features contribute to its emotional impact.
- O **D.** a book comparing two political writers and discussing their overall political viewpoints.

Passage 8 (Questions 43–47)

The debate on domestic spying contains important considerations of both a legal and normative nature. From the legal viewpoint, the Bush administration insisted that it had the power to authorize the wiretapping program under both the U.S. Constitution and the congressional resolution of the Authorization of Military Force that authorized use of wartime powers against those responsible for the 9/11 terrorist attacks. The constitutional powers of the U.S. President as commander-in-chief would allow President Bush to pursue, without explicit congressional permission, any enemy operating inside the U.S. Additionally, the wartime powers of the President would allow him to bypass the courts to spy on Americans without warrants, a Presidential power that not even Congress can restrict, as the President has not only the authority but also the duty to protect the nation. It is further argued that the Congressional resolution on the Authorization of Military Force that passed shortly after 9/11 also granted the President the right to use all 'necessary and appropriate force,' thereby effectively suspending the FISA requirements which are considered outdated and inappropriate in view of the contemporary war on terror. When President Bush in a televised address admitted that he had authorized domestic, warrant-less monitoring of calls involving an overseas party, he defended his actions as crucial to national security.

Opponents argue that the President's expansion of executive power violates constitutionally framed mandates for judicial and congressional oversight. Congress and the courts have a constitutional right and obligation to provide a check against extra-legal activities in the executive branch. The uncovered domestic spying programs, they claim, violate Fourth-Amendment protections against illegal search and seizure. The Supreme Court has likewise held that most surveillance by government agencies must be based on a judicial finding of probable cause of criminal wrongdoing.

Other arguments against domestic spying invoke concerns over two specific federal acts. First, critics say the program violates provisions of the 1978 FISA Act which requires warrants. The USA PATRIOT Act only allows for the collection of data for up to 72 hours before a warrant must be requested from the courts, and the Authorization of Military Force resolution does not give the President the power to bypass this law. Second, because only eight members of the House and Senate were briefed about relevant developments, the NSA program violates the National Security Act of 1947 which requires that intelligence oversight committees of Congress be kept informed of U.S. intelligence activities. Absent such congressional approval, prosecutions of captured terrorists may be jeopardized by defendants' claims that the evidence against them was collected illegally. In August 2006, a U.S. District Court ruled the NSA surveillance program to be unconstitutional. At this writing, an appeal is still pending.

Underlying the legal debate on domestic spying are conflicting positions about its normativity. On the one hand, proponents suggest that special surveillance programs are necessary because of the severity and nature of the current terrorist threat and, moreover, that they have effectively prevented other terrorist attacks on U.S. soil. Under present-day circumstances, they claim, most Americans would agree that some of their rights have to be sacrificed in order to preserve national security. On the other hand, opponents argue measures implemented against terrorist groups should not curb civil rights, which are an essential part of a free and open society. Making exceptions on constitutional restrictions on presidential power in the area of counter-terrorism might lead to wrongly justify other special provisions, such as on the use of torture and the indefinite detention of citizens. Modernizing the rules of counter-terrorism surveillance in the United States could allow for the use of new means but only within proper limits that prevent innocent citizens from being investigated.

Given the continued anxieties over the terrorist threat and the likewise persistent concerns over civil rights, the debate on domestic spying is likely to stay in the public consciousness for some time in the foreseeable future.

Deflem, M., & Dilks, L. (2008). Terrorism, Domestic Spying. *Encyclopedia of Social Problems*, 931-933. Thousand Oaks, CA: Sage Publications.

Question 43

In context, the debate over whether wiretapping is "normative" refers to what?

- A. Whether wiretapping will become normal or just be a fluke
- B. Whether wiretapping is legal or illegal
- C. Whether it conforms to how things ought to be
- D. Whether it will set a precedent for the future

Question 44

Which of the pieces of hypothetical evidence listed below would diminish the claims of opponents of domestic spying and surveillance?

- A. Some Americans do not care if their communication is monitored by third parties in the government.
- B. Issues of national security are subject to the review of Congress.
- C. Counter-terrorism measures have not led to investigation of innocent people or erosion of civil rights in other areas.
- D. The information collected through surveillance has not been used for any illicit or non-terrorism-related purposes.

Question 45

Both proponents and opponents of domestic spying, in relation to 9/11, rely on certain key assumptions. Proponents insist that domestic spying is necessary for national security purposes while opponents insist domestic spying:

- A. impedes national security.
- B. should be subject to a popular vote before it becomes policy.
- C. is a violation of the US citizens' rights.
- D. targets mostly people who are not guilty of any wrongdoing.

Question 46

How is the author's purpose in writing the passage supported?

- A. Through a focus on the historical sequences of legislation passed concerning domestic spying.
- B. Through a balance of arguments for both sides involved.
- C. Through a focus on the need for tighter security in response to terrorism.
- D. Through real and hypothetical examples and characterizations.

Question 47

The passage emphasizes that domestic spying is a controversial action within the U.S. marked by a debate concerning:

- A. the Fourth Amendment and justice.
- B. civil liberties and personal freedom.
- C. surveillance of criminals and international terrorism.
- D. civil liberties and national security.

Passage 9 (Questions 48–53)

College students majoring in STEM (science, technology, engineering, and mathematics) fields study a relatively well-defined mathematics curriculum, which usually includes calculus-based skills that they will use regularly in their careers. Recently, there has been tremendous attention and funding directed toward students in these majors, in particular those who are enrolled in "gateway" courses such as first-semester calculus. But what of the rest of the students, those who have chosen a major outside of STEM? These students greatly outnumber their STEM peers among all college students.

Of these students, who among them are required to take a single semester-long mathematics course for the sole purpose of fulfilling their general education requirements? This population of students comprises a large proportion of the student body at colleges and universities. Many colleges and universities have specific courses that are designed to address the needs of these students. Usually, this type of course is a single-semester (or quarter) course specifically intended for "liberal arts" majors to fulfill a general education (GE) requirement. For many of these students, this is the last formal exposure that they will have to mathematics. As educators, this is one of the last settings that we have to expose students to the beauty of mathematics, its relevance to daily life regardless of career choice, and the joy that can be found in problem solving. The impressions and perceptions formed by students in such a terminal course in a bachelor's degree program may influence their attitude towards mathematics for the rest of their lives, and in turn, the lives of their children.

In this paper, I study the effect that such a course has on students. I ask: Does a positive experience in the course correlate with a positive change in the students' attitudes towards mathematics? What aspects of such a course can influence such a change? Effecting such a change in attitude is particularly difficult. Clearly students majoring in a non-STEM discipline who need to fulfill their mathematics GE requirements are the raison d'etre for such a course. But it is quite common that the typical student in such a context had a bad experience with math at some point in the past, be it with a math teacher or a particularly difficult concept, or just has a feeling of having "fallen off the wagon" and being unable to ever get back on.

The single most important course aspect identified by students as having a positive or very positive effect on their course experience was the teacher or professor. This was true in both the Likert-style section about different course aspects, and in analyzing the free responses written by students. Other factors that students identified as especially important for success were course difficulty and workload. The strong direct correlations between these course aspects and students' overall experience show that focusing on improving these aspects of the course will have the most pronounced positive effect on students. Although students reported that time working in groups and online homework affected them negatively, there was no significant correlation observed between these course aspects and reported overall course experience. Therefore, we conclude that while many course aspects were reported as having either a positive or negative effect on the student, the aspects of professor/teacher, course difficulty, and workload yielded the most significant correlations with overall experience.

Although it was not intentionally addressed in the research question, we did find that students' responses to questions about confidence in solving mathematics problems in general is different from their responses to "I identify myself as a math person." This shows that on average, even if a student feels confident solving mathematics problems and feels that they are able to "do math," they still do not identify themselves as a "math person"! This corroborates the perception that there are people who have a "math brain" and other people who simply do not. Indeed, even if a student specifically feels that they have the ability to "do math," they will not self-identify as a "math person." This dichotomous perception is one of the most deep-seated beliefs held by students about their so-called mathematical abilities.

Clinkenbeard, J. (2015). Attitudes and Experiences in Liberal Arts Mathematics. *Journal of Humanistic Mathematics,5*(2), 26-50. doi:10.5642/jhummath.201502.04

Question 48

According to passage information, potential problems facing math educators include all of the following EXCEPT:

- ○ **A.** students who do not identify with the subject matter.
- ○ **B.** students who have had bad experiences in the past with the subject matter.
- ○ **C.** courses which are not designed for the type of student who actually takes it.
- ○ **D.** students who find the subject matter too hard.

Question 49

An assumption of the writer about math skills is that:

- ○ **A.** students who have a negative attitude to math will never learn to do it well.
- ○ **B.** ability and appreciation for math is within reach of everyone, just a particular type.
- ○ **C.** mathematics should be learned primarily for its practical benefits in life and the workplace.
- ○ **D.** mathematics is a uniquely difficult subject to teach because student reactions are largely shaped by the difficulty of the material.

Question 50

The main purpose of the passage is to:

- ○ **A.** explain how math can be made more appealing to liberal students.
- ○ **B.** detail the difficulties college math teachers have getting through to students.
- ○ **C.** describe a study that was conducted on making college math courses for liberal arts students more effective.
- ○ **D.** argue that poor teaching is a key element in making students resistant to math.

Question 51

Based on passage information, we might expect teachers trying to follow the writer's advice to:

I. focus on building confidence.
II. instill ability in basic skills by assigning extensive drills and homework.
III. tailor the difficulty level to students' actual abilities.

- ○ **A.** I
- ○ **B.** I and II
- ○ **C.** II and III
- ○ **D.** I and III

Question 52

Based on passage information, we might expect STEM majors to struggle in humanities courses if they do any of the following EXCEPT:

- ○ **A.** believe succeeding in humanities classes requires a unique form of creativity.
- ○ **B.** are assigned papers that are much longer and require more research than any they have ever written before.
- ○ **C.** have not taken a humanities class in a long time.
- ○ **D.** know that the course they are taking will be their last in the subject area.

Question 53

The author's final point in paragraph 5 is introduced mainly to suggest that:

- ○ **A.** students must abandon the idea that math requires a "math brain" to do well in the subject.
- ○ **B.** it is surprising that even confident students may consider themselves separate from truly skilled math students.
- ○ **C.** the study should have addressed the question of whether successful students identify as "math people."
- ○ **D.** some educators mistakenly believe that students must possess a "math brain" to do well in the subject.

CANDIDATE'S NAME ___________________________

RAW SCORE AND SCALED SCORE ___________________

GS-5
Mock Exam 5 of 7
Solutions at MCAT-prep.com

GS-5 Section III: Biological and Biochemical Foundations of Living Systems

Questions: 1-59
Time: 95 minutes

INSTRUCTIONS: Of all the questions on this test, most are organized into groups preceded by a passage. After evaluating the passage, select the best answer to each question in the group. Fifteen questions are independent of any descriptive passage or each other. Similarly, select the best answer to these questions. If you are unsure of an answer, eliminate the alternatives that you know to be incorrect and select an answer from the remaining alternatives. To indicate your selection, use a pencil to blacken the corresponding circle next to the answer choice and/or you can use the answer document at the back of this book. No marks are deducted for wrong answers.

The computer-based real MCAT has an on-screen highlighter function and ~~STRIKEOUT~~ function. These tools help to spotlight text or assist in the process of elimination. You may use a yellow highlighter for this paper-based exam and/or a pen (or preferably a pencil to make it easier should you change your mind) to mark text. At the time of publishing, both highlighting and strikeout functions can be used for passages, questions and answer choices. You can also flag a question to review later should time remain.

For the real exam, you will be provided with a dry erase board which is a white laminated noteboard booklet accompanied by a fine point marker. The noteboard includes 9 graph-lined pages for you to write though you cannot erase. You can simulate the experience with a fine point marker on a noteboard or with 8” x 14” plain graph paper.

You may consult the periodic table at any point during the science subtests.

Please note: For the real MCAT, a small number of field-tested questions will remain unscored.

This practice test has been designed exclusively to test knowledge and thinking skills. This exam may contain hypothetical statements and/or express controversial ideas. Statements contained herein do not necessarily reflect the policy, position, or view of RuveneCo Inc. or MCAT-prep.com.

START EXAM ONLY WHEN TIMER IS READY.

Passage 1 (Questions 1–5)

Proteases have been discovered in every kingdom in nature, and many have been characterized in terms of form and function over the last few decades. These enzymes fall into six broad groups, and differ widely not only structurally, but also mechanistically. However, all have one thing in common - proteases are able to perform proteolysis, a process that involves the hydrolysis of the peptide bond between specific amino acids in a polypeptide chain.

Thus proteases engage in protein catabolism by digesting longer molecular chains into shorter fragments. Some proteases detach the terminal amino acids from a polypeptide chain (exopeptidases, such as aminopeptidases, carboxypeptidase A); others attack internal peptide bonds of a polypeptide chain (endopeptidases, such as chymotrypsin, and the other proteases shown in Table 1).

Depending on the enzyme, the specificity of proteases ranges significantly but all proteases cleave peptide bonds at specific locations. Some require a specific amino acid sequence or motif, while others will cleave indiscriminately at certain residues - trypsin, for example, targets exposed lysines and arginines.

Table 1 shows a list of proteases commonly used in the laboratory. Each cleavage site is marked with the symbol •. Different cleavage sites are separated by commas (,), while continuous sequences are marked by hyphens (-). "X" denotes any amino acid.

Table 1 Common proteases and their associated cleavage sites

Protease	Cleavage Sites
Chymotrypsin	Trp•-X, Tyr•-X, Phe•-X, Leu•-X
Cyanogen bromide	Met•-X
Papain	[Hydrophobic]-[Arg OR Lys] •-[Any amino acid except Val]
Thrombin	Arg•-Gly
Trypsin	Lys•-X, Arg•-X

Figure 1 Examples of hydrolysis sites for two proteases

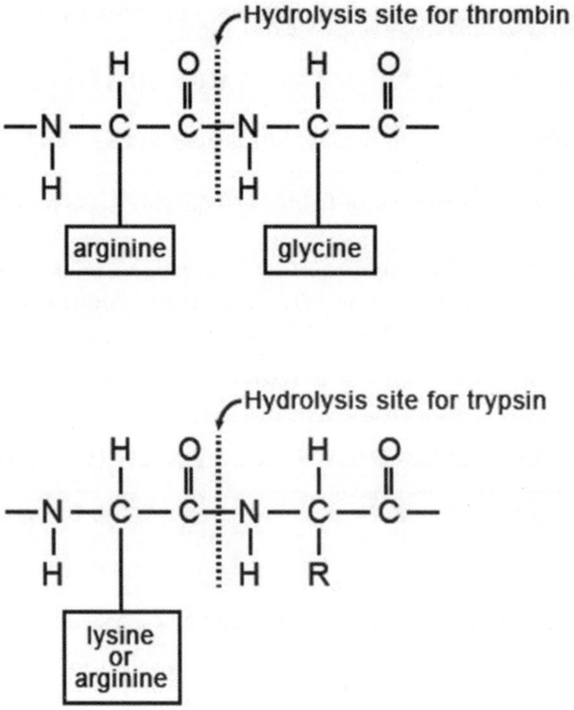

Question 1

Proteases function by:

- O **A.** dehydrating a peptide bond.
- O **B.** attacking hydrogen bonds.
- O **C.** adding a water molecule to the carbon in a peptide bond.
- O **D.** separating hydroxyls.

Question 2

Chymotrypsin cleaves:

- O **A.** at the C-terminal side of tyrosine.
- O **B.** at the N-terminal side of tryptophan but not the C-terminal side.
- O **C.** between adjacent tryptophan and tyrosine residues only.
- O **D.** preferentially at charged residues.

Question 3

Which of the following sequences would be digested by papain?

- O **A.** Ala-Lys-Val
- O **B.** Val-Lys-Val
- O **C.** Phe-Arg-Trp
- O **D.** Lys-Arg-Trp

Question 4

The following peptide is digested with both cyanogen bromide and trypsin: Ala-Phe-Ile-Met-Gln-Gln-Met-Arg-Val-Lys-Ser-Thr-Arg-Glu-Asn-Cys-Gly

How many fragments will result?

- O **A.** 4
- O **B.** 5
- O **C.** 6
- O **D.** 7

Question 5

An octopeptide was analyzed and found to contain the following amino acids: 2 Arg, 1 Glu, 1 Ser, 1 Met, 1 Trp, 1 Lys, 1 Gly

The native octopeptide was first digested with papain, which resulted in a pentapeptide and a tripeptide. UV analysis showed that the pentapeptide was the only fragment that contained an aromatic ring. Another test, which specifically stains for carboxylic acids, shows that only the tripeptide contains an additional carboxylic acid functional group, and analysis demonstrated that glycine was in the third position of the tripeptide. Further digestion with trypsin yielded four fragments of varying sizes: 2 monopeptides, 1 dipeptide, and 1 tetrapeptide. Finally, all fragments were digested with cyanogen bromide, which resulted in 5 total fragments: 2 monopeptides and 3 dipeptides.

The native sequence would be most consistent with which of the following?

- O **A.** Met-Arg-Ser-Trp-Lys-Glu-Gly-Arg
- O **B.** Arg-Ser-Met-Trp-Lys-Glu-Arg-Gly
- O **C.** Arg-Arg-Gly-Lys-Glu-Met-Ser-Trp
- O **D.** Trp-Arg-Gly-Met-Ser-Trp-Lys-Arg

Passage 2 (Questions 6–9)

Many forms of cancer have been discovered to be caused by exposure to chemicals and as such have been termed carcinogens. Approximately 80% of all human cancers are caused by carcinogens. These chemical agents may act in several different mechanisms to alter the state of the cell and allow unlimited cell proliferation. Some chemicals are able to mutate essential enzymes of the cell, but the most common mechanism of carcinogens involves intercalation into DNA.

One of the most rapid and effective bacterial assays to test for carcinogenicity is known as the Ames test, developed by Bruce Ames. This test uses special strains of Salmonella typhimurium which are incapable of synthesising histidine, so that they are unable to grow in the absence of histidine as a nutrient. In addition, their DNA repair mechanisms are also rendered inactive.

The Ames test uses approximately 10^9 bacteria, which are spread on a culture plate that lacks histidine. The carcinogen to be tested is then applied to the culture plate and will cause some of the histidine-deficient bacteria to revert back to being able to synthesise histidine. These bacteria will grow to form visible colonies on the plate. The mutagenicity of a chemical can thus be calculated as the number of these colonies minus the number of colonies that spontaneously revert on a culture plate lacking the mutagen.

Figure 1 illustrates the Ames test performed on 3 different carcinogens (plates 1-3).

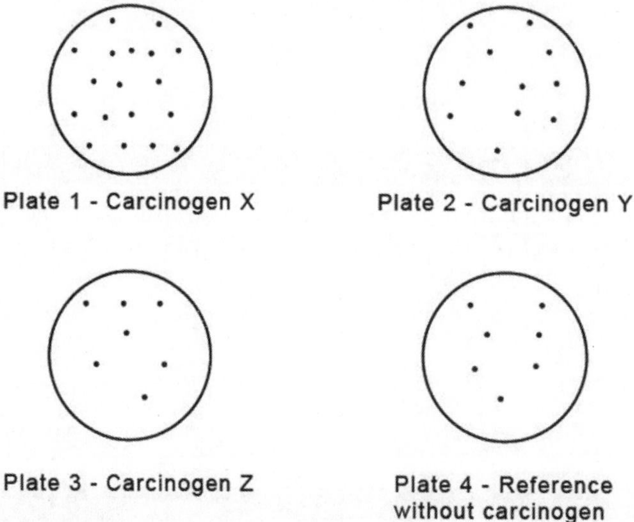

Figure 1 Experiment using the Ames test with carcinogens X, Y, Z on plates 1, 2, 3, respectively.

Question 6

If the DNA repair mechanism of the bacteria was NOT rendered inactive how would the results change?

○ **A.** There would be more colonies than what is observed.
○ **B.** There would be fewer colonies than what is observed.
○ **C.** There would be no change in the number of colonies.
○ **D.** There would be more colonies only on Plate 4.

Question 7

The Ames test relies largely on the fact that the carcinogen:

○ **A.** will mutate the gene responsible for histidine synthesis back to its original form.
○ **B.** will create a new enzyme capable of synthesising histidine.
○ **C.** will further mutate the enzyme responsible for histidine synthesis.
○ **D.** will mutate the protein responsible for histidine synthesis back to its original form.

Question 8

Which carcinogen has the highest mutagenicity?

- O **A.** Carcinogen X
- O **B.** Carcinogen Y
- O **C.** Carcinogen Z
- O **D.** All are equally mutagenic.

Question 9

What is the driving force behind the colonies formed in Plate 4?

- O **A.** Carcinogens in the culture media
- O **B.** Random spontaneous mutations in bacteria
- O **C.** Carcinogens arising from the decomposition of some of the bacteria
- O **D.** Reactivation of the DNA repair mechanism

The following questions are NOT based on a descriptive passage (Questions 10–13).

Question 10

Consider Figure 1.

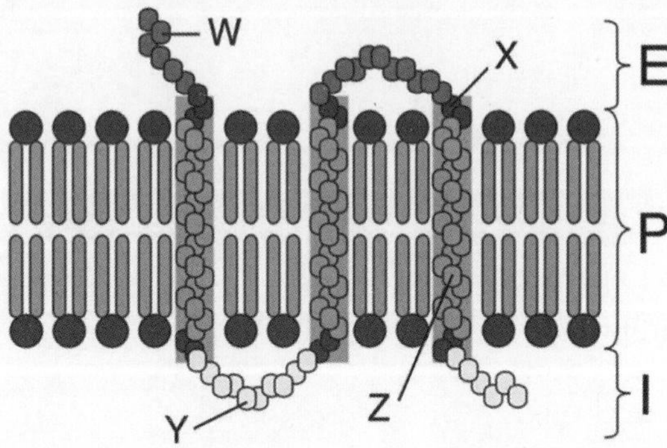

Figure 1 Transmembrane receptor in its native state with four zones indicated as W, X, Y and Z. E = extracellular space; P = plasma membrane; I = intracellular space

If mutants were evaluated which resulted in the substitution of a single amino acid, which of the following zones is paired with a change that would result in the largest decrease in entropic penalty?

- O **A.** Zone W: Glu to Tyr
- O **B.** Zone X: Pro to Gly
- O **C.** Zone Y: Phe to Lys
- O **D.** Zone Z: Asn to Thr

Question 11

In the process of osmosis, the net flow of water molecules into or out of the cell depends primarily on the differences in the:

- O **A.** concentration of protein on either side of the cell membrane.
- O **B.** concentration of solute molecules on either side of the cell membrane.
- O **C.** rate of molecular transport on either side of the cell membrane.
- O **D.** rate of movement of ions inside the cell.

Question 12

Consider the following diagram.

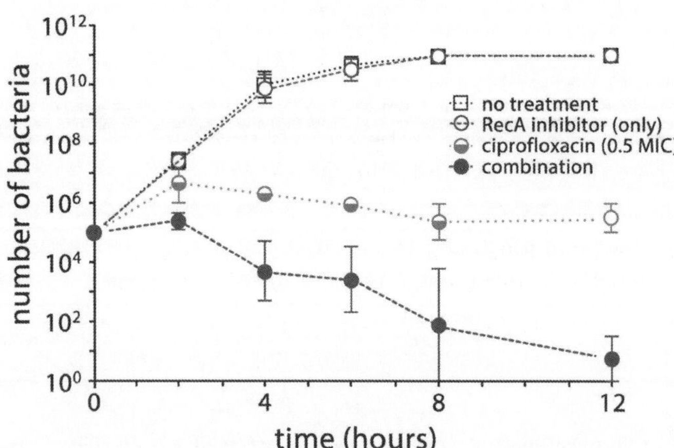

Figure 1 Synergy between the antibiotic ciprofloxacin and a RecA inhibitor in killing *E. coli* bacteria.

The greatest decline in *E. coli* numbers occurs between hour 2 and hour 8 in which of the following trials?

- O **A.** No treatment
- O **B.** RecA inhibitor (only)
- O **C.** Ciprofloxacin (0.5 MIC)
- O **D.** Combination

Question 13

Which of the following are LEAST appropriately matched?

- O **A.** Activation energy - entropy
- O **B.** Endergonic reaction - anabolism
- O **C.** Reduction - gain of an electron
- O **D.** Anabolic reactions - expend energy

Passage 3 (Questions 14–17)

Antigens are chemical substances (usually proteins) that when introduced into the body cause an immune response. Lymphocytes are responsible for much of the body's immunity; they differentiate into B cells and T cells. Some B cells differentiate into antibody producing plasma cells. Antibodies combine with antigens to form an antibody-antigen complex.

Some T cells differentiate into cytotoxic T cells which engulf and destroy antibody-antigen complexes.

Three experiments were performed to study the effect of the thymus gland on the development of immune system cells in mice.

Experiment 1

The thymuses of newborn mice were radiolabeled and transplanted into unradiolabeled newborns whose thymuses had been removed. Within one week, 90% of the radiolabel was located in the lymphatic tissue (connective tissue that contains large numbers of lymphocytes; functions in the surveillance and defense from foreign materials) of the transplant recipient mice.

Experiment 2

Thymus cells were removed from nine day old and fifteen day old mice. The cells were grown in culture, and checked every day for T cell development. T cells only developed in the fifteen day old mice.

Experiment 3

A thymectomy (thymus removal) was performed on both newborn and adult mice. The table below shows the results on both sample groups following the procedure.

	newborns	adults
Able to produce some T cells	no	yes
Able to produce all T cells	no	yes
Able to produce some antibodies	yes	yes
Able to produce all antibodies	no	yes
Able to reject foreign tissue	no	yes

Question 14

Which of the following experiments directly supports the conclusion that the immune system of newborn mice is compromised by the removal of the thymus?

- O **A.** 1 only
- O **B.** 3 only
- O **C.** 1 and 3 only
- O **D.** 2 and 3 only

Question 15

All of the following are implicit assumptions of Experiment 2, EXCEPT which of the following?

- O **A.** Growing cells in culture, as opposed to *in vivo*, will not have a deleterious effect.
- O **B.** Nine day old and fifteen day old cells develop in equivalent stages.
- O **C.** The concentration of cells removed from the thymuses were equivalent.
- O **D.** A total time period of two weeks is an adequate period of time for the nine day old cells to differentiate into T cells.

Question 16

Experiment 1 assumes that the thymuses were NOT affected by:

I. the transplantation.
II. the radiolabel.
III. the age of the mice.

- O **A.** I and II only
- O **B.** II and III only
- O **C.** I and III only
- O **D.** I, II , and III

Question 17

All of the following could explain the rejection of foreign tissue by the bodies of adult mice, **EXCEPT**:

- O **A.** uncontrolled cell growth at the site of tissue transplantation.
- O **B.** antibody-antigen complex formation.
- O **C.** phagocytosis by neutrophils.
- O **D.** phagocytosis by macrophages.

Passage 4 (Questions 18–21)

Phenylketonuria, or PKU disease, is a recessive autosomal genetic condition which involves symptoms of mental retardation, short stature, and lack of pigment. The normal gene at the PKU locus produces the liver enzyme phenylalanine hydroxylase, which is required for the metabolism of the amino acid phenylalanine into tyrosine.

Individuals homozygous for the PKU gene cannot produce this enzyme. Given a diet which contains normal levels of phenylalanine, the serum levels of phenylalanine in individuals with PKU rises dramatically. Excess phenylalanine interferes with the production of the myelin sheath of the nerve cells in the brain.

DNA sequence analysis of the normal and abnormal alleles has been done. Only four alleles would need to be identified in order to detect 50% of the PKU cases in the United States. Tests for PKU could be carried out by a single, automated DNA-based method as opposed to current methods which require a variety of technical skills and interpretive abilities. Once the alleles have been identified, the disease's effect can be avoided if a diet low in phenylalanine is provided.

Question 18

Destruction of the myelin sheath would have which of the following effects?

- O **A.** Decrease in the movement of potassium ions into the nerve cell
- O **B.** Decrease in the potentiation of neural impulses
- O **C.** Increase in the cellular metabolism of Schwann cells
- O **D.** Increase in the level of neurotransmitters in nerve cells

Question 19

If individuals with PKU disease lack the protein phenylalanine hydroxylase, what would best explain their being able to metabolize small amounts of phenylalanine?

- O **A.** Non-specific enzymes cleave phenylalanine.
- O **B.** Phenylalanine catalyzes reactions in the liver.
- O **C.** Phenylalanine is broken down mechanically in the formation of chyme in the stomach.
- O **D.** Phenylalanine is defecated from the body.

Question 20

Phenylalanine hydroxylase most likely:

- O **A.** cleaves a $-OCH_3$ group from phenylalanine.
- O **B.** adds a $-OCH_3$ group to phenylalanine.
- O **C.** cleaves a $-OH_2$ group from phenylalanine.
- O **D.** adds a -OH group to phenylalanine.

Question 21

DNA isolated from parents reacted with normal specific and abnormal specific probes in the following manner:

	normal specific	abnormal specific
mother	reaction	reaction
father	no reaction	reaction

A male offspring of the couple represented in the table above could potentially be which of the following?

I. PKU disease positive
II. PKU disease negative, PKU gene carrier
III. PKU disease negative, PKU gene non-carrier

- O **A.** I only
- O **B.** I and II only
- O **C.** I and III only
- O **D.** II and III only

Passage 5 (Questions 22–27)

Glycogen is a branched polysaccharide built of D-glucose monosaccharides. Glycogen serves as the main carbohydrate storage in animal cells. In humans, glycogen is stored in the liver and in the muscles. When the body needs energy, glycogen is broken down to glucose monomers, which are utilized during cell respiration to produce ATP. Glycogen phosphorylase (GP) is an enzyme that catalyzes phosphorolysis, a rate-limiting step of glycogen degradation. During phosphorolysis, α-1,4-glucose (α-1,4-Glc) residues are phosphorylated to form α-D-glucose-1-phosphate (Glc-1-P), which could serve as a readout when measuring GP activity (*see* Figure 1).

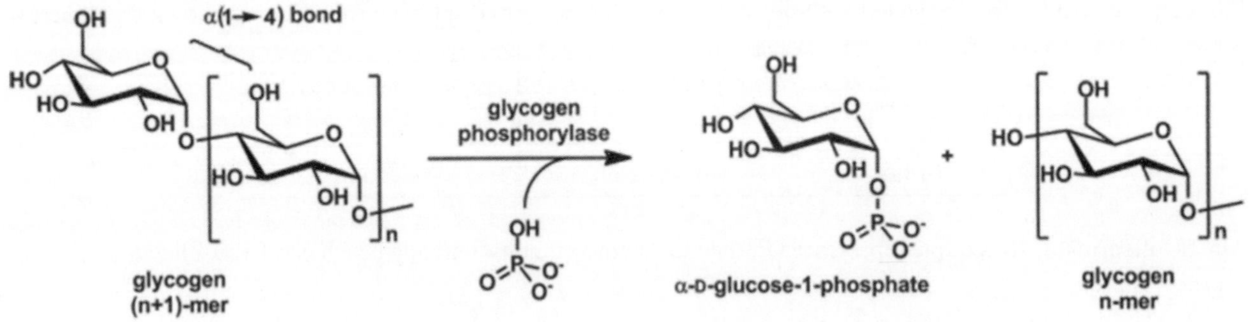

α(1→4) bond

glycogen (n+1)-mer

glycogen phosphorylase

α-D-glucose-1-phosphate

glycogen n-mer

Figure 1 A phosphorolysis reaction catalyzed by glycogen phosphorylase. An inorganic phosphate (P_i) is used in this reaction.

GP consists of two identical subunits and each subunit has two distinct maltooligosaccharide binding sites: a storage site and a catalytic site (note: a maltooligosaccharide is any oligosaccharide derived from glucose monomers linked as in maltose, an α-D-1,4 disaccharide of glucose). The storage site can bind both glycogen and maltooligosaccharide, while the catalytic site only binds to maltooligosaccharide. The storage site is about 30 Å away from the catalytic site and possesses about a 20 times higher affinity for maltooligosaccharide with K_d ~ 1mM as compared to the catalytic site. Thus, GP exhibits two distinct activities: A_s for the storage site characterized by glycogen-binding activity and A_c for the catalytic site, which is characterized by the phosphorolysis activity. In standard assays, it is difficult to differentiate between these two activities because normally, the storage site is saturated with the maltooligosyl used as a substrate.

Experiment: Determination of GP Regulation

It has been speculated that the activity of GP might be regulated by its glycogen-binding storage site. However, due to the proximity of the storage and the catalytic sites, the experimental assessment of this hypothesis was technically challenging. To address the mechanism of GP activity regulation, cyclodextrins (CDs) were used as GP inhibitors. CDs have K_i values within the millimolar range (*see* Table 1). CDs bind directly to the storage sites of GP causing a small alteration in the molecular structure of the enzyme. Three different CD isoforms were used: alpha, beta and gamma: α-CD, β-CD, and γ-CD.

Table 1 The inhibitory constant values for the CDs used in this study

Cyclodextrins	Reported K_i values (mM)
α-CD	8.5
β-CD	7.0
γ-CD	9.5

It was shown that the GP-catalyzed reaction behaves according to Michaelis-Menten kinetics and might depend on the ionic strength of the medium. The K_m and V_{max} values for GP-catalyzed reactions were measured in the presence of inorganic phosphate P_i and one equivalent of cyclic AMP as an allosteric activator of GP. A variation of maltooligosaccharide - pyridylaminated (PA-) maltohexaose - was used as a GP substrate at a concentration of 5 μM. The CD concentration ranged between 0-10 mM.

Table 2 The effect of CDs on GP activity. The GP activity was measured in the presence of 5 μM of PA-maltohexaose as a substrate, inorganic phosphate and cyclic AMP.

Additive (10mM)	Relative GP activity
None	1.00 ± 0.03
α-CD	0.96 ± 0.03
β-CD	0.97 ± 0.03
γ CD	0.96 ± 0.03

Table 3 The effect of CDs on the kinetics of GP from muscle cells. The GP activity was measured in the presence of 5 μM of PA-maltohexaose as a substrate, inorganic phosphate and cyclic AMP.

Additive (10mM)	Apparent K_m (mM)	Apparent V_{max} (μmol/min/mg)
None	14 ± 2	17 ± 2
α-CD	13 ± 2	15 ± 2
β-CD	14 ± 2	16 ± 2
γ-CD	13 ± 2	15 ± 2

Figure 2 The effect of ionic strength of the medium on GP activity. GP activity was assayed by measuring the accumulation of a final product Glc-1-P: solid line corresponds to glycogen; dotted line corresponds to maltohexaose. The maltohexaose degradation was assayed in the presence of 10 mM of γ-CD.

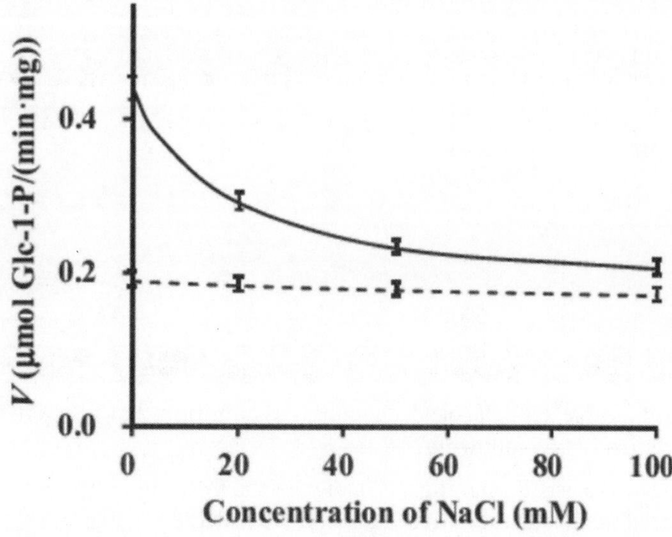

Adapted from Yasushi Makino, Yuta Fujii and Motoi Taniguchi. Properties and functions of the storage sites of glycogen phosphorylase. 2015. J Biochem. 157(6): 451–458

Question 22

Consider the following 3 disaccharides.

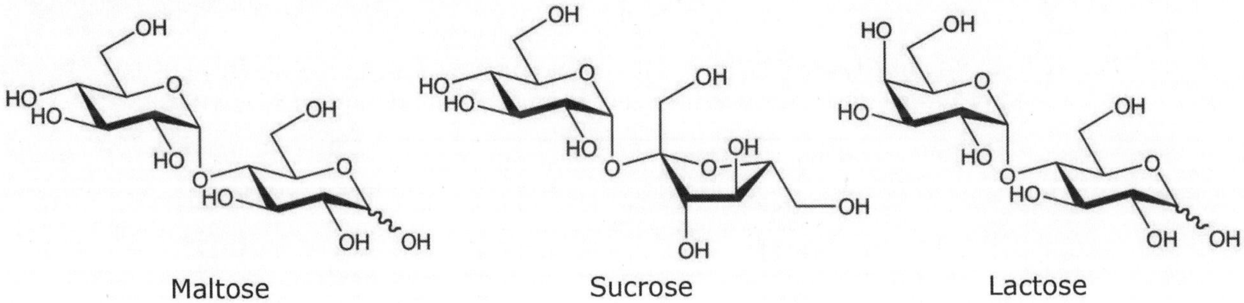

Maltose Sucrose Lactose

In the presence of Ag_2O in ammonia (Tollen's reagent), which of the following would NOT form a silver mirror on clean glassware?

- O **A.** Maltose
- O **B.** Sucrose
- O **C.** Lactose
- O **D.** More than one of the above

Question 23

The K_a value for the catalytic site of GP should be:

- O **A.** 5 mM^{-1}.
- O **B.** 20 mM^{-1}.
- O **C.** 0.05 mM^{-1}.
- O **D.** 100 mM^{-1}.

Question 24

The reason for using a very low substrate concentration (5 μM) when measuring GP activity in the presence of CDs as shown in Table 2 is:

I. to ensure that the reaction proceeds to V_{max}.
II. to ensure the saturation of the storage sites on GP by the CDs, which will allow the measuring of the GP catalytic site activity.
III. to avoid the high ionic strength in the medium.

- O **A.** I only
- O **B.** II only
- O **C.** I and III only
- O **D.** I, II and III

Question 25

Based on the data presented in Table 2 and Table 3, the initial assumption that GP activity is regulated through its glycogen-binding site is which of the following?

- O **A.** Incorrect, because there was no significant change in the GP catalytic activity and the apparent V_{max} while the catalytic activity was measured independently of the storage site activity.
- O **B.** Only partially true, because there was a slight reduction in the GP catalytic activity and the apparent V_{max} while the catalytic site activity was measured independently of the storage site activity.
- O **C.** Incorrect, because there was no significant change in the GP catalytic activity and in the K_m while the catalytic site activity was measured along with the storage site activity.
- O **D.** Correct, because there was a reduction in the GP catalytic activity and the apparent V_{max} while the catalytic site activity was measured along with the storage site activity.

Question 26

During intense physical activity, such as sport exercise, GP is activated in muscle to increase glycogen breakdown. The possible mechanism of GP activation is most likely to involve which of the following?

- A. A reduction in oxygen levels during intense cell respiration to produce more ATP.
- B. An accumulation of lactic acid, which could serve as an allosteric regulator of GP.
- C. An increase in cyclic AMP level, which could serve as an allosteric regulator of GP.
- D. An elevation of CO_2 levels during intense cell respiration to produce more ATP.

Question 27

The ionic strength of the medium affects the activity of which of the following sites of GP?

- A. The storage site only
- B. The catalytic site only
- C. Both the storage and the catalytic sites
- D. Neither of the two sites

The following questions are NOT based on a descriptive passage (Questions 28–31).

Question 28

Von Willebrand's disease (VWD) is an autosomal dominant disorder caused by a missing or defective von Willebrand factor, a clotting protein. Consider a woman who does not have the disease but has two children with a man who is heterozygous for the condition. If the first child expresses VWD, what is the probability that the second child will have the disease?

- A. 0.25
- B. 0.50
- C. 0.90
- D. 1.00

Question 29

The structure of β-D-glucose is shown below in two different projection systems. The circled hydroxyl group in Figure 1 would be located at which position in the modified Fischer projection depicted in Figure 2?

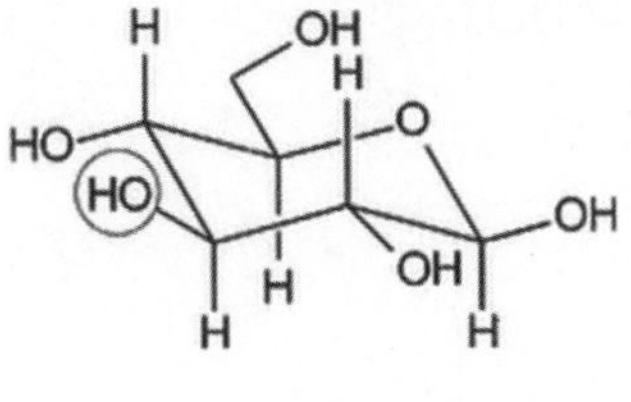

Figure 1

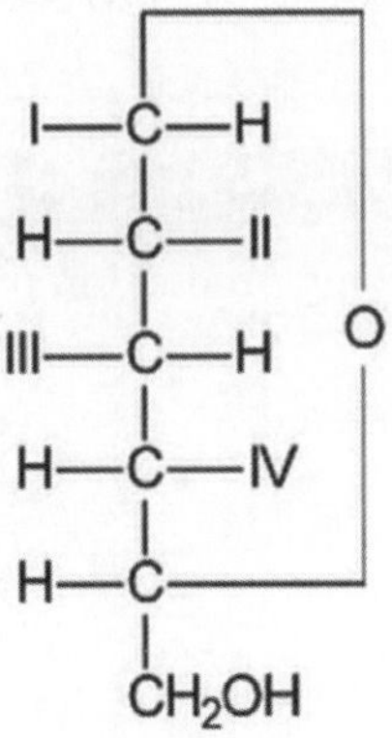

Figure 2

- A. I
- B. II
- C. III
- D. IV

Question 30

Which of the following is NOT a product of glycolysis:

- ○ **A.** a net 2 ATP.
- ○ **B.** acetyl-CoA.
- ○ **C.** pyruvate.
- ○ **D.** reducing equivalents.

Question 31

Identify the smallest unit of the urinary system capable of forming urine.

- ○ **A.** Minor calyx
- ○ **B.** Glomerulus
- ○ **C.** Bowman's capsule
- ○ **D.** Nephron

Passage 6 (Questions 32–36)

The infertility rate of married couples is about 14% in the United States. The number of infertile men and women is about equal. In almost 90% of cases of infertility, successful therapy is possible with medications, artificial insemination or corrective surgery. A combination is used in the technique of *in vitro* fertilization.

The procedure begins by injecting the woman with medications which stimulate multiple egg production in the ovary. Immediately prior to ovulation, a needle is usually inserted into the ovary via the abdominal wall thus extracting at least one egg. The egg is then incubated for days with the sperm of the male partner. Once the zygote has developed into a cluster of two to eight cells, it is transferred to the woman's uterus. Studies using this technique have demonstrated success rates from 20% to 30% and progress continues to be made.

For many socioeconomic reasons, the choice by women to delay childbearing until their thirties has been on the rise. Fertility in women likely peaks in the late teens and early twenties. The risk of many chromosomal abnormalities, including Down's syndrome, increases with advancing maternal age.

Of interest, many recent studies have clearly demonstrated that women over 30 did not have an increased risk of an infant who either died in the perinatal period, or was small for gestational age, or had a low Apgar score (a 10-point scale used to assess the appearance and responsiveness of a newborn).

Question 32

Drugs that stimulate multiple egg production probably contain, or increase the production of, which of the following hormones?

I. LH
II. FSH
III. ACTH
IV. Estrogen

- ○ **A.** I only
- ○ **B.** IV only
- ○ **C.** I, II and IV only
- ○ **D.** I, II, III and IV

Question 33

In the process of *in vitro* fertilization, the egg is removed from the ovary BEFORE fertilization in order to:

- O **A.** ensure that follicular atresia can occur.
- O **B.** ensure that menses does not begin in the luteal phase before *in vitro* fertilization is complete.
- O **C.** leave open the possibility of natural fertilization occurring.
- O **D.** prevent ovulation from occurring.

Question 34

The cell cluster that is transferred to the woman's uterus is referred to as:

- O **A.** neurula.
- O **B.** morula.
- O **C.** blastomere.
- O **D.** blastocyst.

Question 35

Down's syndrome, in which 2N = 47, is one of the most common forms of chromosomal abnormalities. This results from the failure of one pair of homologous chromosomes to separate during meiosis. During which of the meiotic phases would this likely occur?

- O **A.** Metaphase I
- O **B.** Metaphase II
- O **C.** Anaphase I
- O **D.** Anaphase II

Question 36

The most likely reason that an infant would have a low Apgar score is because:

- O **A.** going through the birth canal can be quite traumatic.
- O **B.** the infant was conceived via *in vitro* fertilization.
- O **C.** a synthetic version of oxytocin was used to induce delivery.
- O **D.** the infant's arterial partial pressure of O_2 dropped significantly for a prolonged period.

Passage 7 (Questions 37–40)

The transportation of respiratory gases (O_2 and CO_2) between the lungs and body tissues is a function of the blood and the circulatory system. Active cells require oxygen for metabolism. 97% of oxygen in blood is carried by hemoglobin (Hb) molecules in red blood cells. Each hemoglobin molecule contains four atoms of iron each capable of combining with a molecule of oxygen.

$$Hb + O_2 \leftrightarrow HbO_2$$

When Hb is completely converted to HbO_2, hemoglobin is fully saturated. When there exists a combination of Hb and HbO_2, hemoglobin is said to be partially saturated. The percent saturation of hemoglobin is a product of the following fraction of concentrations:

$$[HbO_2] / ([Hb] + [HbO_2])$$

The partial pressure of oxygen in blood (pO_2) is a major determinant of how much oxygen combines with hemoglobin.

pO_2 (mmHg)	% saturation of Hb
0	0
20	35
40	75
60	90
80	95
100	97

Other factors include pH, temperature, and 2,3 - diphosphoglycerate (DPG), a substance found in red blood cells during glycolysis.

Question 37

Which of the following best explains why 97% of oxygen in blood is in the HbO_2 form?

- ○ **A.** Oxygen binds irreversibly to the iron atoms in hemoglobin.
- ○ **B.** Oxygen does not dissolve well in blood plasma.
- ○ **C.** There are allosteric interactions involving oxygen and hemoglobin subunits.
- ○ **D.** Hemoglobin consists of four proteinacious subunits.

Question 38

Which of the following graphs best represents the relationship between percent saturation of hemoglobin and pO_2 (mmHg) at different temperatures?

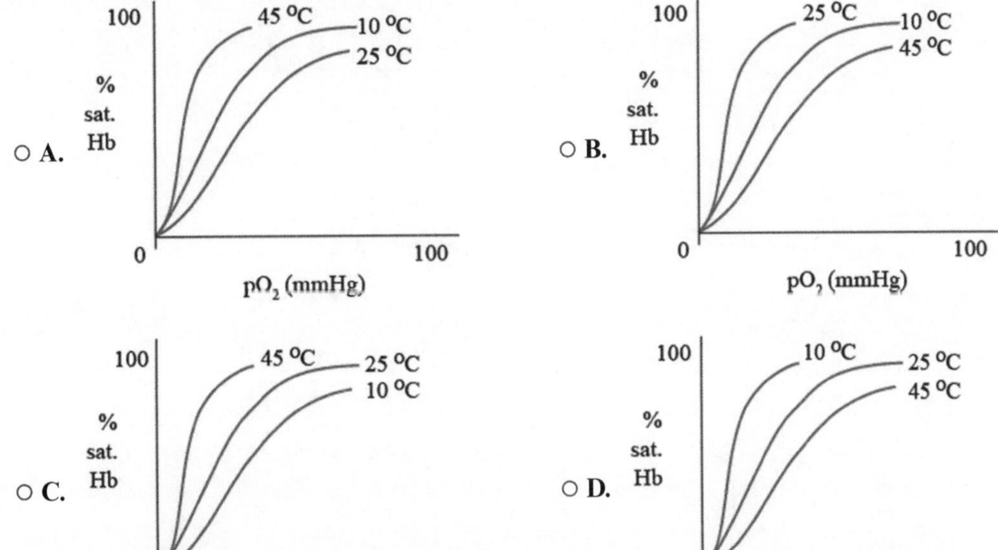

Question 39

In which of the following blood vessels would pO_2 be the highest?

- O **A.** Aorta
- O **B.** Left pulmonary artery
- O **C.** Renal vein
- O **D.** Inferior vena cava

Question 40

Which of the following would NOT result in a decrease in the exchange of oxygen and carbon dioxide between alveoli of the lungs and pulmonary blood capillaries?

- O **A.** A decrease in the overall surface area of the alveoli
- O **B.** Respiring at a higher altitude
- O **C.** A decrease in respiratory rate
- O **D.** A decrease in capillary thickness

Passage 8 (Questions 41–44)

Aromatase enzymes are utilized in the endogenous sex hormone pathway and are used to convert androstenedione to estrone and testosterone to estradiol (*see* Figure 1).

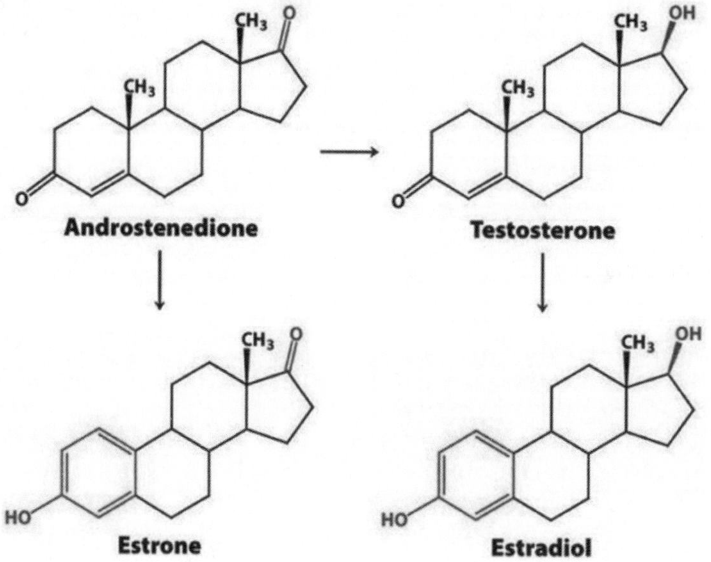

Androstenedione → Testosterone

Androstenedione ↓ Estrone

Testosterone ↓ Estradiol

Figure 1 Aromatase activity for steroidogenesis

Aromatase is in the cytochrome P450 enzyme super family (CYP19A1) and its activity is aimed at a heme protein core (*see* Figure 2). The active site of the heme protein for reactions within the CYP family is the iron moiety centered in the polyporphyrin ring structure.

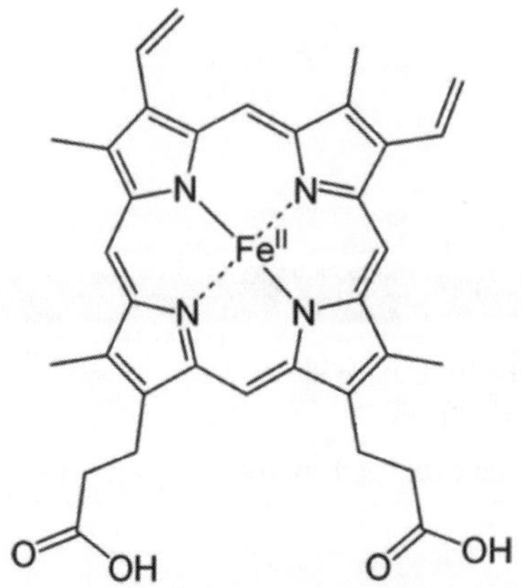

Figure 2 Heme group

For CYP19A1, the main cofactors for the reaction are molecular oxygen (O_2) and the redox agent NADPH. The main areas of density for this enzyme includes the gonads, brain, adipose tissue, placenta, blood vessels and bone. In abnormal cell development in certain tissue types, aromatase can be upregulated. This is true for breast and endometrial cancers.

Medications called aromatase inhibitors are used to combat the overexpression of aromatase in estrogen sensitive cancers like certain types of breast cancer. This lowers the level of estrogens thus slowing the tumor growth. For example, the medication Aromasin is used in therapy for estrogen receptor (ER) positive breast cancer (*see* Figure 3). It has been shown to decrease circulating levels of both estrone and estradiol in clinical studies through irreversible inactivation of aromatase via an intermediate formed through processing of the medication by the enzyme.

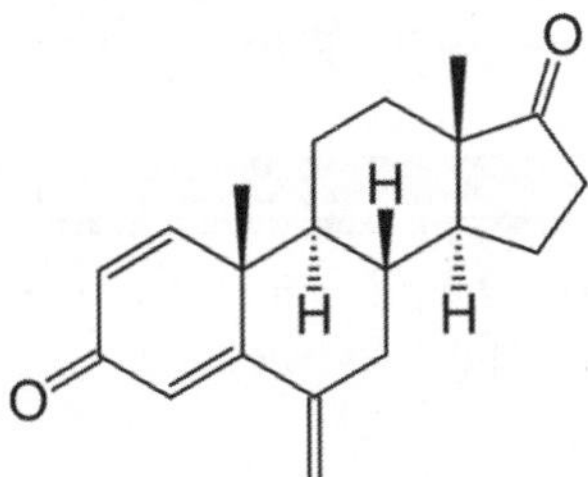

Figure 3 The molecular structure of Aromasin

Question 41

The action of aromatase begins at the lone methyl group on the A-to-B-ring bridgehead carbon using O_2 and NADPH as cofactors to eventually create an aromatic ring. Byproducts include water, $NADP^+$ and methanoate. What best describes likely enzymatic steps involved in the conversion of testosterone to estradiol?

- O **A.** Reduction of the methyl group followed by enolization
- O **B.** Oxidation of the methyl group followed by enolization
- O **C.** Hydrolysis of the methyl group followed by S_N2
- O **D.** Reduction of the methyl group followed by aromatization

Question 42

Which of the following is likely to be true regarding androstenedione?

I. Cholesterol is the precursor of androstenedione.
II. Androstenedione is the common precursor of male and female sex hormones.
III. In males, conversion of androstenedione to testosterone requires the enzyme hydroxysteroid dehydrogenase.

- O **A.** I only
- O **B.** II only
- O **C.** I and II only
- O **D.** I, II, III

Question 43

A lab is hired to process sex hormone samples from a local clinical trial for a new drug. The sample needs to be tested for serum levels of estrone, estradiol, and testosterone, which will utilize high performance liquid chromatography (HPLC). The column is nonpolar and the mobile phase is polar, following a reverse-phase design (RP-HPLC). What is the relative order that will elute to the detector?

- O **A.** Estrone, testosterone, estradiol
- O **B.** Testosterone, estrone, estradiol
- O **C.** Estrone, estradiol, testosterone
- O **D.** Testosterone, estradiol, estrone

Question 44

Consider an *in vitro* biochemical experiment evaluating aromatase enzyme kinetics and Arosamin in ER positive breast cancer cells. Data without the drug reveals that the Vmax is 200 and Km is 0.0001 M. After adding Aromasin to the *in vitro* assay, there was no change in Km but Vmax has significantly decreased. What mechanism most likely explains Aromasin's effect on aromatase?

- O **A.** Non-competitive inhibition
- O **B.** Anti-competitive (uncompetitive) inhibition
- O **C.** Competitive inhibition
- O **D.** Reactive inhibition

The following questions are NOT based on a descriptive passage (Questions 45–48).

Question 45

If increasing the concentration gradient across the plasma membrane increases the rate of transport until a maximum rate is reached, this would be convincing evidence for:

- O **A.** simple diffusion.
- O **B.** carrier-mediated transport.
- O **C.** a completely permeable membrane.
- O **D.** osmosis.

Question 46

The structure of lysine is given below.

$$H_2N-CH_2-CH_2-CH_2-CH_2-\underset{}{\overset{NH_2}{\overset{|}{C}H}}-CO_2H$$

If an electrical potential is placed across two electrodes in a lysine solution, lysine will migrate to the cathode or to the anode depending on the pH. It is reasonable to assume that at the isoelectric point:

- O **A.** the pH would be above 7 and the net migration of lysine would be toward the cathode.
- O **B.** the pH would be above 7 and there would be no net migration of lysine.
- O **C.** the pH would be below 7 and the net migration of lysine would be toward the cathode.
- O **D.** the pH would be below 7 and there would be no net migration of lysine.

Question 47

Consider the following diagram illustrating the binding of substrate C to active site A of enzyme E with allosteric site B.

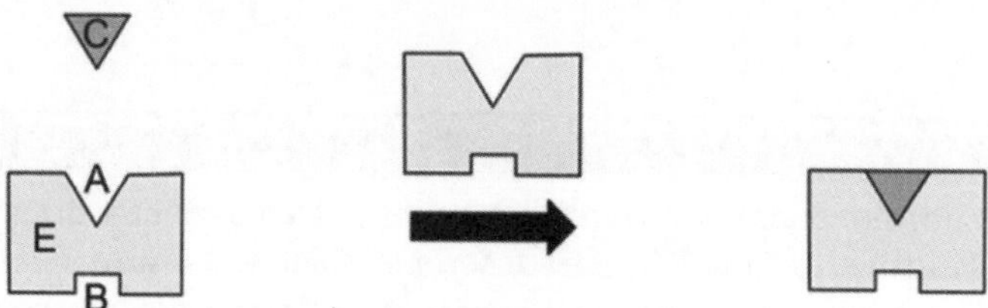

Consider the following diagram which introduces the molecule D.

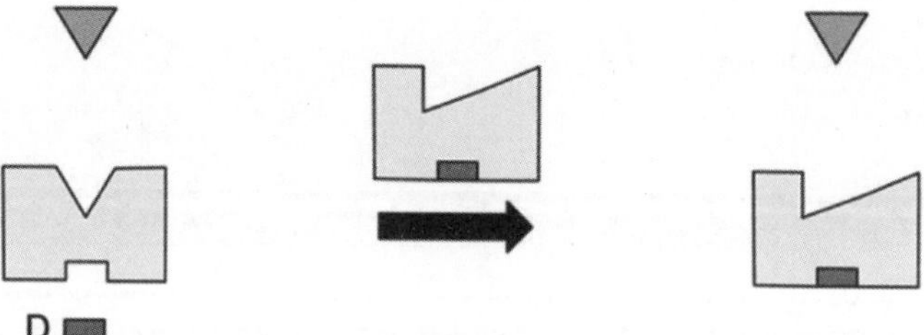

What does D likely represent?

- O **A.** Uncompetitive inhibitor
- O **B.** Competitive inhibitor
- O **C.** Positive effector
- O **D.** Negative effector

Question 48

It has been well established that disulfide bonds are formed between cysteine side chains during protein folding. The adding of beta-mercaptoethanol to a solution results in the cleavage of disulfide bonds and protein misfolding because beta-mercaptoethanol:

- O **A.** contains ethanol which means hydroxyl groups that can interfere with proper disulfide bond formation.
- O **B.** provides reducing power restoring the SH groups on cysteine side chains.
- O **C.** binds to the SH groups of cysteine side chains.
- O **D.** acts as an oxidizing agent removing the SH groups from cysteine side chains.

Passage 9 (Questions 49–52)

Hemophilia is a sex-linked disorder caused by a deficiency of the soluble blood clotting protein, Factor VIII. This protein is essential for the ability of blood to clot and individuals lacking such a factor reveal excess bleeding, sometimes to the point of being lethal. Factor VIII is produced by the hepatocytes and secreted into the bloodstream in response to injury.

When injury to a blood vessel disrupts the endothelium and allows the blood to contact the underlying tissue, a cascade of chemical mechanisms is initiated. The cascade will cause the plasma protein prothrombin to be converted to the enzyme thrombin. Thrombin is responsible for the activation of Factor VIII. Thrombin will also catalyze the cleavage of another plasma protein, fibrinogen, at several different sites. The now activated fibrinogen molecules will bind to each other to form a mesh of interlacing strands called fibrin. Fibrin quickly stabilizes by specific transamidation reactions which form covalent cross-links. These cross-links are catalyzed by Factor XIIIa. As fibrin polymerizes to plug the wound, many erythrocytes and other cells are trapped in the blood clot.

Several different mutations such as nonsense mutations which result in a premature stop codon, and frame shift mutations have been found in the Factor VIII gene. Since hemophilia is a sex-linked recessive disorder, the frequency of males with the disorder is much higher than in females.

Figure 1 is a pedigree which displays the phenotypic inheritance of hemophilia for a certain family.

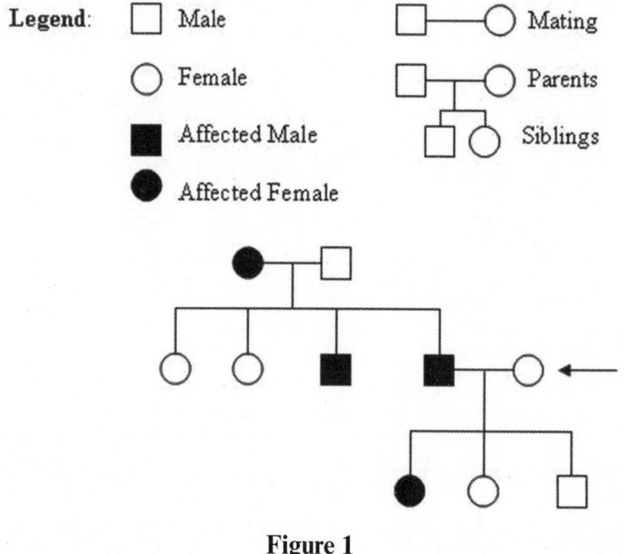

Figure 1

Question 49

Which of the following claims best supports the fact that hemophilia is caused by a deficiency in functional Factor VIII?

- ○ **A.** Factor VIII is found in the bloodstream.
- ○ **B.** The gene for Factor VIII is found on the X chromosome.
- ○ **C.** Individuals with mutated Factor VIII genes or proteins reveal traits of hemophilia.
- ○ **D.** Inhibition of thrombin hinders the activation of Factor VIII and induces hemophilia.

Question 50

Nonsense mutations and frame shift mutations sometimes found in the Factor VIII gene would most likely originate during:

- A. DNA replication.
- B. transcription.
- C. translation.
- D. splicing.

Question 51

According to the pedigree in Figure 1, what is the probability of obtaining a female with hemophilia in the 2nd generation?

- A. 0%
- B. 25%
- C. 50%
- D. 100%

Question 52

What is the genotype of the female pointed to in Figure 1 (H= dominant allele for hemophilia, h= recessive allele for hemophilia)?

- A. X^hY
- B. X^hX^H
- C. X^HX^H
- D. X^hX^h

Passage 10 (Questions 53–56)

Histones are highly alkaline proteins found in eukaryotic cell nuclei that package and order the DNA into structural units called nucleosomes. In general, genes that are active have less bound histones, while inactive genes are highly associated with histones. Histone deacetylases (HDAC) are a class of enzymes that permit histones to wrap the DNA more tightly. Since DNA is wrapped around histones, DNA expression is regulated by acetylation and deacetylation.

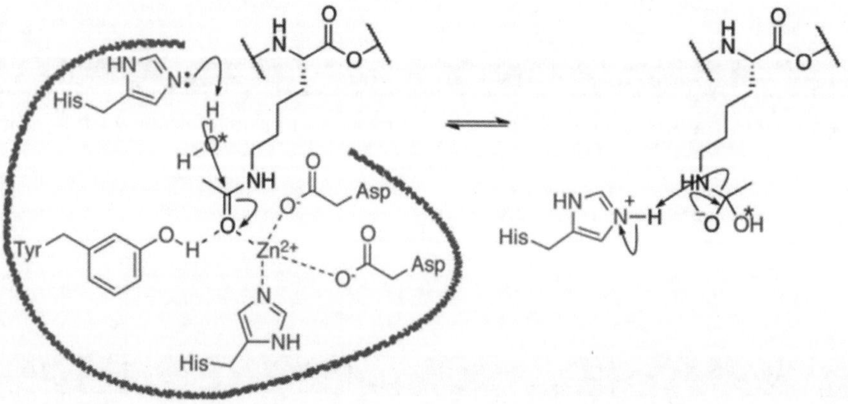

Figure 1 Mechanism of histone deacetylation within the active site of HDAC in gray leading to gene inactivation. Asterisk represents isotopically labeled oxygen in water.

Deacetylation can be important for the health of the cell. Mutations of the HDAC genes stimulate tumor development by inducing the aberrant transcription of key genes that regulate important cellular functions such as cell proliferation, cell-cycle regulation, and apoptosis. On the other hand, increased activity of HDAC genes have been shown to be carcinogenic in specific cell lines. As a consequence to the latter, a new generation of chemotherapeutic medications have been created which target HDACs including the following compounds which are currently undergoing clinical trials: vorinostat, belinostat and panobinostat; and the benzamides, entinostat and mocetinostat (Figure 2).

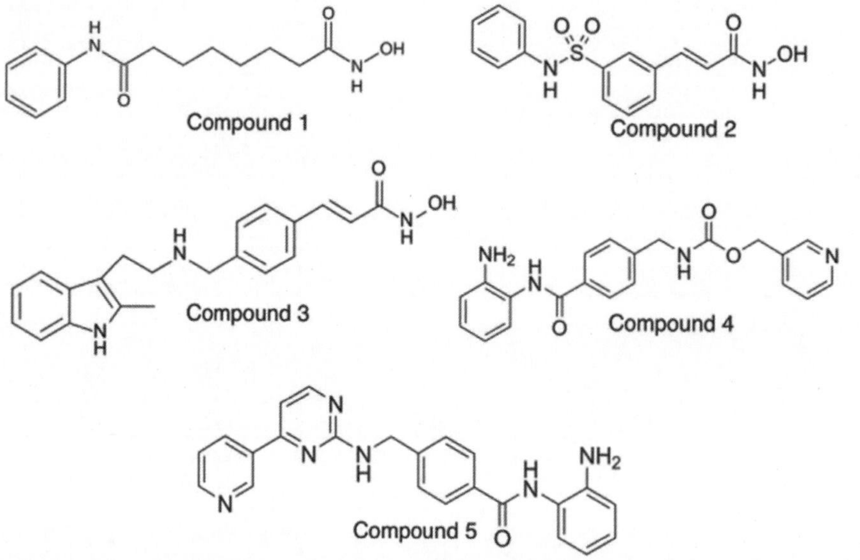

Compound 1

Compound 2

Compound 3

Compound 4

Compound 5

Figure 2 Compounds that target HDACs, from top to bottom: Compound 1 (vorinostat), Compound 2 (belinostat), Compound 3 (panobinostat), Compound 4 (entinostat) and Compound 5 (mocetinostat). Note that Compound 1 has a hydrogen bond donor count of 3 (meaning that there are 3 very electronegative atoms, i.e. 2 nitrogens and 1 oxygen, that are attached to at least one hydrogen), and a hydrogen bond acceptor count of 3 (meaning that there are 3 very electronegative atoms, the 3 oxygens, that have lone pair electrons available for bonding).

Studies were carried out to determine the dissociation constant Ki for several of the medications under study from Figure 2 and the results are listed in Table 1.

Table 1 K_i for mocetinostat, belinostat, and entinostat

Drug	K_i
Mocetinostat	0.009 μM
Belinostat	0.00085 μM
Entinostat	0.022 μM

Question 53

Which of the following amino acid residues are likely to be most important for high affinity binding of histone to DNA?

- ○ **A.** C and M
- ○ **B.** D and E
- ○ **C.** Y and W
- ○ **D.** R and K

Question 54

Based on the information provided in the passage, which of the following is likely to be true?

I. The key step in histone deacetylation involves the removal of three carbons.
II. Acetylation of specific lysine residues in histone is associated with gene activation.
III. Histidine, tyrosine and aspartate are key residues in the substrate for HDAC.

- ○ **A.** I only
- ○ **B.** II only
- ○ **C.** I and III only
- ○ **D.** I, II, III

Question 55

Researchers used a reversed phase HPLC assay separating the molecules in Figure 2 via a C18 column. The latter is a hydrophobic column (stationary phase) with an added agent possessing hydrogen bond donating capability. What order would the molecules elute under these conditions?

- ○ **A.** Vorinostat, belinostat, panobinostat, entinostat, mocetinostat
- ○ **B.** Vorinostat, panobinostat, entinostat, belinostat, mocetinostat
- ○ **C.** Panobinostat, entinostat, vorinostat, belinostat, mocetinostat
- ○ **D.** Panobinostat, entinostat, belinostat, vorinostat, mocetinostat

Question 56

Consider the data provided in Table 1 in the passage. Given only the potency of binding/inhibition per 100 mg dose, what is the most potent inhibitor and what would the other compounds' dose need to be to equal a similar dose of the most potent inhibitor?

- ○ **A.** Belinostat; mocetinostat 1058 mg; entinostat 2588 mg
- ○ **B.** Entinostat; mocetinostat 1058 mg; belinostat 2588 mg
- ○ **C.** Belinostat; mocetinostat 106 mg; entinostat 259 mg
- ○ **D.** Entinostat; mocetinostat 244 mg; belinostat 258 mg

The following questions are NOT based on a descriptive passage (Questions 57–59).

Question 57

Consider the data in Table 1.

Table 1 The pKa values for glutamic acid: pKa_1= α-carboxyl group, pKa_2 = α-ammonium ion, and pKa_3 = side chain group

pKa_1	pKa_2	pKa_3
2.19	9.67	4.25

The isoelectric point of glutamic acid is:

- ○ **A.** between pH 2 and 3.
- ○ **B.** between pH 3 and 4.
- ○ **C.** between pH 4 and 5.
- ○ **D.** between pH 5 and 6.

Question 58

Suppose that the oxygen supply to continuously contracting red muscles fibers is abruptly cut off. Which of the following processes would occur in the muscles?

- ○ **A.** Increased rate of synthesis of muscle glycogen
- ○ **B.** Increased rate of production of ATP
- ○ **C.** Increased rate of production of carbon dioxide
- ○ **D.** Increased rate of production of lactic acid

Question 59

Penicillin is a β-lactam antibiotic used in the treatment of bacterial infections caused by susceptible, usually Gram-positive, organisms. Beta-lactamases are enzymes produced by some bacteria that provide resistance to β-lactam antibiotics by breaking the antibiotic's structure.

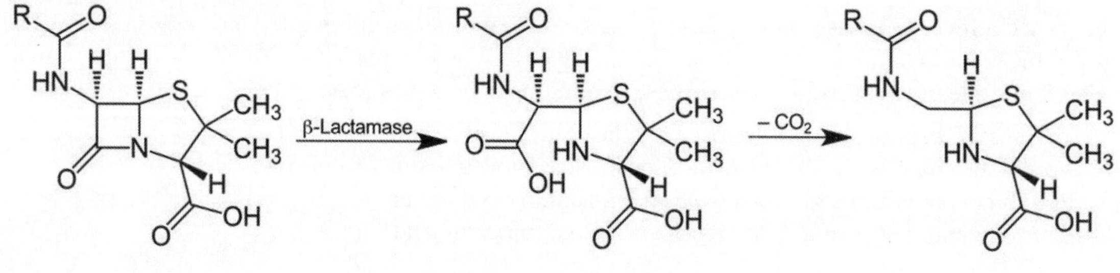

Beta-lactamase is best described as which of the following?

- ○ **A.** Hydroxylase
- ○ **B.** Hydrolase
- ○ **C.** Decarboxylase
- ○ **D.** Oxireductase

CANDIDATE'S NAME ______________________________

RAW SCORE AND SCALED SCORE ______________________

GS-5 Section IV: Psychological, Social, and Biological Foundations of Behavior

Questions: 1-59
Time: 95 minutes

INSTRUCTIONS: Of all the questions on this test, most are organized into groups preceded by a passage. After evaluating the passage, select the best answer to each question in the group. Fifteen questions are independent of any descriptive passage or each other. Similarly, select the best answer to these questions. If you are unsure of an answer, eliminate the alternatives that you know to be incorrect and select an answer from the remaining alternatives. To indicate your selection, use a pencil to blacken the corresponding circle next to the answer choice and/or you can use the answer document at the back of this book. No marks are deducted for wrong answers.

The computer-based real MCAT has an on-screen highlighter function and ~~STRIKEOUT~~ function. These tools help to spotlight text or assist in the process of elimination. You may use a yellow highlighter for this paper-based exam and/or a pen (or preferably a pencil to make it easier should you change your mind) to mark text. At the time of publishing, both highlighting and strikeout functions can be used for passages, questions and answer choices. You can also flag a question to review later should time remain.

For the real exam, you will be provided with a dry erase board which is a white laminated noteboard booklet accompanied by a fine point marker. The noteboard includes 9 graph-lined pages for you to write though you cannot erase. You can simulate the experience with a fine point marker on a noteboard or with 8" x 14" plain graph paper.

Please note: For the real MCAT, a small number of field-tested questions will remain unscored.

This practice test has been designed exclusively to test knowledge and thinking skills. This exam may contain hypothetical statements and/or express controversial ideas. Statements contained herein do not necessarily reflect the policy, position, or view of RuveneCo Inc. or MCAT-prep.com.

START EXAM ONLY WHEN TIMER IS READY.

Passage 1 (Questions 1–4)

The rise of new technologies has expanded people's choices in how information is consumed. Paper books, e-books, personal computers, phones, tablet screens, or audio books: these are some of the new possibilities.

This has led to a stream of research that investigates how those various ways of consuming information influence our attention and how we process information. For example, a study was conducted at the University of Waterloo to find out how the mind responds to material that is presented in different ways. There were three conditions. Firstly, participants had to read a passage silently. This is perceived as the most common way of processing written information. In addition, participants had to listen to an audio recording and to read a passage aloud. For each passage reading instance, participants described whether they had been mind-wandering or not. Furthermore, they were asked to rate their interest in the passage on a five-point scale, and their memory was tested with a multiple-choice comprehension test. The results are displayed in Table 1.

Table 1 Pearson Product-Moment Correlations of Proportion of Mind Wandering (Mind Wandering), Memory Test Proportion Correct (Memory), and Interest Rating (Interest), for Each Encounter Type and Sample

	Sample 1		Sample 2	
Encounter type	Memory	Interest	Memory	Interest
READING ALOUD				
Mind wandering	−0.08	−0.20*	0.01	−0.36***
Memory		0.14		0.23*
READING SILENTLY				
Mind wandering	−0.36***	−0.43***	−0.22*	−0.42***
Memory		0.40***		0.33***
LISTENING				
Mind wandering	−0.25**	−0.51***	−0.43***	−0.65***
Memory		0.33***		0.43***

****$p < 0.001$, ***$p = 0.01$, *$p < 0.05$.*

Although choices have become more varied, many people still seem to prefer reading a paper book rather than an e-book. It has been argued that the way one is presented with the information affects attention and information processing differently and that our brains naturally retain information better from a paper book. Other scholars have argued that the reason behind the paper books' preference is unrelated to information processing efficiency. Instead, this preference can be better explained by the longtime cultural dominance and the values that we associate with reading a paper book.

Source: Adapted from T.L. Varao Sousa, J.S.A. Carriere, and D. Smilek, "The Way We Encounter Reading Material Influences How Frequently We Mind Wander." Copyright 2013 Perception Science.

Question 1

Which of the following conclusions is LEAST supported by the data in Table 1?

- O **A.** Mind wandering decreases as interest increases.
- O **B.** Memory performance improves as interest increases.
- O **C.** Mind wandering either does not affect or hinders memory performance.
- O **D.** The relationships between memory, interest, and mind wandering are strongest in the reading out loud condition.

Question 2

The study tested three different ways of obtaining information from a text: reading aloud, reading silently, and listening. Reading silently most likely served as:

- O **A.** a baseline condition.
- O **B.** a screening condition.
- O **C.** a moderating variable.
- O **D.** a confounding variable.

Question 3

What could the researchers have encountered while measuring mind wandering?

- O **A.** Extreme response style
- O **B.** Social desirability bias
- O **C.** Bradley effect
- O **D.** Moderacy bias

Question 4

Designers are working on e-books that imitate the visual page appearance of paper books. What are they probably trying to achieve?

- O **A.** Emulation of tactile representation
- O **B.** Activation of physical landmark processing
- O **C.** Enhancement of focal attention
- O **D.** Activation of the ventral pathway

Passage 2 (Questions 5–9)

The Western biomedical model emphasizes the importance of full disclosure of medical information so that patients and their families can make informed choices about their treatment. It is premised on the assumption that a realistic assessment is vital and that truth-telling is at the heart of the doctor–patient relationship. However, this is a Western norm, and in other cultures, being explicit in breaking bad news like death may be culturally dissonant to patients and their family members. For example, in some Asian cultures, direct communication is perceived as rude, and indirect ways of communicating such as employing euphemisms are preferred. In some Native American groups, some believe that language can inform reality, and consequently to talk about death would be taboo.

Breaking bad news to patients and their family members is one of the most challenging tasks a physician has. There are three stages in the breaking bad news process: first, the "pre-delivery phase" is the beginning of the consultation up to the first utterance of the deliverance of the bad news. Second, the "delivery phase" is the period that consists of the speech in which the doctor delivers the bad news. Finally, the "post-delivery" stage is the time of the first utterance following the disclosure of the bad news to the end of the consultation.

A study found three different delivery styles of breaking bad news of sudden death after a sample of physicians were given a scenario and asked to give the bad news to a trained actor. A blunt style consists of delivering the bad news within 30 seconds of the interaction between the doctor and the patient. A forecasting style is one that delivers the news within the first two minutes, with the news is couched in context. Finally, a stalling style waits to deliver the bad news for more than two minutes. The stalling style relies on the patient to reach a conclusion without the physician's direct and explicit communication of the news.

In a study that evaluated training of medical residents in delivering bad news, those who were trained used more supportive utterances, checking-in questions, and assessment questions than those residents who were not trained. In a similar study, physicians were specifically trained to provide culture-shaped utterances that demonstrated the ability to communicate with patients from diverse cultural backgrounds. They improved in several domains. Figure 1 displays the results.

Scale	Pretest ± SD	Posttest ± SD	P
Compassionate Counseling	4.33 ± 0.60	4.56 ± 0.50	0.32
Open-Ended Questions	3.39 ± 1.17	3.72 ± 1.30	0.39
Health Benefits/Barriers	3.22 ± 0.57	3.94 ± 0.95	0.03
Cultural Norms	2.56 ± 0.88	3.44 ± 0.88	<.01
Screening	2.83 ± 0.97	3.44 ± 1.26	0.17
Emotional Talk	3.44 ± 0.74	4.19 ± 0.58	0.01
Literacy Skills	3.11 ± 1.01	3.52 ± 0.73	0.26
Cultural Beliefs	2.67 ± 1.09	3.89 ± 0.78	<.01
Health Beliefs	3.33 ± 0.69	3.85 ± 0.71	0.09
Emotional Adjustment	2.78 ± 1.09	3.78 ± 1.20	<.01
Negotiation	2.78 ± 0.67	3.78 ± 1.20	0.03
Partnership Building	3.89 ± 0.78	4.56 ± 0.53	0.02
Empower	3.50 ± 0.61	4.00 ± 0.83	0.15

Figure 1 Physicians' scores on different skills and knowledge after cultural based intervention participation

Source: Adapted from M.Y. Martin, W. Keys, S.D. Person et al., "Enhancing Patient-physician Communication: A Community and Culturally Based Approach." Copyright 2005 Journal of Cancer Education.

Question 5

The Western biomedical model of disclosing explicit information about the prognosis of an illness is based on:

- O **A.** patient-centered communication.
- O **B.** justice.
- O **C.** collectivism.
- O **D.** autonomy.

Question 6

When the statistical analysis was run using the variable "physicians' level of experience" and the variable "delivery style of bad news," the result was $\chi^2 = 0.433$; $p = 0.86$. What can be concluded?

- O **A.** There is no significant statistical difference in level of physicians' experience and delivery style of bad news.
- O **B.** There is a slight difference in how level of experience affected delivery style, as it is approaching statistical significance.
- O **C.** There is a significant statistical difference in level of physicians' experience and delivery style of bad news.
- O **D.** It is necessary to reject the null hypothesis that there is a statistical difference in level of physicians' experience and delivery style of bad news.

Question 7

How would conflict theory most likely operationalize physician-patient communication in the three phases of bad news delivery?

- O **A.** Measuring each party's level of conformity to its roles and the tasks and activities associated with the respective roles.
- O **B.** Measuring verbal dominance during physician–patient interaction (e.g., ratio of physician talk to patient talk).
- O **C.** Measuring patients' views about their beliefs about their symptoms, illness experience, and expectations of what should be done.
- O **D.** Measuring the rational exchange and cost of services between the physician and patient.

Question 8

In the ten minutes available for an appointment, a doctor employs extensive medical and technical language while communicating a breast cancer diagnosis. The patient is slightly bewildered and remains silent until the end. This approach to the delivery of the medical news most likely is:

- O **A.** compliance rooted.
- O **B.** action oriented.
- O **C.** consumer focused.
- O **D.** paternalistic oriented.

Question 9

What would interest Carol Gilligan the most when looking at some of the statistically significant results in Table 1 related to communicating?

- O **A.** The number of women who participated in the study, because female physicians are more focused on ethics of care
- O **B.** Whether there was an equal distribution of research subjects in the study across age groups in order to ensure generalizability of findings
- O **C.** Interviewing procedures in order to draw hypotheses related to the adherence to social roles and conventions during data collection
- O **D.** Research participants' nationalities and likely level of adherence to individualistic and collectivistic orientations

The following questions are NOT based on a descriptive passage (Questions 10–13).

Question 10

What hypothesis are the researchers likely investigating if they employ an instrument consisting of a list of adjectives and photos of different body types and ask participants to indicate the top three adjectives that describe each one of the photos?

- O **A.** High vs. average BMI individuals are more likely to be described as strong, courageous, and assertive.
- O **B.** Mesomorphs are more likely to be described as confident, powerful, and adventurous compared with ectomorphs.
- O **C.** Ectomorphs are more likely to be described as confident, powerful, and adventurous compared with their mesomorph counterparts.
- O **D.** Endomorphs are more likely to be described as shy, awkward, and tense compared with their ectomorph counterparts.

Question 11

While being scanned for MRI, research subjects were given the choice of immediately receiving a $10 gift certificate, or wait two weeks for a $25 gift certificate. The MRIs of those who opted for the $10 gift certificate, as compared to that of those who opted for the $25 give certificate, likely showed greater activity in the:

- O **A.** dorsolateral prefrontal cortex.
- O **B.** pons.
- O **C.** limbic system.
- O **D.** Broca's area.

Question 12

To study specific traits and qualities of histrionic personalities under an idiographic perspective, the most appropriate method is:

- O **A.** a quasi-experimental method.
- O **B.** a case study method.
- O **C.** a longitudinal survey method.
- O **D.** focus groups.

Question 13

A researcher went off book when suddenly deciding to jot down license plate numbers, as the face-to-face research subjects drove away, just in case there were follow-up questions. What would be the primary ethical issue with such procedure?

- O **A.** The sample was skewed because research subjects were car owners and potentially more well-to-do.
- O **B.** Face-to-face interviews can place research subjects at emotional, psychological, and social risks. Mailing surveys should have been preferred for data collection method.
- O **C.** Face-to-face interviews should never lead to follow-up questions. They should focus on participants' views on a specific point in time.
- O **D.** The participants were unaware that their license plates were being registered. They should have been informed and asked for permission beforehand.

Note: This page is left blank so that the passage would be visible without turning pages while assessing the passage-based questions.

Passage 3 (Questions 14–17)

Personality researchers commonly adopt a psychometric approach. Capturing interindividual differences, there are two main types of personality measures: structured (objective, paper-and-pencil) and non-structured (subjective, projective) tests. These are important tools that allow practicing psychologists to perform tasks such as recruitment, criminal profiling, clinical evaluation, and research.

An example of a paper-and-pencil test is Raymond Cattell's 16 Personality Factors (16PF) test. Answers are provided via a five-point Likert-like scale. Sixteen personality factors are assessed. Low or high saturations in each factor are associated with different personality traits. For example, the factor "abstractedness" varies from a high saturation, translating to an imaginative personality trait, to a low saturation, translating to a practical personality trait. Similarly, the "dominance" factor varies from "forceful" (high saturation) to "submissive" (low saturation).

The 16PF is linked to the Big Five personality theory, which identifies five main personality dimensions: extroversion, neuroticism, agreeableness, conscientiousness, and openness to experience. This very same factorial structure is often found to underlie results obtained via the Big Five's assessment tools and other personality evaluation tools such as self-description and the 16PF.

These structured personality measures have been criticized. For example, they count on individuals' self-awareness and acceptance of their own personality traits and honesty. A varied set of psychometric measures, such as validity scales and statistical methods, was developed to address such criticism. For example, the 16PF has three hidden scales (impression management, acquiescence, and infrequency), which aim at detecting random responding, indecisiveness, and distortions caused by mechanisms like the social desirability bias.

Widely used alternative projective measures aim at revealing individuals' conscious and unconscious needs, motivations, desires, and conflicts, while reducing answering biases that affect objective measures (e.g., social desirability, verbal skills, and self-awareness). Examples are the Rorschach inkblot test and the Thematic Apperception Test (TAT). The Rorschach measures people's spontaneous verbalizations about what 10 ambiguous ink blots represent. The TAT evaluates the way people give meaning to or interpret a set of 32 cartoons. People must describe what, in their opinion, in being narrated by the cartoons.

Source: Adapted from H. Gleitman, "Basic Psychology." Copyright 1992 Norton; D.P. MacAdams, "The Five-Factor Model in Personality: A Critical Appraisal." Copyright 1992 Duke University Press.

Question 14

Which of the following 16PF scales would most probably show the highest negative correlation with the extroversion dimension of the Big Five factor model (personality traits in parenthesis, varying from high—low, respectively)?

- ○ **A.** Abstractedness (imaginative—practical)
- ○ **B.** Self-reliance (self-sufficient—dependent)
- ○ **C.** Sensitivity (tenderhearted—tough-minded)
- ○ **D.** Privateness (discreet—forthright)

Question 15

OCEAN is the acronym for the Big Five's dimensions. From the options below, which is the LEAST informative and helpful definition of what an acronym is?

- O **A.** It is a memorization technique that aids the retrieval of information.
- O **B.** It is a particular type of mnemonic that supports the storing and retrieval of large amounts of information.
- O **C.** It is an abbreviation of a string of words that is constituted by joining together the first letters of the string of words.
- O **D.** It is an experimental procedure used to demonstrate the importance of deep processing for memory and recall.

Question 16

According to the information described in the passage, which of the following personality theories could more adequately be associated with the 16PF and with the Rorschach test (16PF; Rorschach, respectively)?

- O **A.** Behavioral theory; Humanistic theory
- O **B.** Trait theory; Psychodynamic theory
- O **C.** Behavioral theory; Psychodynamic theory
- O **D.** Trait theory; Sociocultural theory

Question 17

Consider a Likert-like scale varying from 1 (false) to 5 (true). Which of the following items and associated rating would most probably reveal the social desirability bias detected by the impression measurement scale of the 16PF (item; response)?

- O **A.** "I always wash my hands after using the bathroom."; 5
- O **B.** "I never lie."; 4
- O **C.** "Seldom am I late."; 4
- O **D.** "I have never used illicit drugs like marijuana."; 2

Passage 4 (Questions 18–22)

Pregnancy and the prenate's development are affected by genetic aspects, the womb's environment, and the mothers' biopsychosocial state. For example, there is some evidence supporting the relationship between stress and spontaneous abortion, preterm births, and infertility.

In addition, the mothers' depression during pregnancy has been strongly linked to prenatal, perinatal, and postnatal complications. Fetal activity was more intense, growth was delayed, and prematurity and low birth weight occurred more frequently. Newborns of depressed mothers showed less positive affect and performed worse on behavioral tests. Moreover, their biochemical profile mimicked that of their mothers (elevated cortisol, lower levels of dopamine and serotonin, greater relative right frontal EEG activation, and lower vagal tone).

Equally important is the prenate or neonate's exposure to the mother's voice. Ultrasound studies have shown that the mothers' voices were heard in the womb with the same or greater intensity than outside the womb and lead to heart rate increases. The authors argued that these findings were evidence of "fetal voice processing." The beneficial effects of mothers' voices were further detected in a sample using preterms. While exposed to their mothers' voices and singing, the preterms experienced fewer critical events and had a significantly greater oxygen saturation level and heart rate.

In line with the mothers' voice and singing study, a recent experiment tested the effects of music exposure during pregnancy on neonates' development. Singleton pregnant mothers, at 20 weeks of gestation or less, were randomly assigned to two conditions: music and control. Both groups received the standard prenatal care, but the music group listened to a prerecorded music cassette for approximately one hour a day. Newborns were then assessed via the most widely used infant development assessment scale, the Brazelton Neonatal Behavioral Assessment Scale (BNBAS). It was found that the group that had been exposed to music performed statistically significantly better on several of the BNBAS clusters. The findings are described in Table 1.

Table 1 Comparison of BNBAS Clusters Scores between Music and Control Groups

Cluster	MC mean (± SD) N=126	CC mean (± SD) N=134	Effect size (95% CI)	Statistical test result results	p-value
Habituation	5.72 ± 1.9	4.67 ± 2.3	1.05 (0.53, 1.57)	t (258) = 3.999	0.0001
Orientation	6.51 ± 1.1	5.38 ± 1.4	1.13 (0.82, 1.44)	t (258) = 7.207	<0.0001
Motor performance	4.56 ± 1.2	4.31 ± 0.8	0.25 (0.00, 0.50)	t (258) = 1.98	0.0479
Range of state	4.35 ± 0.5	4.04 ± 0.6	0.31 (0.17, 0.45)	t (258) = 4.511	<0.0001
Regulation of state	4.33 ± 1.0	3.79 ± 1.1	0.54 (0.28, 0.80)	t (258) = 4.134	<0.0001
Autonomic stability	5.88 ± 0.70	5.62 ± 0.9	0.26 (0.06, 0.46)	t (258) = 2.589	0.0102
Reflexes	5.19 ± 1.9	5.24 ± 2.4	−0.05 (−0.58, 0.48)	t (258) = −0.185	0.8530
Notes MC: music condition, CC: control condition, SD: standard deviation, CI: confidence interval					

Sources: P.G. Heppera, and B.S. Shahidullaha, "The Development of Fetal Hearing." Copyright 1994 Fetal and Maternal Medicine Review; A.J. Decasper, J.-P. Lecanuet, M.-C. Busnel et al., "Fetal Reactions to Recurrent Maternal Speech." Copyright 1994 Infant Behavior and Development; R. Arya, M. Chansoria, R. Konanki, and D.K. Tiwari, "Maternal Music Exposure during Pregnancy Influences Neonatal Behaviour: An Open-Label Randomized Controlled Trial." Copyright 2012 International Journal of Pediatrics; B.S. Kisilevsky, S.M.J. Hains, K. Lee et al, "Effects of Experience on Fetal Voice Recognition." Copyright 2003 Psychological Science; T. Field, M. Diego, and M. Hernandez-Reif, "Prenatal Depression Effects on the Fetus and Newborn: A Review." Copyright 2006 Infant Behavior and Development; M. Filippa, E. Devouche, C. Arioni et al., "Live maternal speech and singing have beneficial effects on hospitalized preterm infants." Copyright 2013 Foundation Acta Pædiatrica.

Question 18

According to Table 1, which developmental skills were not statistically significantly positively affected by music exposure during pregnancy, at a confidence level of 99%?

- ○ **A.** Habituation, orientation, range of state, regulation of state
- ○ **B.** Motor performance, autonomic stability, and reflexes
- ○ **C.** Habituation, orientation, range of state, regulation of state, and autonomic stability
- ○ **D.** Motor performance and reflexes

Question 19

The motor reflexes of a full-term singleton were tested two days after birth. Which of the following reflexes was probably NOT assessed at that time?

- ○ **A.** Plantar grasp reflex
- ○ **B.** Babinski reflex
- ○ **C.** Sucking reflex
- ○ **D.** Fight-or-flight reflex

Question 20

From the viewpoint of current knowledge, it can be stated that the autonomic nervous system does NOT:

- ○ **A.** regulate visceral organs, such as the heart and the smooth muscles, and the release of hormones.
- ○ **B.** divide into two subsystems: the sympathetic and the parasympathetic.
- ○ **C.** become active in emergency and non-emergency situations alike.
- ○ **D.** adjust the size of the pupils to light.

Question 21

The passage describes how there is mimicry in the "biochemical profiles" of the depressed mother and the infant. This probably means that:

- ○ **A.** there was a similarity between baby and mother's internal biological states.
- ○ **B.** the baby inherited depression genes, and therefore shows a similar biochemical profiles.
- ○ **C.** the baby looks up to the mother and wants to resemble the mother inasmuch as possible. Therefore he/she mimics everything she does and feels.
- ○ **D.** the baby received the mother's chemicals via the umbilical cord.

Question 22

Biologically speaking, pregnancy starts when:

- ○ **A.** the embryo becomes a fetus.
- ○ **B.** the zygote is formed.
- ○ **C.** abortion becomes illegal.
- ○ **D.** the heart starts beating.

Passage 5 (Questions 23–27)

Traveling for leisure for the most part is highly desirable for most people. Some are motivated because they view traveling as part of their lifelong learning journey. Some desire new scenery and appreciate the novelty offered during traveling. In studying the motivations for travel, a model depicting a ladder was formulated in which the rungs represented different hierarchical levels of needs for travel. The ladder starts with relaxation needs at the bottom rung, followed by stimulation, relationship, and self-esteem and development, and ends with fulfillment needs at the highest rung. Baby boomers are one of the largest segments of the population that travels for leisure and that are targeted by marketers. The millennial generation, those born after 1980, is another large demographic segment of the population that enjoys traveling; however, advertisers and marketers tend to focus on baby boomers.

Over the years, much research has been conducted to understand traveling and travelers. Plog's tourist or traveler typology attempts to capture a traveler's personality. On a continuum, there first are the travelers, who tend to go on short journeys and prefer structured trips. On the other end of the spectrum are the venturers, who take much longer and generally unstructured trips, and desire to explore the world. However, the majority of travelers fall in the middle of this continuum.

An alternative typology has been formulated. It has four dimensions, and these dimensions are not placed along a continuum. The categories are: nostalgics, friendlies, learners, and escapists. Nostalgics desire to visit familiar places and visit family. Friendlies want to meet new people, and learners want to go to new destinations in order to broaden their horizons. As the name implies, escapists are motivated to escape from daily life and responsibilities. Not surprisingly, studies have shown that this classification of travelers is correlated with the sensation seeking personality trait.

Question 23

Which theory does the hierarchical levels of needs for travel resemble the most?

- ○ **A.** Maslow's self-actualization theory
- ○ **B.** Carl Roger's humanistic theory
- ○ **C.** Carl Jung's archetypes
- ○ **D.** Erik Erikson's ego integrity versus despair

Question 24

What theory would best explain why actors who relax the muscles of the jaw and then smile may end up actually feeling happy subjectively?

- ○ **A.** Arousal theory
- ○ **B.** Cannon–Bard theory
- ○ **C.** James–Lange theory
- ○ **D.** Facial feedback theory

Question 25

Which statement is most likely NOT true of the "venturer" type of traveler who likes adventure and unstructured, exotic travel?

- ○ **A.** They are more likely to engage in smoking and impulsive decision making.
- ○ **B.** They demonstrate a weak orienting response to the presentation of new stimuli and therefore higher levels of melatonin secretion.
- ○ **C.** They show higher activation in the brain regions of the right insula and posterior orbitofrontal cortex.
- ○ **D.** They exhibit blunted cortisol responses to stressors.

Question 26

A study utilized Form V of the Sensation Seeking Scale, which has an internal consistency of 0.76. What does this suggest?

- O **A.** The instrument has high predictive ecological validity and can be utilized in real life and not just in the laboratory.
- O **B.** The instrument can capture and hold the test takers' attention and imagination given the topic, and as a result, the response rate will be high.
- O **C.** The instrument measures sensation seeking well as a construct, and the scores from instrument are reliable.
- O **D.** The instrument needs to be further pilot tested to ensure that the item sensitivity threshold is met for this particular study population.

Question 27

Which sensory receptors are most activated when entering a place with a great variety of smells?

- O **A.** Terminal receptors
- O **B.** Thermoreceptors
- O **C.** Mechanoreceptors
- O **D.** Chemoreceptors

The following questions are NOT based on a descriptive passage (Questions 28–31).

Question 28

Which of the following sleep disorders involves the destruction of hypocretin and causes individuals to seem to have fallen asleep unexpectedly right in the middle of an ongoing interactive action, such as a conversation?

- O **A.** Narcolepsy
- O **B.** Hypersomnia
- O **C.** Apnea
- O **D.** Somnambulism

Question 29

How is an interviewee, who cycles between constant brief speech pauses, intermittent squeaks, and excessively quick verbal discourse during a phone interview, most likely expressing the experienced nervousness?

- O **A.** Through paralinguistic communication
- O **B.** Through metacognitive verbalizations
- O **C.** Through intuitive verbalizations
- O **D.** Through haptic communication

Question 30

If a patient decides not to get the EEG examination recommended by the doctor, what principle are they invoking, but simultaneously what role are they violating?

- O **A.** They are invoking their privacy rights and violating the justice role.
- O **B.** They are invoking their consumerism rights and violating the paternalized role.
- O **C.** They are invoking their autonomy rights and violating the sick role.
- O **D.** They are invoking their discretion rights and violating the doctor–patient communication role.

Question 31

The regular use of Cannabis sativa is associated with several short-term and long-term negative biopsychosocial effects, such as early onset of psychosis, poor motor coordination, attentional difficulties, and lung cancer. Which of the following is probably NOT a drug abuse cause?

- O **A.** Peer pressure
- O **B.** Neuronal reward pathway
- O **C.** Social isolation
- O **D.** Wealth

Passage 6 (Questions 32–35)

The way we perceive breast cancer and how we deal with it in society has significantly changed. Mammography has been used since the 1950s. In those early years having breast cancer was seen as a social stigma that women needed to hide. It was very common that women who were diagnosed with breast cancer underwent mastectomy on the very same day as their diagnosis, often directly after biopsy when the women were still under anesthesia.

In the 1970s a social movement formed that addressed those issues within the medical field and the larger society. Its main aims were to raise awareness for breast cancer and how many women it affects, and to find better treatment, prevention, and funding for it, but also to change the social perception of breast cancer.

The breast cancer movement had its strongest impact in the 1980s and 1990s. Women affected by breast cancer began to be seen as "survivors" rather than "victims." At this time the movement was accompanied by large, well-funded breast cancer organizations and a development of corporate interest in the disease. A new public culture emerged that showed support for the cause. The movement managed to ensure changes in the allocation of research funds and the conduct of clinical trials and helped patients to better participate in clinical decision making. The emergence of large corporate and public support is the most likely explanation for the movement's success over the years.

Social movements have played a significant role in changing discourse in the medical field. Another, for example, is the AIDS movement. Social movements in medicine challenge the sick role and critically engage with disease regimes. Their scope ranges from improving situations for single individuals to demanding radical changes not only for patients but for society as a whole.

Source: Adapted from M. Klawiter, "Breast Cancer in Two Regimes: The Impact of Social Movements on Illness Experience." Copyright 2004 Sociology of Health & Illness.

Question 32

The description of the breast cancer movement in the passage is derived from:

- O **A.** collective behavior theory.
- O **B.** resource mobilization theory.
- O **C.** relative deprivation theory.
- O **D.** transformative discourse theory.

Question 33

The breast cancer movement has been criticized for focusing on one social issue, while neglecting the larger health, health care, and social contexts. This type of criticism is often voiced toward:

- O **A.** reformative social movements.
- O **B.** redemptive social movements.
- O **C.** alternative social movements.
- O **D.** revolutionary social movements.

Question 34

Which of the following types of ethical principles was most likely violated by the one-step procedure requiring patients to authorize the surgeon to perform a mastectomy before cancer was diagnosed?

- O **A.** Justice
- O **B.** Beneficence
- O **C.** Non-maleficence
- O **D.** Autonomy

Question 35

Framing plays an important part in understanding the success and failure of social movements and how they affect society as a whole. An example of framing that occurred in the breast cancer movement is:

- O **A.** involving the public and raising donations for better research.
- O **B.** integrating patients in clinical decision making processes.
- O **C.** changing the sick role of women with breast cancer.
- O **D.** more women undergoing screening procedures earlier.

Passage 7 (Questions 36–39)

It is difficult to clearly pin down the number of illicit drug addicts in a society. The reason is that addiction and dependency are very fluid concepts that are often used inconsistently. From a purely biological perspective it is possible to pin down the effects and consequences of addiction, but those are mediated by social perceptions, reactions, situations, and ties.

The discourse around addiction tends to emphasize the dangerous biological effects and chronic condition of addiction. These pathology-oriented views either believe that drug users have abnormal personalities and therefore engage in drug consumption, or that the drug itself makes people develop an abnormal personality. However, there are theories that contradict this view. They emphasize the role that political and social systems, conditions, and contexts as well as cognitive processes play in drug consumption patterns. This perspective would explain why social class seems to play a role when it comes to drug use.

Specifically, the danger of addiction is there for any class, but the types of drugs and degrees of addiction vary between classes. Middle-class and upper-middle-class citizens seem to engage more in recreational drug use. Overall they do not engage less in drug consumption, but their use is more episodic or more controlled. Lower-class citizens are more at risk of chronic, compulsive, and heavy use.

Terminating drug use habits is usually is a hazardous, strenuous, and long-term process. Withdrawal symptoms have biological and psychological causes, but the severity and significance of the detoxification process can vary greatly depending on the social circumstances. Drug users are further required to change the roles and identities they have adopted for themselves and others.

Source: Adapted from E. Goode, "The Sociology of Drug Use" in 21st Century Sociology. *Copyright 2006 Sage Publications.*

Question 36

What assumption do the pathology approach and the social condition approach share?

- ○ **A.** Drug users are mentally ill.
- ○ **B.** Drugs make people act against their will.
- ○ **C.** Neighborhoods play a role in determining what drugs are used.
- ○ **D.** Taking drugs is deviant, abnormal behavior.

Question 37

Symbolic interactionism might propose that social interventions sometimes reinforce or increase users' drug abuse behavior because:

- ○ **A.** outgroups have no impact on individual users.
- ○ **B.** users enact the negative meanings assigned to them by society.
- ○ **C.** users lose the connection to the conventional world.
- ○ **D.** society overvalues problematic cases, which amplifies marginalization.

Question 38

Richard J. Herrnstein and Charles Murray explained the higher drug use and dependency risk associated with lower-class citizens in their book The Bell Curve, which was published in 1994. They controversially claimed that the underlying reason for those differences is that poor people on average:

- ○ **A.** have better access to drugs than rich people.
- ○ **B.** are less concerned about their health than rich people.
- ○ **C.** have lower intelligence coefficients than rich people.
- ○ **D.** live in more deprived areas than rich people.

Question 39

According to social support theories, why might it be easier for someone from upper classes than for someone from lower social classes to fight addiction?

- O **A.** Upper-class people have more supportive networks, more education, and more access to knowledge.
- O **B.** Lower-class people have social networks with better access to drugs.
- O **C.** Lower-class people face an increased risk of biopsychosocial harm following drug abuse.
- O **D.** Upper-class people find it easier to form a mutually supportive counterculture.

Passage 8 (Questions 40–44)

We hold to the belief that voting is a rational process. We also believe people are motivated to vote because they assume voting will make a difference, as everyone is going through a rational decision-making process. The reality is that we often make voting decisions based on emotions or are influenced by factors that are outside of our control (e.g., polling locations). In addition, we tend to vote because of the desire to feel good about ourselves. We want to enhance our self-concepts or self-image; for example, we want to feel that we have performed our civic duty.

Researchers have considered voting as a prosocial behavior because the probability of one voter affecting the outcome of elections and positively influence events is negligible. Voting is only meaningful as a collective action, and, as such, can be regarded as a prosocial, non-individualistic action, which is performed for the greater good. In a study using registered voter data, registered individuals were randomly assigned to three conditions. In the first condition, research subjects simply received a letter in the mail that reminded them about the upcoming election and to vote. In the second condition, research subjects received a letter that thanked them for voting in the last election and encouraged them to vote in the upcoming election. The third condition was the control condition, and research subjects did not receive anything. After the election, the researchers obtained the voter turnout data. The findings indicated that those who were sent the thank-you reminder turned out to vote at statistically significantly higher rates relative to the control group or the no-gratitude condition. The researchers concluded that the motivation to vote is in part influenced by emotions such as gratitude and that the acknowledgment and expression of gratitude reinforces altruistic or philanthropic behavior like voting.

Question 40

What is the campaign manager of a candidate with controversial views on euthanasia likely attempting to do when looking for funeral homes interested in being a polling location?

- ○ **A.** He is regulating affective states such as compassion or grief so that voters become more likely to sympathize with the candidate.
- ○ **B.** He is stimulating salient partisan knowledge and communal orientation so as to foster altruism.
- ○ **C.** He is exposing a stimulus capable of stirring up voters' repressed anxiety about death to the threshold of conscious awareness.
- ○ **D.** He is priming individuals to think about mortality since the candidate is known for his controversial stance on euthanasia.

Question 41

What variables might be included in a study seeking to understand how social capital plays a role in the relationship between religious affiliation and political participation?

- ○ **A.** Research participants' level of communication and risk taking
- ○ **B.** Research participants' level of education and involvement in the community
- ○ **C.** Number of children that research participants have and home ownership
- ○ **D.** Research participants' level of adherence to ideologies of individualism and work ethic

Question 42

Which empirical finding in a study about voting is best explained by cognitive dissonance theory?

- ○ **A.** People have more positive attitudes toward the winning candidate they did not vote for after the election.
- ○ **B.** People vote for the candidate who is likely to win according to the polls.
- ○ **C.** Individuals who tend not to vote will adjust their level of voting participation to conform to their partners' habits.
- ○ **D.** Monetary voting incentives are counterproductive because voters find the voting process inherently satisfying.

Question 43

In one study comparing voting in the married vs. non-married group (joining single, divorced, or windowed together), t-test statistical results were: $t(98)=3.013$; $p=0\ .003$. Which of the following conclusions is most accurate?

- ○ **A.** When looking at the p value, one should accept the null hypothesis.
- ○ **B.** Age is confounding variable, for those who are widowed may be homebound and unable to get out to vote.
- ○ **C.** It is not possible to conclude that marital status causes voting turnout.
- ○ **D.** Being married causes one's belief systems to change and also affects political participation.

Question 44

Some states rotate their ballot order district by district because rotating the balloons minimizes the effects of:

- ○ **A.** discrimination biases.
- ○ **B.** stabilizes descriptive social norms of voters.
- ○ **C.** right-side brain dominance.
- ○ **D.** response-order biases.

The following questions are NOT based on a descriptive passage (Questions 45–48).

Question 45

Which memory retrieval model states that concepts are represented by nodes and associations are represented by links?

- ○ **A.** Insight
- ○ **B.** Transfer appropriate processing
- ○ **C.** Spreading activation
- ○ **D.** Encoding specificity

Question 46

From the viewpoint of cognitive attention models, what function would most likely make a patient remember only two of the available therapies after having just been informed about the disease, mortality rates, three available therapies, and their complications?

- ○ **A.** Focused attention
- ○ **B.** Attention deficit
- ○ **C.** Divided attention
- ○ **D.** Selective attention

Question 47

What name did Wolfgang Kohler give to the cognitive process behind chimpanzees' ability to use two bamboo sticks together to suddenly succeed at grabbing the bananas that had been placed outside the cage?

- ○ **A.** Bottom-up learning
- ○ **B.** Insight learning
- ○ **C.** Observational learning
- ○ **D.** Operant conditioning

Question 48

According to Ferdinand Tönnies and Émile Durkheim, modernity (the era of industrial societies) is essentially shaped by:

- ○ **A.** the process of rationalization that replaced traditional worldviews.
- ○ **B.** an increased division of labor that led to highly specific roles for each individual.
- ○ **C.** the rise of capitalism that increased social stratification and led to class society.
- ○ **D.** the decline of small communities that offered a sense of purpose and belonging to their members.

Passage 9 (Questions 49–52)

Generally, sports participation in school's athletic teams is socially perceived as highly desirable. Associated with sports participation are health benefits and positive psychosocial outcomes. There is also research suggesting that participation in athletic teams serves as a protective mechanism against smoking and alcohol use. However, it may only serve as a protective factor for younger youths. For adolescents, it may serve as a risk factor. In addition to age, the type of sports (team vs. individual) is also an influent variable. For example, a study showed that blood-alcohol content levels and weekly alcohol use was lower among high school athletes in individual sports compared with those in team sports or those in a combination.

Participation in sports and school athletics is influenced by a host of psychological factors such as level of motivation and persistence. Sports participation is also related to demographic factors such as household income, parental education, race and ethnicity, and mother employment. See Figure 1, which shows 8th, 10th, and 12th graders' school athletic participation based on parental educational levels.

Many parents like the idea of their children being engaged in sports because of possible positive role modeling. A coach, for example, may serve as an influential force on their character development, and well-known athletes may serve as role models because of their sporting behavior such as skills or endurance.

However, there is also the argument that the sports' environment fosters aggression by emphasizing competition, "win at all costs" attitudes, and hypermasculine norms. Despite adult figures like parents or coaches denouncing aggressive behavior, when the youth is out on the field playing, the use of aggressive behavior in competition may be subtly legitimized. Furthermore, when youths watch sporting events such as ice hockey on television, they see how players display both verbal and physical aggressive behaviors in the rink and how the crowds incite these negative behaviors or, in certain cases, how the crowds themselves become physically aggressive. Socially then, the use of aggressiveness in the fields is also indirectly legitimized.

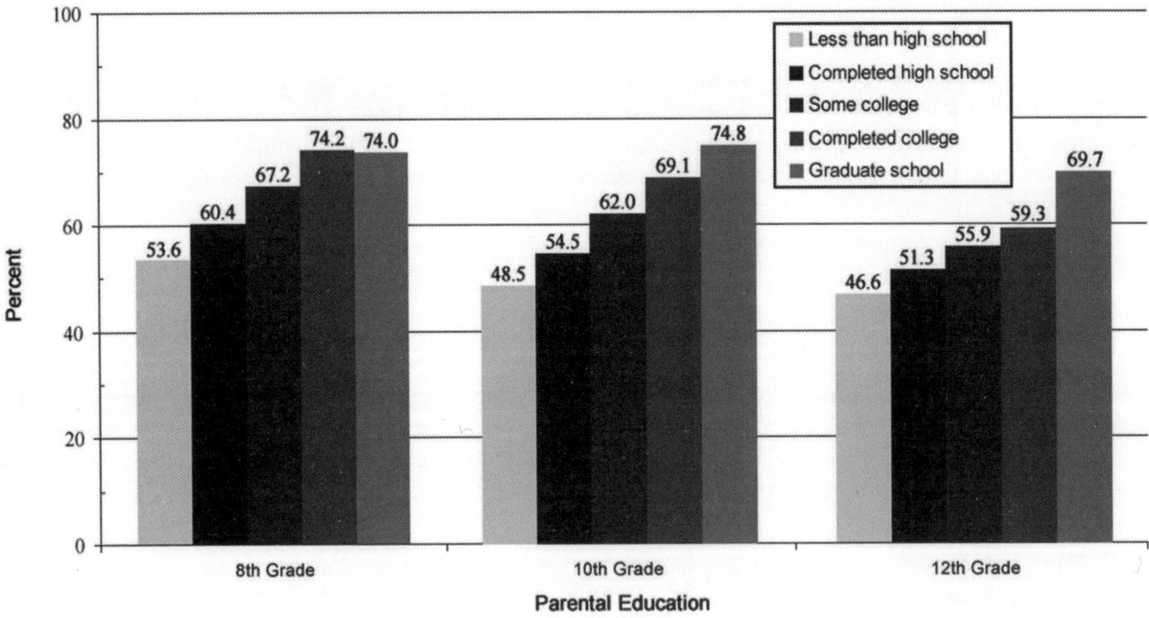

Figure 1 Percentage of 8th-, 10th-, and 12th-grade students who participated in school athletics, by parental education, 2011

Source: Adapted from Child Trends, "Participation in School Athletics." Copyright 2013 http://www.childtrends.org.

Question 49

Which of the following methodological reasons more strongly justifies the use of archival data (e.g., official penalty records) while studying sports-related aggression behavior? In comparison with self-report measures, archival data:

- ○ **A.** widens the number of variables and the variety of their roles (e.g., independent, moderating, mediating, and dependent) during statistical analysis.
- ○ **B.** resolves research respondent participation and increases sample sizes.
- ○ **C.** helps to improve studies' ecological validity.
- ○ **D.** helps to improve the sometimes low inter-rater reliability associated with self-report measures.

Question 50

A girl, interested in basketball since the fourth grade, feels proud of her performance and wants to continue training. On the other hand, her friend quits because her parents will not like her better just because she is doing sports. What do their drives to play sports display?

- ○ **A.** The girl is guided by a compass that revolves around consistency, while her friend is guided by bounded rationality.
- ○ **B.** The girl is influenced by low arousal states, while her friend is influenced by high arousal states.
- ○ **C.** The girl is influenced by an authoritarian personality orientation, while her friend is more concerned with relatedness.
- ○ **D.** The girl is influenced by intrinsic motivation, while her friend is influenced by extrinsic motivation.

Question 51

Which demographic variable, if replaced by parental education, would most likely produce similar findings to those displayed in Figure 1?

- ○ **A.** Goal directedness
- ○ **B.** Household income
- ○ **C.** Parental marital status
- ○ **D.** Religious affiliation

Question 52

When exploring the concept of coaches as role models under social learning theory, what research question might be asked?

- ○ **A.** How does motivation of players influence conforming to the coach's instructions?
- ○ **B.** How does observation of an identified exemplary player influence coaching style?
- ○ **C.** How does socialization by a coach affect the performance of players?
- ○ **D.** How do learning styles of the players influence types of persuasive tactics used by the coach?

Passage 10 (Questions 53–56)

Awareness is increasing as to the importance of work–family conflict. The number of couples performing simultaneously career and household–managing tasks has grown considerably since World War II. Although sometimes work and family may function as allies, their conjugation is often distressing. Research in this area has mainly focused on the negative consequences of work–family conflict.

Table 1 compiles a simplified version of the statistical results of a meta-analysis conducted in 2000 about the effect sizes of known negative outcomes of the family-work conflict by outcome domain (work-related, non-work, and stress related). It shows the weighted mean of the effect sizes associated with each outcome.

Table 1 Effect sizes of studies reporting work–family conflict outcomes

Outcomes	Sample groups	Weighted correlations mean	Range
Work outcomes			
Job satisfaction	38	-0.24	0.14 to -0.47
Career satisfaction	2	-0.04	-0.07 to 0.47
Organizational commitment	6	-0.23	-0.06 to -0.42
Intention to turnover	10	0.29	0.03 to 0.50
Absenteeism	2	-0.02	0.00 to -0.13
Job performance	4	-0.12	0.00 to -0.26
Non-work outcomes			
Life satisfaction	18	-0.28	-0.09 to -0.53
Marital satisfaction	14	-0.23	-0.01 to -0.49
Family satisfaction	7	-0.17	-0.02 to -0.27
Stress outcomes			
General psychological strain	13	0.29	0.16 to 0.57
Somatic/physical symptoms	17	0.29	0.08 to 0.53
Depression	11	0.32	0.20 to 0.51
Alcohol abuse	3	0.13	0.12 to 0.14
Burnout	10	0.42	0.08 to 0.57
Work-related stress	15	0.41	0.12 to 0.56
Family-related stress	6	0.31	0.20 to 0.51

There are some theoretical models that attempt to explain work–family conflict and how its negative outcomes come about. An example is the attribution model, which posits that people make causal attributions to the conflict. These attributions provoke various emotional reactions (e.g., guilt, shame, and anger), which then result in resorting to either maladaptive (e.g., withdrawal, aggression, turnover) or adaptive (e.g., job crafting, self-development) behavioral reactions. Adaptive reactions are regarded as those that can minimize the stress experienced when juggling family and work, and its negative consequences. Some gender differences were observed in several studies. For example, the solutions that seem to protect men against the negative consequences of the conflict are decision latitude and organizational social support. Those that seem to protect women are domestic help.

A more recent 2011 meta-analysis analyzed separately work vs. family interferences. Table 2 summarizes results. There, the negative outcomes of the conflict are also organized by domain (work-related, family-related, and domain-unspecific). Findings showed that the outcomes in areas other than family and work were more statistically significant than those associated with family and work.

Perhaps as a spontaneous reaction to work–family conflict and its consequences, and alongside the great socio-technological developments, people have begun adopting a work-from-home solution. The 2000 and 2010 census comparison between Americans who reported working from home, by occupation, showed such a change as a clear general rising trend. Yet this solution does not necessarily resolve work–family conflict. Some studies suggest that, beyond its many advantages, work–family boundaries may be more tenuous when people work from home, and their stress thereby may increase.

Table 2 Results of the Meta-Analysis for Work Interference with Family, Work, and Domain-unspecific outcomes

Outcomes	Sample groups	Weighted correlations mean	Confidence Interval
Work-related outcomes	89	-0.29	[-0.303, -0.285]
Work satisfaction	54	-0.26	[-0.148, -0.120]
Organizational commitment	14	-0.17	[-0.187, -0.142]
Intention to turnover	24	0.21	[0.191, 0.227]
Burnout/exhaustion	15	0.38	[0.361, 0.396]
Absenteeism	5	0.03	[0.007, 0.056]
Work-related performance	10	-0.11	[-0.149, -0.668]
Work-related stress	16	0.49	[0.477, 0.510]
Career satisfaction	4	-0.09	[-0.141, -0.036]
OCD	3	-0.63	[-0.679, -0.578]
Family-related outcomes	31	-0.18	[-0.194, -0.163]
Marital satisfaction	12	-0.17	[-0.192, -0.146]
Family satisfaction	13	-0.18	[-0.199, -0.153]
Family-related performance	3	-0.18	[-0.646, -0.111]
Family-related stress	7	0.23	[0.184, -0.279]
Domain-unspecific outcomes	56	-0.32	[0.328, 0.308]
Life satisfaction	12	-0.31	[-0.338, -0.257]
Health problems	4	0.28	[0.253, 0.304]
Psychological strain	18	0.35	[0.326, 0.365]
Somatic/Physical symptoms	18	0.29	[0.268, 0.306]
Depression	14	0.23	[0.209, 0.347]
Substance use/abuse	3	0.08	[0. 048, 0.104]
Stress	6	0.54	[0.515, 0.553]
Anxiety	3	0.14	[0.111, 0.167]

For full references for this passage, see over (after Question 56).

Question 53

Which one of the following identifies correctly the passage Table where absenteeism findings, explainable via conformity theory, are presented? (Table; finding; explanation, respectively)?

○ **A.** Table 2; work–family conflict does not lead to absenteeism; employees tend to attend their jobs regularly, possibly because feel they are performing personally and socially meaningful work outside their homes.
○ **B.** Table 1; work–family conflict leads to absenteeism; employees tend to stay away from work, possibly because they feel they are not being fairly rewarded for their efforts while at work.
○ **C.** Table 2; work–family conflict is related to absenteeism positively and very weakly; employees tend to stay away from their jobs, possibly because family demands are more important to them than their jobs.
○ **D.** Table 1; work–family conflict is related to absenteeism negatively and very weakly; employees tend to attend their jobs regularly, possibly because they want to succeed at managing their work and family demands as much as any other employee.

Question 54

While comparing the studies illustrated in Table 1 (study A) and Table 2 (study B), which of the following observations most probably is NOT correct?

○ **A.** There seems to be convergent validity; the effect sizes of many variables are fairly similar across studies, and the direction of relationships is maintained for the greater part of the variables.
○ **B.** Since the aim of Studies A and B was to longitudinally compare their results, the same variables were studied and the same research procedures were adopted.
○ **C.** The number of studies in Study B is equal to or greater than those in Study A, thus Study B likely has greater external validity.
○ **D.** Study B has a few new variables, probably because since the conduction of study A, new variables were found to be affected by or related to the work-family conflict.

Question 55

Which one of the following would NOT be a primary prevention organizational program, implemented to minimize the odds of workers' "burnout" (i.e., long-term physical and psychological exhaustion related to chronic professional stress and work-family conflict)?

- ○ **A.** Holding individual and group meetings among employees, wherein work and family responsibilities could be informally discussed
- ○ **B.** Creating regular and voluntary mild exercise programs such as walks in the nearest park
- ○ **C.** Offering appealing and expenses-paid vacation opportunities to employees
- ○ **D.** Offering therapy sessions to burned-out employees, wherein coping strategies could be discussed

Question 56

According to the information provided in the passage, how could the identified gender differences associated with the work–family conflict be explained?

- ○ **A.** The coping strategies that are more helpful for each gender target the areas that each gender generally masters less.
- ○ **B.** The masculine gender is more prone to experiencing negative emotions, and as such more often resorts to maladaptative coping strategies when dealing with the family-work conflict.
- ○ **C.** The coping strategies that are more helpful for each gender are congruent with gender-role expectations.
- ○ **D.** Since women are more often discriminated against in the work place, they are those who suffer most with the family-work conflict.

Sources: *T.D. Allen, D. Herst, C. Bruck, and M. Sutton, "Consequences Associated with Work-to-family Conflict: A Review and Agenda for Future Research." Copyright 2000 Journal of Occupational Health Psychology; F.T. Amstad, L.L. Meier, U. Fasel et al., "A Meta-analysis of Work–family Conflict and Various Outcomes with a Special Emphasis on Cross-domain versus Matching-domain Relations." Copyright 2011 Journal of Occupational Health Psychology; U.S. Census Bureau 2010, "Out of Office." Copyright 2010 The Wall Street Journal; A.L. Cox, J. Bird, N. Mauthner et al., "Socio-technical Practices and Work-Home Boundaries." Copyright 2014 MobileHCI; N. Jansen, I.J. Kant, T.S. Kristensen, and F.J.N. Nijhuis, "Antecedents and Consequences of Work–Family Conflict: A Prospective Cohort Study." Copyright 2003 The American College of Occupational and Environmental Medicine; R. Ilies, I.E. De Pater, S. Lim, and C. Binnewies, "Attributed Causes for Work–Family Conflict: Emotional and Behavioral Outcomes." Copyright 2012 Organizational Psychology Review; R.S. Gajendran and D.A. Harrison, "The Good, the Bad, and the Unknown About Telecommuting: Meta-Analysis of Psychological Mediators and Individual Consequences." Copyright 2007 Journal of Applied Psychology.*

The following questions are NOT based on a descriptive passage (Questions 57–59).

Question 57

Which statement below is the most consistent with the Pygmalion effect hypothesis in explaining the home advantage (i.e., winning more often when competing at home vs. elsewhere) observed in certain sports?

- ○ **A.** Referees tend to unconsciously and biasedly favor home teams (vs. visiting teams) because they have an a priori expectation that that team will perform better.
- ○ **B.** Home teams feel more confident, secure, and dominant in a familiar (vs. unfamiliar) environment, and consequently play more aggressively and competitively.
- ○ **C.** Home (vs. visiting) teams tend to have bigger crowds of cheering viewers and are spurred to exhibit more competitive and aggressive behaviors.
- ○ **D.** Home team (vs. visiting) coaches are more financially and emotionally pressed by sponsors, and thus more actively inspire cooperative behaviors among players.

Question 58

Pheromones are NOT usually regarded as possessing which of the following characteristics?

- ○ **A.** They increase gonadotropin-releasing hormone secretion.
- ○ **B.** They cannot be artificially synthesized and bought.
- ○ **C.** They are a nonverbal form of communicating.
- ○ **D.** They are sensed by Bowman's glands.

Question 59

What sociological explanation can be used to understand why butcher shoppers tend to expect butchers to NOT use their knives to harm them?

- ○ **A.** Max Weber's theory of Protestant ethic
- ○ **B.** Jean Baudrillard's object value system theory
- ○ **C.** Georg Simmel's concept of the stranger
- ○ **D.** Emile Durkheim's notion of collective consciousness

CANDIDATE'S NAME ______________________________

TOTAL SCORE (conversions at MCAT-prep.com) ________ / 528

GS-1
Mock Exam 1 of 7
Solutions at MCAT-prep.com

Section I: Chemical and Physical Foundations of Biological Systems

	A B C D		A B C D		A B C D
1	(A)(B)(C)(D)	26	(A)(B)(C)(D)	51	(A)(B)(C)(D)
2	(A)(B)(C)(D)	27	(A)(B)(C)(D)	52	(A)(B)(C)(D)
3	(A)(B)(C)(D)	28	(A)(B)(C)(D)	53	(A)(B)(C)(D)
4	(A)(B)(C)(D)	29	(A)(B)(C)(D)	54	(A)(B)(C)(D)
5	(A)(B)(C)(D)	30	(A)(B)(C)(D)	55	(A)(B)(C)(D)
6	(A)(B)(C)(D)	31	(A)(B)(C)(D)	56	(A)(B)(C)(D)
7	(A)(B)(C)(D)	32	(A)(B)(C)(D)	57	(A)(B)(C)(D)
8	(A)(B)(C)(D)	33	(A)(B)(C)(D)	58	(A)(B)(C)(D)
9	(A)(B)(C)(D)	34	(A)(B)(C)(D)	59	(A)(B)(C)(D)
10	(A)(B)(C)(D)	35	(A)(B)(C)(D)		
11	(A)(B)(C)(D)	36	(A)(B)(C)(D)		
12	(A)(B)(C)(D)	37	(A)(B)(C)(D)		
13	(A)(B)(C)(D)	38	(A)(B)(C)(D)		
14	(A)(B)(C)(D)	39	(A)(B)(C)(D)		
15	(A)(B)(C)(D)	40	(A)(B)(C)(D)		
16	(A)(B)(C)(D)	41	(A)(B)(C)(D)		
17	(A)(B)(C)(D)	42	(A)(B)(C)(D)		
18	(A)(B)(C)(D)	43	(A)(B)(C)(D)		
19	(A)(B)(C)(D)	44	(A)(B)(C)(D)		
20	(A)(B)(C)(D)	45	(A)(B)(C)(D)		
21	(A)(B)(C)(D)	46	(A)(B)(C)(D)		
22	(A)(B)(C)(D)	47	(A)(B)(C)(D)		
23	(A)(B)(C)(D)	48	(A)(B)(C)(D)		
24	(A)(B)(C)(D)	49	(A)(B)(C)(D)		
25	(A)(B)(C)(D)	50	(A)(B)(C)(D)		

Raw Score / 59

Scaled Score / 132

Section II: Critical Analysis and Reasoning Skills (CARS)

	A B C D		A B C D		A B C D
1	(A)(B)(C)(D)	26	(A)(B)(C)(D)	51	(A)(B)(C)(D)
2	(A)(B)(C)(D)	27	(A)(B)(C)(D)	52	(A)(B)(C)(D)
3	(A)(B)(C)(D)	28	(A)(B)(C)(D)	53	(A)(B)(C)(D)
4	(A)(B)(C)(D)	29	(A)(B)(C)(D)		
5	(A)(B)(C)(D)	30	(A)(B)(C)(D)		
6	(A)(B)(C)(D)	31	(A)(B)(C)(D)		
7	(A)(B)(C)(D)	32	(A)(B)(C)(D)		
8	(A)(B)(C)(D)	33	(A)(B)(C)(D)		
9	(A)(B)(C)(D)	34	(A)(B)(C)(D)		
10	(A)(B)(C)(D)	35	(A)(B)(C)(D)		
11	(A)(B)(C)(D)	36	(A)(B)(C)(D)		
12	(A)(B)(C)(D)	37	(A)(B)(C)(D)		
13	(A)(B)(C)(D)	38	(A)(B)(C)(D)		
14	(A)(B)(C)(D)	39	(A)(B)(C)(D)		
15	(A)(B)(C)(D)	40	(A)(B)(C)(D)		
16	(A)(B)(C)(D)	41	(A)(B)(C)(D)		
17	(A)(B)(C)(D)	42	(A)(B)(C)(D)		
18	(A)(B)(C)(D)	43	(A)(B)(C)(D)		
19	(A)(B)(C)(D)	44	(A)(B)(C)(D)		
20	(A)(B)(C)(D)	45	(A)(B)(C)(D)		
21	(A)(B)(C)(D)	46	(A)(B)(C)(D)		
22	(A)(B)(C)(D)	47	(A)(B)(C)(D)		
23	(A)(B)(C)(D)	48	(A)(B)(C)(D)		
24	(A)(B)(C)(D)	49	(A)(B)(C)(D)		
25	(A)(B)(C)(D)	50	(A)(B)(C)(D)		

Raw Score / 53

Scaled Score / 132

Section III: Biological and Biochemical Foundations of Living Systems

	A B C D		A B C D		A B C D
1	(A)(B)(C)(D)	26	(A)(B)(C)(D)	51	(A)(B)(C)(D)
2	(A)(B)(C)(D)	27	(A)(B)(C)(D)	52	(A)(B)(C)(D)
3	(A)(B)(C)(D)	28	(A)(B)(C)(D)	53	(A)(B)(C)(D)
4	(A)(B)(C)(D)	29	(A)(B)(C)(D)	54	(A)(B)(C)(D)
5	(A)(B)(C)(D)	30	(A)(B)(C)(D)	55	(A)(B)(C)(D)
6	(A)(B)(C)(D)	31	(A)(B)(C)(D)	56	(A)(B)(C)(D)
7	(A)(B)(C)(D)	32	(A)(B)(C)(D)	57	(A)(B)(C)(D)
8	(A)(B)(C)(D)	33	(A)(B)(C)(D)	58	(A)(B)(C)(D)
9	(A)(B)(C)(D)	34	(A)(B)(C)(D)	59	(A)(B)(C)(D)
10	(A)(B)(C)(D)	35	(A)(B)(C)(D)		
11	(A)(B)(C)(D)	36	(A)(B)(C)(D)		
12	(A)(B)(C)(D)	37	(A)(B)(C)(D)		
13	(A)(B)(C)(D)	38	(A)(B)(C)(D)		
14	(A)(B)(C)(D)	39	(A)(B)(C)(D)		
15	(A)(B)(C)(D)	40	(A)(B)(C)(D)		
16	(A)(B)(C)(D)	41	(A)(B)(C)(D)		
17	(A)(B)(C)(D)	42	(A)(B)(C)(D)		
18	(A)(B)(C)(D)	43	(A)(B)(C)(D)		
19	(A)(B)(C)(D)	44	(A)(B)(C)(D)		
20	(A)(B)(C)(D)	45	(A)(B)(C)(D)		
21	(A)(B)(C)(D)	46	(A)(B)(C)(D)		
22	(A)(B)(C)(D)	47	(A)(B)(C)(D)		
23	(A)(B)(C)(D)	48	(A)(B)(C)(D)		
24	(A)(B)(C)(D)	49	(A)(B)(C)(D)		
25	(A)(B)(C)(D)	50	(A)(B)(C)(D)		

Raw Score / 59

Scaled Score / 132

Section IV: Psychological, Social, and Biological Foundations of Behavior

	A B C D		A B C D		A B C D
1	(A)(B)(C)(D)	26	(A)(B)(C)(D)	51	(A)(B)(C)(D)
2	(A)(B)(C)(D)	27	(A)(B)(C)(D)	52	(A)(B)(C)(D)
3	(A)(B)(C)(D)	28	(A)(B)(C)(D)	53	(A)(B)(C)(D)
4	(A)(B)(C)(D)	29	(A)(B)(C)(D)	54	(A)(B)(C)(D)
5	(A)(B)(C)(D)	30	(A)(B)(C)(D)	55	(A)(B)(C)(D)
6	(A)(B)(C)(D)	31	(A)(B)(C)(D)	56	(A)(B)(C)(D)
7	(A)(B)(C)(D)	32	(A)(B)(C)(D)	57	(A)(B)(C)(D)
8	(A)(B)(C)(D)	33	(A)(B)(C)(D)	58	(A)(B)(C)(D)
9	(A)(B)(C)(D)	34	(A)(B)(C)(D)	59	(A)(B)(C)(D)
10	(A)(B)(C)(D)	35	(A)(B)(C)(D)		
11	(A)(B)(C)(D)	36	(A)(B)(C)(D)		
12	(A)(B)(C)(D)	37	(A)(B)(C)(D)		
13	(A)(B)(C)(D)	38	(A)(B)(C)(D)		
14	(A)(B)(C)(D)	39	(A)(B)(C)(D)		
15	(A)(B)(C)(D)	40	(A)(B)(C)(D)		
16	(A)(B)(C)(D)	41	(A)(B)(C)(D)		
17	(A)(B)(C)(D)	42	(A)(B)(C)(D)		
18	(A)(B)(C)(D)	43	(A)(B)(C)(D)		
19	(A)(B)(C)(D)	44	(A)(B)(C)(D)		
20	(A)(B)(C)(D)	45	(A)(B)(C)(D)		
21	(A)(B)(C)(D)	46	(A)(B)(C)(D)		
22	(A)(B)(C)(D)	47	(A)(B)(C)(D)		
23	(A)(B)(C)(D)	48	(A)(B)(C)(D)		
24	(A)(B)(C)(D)	49	(A)(B)(C)(D)		
25	(A)(B)(C)(D)	50	(A)(B)(C)(D)		

Raw Score / 59

Scaled Score / 132

CANDIDATE'S NAME ______________________________

TOTAL SCORE (conversions at MCAT-prep.com) ____________ / 528

GS-2
Mock Exam 2 of 7
Solutions at MCAT-prep.com

Section I:
Chemical and Physical Foundations of Biological Systems

	A	B	C	D		A	B	C	D		A	B	C	D
1	A	B	C	D	26	A	B	C	D	51	A	B	C	D
2	A	B	C	D	27	A	B	C	D	52	A	B	C	D
3	A	B	C	D	28	A	B	C	D	53	A	B	C	D
4	A	B	C	D	29	A	B	C	D	54	A	B	C	D
5	A	B	C	D	30	A	B	C	D	55	A	B	C	D
6	A	B	C	D	31	A	B	C	D	56	A	B	C	D
7	A	B	C	D	32	A	B	C	D	57	A	B	C	D
8	A	B	C	D	33	A	B	C	D	58	A	B	C	D
9	A	B	C	D	34	A	B	C	D	59	A	B	C	D
10	A	B	C	D	35	A	B	C	D					
11	A	B	C	D	36	A	B	C	D					
12	A	B	C	D	37	A	B	C	D					
13	A	B	C	D	38	A	B	C	D					
14	A	B	C	D	39	A	B	C	D					
15	A	B	C	D	40	A	B	C	D					
16	A	B	C	D	41	A	B	C	D					
17	A	B	C	D	42	A	B	C	D					
18	A	B	C	D	43	A	B	C	D					
19	A	B	C	D	44	A	B	C	D					
20	A	B	C	D	45	A	B	C	D					
21	A	B	C	D	46	A	B	C	D					
22	A	B	C	D	47	A	B	C	D					
23	A	B	C	D	48	A	B	C	D					
24	A	B	C	D	49	A	B	C	D					
25	A	B	C	D	50	A	B	C	D					

Raw Score / 59

Scaled Score / 132

Section II:
Critical Analysis and Reasoning Skills (CARS)

	A	B	C	D		A	B	C	D		A	B	C	D
1	A	B	C	D	26	A	B	C	D	51	A	B	C	D
2	A	B	C	D	27	A	B	C	D	52	A	B	C	D
3	A	B	C	D	28	A	B	C	D	53	A	B	C	D
4	A	B	C	D	29	A	B	C	D					
5	A	B	C	D	30	A	B	C	D					
6	A	B	C	D	31	A	B	C	D					
7	A	B	C	D	32	A	B	C	D					
8	A	B	C	D	33	A	B	C	D					
9	A	B	C	D	34	A	B	C	D					
10	A	B	C	D	35	A	B	C	D					
11	A	B	C	D	36	A	B	C	D					
12	A	B	C	D	37	A	B	C	D					
13	A	B	C	D	38	A	B	C	D					
14	A	B	C	D	39	A	B	C	D					
15	A	B	C	D	40	A	B	C	D					
16	A	B	C	D	41	A	B	C	D					
17	A	B	C	D	42	A	B	C	D					
18	A	B	C	D	43	A	B	C	D					
19	A	B	C	D	44	A	B	C	D					
20	A	B	C	D	45	A	B	C	D					
21	A	B	C	D	46	A	B	C	D					
22	A	B	C	D	47	A	B	C	D					
23	A	B	C	D	48	A	B	C	D					
24	A	B	C	D	49	A	B	C	D					
25	A	B	C	D	50	A	B	C	D					

Raw Score / 53

Scaled Score / 132

Section III:
Biological and Biochemical Foundations of Living Systems

	A	B	C	D		A	B	C	D		A	B	C	D
1	A	B	C	D	26	A	B	C	D	51	A	B	C	D
2	A	B	C	D	27	A	B	C	D	52	A	B	C	D
3	A	B	C	D	28	A	B	C	D	53	A	B	C	D
4	A	B	C	D	29	A	B	C	D	54	A	B	C	D
5	A	B	C	D	30	A	B	C	D	55	A	B	C	D
6	A	B	C	D	31	A	B	C	D	56	A	B	C	D
7	A	B	C	D	32	A	B	C	D	57	A	B	C	D
8	A	B	C	D	33	A	B	C	D	58	A	B	C	D
9	A	B	C	D	34	A	B	C	D	59	A	B	C	D
10	A	B	C	D	35	A	B	C	D					
11	A	B	C	D	36	A	B	C	D					
12	A	B	C	D	37	A	B	C	D					
13	A	B	C	D	38	A	B	C	D					
14	A	B	C	D	39	A	B	C	D					
15	A	B	C	D	40	A	B	C	D					
16	A	B	C	D	41	A	B	C	D					
17	A	B	C	D	42	A	B	C	D					
18	A	B	C	D	43	A	B	C	D					
19	A	B	C	D	44	A	B	C	D					
20	A	B	C	D	45	A	B	C	D					
21	A	B	C	D	46	A	B	C	D					
22	A	B	C	D	47	A	B	C	D					
23	A	B	C	D	48	A	B	C	D					
24	A	B	C	D	49	A	B	C	D					
25	A	B	C	D	50	A	B	C	D					

Raw Score / 59

Scaled Score / 132

Section IV:
Psychological, Social, and Biological Foundations of Behavior

	A	B	C	D		A	B	C	D		A	B	C	D
1	A	B	C	D	26	A	B	C	D	51	A	B	C	D
2	A	B	C	D	27	A	B	C	D	52	A	B	C	D
3	A	B	C	D	28	A	B	C	D	53	A	B	C	D
4	A	B	C	D	29	A	B	C	D	54	A	B	C	D
5	A	B	C	D	30	A	B	C	D	55	A	B	C	D
6	A	B	C	D	31	A	B	C	D	56	A	B	C	D
7	A	B	C	D	32	A	B	C	D	57	A	B	C	D
8	A	B	C	D	33	A	B	C	D	58	A	B	C	D
9	A	B	C	D	34	A	B	C	D	59	A	B	C	D
10	A	B	C	D	35	A	B	C	D					
11	A	B	C	D	36	A	B	C	D					
12	A	B	C	D	37	A	B	C	D					
13	A	B	C	D	38	A	B	C	D					
14	A	B	C	D	39	A	B	C	D					
15	A	B	C	D	40	A	B	C	D					
16	A	B	C	D	41	A	B	C	D					
17	A	B	C	D	42	A	B	C	D					
18	A	B	C	D	43	A	B	C	D					
19	A	B	C	D	44	A	B	C	D					
20	A	B	C	D	45	A	B	C	D					
21	A	B	C	D	46	A	B	C	D					
22	A	B	C	D	47	A	B	C	D					
23	A	B	C	D	48	A	B	C	D					
24	A	B	C	D	49	A	B	C	D					
25	A	B	C	D	50	A	B	C	D					

Raw Score / 59

Scaled Score / 132

CANDIDATE'S NAME ______________________

TOTAL SCORE (conversions at MCAT-prep.com) ________ / 528

GS-3
Mock Exam 3 of 7
Solutions at MCAT-prep.com

Section I: Chemical and Physical Foundations of Biological Systems

	A B C D		A B C D		A B C D
1	(A)(B)(C)(D)	26	(A)(B)(C)(D)	51	(A)(B)(C)(D)
2	(A)(B)(C)(D)	27	(A)(B)(C)(D)	52	(A)(B)(C)(D)
3	(A)(B)(C)(D)	28	(A)(B)(C)(D)	53	(A)(B)(C)(D)
4	(A)(B)(C)(D)	29	(A)(B)(C)(D)	54	(A)(B)(C)(D)
5	(A)(B)(C)(D)	30	(A)(B)(C)(D)	55	(A)(B)(C)(D)
6	(A)(B)(C)(D)	31	(A)(B)(C)(D)	56	(A)(B)(C)(D)
7	(A)(B)(C)(D)	32	(A)(B)(C)(D)	57	(A)(B)(C)(D)
8	(A)(B)(C)(D)	33	(A)(B)(C)(D)	58	(A)(B)(C)(D)
9	(A)(B)(C)(D)	34	(A)(B)(C)(D)	59	(A)(B)(C)(D)
10	(A)(B)(C)(D)	35	(A)(B)(C)(D)		
11	(A)(B)(C)(D)	36	(A)(B)(C)(D)		
12	(A)(B)(C)(D)	37	(A)(B)(C)(D)		
13	(A)(B)(C)(D)	38	(A)(B)(C)(D)		
14	(A)(B)(C)(D)	39	(A)(B)(C)(D)		
15	(A)(B)(C)(D)	40	(A)(B)(C)(D)		
16	(A)(B)(C)(D)	41	(A)(B)(C)(D)		
17	(A)(B)(C)(D)	42	(A)(B)(C)(D)		
18	(A)(B)(C)(D)	43	(A)(B)(C)(D)		
19	(A)(B)(C)(D)	44	(A)(B)(C)(D)		
20	(A)(B)(C)(D)	45	(A)(B)(C)(D)		
21	(A)(B)(C)(D)	46	(A)(B)(C)(D)		
22	(A)(B)(C)(D)	47	(A)(B)(C)(D)		
23	(A)(B)(C)(D)	48	(A)(B)(C)(D)		
24	(A)(B)(C)(D)	49	(A)(B)(C)(D)		
25	(A)(B)(C)(D)	50	(A)(B)(C)(D)		

Raw Score / 59

Scaled Score / 132

Section II: Critical Analysis and Reasoning Skills (CARS)

	A B C D		A B C D		A B C D
1	(A)(B)(C)(D)	26	(A)(B)(C)(D)	51	(A)(B)(C)(D)
2	(A)(B)(C)(D)	27	(A)(B)(C)(D)	52	(A)(B)(C)(D)
3	(A)(B)(C)(D)	28	(A)(B)(C)(D)	53	(A)(B)(C)(D)
4	(A)(B)(C)(D)	29	(A)(B)(C)(D)		
5	(A)(B)(C)(D)	30	(A)(B)(C)(D)		
6	(A)(B)(C)(D)	31	(A)(B)(C)(D)		
7	(A)(B)(C)(D)	32	(A)(B)(C)(D)		
8	(A)(B)(C)(D)	33	(A)(B)(C)(D)		
9	(A)(B)(C)(D)	34	(A)(B)(C)(D)		
10	(A)(B)(C)(D)	35	(A)(B)(C)(D)		
11	(A)(B)(C)(D)	36	(A)(B)(C)(D)		
12	(A)(B)(C)(D)	37	(A)(B)(C)(D)		
13	(A)(B)(C)(D)	38	(A)(B)(C)(D)		
14	(A)(B)(C)(D)	39	(A)(B)(C)(D)		
15	(A)(B)(C)(D)	40	(A)(B)(C)(D)		
16	(A)(B)(C)(D)	41	(A)(B)(C)(D)		
17	(A)(B)(C)(D)	42	(A)(B)(C)(D)		
18	(A)(B)(C)(D)	43	(A)(B)(C)(D)		
19	(A)(B)(C)(D)	44	(A)(B)(C)(D)		
20	(A)(B)(C)(D)	45	(A)(B)(C)(D)		
21	(A)(B)(C)(D)	46	(A)(B)(C)(D)		
22	(A)(B)(C)(D)	47	(A)(B)(C)(D)		
23	(A)(B)(C)(D)	48	(A)(B)(C)(D)		
24	(A)(B)(C)(D)	49	(A)(B)(C)(D)		
25	(A)(B)(C)(D)	50	(A)(B)(C)(D)		

Raw Score / 53

Scaled Score / 132

Section III: Biological and Biochemical Foundations of Living Systems

	A B C D		A B C D		A B C D
1	(A)(B)(C)(D)	26	(A)(B)(C)(D)	51	(A)(B)(C)(D)
2	(A)(B)(C)(D)	27	(A)(B)(C)(D)	52	(A)(B)(C)(D)
3	(A)(B)(C)(D)	28	(A)(B)(C)(D)	53	(A)(B)(C)(D)
4	(A)(B)(C)(D)	29	(A)(B)(C)(D)	54	(A)(B)(C)(D)
5	(A)(B)(C)(D)	30	(A)(B)(C)(D)	55	(A)(B)(C)(D)
6	(A)(B)(C)(D)	31	(A)(B)(C)(D)	56	(A)(B)(C)(D)
7	(A)(B)(C)(D)	32	(A)(B)(C)(D)	57	(A)(B)(C)(D)
8	(A)(B)(C)(D)	33	(A)(B)(C)(D)	58	(A)(B)(C)(D)
9	(A)(B)(C)(D)	34	(A)(B)(C)(D)	59	(A)(B)(C)(D)
10	(A)(B)(C)(D)	35	(A)(B)(C)(D)		
11	(A)(B)(C)(D)	36	(A)(B)(C)(D)		
12	(A)(B)(C)(D)	37	(A)(B)(C)(D)		
13	(A)(B)(C)(D)	38	(A)(B)(C)(D)		
14	(A)(B)(C)(D)	39	(A)(B)(C)(D)		
15	(A)(B)(C)(D)	40	(A)(B)(C)(D)		
16	(A)(B)(C)(D)	41	(A)(B)(C)(D)		
17	(A)(B)(C)(D)	42	(A)(B)(C)(D)		
18	(A)(B)(C)(D)	43	(A)(B)(C)(D)		
19	(A)(B)(C)(D)	44	(A)(B)(C)(D)		
20	(A)(B)(C)(D)	45	(A)(B)(C)(D)		
21	(A)(B)(C)(D)	46	(A)(B)(C)(D)		
22	(A)(B)(C)(D)	47	(A)(B)(C)(D)		
23	(A)(B)(C)(D)	48	(A)(B)(C)(D)		
24	(A)(B)(C)(D)	49	(A)(B)(C)(D)		
25	(A)(B)(C)(D)	50	(A)(B)(C)(D)		

Raw Score / 59

Scaled Score / 132

Section IV: Psychological, Social, and Biological Foundations of Behavior

	A B C D		A B C D		A B C D
1	(A)(B)(C)(D)	26	(A)(B)(C)(D)	51	(A)(B)(C)(D)
2	(A)(B)(C)(D)	27	(A)(B)(C)(D)	52	(A)(B)(C)(D)
3	(A)(B)(C)(D)	28	(A)(B)(C)(D)	53	(A)(B)(C)(D)
4	(A)(B)(C)(D)	29	(A)(B)(C)(D)	54	(A)(B)(C)(D)
5	(A)(B)(C)(D)	30	(A)(B)(C)(D)	55	(A)(B)(C)(D)
6	(A)(B)(C)(D)	31	(A)(B)(C)(D)	56	(A)(B)(C)(D)
7	(A)(B)(C)(D)	32	(A)(B)(C)(D)	57	(A)(B)(C)(D)
8	(A)(B)(C)(D)	33	(A)(B)(C)(D)	58	(A)(B)(C)(D)
9	(A)(B)(C)(D)	34	(A)(B)(C)(D)	59	(A)(B)(C)(D)
10	(A)(B)(C)(D)	35	(A)(B)(C)(D)		
11	(A)(B)(C)(D)	36	(A)(B)(C)(D)		
12	(A)(B)(C)(D)	37	(A)(B)(C)(D)		
13	(A)(B)(C)(D)	38	(A)(B)(C)(D)		
14	(A)(B)(C)(D)	39	(A)(B)(C)(D)		
15	(A)(B)(C)(D)	40	(A)(B)(C)(D)		
16	(A)(B)(C)(D)	41	(A)(B)(C)(D)		
17	(A)(B)(C)(D)	42	(A)(B)(C)(D)		
18	(A)(B)(C)(D)	43	(A)(B)(C)(D)		
19	(A)(B)(C)(D)	44	(A)(B)(C)(D)		
20	(A)(B)(C)(D)	45	(A)(B)(C)(D)		
21	(A)(B)(C)(D)	46	(A)(B)(C)(D)		
22	(A)(B)(C)(D)	47	(A)(B)(C)(D)		
23	(A)(B)(C)(D)	48	(A)(B)(C)(D)		
24	(A)(B)(C)(D)	49	(A)(B)(C)(D)		
25	(A)(B)(C)(D)	50	(A)(B)(C)(D)		

Raw Score / 59

Scaled Score / 132

CANDIDATE'S NAME ______________________

TOTAL SCORE (conversions at MCAT-prep.com) ________ / 528

GS-4
Mock Exam 4 of 7
Solutions at MCAT-prep.com

Section I: Chemical and Physical Foundations of Biological Systems

	A	B	C	D		A	B	C	D		A	B	C	D
1	A	B	C	D	26	A	B	C	D	51	A	B	C	D
2	A	B	C	D	27	A	B	C	D	52	A	B	C	D
3	A	B	C	D	28	A	B	C	D	53	A	B	C	D
4	A	B	C	D	29	A	B	C	D	54	A	B	C	D
5	A	B	C	D	30	A	B	C	D	55	A	B	C	D
6	A	B	C	D	31	A	B	C	D	56	A	B	C	D
7	A	B	C	D	32	A	B	C	D	57	A	B	C	D
8	A	B	C	D	33	A	B	C	D	58	A	B	C	D
9	A	B	C	D	34	A	B	C	D	59	A	B	C	D
10	A	B	C	D	35	A	B	C	D					
11	A	B	C	D	36	A	B	C	D					
12	A	B	C	D	37	A	B	C	D					
13	A	B	C	D	38	A	B	C	D					
14	A	B	C	D	39	A	B	C	D					
15	A	B	C	D	40	A	B	C	D					
16	A	B	C	D	41	A	B	C	D					
17	A	B	C	D	42	A	B	C	D					
18	A	B	C	D	43	A	B	C	D					
19	A	B	C	D	44	A	B	C	D					
20	A	B	C	D	45	A	B	C	D					
21	A	B	C	D	46	A	B	C	D					
22	A	B	C	D	47	A	B	C	D					
23	A	B	C	D	48	A	B	C	D					
24	A	B	C	D	49	A	B	C	D					
25	A	B	C	D	50	A	B	C	D					

Raw Score / 59

Scaled Score / 132

Section II: Critical Analysis and Reasoning Skills (CARS)

	A	B	C	D		A	B	C	D		A	B	C	D
1	A	B	C	D	26	A	B	C	D	51	A	B	C	D
2	A	B	C	D	27	A	B	C	D	52	A	B	C	D
3	A	B	C	D	28	A	B	C	D	53	A	B	C	D
4	A	B	C	D	29	A	B	C	D					
5	A	B	C	D	30	A	B	C	D					
6	A	B	C	D	31	A	B	C	D					
7	A	B	C	D	32	A	B	C	D					
8	A	B	C	D	33	A	B	C	D					
9	A	B	C	D	34	A	B	C	D					
10	A	B	C	D	35	A	B	C	D					
11	A	B	C	D	36	A	B	C	D					
12	A	B	C	D	37	A	B	C	D					
13	A	B	C	D	38	A	B	C	D					
14	A	B	C	D	39	A	B	C	D					
15	A	B	C	D	40	A	B	C	D					
16	A	B	C	D	41	A	B	C	D					
17	A	B	C	D	42	A	B	C	D					
18	A	B	C	D	43	A	B	C	D					
19	A	B	C	D	44	A	B	C	D					
20	A	B	C	D	45	A	B	C	D					
21	A	B	C	D	46	A	B	C	D					
22	A	B	C	D	47	A	B	C	D					
23	A	B	C	D	48	A	B	C	D					
24	A	B	C	D	49	A	B	C	D					
25	A	B	C	D	50	A	B	C	D					

Raw Score / 53

Scaled Score / 132

Section III: Biological and Biochemical Foundations of Living Systems

	A	B	C	D		A	B	C	D		A	B	C	D
1	A	B	C	D	26	A	B	C	D	51	A	B	C	D
2	A	B	C	D	27	A	B	C	D	52	A	B	C	D
3	A	B	C	D	28	A	B	C	D	53	A	B	C	D
4	A	B	C	D	29	A	B	C	D	54	A	B	C	D
5	A	B	C	D	30	A	B	C	D	55	A	B	C	D
6	A	B	C	D	31	A	B	C	D	56	A	B	C	D
7	A	B	C	D	32	A	B	C	D	57	A	B	C	D
8	A	B	C	D	33	A	B	C	D	58	A	B	C	D
9	A	B	C	D	34	A	B	C	D	59	A	B	C	D
10	A	B	C	D	35	A	B	C	D					
11	A	B	C	D	36	A	B	C	D					
12	A	B	C	D	37	A	B	C	D					
13	A	B	C	D	38	A	B	C	D					
14	A	B	C	D	39	A	B	C	D					
15	A	B	C	D	40	A	B	C	D					
16	A	B	C	D	41	A	B	C	D					
17	A	B	C	D	42	A	B	C	D					
18	A	B	C	D	43	A	B	C	D					
19	A	B	C	D	44	A	B	C	D					
20	A	B	C	D	45	A	B	C	D					
21	A	B	C	D	46	A	B	C	D					
22	A	B	C	D	47	A	B	C	D					
23	A	B	C	D	48	A	B	C	D					
24	A	B	C	D	49	A	B	C	D					
25	A	B	C	D	50	A	B	C	D					

Raw Score / 59

Scaled Score / 132

Section IV: Psychological, Social, and Biological Foundations of Behavior

	A	B	C	D		A	B	C	D		A	B	C	D
1	A	B	C	D	26	A	B	C	D	51	A	B	C	D
2	A	B	C	D	27	A	B	C	D	52	A	B	C	D
3	A	B	C	D	28	A	B	C	D	53	A	B	C	D
4	A	B	C	D	29	A	B	C	D	54	A	B	C	D
5	A	B	C	D	30	A	B	C	D	55	A	B	C	D
6	A	B	C	D	31	A	B	C	D	56	A	B	C	D
7	A	B	C	D	32	A	B	C	D	57	A	B	C	D
8	A	B	C	D	33	A	B	C	D	58	A	B	C	D
9	A	B	C	D	34	A	B	C	D	59	A	B	C	D
10	A	B	C	D	35	A	B	C	D					
11	A	B	C	D	36	A	B	C	D					
12	A	B	C	D	37	A	B	C	D					
13	A	B	C	D	38	A	B	C	D					
14	A	B	C	D	39	A	B	C	D					
15	A	B	C	D	40	A	B	C	D					
16	A	B	C	D	41	A	B	C	D					
17	A	B	C	D	42	A	B	C	D					
18	A	B	C	D	43	A	B	C	D					
19	A	B	C	D	44	A	B	C	D					
20	A	B	C	D	45	A	B	C	D					
21	A	B	C	D	46	A	B	C	D					
22	A	B	C	D	47	A	B	C	D					
23	A	B	C	D	48	A	B	C	D					
24	A	B	C	D	49	A	B	C	D					
25	A	B	C	D	50	A	B	C	D					

Raw Score / 59

Scaled Score / 132

CANDIDATE'S NAME ______________________________

TOTAL SCORE (conversions at MCAT-prep.com) ____________ / 528

GS-5
Mock Exam 5 of 7
Solutions at MCAT-prep.com

Section I: Chemical and Physical Foundations of Biological Systems

	A B C D		A B C D		A B C D
1	A B C D	26	A B C D	51	A B C D
2	A B C D	27	A B C D	52	A B C D
3	A B C D	28	A B C D	53	A B C D
4	A B C D	29	A B C D	54	A B C D
5	A B C D	30	A B C D	55	A B C D
6	A B C D	31	A B C D	56	A B C D
7	A B C D	32	A B C D	57	A B C D
8	A B C D	33	A B C D	58	A B C D
9	A B C D	34	A B C D	59	A B C D
10	A B C D	35	A B C D		
11	A B C D	36	A B C D		
12	A B C D	37	A B C D		
13	A B C D	38	A B C D		
14	A B C D	39	A B C D		
15	A B C D	40	A B C D		
16	A B C D	41	A B C D		
17	A B C D	42	A B C D		
18	A B C D	43	A B C D		
19	A B C D	44	A B C D		
20	A B C D	45	A B C D		
21	A B C D	46	A B C D		
22	A B C D	47	A B C D		
23	A B C D	48	A B C D		
24	A B C D	49	A B C D		
25	A B C D	50	A B C D		

Raw Score / 59

Scaled Score / 132

Section II: Critical Analysis and Reasoning Skills (CARS)

	A B C D		A B C D		A B C D
1	A B C D	26	A B C D	51	A B C D
2	A B C D	27	A B C D	52	A B C D
3	A B C D	28	A B C D	53	A B C D
4	A B C D	29	A B C D		
5	A B C D	30	A B C D		
6	A B C D	31	A B C D		
7	A B C D	32	A B C D		
8	A B C D	33	A B C D		
9	A B C D	34	A B C D		
10	A B C D	35	A B C D		
11	A B C D	36	A B C D		
12	A B C D	37	A B C D		
13	A B C D	38	A B C D		
14	A B C D	39	A B C D		
15	A B C D	40	A B C D		
16	A B C D	41	A B C D		
17	A B C D	42	A B C D		
18	A B C D	43	A B C D		
19	A B C D	44	A B C D		
20	A B C D	45	A B C D		
21	A B C D	46	A B C D		
22	A B C D	47	A B C D		
23	A B C D	48	A B C D		
24	A B C D	49	A B C D		
25	A B C D	50	A B C D		

Raw Score / 53

Scaled Score / 132

Section III: Biological and Biochemical Foundations of Living Systems

	A B C D		A B C D		A B C D
1	A B C D	26	A B C D	51	A B C D
2	A B C D	27	A B C D	52	A B C D
3	A B C D	28	A B C D	53	A B C D
4	A B C D	29	A B C D	54	A B C D
5	A B C D	30	A B C D	55	A B C D
6	A B C D	31	A B C D	56	A B C D
7	A B C D	32	A B C D	57	A B C D
8	A B C D	33	A B C D	58	A B C D
9	A B C D	34	A B C D	59	A B C D
10	A B C D	35	A B C D		
11	A B C D	36	A B C D		
12	A B C D	37	A B C D		
13	A B C D	38	A B C D		
14	A B C D	39	A B C D		
15	A B C D	40	A B C D		
16	A B C D	41	A B C D		
17	A B C D	42	A B C D		
18	A B C D	43	A B C D		
19	A B C D	44	A B C D		
20	A B C D	45	A B C D		
21	A B C D	46	A B C D		
22	A B C D	47	A B C D		
23	A B C D	48	A B C D		
24	A B C D	49	A B C D		
25	A B C D	50	A B C D		

Raw Score / 59

Scaled Score / 132

Section IV: Psychological, Social, and Biological Foundations of Behavior

	A B C D		A B C D		A B C D
1	A B C D	26	A B C D	51	A B C D
2	A B C D	27	A B C D	52	A B C D
3	A B C D	28	A B C D	53	A B C D
4	A B C D	29	A B C D	54	A B C D
5	A B C D	30	A B C D	55	A B C D
6	A B C D	31	A B C D	56	A B C D
7	A B C D	32	A B C D	57	A B C D
8	A B C D	33	A B C D	58	A B C D
9	A B C D	34	A B C D	59	A B C D
10	A B C D	35	A B C D		
11	A B C D	36	A B C D		
12	A B C D	37	A B C D		
13	A B C D	38	A B C D		
14	A B C D	39	A B C D		
15	A B C D	40	A B C D		
16	A B C D	41	A B C D		
17	A B C D	42	A B C D		
18	A B C D	43	A B C D		
19	A B C D	44	A B C D		
20	A B C D	45	A B C D		
21	A B C D	46	A B C D		
22	A B C D	47	A B C D		
23	A B C D	48	A B C D		
24	A B C D	49	A B C D		
25	A B C D	50	A B C D		

Raw Score / 59

Scaled Score / 132

Note: Summaries are only useful post-content review.

Gold Standard MCAT Physics Equations - Memorize

Translational motion	$x = x_o + v_o t + 1/2at^2$ | $(V_f)^2 = (V_o)^2 + 2ax$	$V_f = V_o + at$
Frictional force	$f_{max} = \mu N$	$\mu_k < \mu_s$ always
Uniform circular motion*	$F_c = ma_c = mv^2/r$	$a_c = v^2/r$
Momentum, Impulse*	$I = F\Delta t = \Delta M$	$M = mv$
Work, Power	$W = F d \cos\theta$	$P = \Delta W/\Delta t$
Energy (conservation)	$E_T = E_k + E_p$	$E = mc^2$
Spring Force, Work	$F = -kx$	$W = kx^2/2$
Continuity (fluids)	$A v = $ const.	$\rho Av = $ const.
Current and Resistance	$I = Q/t$	$R = \rho l/A$
Resistors (series, par.)	$R_{eq} = R_1 + R_2 \ldots$ | $1/R_{eq} = 1/R_1 + 1/R_2$	$R = 1$ / conductance
Capacitors in Ser. and Par.	$1/C_{eq} = 1/C_1 + 1/C_2 + 1/C_3 \ldots$	$C_{eq} = C_1 + C_2 \ldots$
Sound	$dB = 10 \log_{10}(I/I_0)$	beats = Δf
Kirchoff's Laws	$\Sigma i = 0$ at a junction	$\Sigma\Delta V = 0$ in a loop
Thermodynamics	$Q = mc\Delta T$ (*resembles* MCAT !)	$Q = mL$
Torque forces	$L_1 = F_1 \times r_1$ (CCW + ve)	$L_2 = F_2 \times r_2$ (CW - ve)
Torque force at EQ	$\Sigma F_x = 0$ and $\Sigma F_y = 0$	$\Sigma L = 0$
Refraction	$(\sin\theta_1)/(\sin\theta_2) = v_1/v_2 = n_2/n_1 = \lambda_1/\lambda_2$	$n = c/v$

*Not technically in the new MCAT Physics syllabus but since these are simple concepts that have been the source of traditional MCAT questions, we do not believe that they should be discarded from your preparation.

Gold Standard MCAT Physics Equations - Memorize As Pairs

$F = ma$	$F = qE$	Similar Form
$F = K_G(m_1 m_2/r^2)$	$F = k(q_1 q_2/r^2)$	
$V = IR$	$P = IV$	Paired Use
$v_{av} = \Delta d/\Delta t$	$a_{av} = \Delta v/\Delta t$	(avg vel, acc)
$v = \lambda f$	$E = hf$	$(f = 1/T)$
$E_k = 1/2\, mv^2$	$E_p = mgh$	(kin, pot E)
$P = F/A$	$\Delta P = \rho g\Delta h$	(pressure P)
SG = ρ substance / ρ water	$\rho = 1\ g/cm^3 = 10^3\ kg/m^3$	(Spec Grav)
ρ = mass / volume	$F_b = V\rho g = mg$	(buoyant F)
$1/i + 1/o = 1/f = 2/r$ = Power	M = magnification = $-i/o$	Optics
$\Delta G = \Delta H - T\Delta S$	Gibbs Free Energy	$\Delta G° = -RT\ln K_{eq}$

Gold Standard MCAT Physics Equations - Know How to Use - Do Not Memorize

$P + \rho gh + 1/2\,\rho v_2 = $ constant	Bernouilli's Equation	Fluids in Motion
$f_0 = f_s(V \pm V_0)/(V \pm V_s)$	Doppler Effect: when d is decreasing use $+V_0$ and $-V_s$	
$V = Ed$ for a parallel plate capacitor	d = the distance between the plates	
$dF = dq\, v(B\sin\alpha) = I\, dl(B\sin\alpha)$	Laplace's Law	RH rule
Potential Energy (PE) = W = 1/2 QV	Work in Electricity	$W = 1/2\, CV^2$

Gold Standard MCAT Physics Equations - Atomic Nucleus & Electronic Structure

1. Alpha (α) particle = $_2He^4$ (helium nucleus);
2. Beta (β) particle = $_{-1}e^0$ (an electron);
3. A positron = $_{+1}e^0$ (same mass as an electron but opposite charge);
4. Gamma (γ) ray = no mass, no charge, just electromagnetic energy;
5. $\Delta m / \Delta t$ = rate of decay where Δm = change in mass, Δt = change in time.
6. If the number of half-lifes n are known we can calculate the percentage of a pure radioactive sample left after undergoing decay since the fraction remaining = $(1/2)^n$.
7. $N_{electrons} = 2n^2$, where $N_{electrons}$ designates the number of electrons in shell n.
8. The state of each electron is determined by the four quantum numbers:

○ Principal quantum number = n ▪ Determines the number of shells ▪ Possible values are: 1 (K), 2 (L), 3 (M), etc...	○ Magnetic momentum quantum number = m_l ▪ Determines the orbital ▪ Possible values are: ± l , ... , 0
○ Angular momentum quantum number = l ▪ Determines the subshell ▪ Possible values are: 0 (s), 1 (p), 2 (d), 3 (f), n-1, etc...	○ Spin quantum number = m_s ▪ Determines the direction of rotation of the electron ▪ Possible values are: ± 1/2

Gold Standard MCAT Physics Equations - Trigonometry - The Basics

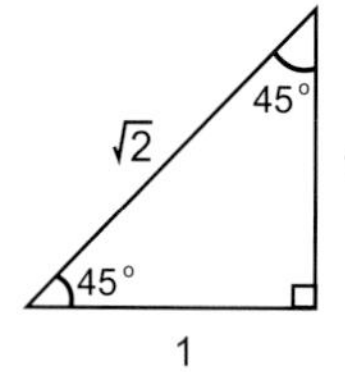

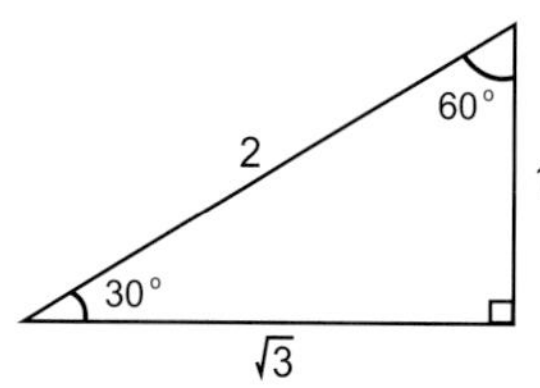

$\sin\theta = \text{opp/hyp}$ $\qquad \theta = \sin^{-1} x$

$\cos\theta = \text{adj/hyp}$ $\qquad \text{arcsec}\,\theta = \sec^{-1}\theta$

$\tan\theta = \text{opp/adj}$ $\qquad r^2 = x^2 + y^2$

- Angle θ may be given in radians (R) where 1 revolution = $2\pi^R = 360°$
- Estimate square root 3 as 1.7 and root 2 as 1.4
- Cross-sectional area of a tube = area of a circle = πr^2 where π can be estimated as 3.14 and r is the radius of the circle; circumference = $2\pi r$

Gold Standard MCAT Physics Equations - Units to Memorize

- Both work and energy are measured in joules where $1\ joule\ (J) = 1\ N \times 1\ m$. {Imperial units: the *foot-pound*, CGS units: the *dyne-centimeter* or *erg* }
- The SI unit for power is the *watt* (W) which equals one *joule per second* (J/s) = *volts* × *amperes.*
- Current is measured in *amperes* = *coulombs/sec*. The units of resistance are ohms, symbolized by Ω (omega), where 1 ohm = 1 volt/ampere.
- The SI unit for pressure is the pascal (1 Pa = 1 N/m^2). Other units are: 1.00 atm = 1.01×10^5 Pa = 1.01 bar = 760 mmHg = 760 torr.
- The SI unit for the magnetic induction vector *B* is the tesla where 1 T = 1 N/(A)(m) = 10^4 gauss.

Gold Standard MCAT General Chemistry Review: Stoichiometry

- Mole - Atomic and Molecular Weights

For element:

$$\text{moles} = \frac{\text{weight of sample in grams}}{\text{GAW}}$$

1 mol = 6.02×10^{23} atoms

For compound:

$$\text{moles} = \frac{\text{weight of sample in grams}}{\text{GMW}}$$

1 mol = 6.02×10^{23} molecules

- Categories of Chemical Reactions

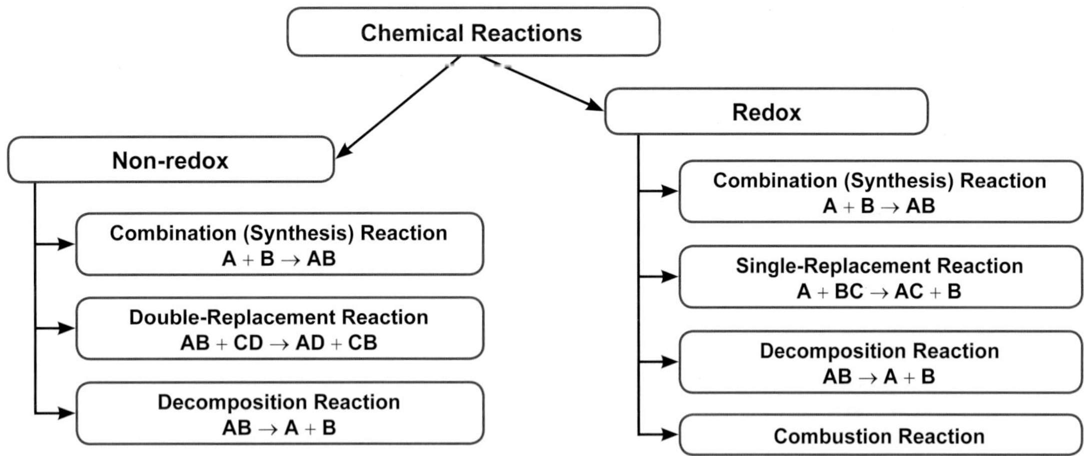

Note: Any reaction that does not involve the transfer of electrons (= change in oxidation numbers) qualifies as a non-redox reaction. Combination reactions qualify as non-redox reactions when all reactants and products are compounds and the oxidation numbers do not change. Decomposition reactions qualify as non-redox reactions when all reactants and products are compounds and the oxidation numbers do not change.

- Oxidation Numbers, Redox Reactions, Oxidizing vs. Reducing Agents
  - Here are the general rules:
    - In elementary substances, the oxidation number of an uncombined element is zero
    - In monatomic ions the oxidation number of the elements that make up this ion is equal to the charge of the ion
    - In a neutral molecule the sum of the oxidation numbers of all the elements that make up the molecule is zero
  - Some useful oxidation numbers to memorize
    - For H: +1, except in metal hydrides where it is equal to -1
    - For O: -2 in most compounds; In peroxides (e.g. in H_2O_2) the oxidation number for O is -1, it is +2 in OF_2 and -1/2 in superoxides
    - For alkali metals: +1
    - For alkaline earth metals: +2
    - Aluminium always has an oxidation number of +3 in all its compounds

Common Redox Agents

Reducing Agents	Oxidizing Agents
* Lithium aluminium hydride ($LiAlH_4$) * Sodium borohydride ($NaBH_4$) * Metals * Ferrous ion (Fe^{2+})	* Iodine (I_2) and other halogens * Permanganate (MnO_4) salts * Peroxide compounds (i.e. H_2O_2) * Ozone (O_3); osmium tetroxide (OsO_4) * Nitric acid (HNO_3); nitrous oxide (N_2O)

- Mixtures

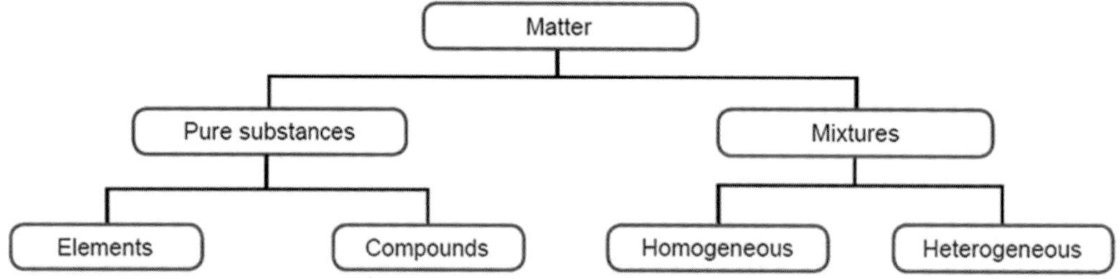

Gold Standard MCAT General Chemistry Review: Electronic Structure & The Periodic Table

- Conventional Notation for Electronic Structure

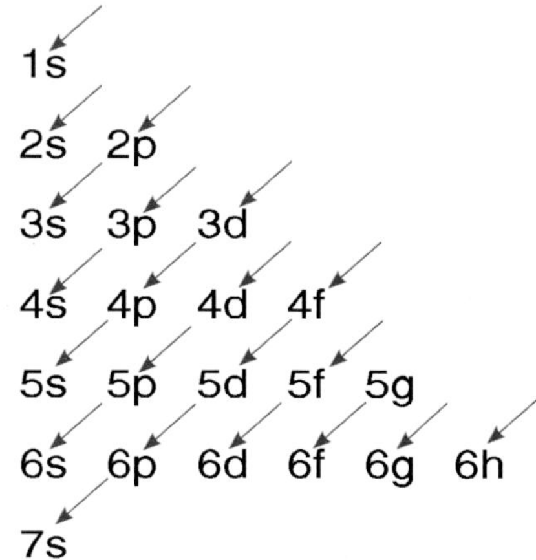

The order for filling atomic orbitals: Follow the direction of successive arrows moving from top to bottom.

- Metals, Nonmetals and Metalloids

*General Characteristics of metals, nonmetals and metalloids

Metals	Nonmetals	Metalloids
Hard and shiny	Gases or dull, brittle solids	Appearance will vary
3 or less valence electrons	5 or more valence electrons	3 to 7 valence electrons
Form + ions by losing e^-	Form − ions by gaining e^-	Form + and/ or − ions
Good conductors of heat and electricity	Poor conductors of heat and electricity	Conduct better than nonmetals, but not as well as metals

*These are general characteristics. There are exceptions beyond the scope of the exam.

Gold Standard MCAT General Chemistry Review: Bonding

- Partial Ionic Character
    - This polar bond will also have a dipole moment given by:

$$D = q \cdot d$$

where q is the charge and d is the distance between these two atoms.

- Lewis Acids and Lewis Bases
    - The Lewis acid BF_3 and the Lewis base NH_3. Notice that the green arrows follow the flow of electron pairs. {Mnemonic: lEwis Acids: Electron pair Acceptors}

- Valence Shell Electronic Pair Repulsions (VSEPR Models)
  - Geometry of simple molecules in which the central atom A has one or more lone pairs of electrons (= e⁻)

Total number of e⁻ pairs	Number of lone pairs	Number of bonding pairs	Electron Geometry, Arrangement of e⁻ pairs	Molecular Geometry (Hybridization State)	Examples
3	1	2	Trigonal planar	Bent (sp^2)	SO_2
4	1	3	Tetrahedral	Trigonal pyramidal (sp^3)	NH_3
4	2	2	Tetrahedral	Bent (sp^3)	H_2O
5	1	4	Trigonal bipyramidal	Seesaw (sp^3d)	SF_4
5	2	3	Trigonal bipyramidal	T-shaped (sp^3d)	ClF_3

Note: dotted lines only represent the overall molecular shape and not molecular bonds. In brackets under "Molecular Geometry" is the hybridization.

linear arrangement of 2 electron pairs around central atom A

trigonal planar arrangement of 3 electron pairs around central atom A

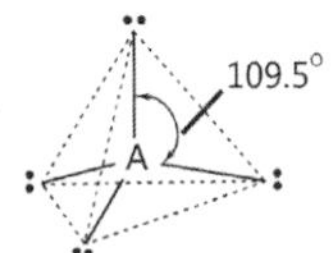

tetrahedral arrangement of 4 electron pairs around central atom A

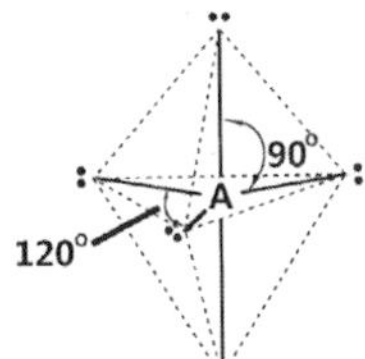

trigonal bipyramidal arrangement of 5 electron pairs around central atom A

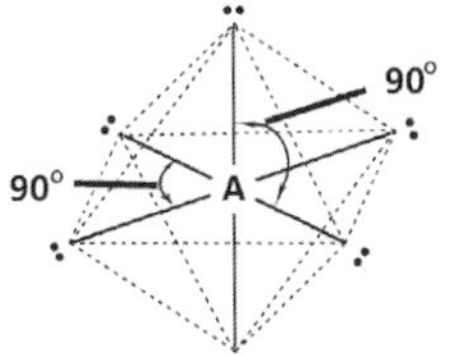

octahedral arrangement of 6 electron pairs around central atom A

Molecular arrangement of electron pairs around a central atom A. Dotted lines only represent the overall molecular shape and not molecular bonds.

Gold Standard MCAT General Chemistry Review: Phases & Phase Equilibria

- Standard Temperature and Pressure, Standard Molar Volume
  - 0 °C (273.15 K) and 1.00 atm (101.33 kPa = 760 mmHg = 760 torr); these conditions are known as the standard temperature and pressure (STP). {Note: the SI unit of pressure is the pascal (Pa).}
  - The volume occupied by one mole of any gas at STP is referred to as the standard molar volume and is equal to 22.4 L.
- Kinetic Molecular Theory of Gases (A Model for Gases)
  - The average kinetic energy of the particles (KE = 1/2 mv^2) increases in direct proportion to the temperature of the gas (KE = 3/2 kT) when the temperature is measured on an absolute scale (i.e. the Kelvin scale) and k is a constant (the Boltzmann constant).

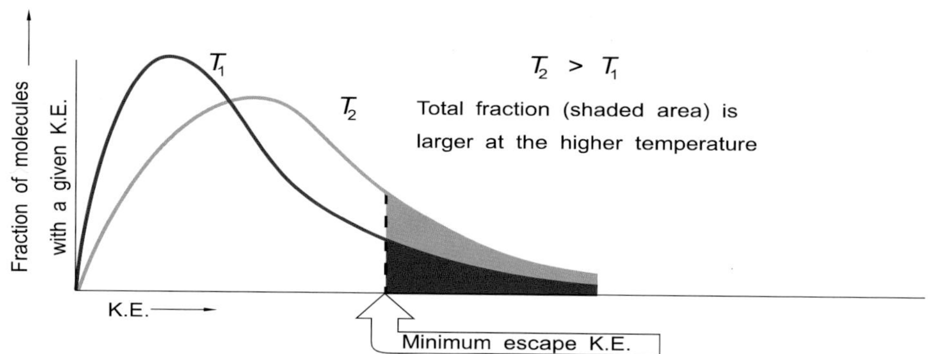

The Maxwell Distribution Plot

Graham's Law (Diffusion and Effusion of Gases)	Combined Gas Law
$\frac{Rate_1}{Rate_2} = \sqrt{\frac{M_2}{M_1}}$	$\frac{P_1V_1}{T_1} = k = \frac{P_2V_2}{T_2}$ (at constant mass)
Charles' Law	**Ideal Gas Law**
$V = Constant \times T$ or $V_1/V_2 = T_1/T_2$	$PV = nRT$ since m/V is the density (d) of the gas: $P = \frac{dRT}{M}$
Boyle's Law	**Partial Pressure and Dalton's Law**
$V = Constant \times 1/P$ or $P_1V_1 = P_2V_2$	$P_T = P_1 + P_2 + \ldots + P_i$ Of course, the sum of all mole fractions in a mixture must equal one: $\Sigma X_1 = 1$
Avogadro's Law	The partial pressure (P_i) of a component of a gas mixture is equal to:
$V/n = Constant$ or $V_1/n_1 = V_2/n_2$	$P_i = X_iP_T$

- Liquid Phase (Intra- and Intermolecular Forces)

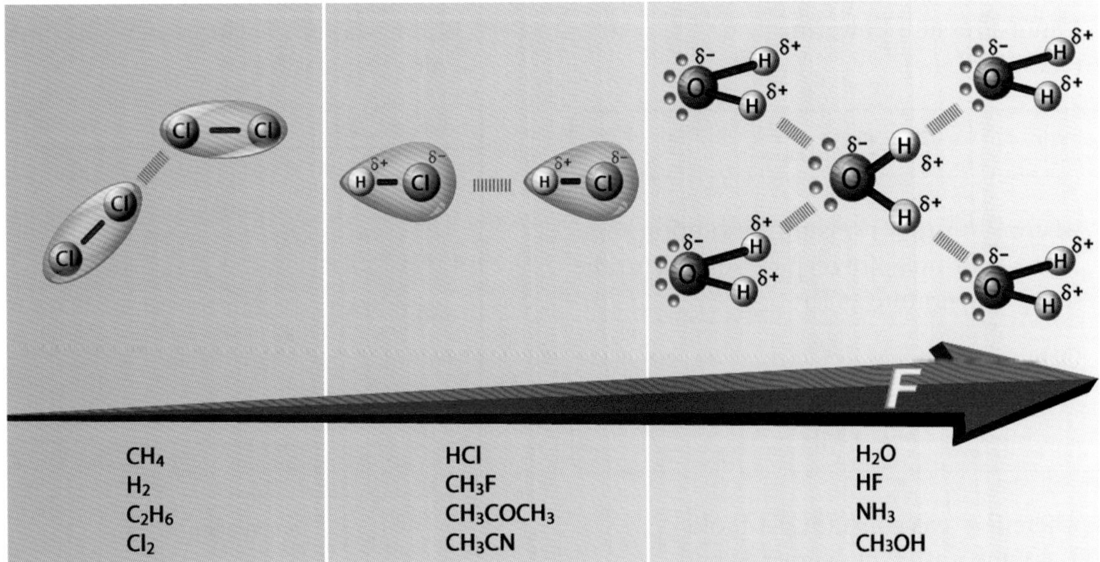

Van Der Waal's forces (weak) and hydrogen bonding (strong). London forces between Cl_2 molecules, dipole-dipole forces between HCl molecules and H-bonding between H_2O molecules. Note that a partial negative charge on an atom is indicated by δ- (delta negative), while a partial positive charge is indicated by δ+ (delta positive). Notice that one H_2O molecule can potentially form 4 H-bonds with surrounding molecules which is highly efficient. The preceding is one key reason that the boiling point of water is higher than that of ammonia, hydrogen fluoride, or methanol.

- Surface Tension
  - PE is directly proportional to the surface area (A)
  - PE = gA; g = surface tension
  - g = F/l; F = force of contraction of surface; l = length along surface

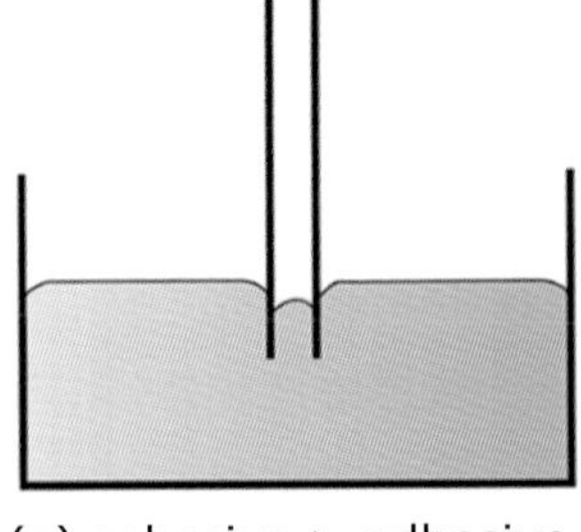
(a) cohesive > adhesive

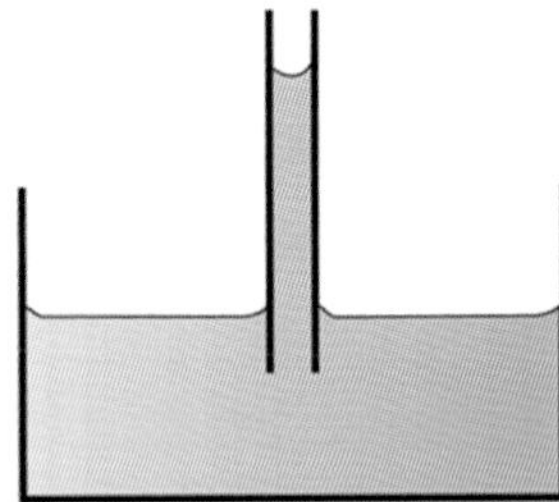
(b) adhesive > cohesive

- Phase Changes

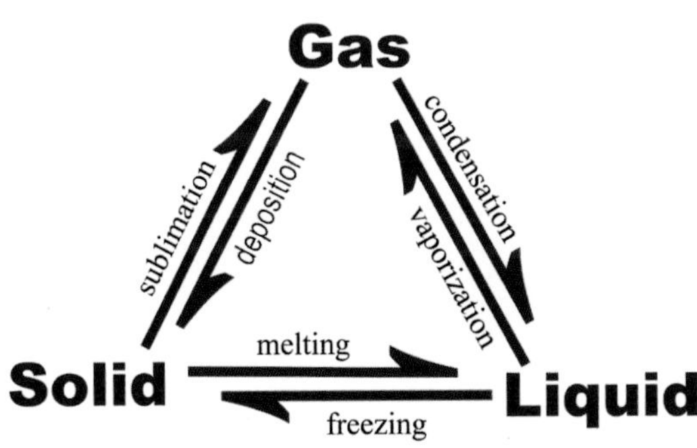

- Phase Diagrams

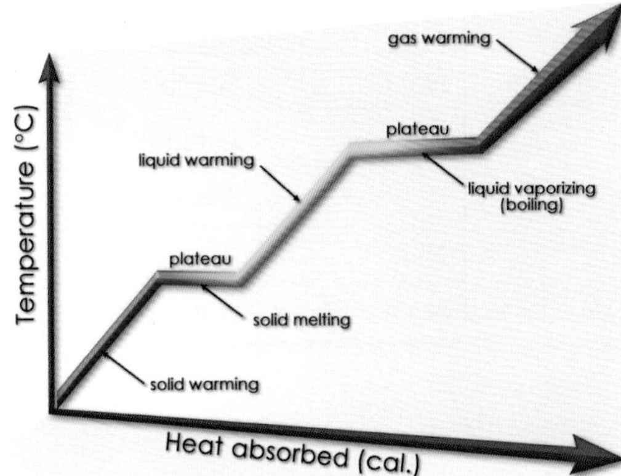

Gold Standard MCAT General Chemistry Review: Solution Chemistry

- Vapor-Pressure Lowering (Raoult's Law)

$$P = P^{\circ}X_{solvent}$$

where P = vapor pressure of solution
P° = vapor pressure of pure solvent (at the same temperature as P)

- Osmotic Pressure

$$\Pi = iMRT$$

where R = gas constant per mole
T = temperature in degrees K and
M = concentration of solute (mole/liter)
i = Van't Hoff factor

- Boiling-Point Elevation and Freezing-Point Depression

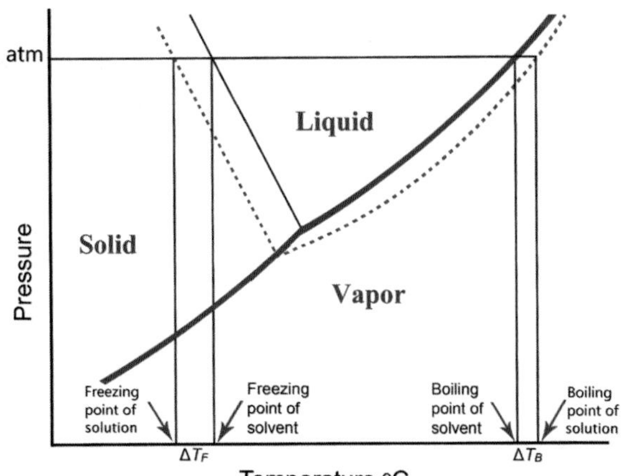

Phase diagram of water demonstrating the effect of the addition of a solute

$\Delta T_B = iK_b m$

$\Delta T_F = iK_F m$

- Ions in Solution
  - Ions that are positively charged = <u>cations</u>; ions that are negatively charged = <u>anions</u>
  - *Mnemonic: a<u>n</u>ions are <u>n</u>egative ions*
  - The word "aqueous" simply means containing or dissolved in water

Common Anions					
F^-	Fluoride	OH^-	Hydroxide	ClO^-	Hypochlorite
Cl^-	Chloride	NO_3^-	Nitrate	ClO_2^-	Chlorite
Br^-	Bromide	NO_2^-	Nitrite	ClO_3^-	Chlorate
I^-	Iodide	CO_3^{2-}	Carbonate	ClO_4^-	Perchlorate
O^{2-}	Oxide	SO_4^{2-}	Sulfate	SO_3^{2-}	Sulfite
S^{2-}	Sulfide	PO_4^{3-}	Phosphate	CN^-	Cyanide
N^{3-}	Nitride	$CH_3CO_2^-$	Acetate	MnO_4^-	Permanganate

Common Cations			
Na^+	Sodium	H^+	Hydrogen
Li^+	Lithium	Ca^{2+}	Calcium
K^+	Potassium	Mg^{2+}	Magnesium
NH_4^+	Ammonium	Fe^{2+}	Iron (II)
H_3O^+	Hydronium	Fe^{3+}	Iron (III)

Common Anions and Cations

- Units of Concentration
  - Molarity (M): moles of solute/liter of solution (solution = solute + solvent)
  - Normality (N): one equivalent per liter
  - Molality (m): one mole/1000g of solvent
  - Molal concentrations are not temperature-dependent as molar and normal concentrations are
  - Density (ρ): Mass per unit volume at the specified temperature
  - Osmole (Osm): The number of moles of particles (molecules or ions) that contribute to the osmotic pressure of a solution
  - Osmolarity: osmoles/liter of solution
  - Osmolality: osmoles/kilogram of solution
  - Mole Fraction: amount of solute (in moles) divided by the total amount of solvent and solute (in moles)
  - Dilution: $M_iV_i = M_fV_f$

- Solubility Product Constant, the Equilibrium Expression

$$AgCl\ (s) \rightleftharpoons Ag^+\ (aq) + Cl^-\ (aq)$$

$$K_{sp} = [Ag^+][Cl^-]$$

Because the K_{sp} product always holds, precipitation will not take place unless the product of $[Ag^+]$ and $[Cl^-]$ exceeds the K_{sp}.

- Solubility Rules
  1. All salts of alkali metals are soluble.
  2. All salts of the ammonium ion are soluble.
  3. All chlorides, bromides and iodides are water soluble, with the exception of Ag^+, Pb^{2+}, and Hg_2^{2+}.
  4. All salts of the sulfate ion (SO_4^{2-}) are water soluble with the exception of Ca^{2+}, Sr^{2+}, Ba^{2+}, and Pb^{2+}.
  5. All metal oxides are insoluble with the exception of the alkali metals and CaO, SrO and BaO.
  6. All hydroxides are insoluble with the exception of the alkali metals and Ca^{2+}, Sr^{2+}, Ba^{2+}.
  7. All carbonates (CO_3^{2-}), phosphates (PO_4^{3-}), sulfides (S^{2-}) and sulfites (SO_3^{2-}) are insoluble, with the exception of the alkali metals and ammonium.

Gold Standard MCAT General Chemistry Review: Acids & Bases

- Acids

$$K_a = [H^+][A^-]/[HA]$$

STRONG	WEAK
Perchloric $HClO_4$	Hydrocyanic HCN
Chloric $HClO_3$	Hypochlorous HClO
Nitric HNO_3	Nitrous HNO_2
Hydrochloric HCl	Hydrofluoric HF
Sulfuric H_2SO_4	Sulfurous H_2SO_3
Hydrobromic HBr	Hydrogen Sulfide H_2S
Hydriodic HI	Phosphoric H_3PO_4
Hydronium Ion H_3O^+	Benzoic, Acetic and other Carboxylic Acids

- Bases

$$K_b = [HB^+][OH^-]/[B]$$

  - Strong bases include any hydroxide of the group 1A metals
  - The most common weak bases are ammonia and any organic amine.

- Conjugate Acid-Base Pairs
  - The acid, HA, and the base produced when it ionizes, A-, are called a conjugate acid-base pair.

- Water Dissociation

$$K_w = [H^+][OH^-] = 1.0 \times 10^{-14}$$

- Salts of Weak Acids and Bases

$$K_a \times K_b = K_w$$

- Buffers

$$pH = pK_a + \log([salt]/[acid])$$

$$pOH = pK_b + \log([salt]/[base])$$

- The pH Scale

$$pH = -\log_{10}[H^+]$$

$$pOH = -\log_{10}[OH^-]$$

at 25°C, pH + pOH = 14.0

- Properties of Logarithms

1. $\log_a a = 1$
2. $\log_a M^k = k \log_a M$
3. $\log_a(MN) = \log_a M + \log_a N$
4. $\log_a(M/N) = \log_a M - \log_a N$
5. $10^{\log_{10}(M)} = M$

Gold Standard MCAT General Chemistry Review: Thermodynamics

- The First Law of Thermodynamics

$$\Delta E = Q - W$$

  - heat absorbed by the system: $Q > 0$
  - heat released by the system: $Q < 0$
  - work done by the system on its surroundings: $W > 0$
  - work done by the surroundings on the system: $W < 0$

- Temperature Scales

$$0 \text{ K} = -273.13 \text{ °C.}$$

$$(X \text{ °F} - 32) \times 5/9 = Y \text{ °C}$$

- State Functions
  - W can be determined experimentally by calculating the area under a pressure-volume curve

	Work	**Heat**	**Changes in internal energy**
1st tranf.	w	0	$-w$
2nd transf.	$W = w + q$	q	$-w$

Gold Standard MCAT General Chemistry Review: Enthalpy & Thermochemistry

- Heat of Reaction: Basic Principles
  - A reaction during which heat is released is said to be exothermic (ΔH is negative).
  - If a reaction requires the supply of a certain amount of heat it is endothermic (ΔH is positive).

$$\Delta H_{OVERALL} = \Delta H_1 + \Delta H_2$$

$$\Delta H^\circ_{reaction} = \Sigma \Delta H_f^\circ{}_{(products)} - \Sigma \Delta H_f^\circ{}_{(reactants)}$$

- Bond Dissociation Energies and Heats of Formation

$$\Delta H^\circ_{(reaction)} = \Sigma \Delta H_{(bonds\ broken)} + \Sigma \Delta H_{(bonds\ formed)}$$
$$= \Sigma BE_{(reactants)} - \Sigma BE_{(products)}$$

- Calorimetry

$$Q = mC(T_2 - T_1)$$

$$Q = m\,L$$

- The Second Law of Thermodynamics
  - For any spontaneous process, the entropy of the universe increases which results in a greater dispersal or randomization of the energy ($\Delta S > 0$).
- Entropy

$$\Delta S^\circ_{reaction} = \Delta S^\circ_{products} - \Delta S^\circ_{reactants}$$

- Free Energy

$$\Delta G = \Delta H - T\,\Delta S$$

  - A reaction carried out at constant pressure is spontaneous if: $\Delta G < 0$
  - It is not spontaneous if: $\Delta G > 0$
  - It is in a state of equilibrium (reaction spontaneous in both directions) if: $\Delta G = 0$

Gold Standard MCAT General Chemistry Review: Rate Processes in Chemical Reactions

- Dependence of Reaction Rates on Concentration of Reactants

$$\text{rate} = k\,[A]^m\,[B]^n$$

  - [ ] is the concentration of the corresponding reactant in moles per liter
  - k is referred to as the rate constant
  - m is the order of the reaction with respect to A
  - n is the order of the reaction with respect to B
  - m+n is the overall reaction order

- Dependence of Reaction Rates upon Temperature

$$k = A\,e^{-Ea/RT}$$

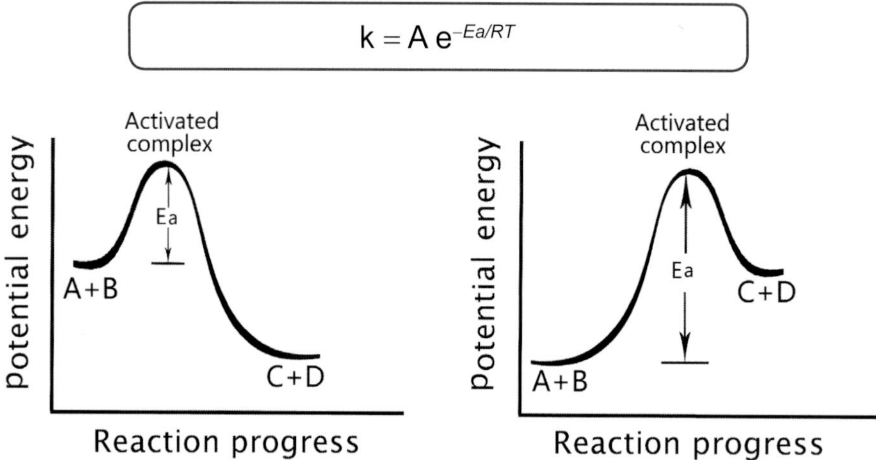

Potential Energy Diagrams: Exothermic vs. Endothermic Reactions

- Catalysis

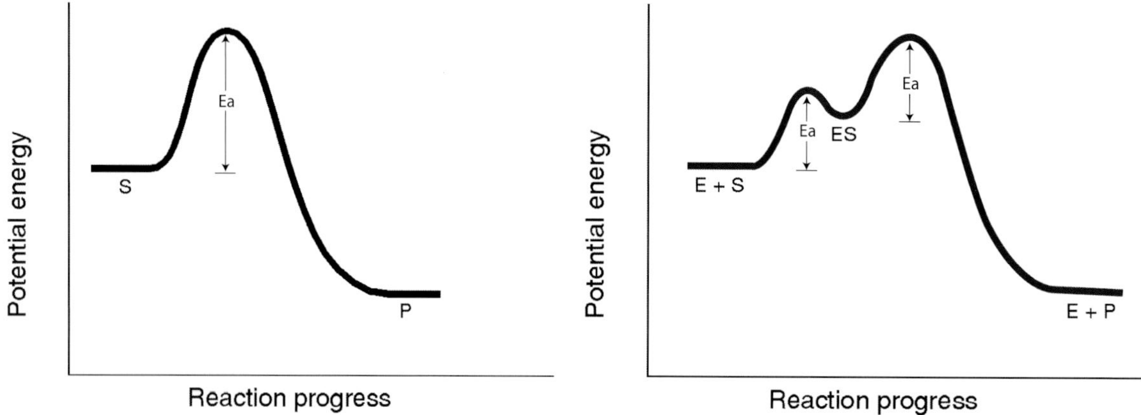

Potential Energy Diagrams: Without and With a Catalyst

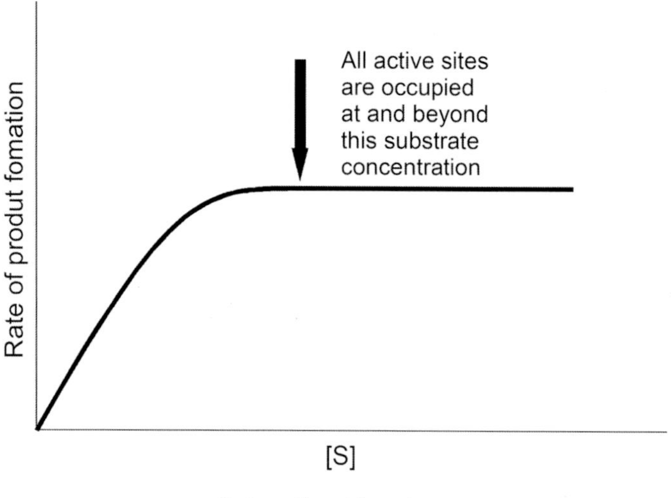

Saturation Kinetics

- Equilibrium in Reversible Chemical Reactions

$$aA + bB \rightleftharpoons cC + dD$$

$$K = \frac{[C]^c\,[D]^d}{[A]^a\,[B]^b}$$

  - {Note: Catalysts speed up the rate of reaction without affecting K_{eq}}

- Le Chatelier's Principle
  - Le Chatelier's principle states that whenever a perturbation is applied to a system at equilibrium, the system evolves in such a way as to compensate for the applied perturbation.
  - Relationship between the Equilibrium Constant and the Change in the Gibbs Free Energy

$$\Delta G^\circ = -R\,T\,ln\,K_{eq}$$

Gold Standard MCAT General Chemistry Review: Electrochemistry

- Generalities
  - The more positive the E° value, the more likely the reaction will occur spontaneously as written.
  - The strongest reducing agents have large negative E° values.
  - The strongest oxidizing agents have large positive E° values.
  - The oxidizing agent is reduced; the reducing agent is oxidized.
- Galvanic Cells
  - Mnemonic: LEO is A GERC
    - Lose Electrons Oxidation is Anode
    - Gain Electrons Reduction at Cathode
- Concentration Cell
  - Nernst equation

$$E_{cell} = E^\circ_{cell} - (RT/nF)(\ln Q)$$

- Faraday's Law
  - Faraday's law relates the amount of elements deposited or gas liberated at an electrode due to current.
  - One mole (= Avogadro's number) of electrons is called a faraday ($\mathfrak{F}$).
  - A faraday is equivalent to 96 500 coulombs.
  - A coulomb is the amount of electricity that is transferred when a current of one ampere flows for one second (1C = 1A . S).

Gold Standard MCAT Organic Chemistry Mechanisms: Summary I

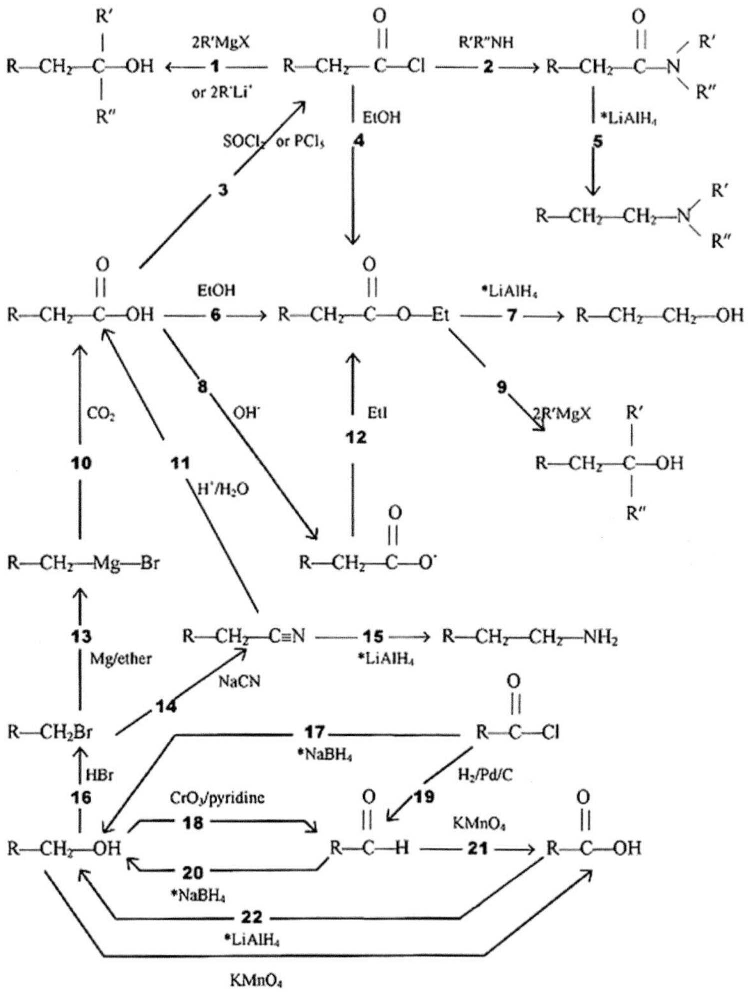

R—CH₂—C(R')(R")—OH ← 1 — 2R'MgX or 2R'Li⁺ — R—CH₂—C(=O)—Cl — 2 → R'R"NH → R—CH₂—C(=O)—N(R')(R")

R—CH₂—C(=O)—N(R')(R") — 5 (*LiAlH₄) → R—CH₂—CH₂—N(R')(R")

R—CH₂—C(=O)—OH — 3 (SOCl₂ or PCl₅) → R—CH₂—C(=O)—Cl

R—CH₂—C(=O)—Cl — 4 (EtOH) → R—CH₂—C(=O)—O—Et

R—CH₂—C(=O)—OH — 6 (EtOH) → R—CH₂—C(=O)—O—Et — 7 (*LiAlH₄) → R—CH₂—CH₂—OH

R—CH₂—C(=O)—O—Et — 9 (2R'MgX) → R—CH₂—C(R')(R")—OH

R—CH₂—C(=O)—OH — 8 (OH⁻) → R—CH₂—C(=O)—O⁻ — 12 (EtI) → R—CH₂—C(=O)—O—Et

R—CH₂—Mg—Br — 10 (CO₂) → R—CH₂—C(=O)—OH

R—CH₂—C≡N — 11 (H⁺/H₂O) → R—CH₂—C(=O)—OH

R—CH₂—C≡N — 15 (*LiAlH₄) → R—CH₂—CH₂—NH₂

R—CH₂Br — 13 (Mg/ether) → R—CH₂—Mg—Br

R—CH₂Br — 14 (NaCN) → R—CH₂—C≡N

R—CH₂—OH — 16 (HBr) → R—CH₂Br

R—C(=O)—Cl — 17 (*NaBH₄) → R—CH₂—OH

R—CH₂—OH — 18 (CrO₃/pyridine) → R—C(=O)—H

R—C(=O)—Cl — 19 (H₂/Pd/C) → R—C(=O)—H

R—C(=O)—H — 20 (*NaBH₄) → R—CH₂—OH

R—C(=O)—H — 21 (KMnO₄) → R—C(=O)—OH

R—C(=O)—OH — 22 (*LiAlH₄) → R—CH₂—OH

R—CH₂—OH — KMnO₄ → R—C(=O)—OH

Gold Standard MCAT Organic Chemistry Mechanisms: Summary II

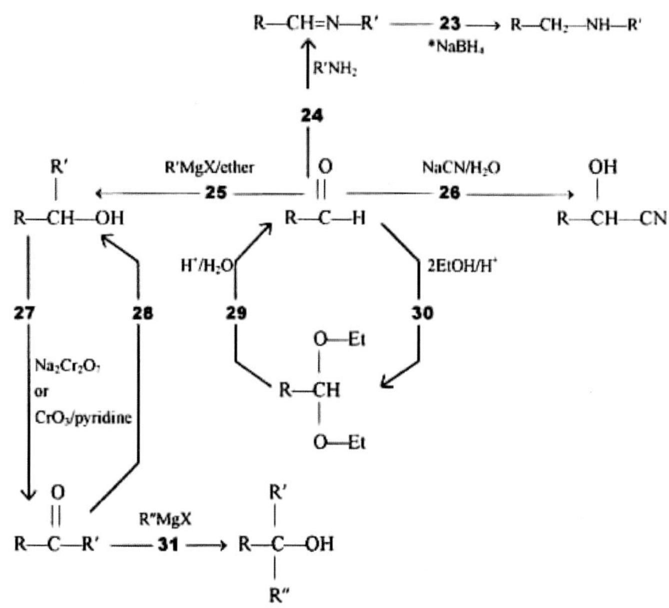

R = alkyl   Et = ethyl   X = halide R^- MgX^+ = Grignard reagent R^- Li^+ = alkyl lithium

Grignard reagents and **alkyl lithiums** are special agents since they can create new C—C bonds (see ORG 1.6).

***Reduction** involves the addition of hydrogen or subtraction of oxygen.

- **Mild reducing agents** add fewer hydrogens/subtract fewer oxygens.
- **Strong reducing agents** add more hydrogens/subtract more oxygens.

Cross-referencing to The Gold Standard MCAT text are found below.

Gold Standard MCAT Organic Chemistry Mechanisms: Basic Principles

Most reactions presented can be derived from basic principles (i.e. ORG 1.6, 7. 1). Many of the reactions are cross-referenced for further information.

1. An acid chloride reacts with a Grignard reagent to produce a tertiary alcohol. See ORG 1.6, 9.1.
2. An acid chloride reacts with a primary or secondary amine to produce an amide. See ORG 9.3 & 11.2.
3. A carboxylic acid reacts with $SOCl_2$ or PCl_5 to produce an acid chloride. See ORG 9.1
4. An acid chloride reacts with an alcohol (e.g. ethanol) to produce an ester. See ORG 9.4.
5. An amide reacts with $LiAlH_4$ to produce an amine. See ORG 8.2, 9.3.
6. A carboxylic acid reacts with an alcohol (e.g. ethanol) to produce an ester. See ORG 8.2.
7. An ester reacts with $LiAlH_4$ to produce a primary alcohol. See ORG 8.2, 9.4.
8. A carboxylic acid reacts with base to produce a carboxylate anion. See CHM 6.3 & ORG 8.1.
9. An ester reacts with a Grignard reagent to produce a tertiary alcohol. See ORG 1.6, 8.1.1, 9.4.
10. A Grignard reagent reacts with carbon dioxide to produce a carboxylic acid. See ORG 8.1.1.
11. A nitrile reacts with aqueous acid to produce a carboxylic acid. See ORG 8.1.1.
12. A carboxylate ion reacts with ethyl iodide to produce an ester.
13. An alkyl halide reacts with Mg/ether to produce a Grignard reagent.
14. An alkyl halide reacts with NaCN to produce a nitrile. See ORG 6.2.3.
15. A nitrile reacts with $LiAlH_4$ to produce an amine. See ORG 8.2.
16. A primary alcohol reacts with HBr to produce an alkyl halide.
17. An acid chloride reacts with $NaBH_4$ to produce a primary alcohol. See ORG 8.2, 9.1.
18. A primary alcohol reacts with CrO_3/pyridine to produce an aldehyde. See ORG 6.2.2, 7.2.1.
19. A acid chloride reacts with H_2/Pd/C to produce an aldehyde. See ORG 7.1, 7.2.1, 9.1.
20. An aldehyde reacts with $NaBH_4$ to produce a primary or secondary alcohol. See ORG 7.1, 8.2.
21. An aldehyde reacts with $KMnO_4$ to produce a carboxylic acid. See ORG 7.2.1, 8.1.1.
22. A carboxylic acid reacts with $LiAlH_4$ to produce a primary alcohol. See ORG 8.2.
23. An imine reacts with $NaBH_4$ to produce a secondary amine. See 7.2.3, 8.2.
24. An aldehyde reacts with a primary amine to produce an imine. See ORG 7.2.3.
25. An aldehyde reacts with a Grignard reagent and ether to produce a secondary alcohol. See ORG 1.6, 7.1.
26. An aldehyde reacts with aqueous NaCN. See ORG 7.1.
27. A secondary alcohol reacts with Na_2CrO_7 or CrO_3/pyridine to produce a ketone. See ORG 6.2.2.
28. A ketone reacts with $NaBH_4$ to produce a secondary alcohol. See ORG 7.2.1.
29. An acetal reacts with aqueous acid to produce an aldehyde. See ORG 7.2.1/2.
30. An aldehyde reacts with an alcohol (e.g. ethanol) and acid to produce an acetal. Note that using with less $EtOH/H^+$, a hemiacetal will form. See ORG 7.2.2.
31. A ketone reacts with a Grignard reagent to produce a tertiary alcohol. See ORG 1.6, 9.

Gold Standard MCAT Organic Chemistry Review: IR Spectroscopy

Memorize at least the following IR spectra data for the MCAT:

- Approx. 3300 cm^{-1} for -OH (alcohol functional group)
- Approx. 1700 cm^{-1} for C=O (carbonyl functional group)

MCAT Biochemistry - Macromolecules, Kinetics, Thermodynamics, & The Plasma Membrane

Building block	Polymerizes to form...	Chemical bonds	Macromolecule
Monomers	Dimer, trimer, tetramer, oligomers, etc.	Covalent* bonds	Polymer
Amino acids	Dipeptide, tripeptide, tetra/oligopeptide, etc	Peptide bonds	Polypeptide, protein (e.g. insulin, hemoglobin)
Monosaccharides ('simple sugars'**)	Disaccharide, tri/tetra/ oligosaccharide, etc.	Glycosidic bonds	Polysaccharide (e.g. starch, glycogen)
Nucleotides	Nucleotide dimer, tri/tetra/oligomer, etc.	Phosphodiester bonds	Polynucleotides, nucleic acids (e.g. DNA, RNA)

*There are exceptions. For example, in certain circumstances polypeptides are considered monomers and they may bond non-covalently to form dimers (i.e. higher orders of protein structure).

**Note that disaccharides are also sugars (i.e. sucrose is a glucose-fructose dimer known as 'table sugar'; lactose is a glucose-galactose known as 'milk sugar').

MCAT Biochemistry Macromolecules: Summary I - Amino Acids & Proteins

The current MCAT regularly has questions which require previous knowledge of the structures, features (including changes in charge with pH), 3- and 1-letter abbreviations of the 20 common protein-generating amino acids, etc.

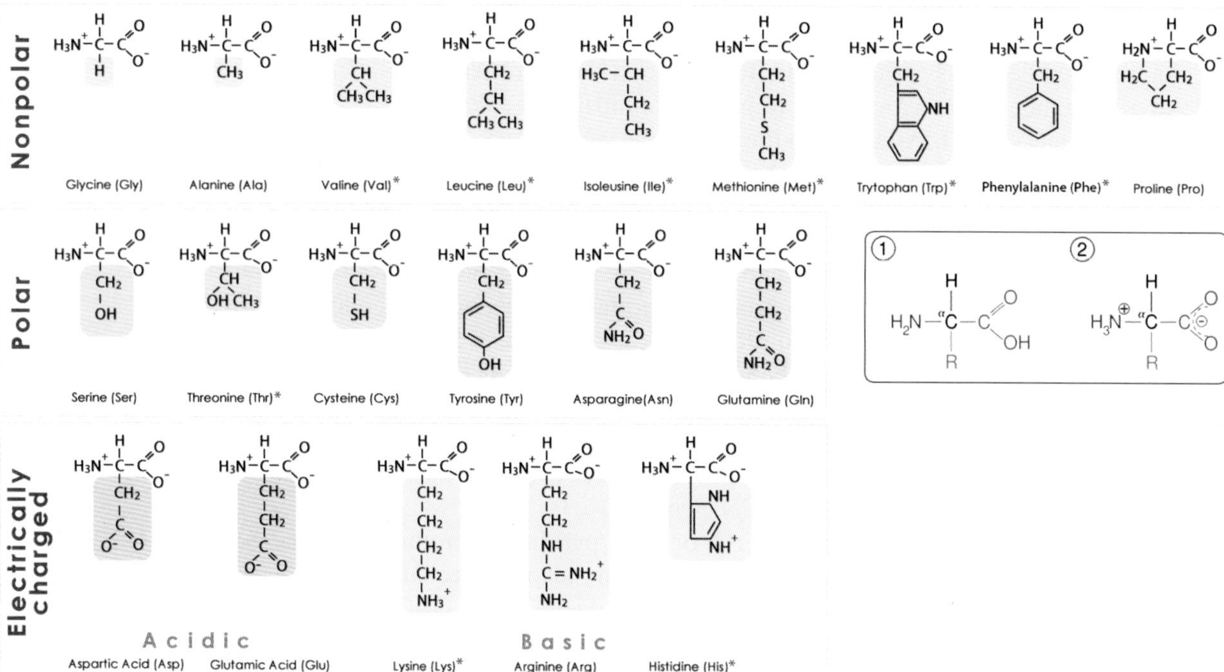

The 20 Standard Amino Acids. A red asterix * is used to indicate the 9 essential amino acids.
Notice that if the acidic electrically charged amino acids are fully protonated, the overall charge would be +1 but if fully deprotonated, the overall charge would be -2. The opposite being true for basic amino acids: If fully protonated, the overall charge would be +2 but if fully deprotonated, the overall charge would be -1. These cases are different than for the average amino acid.

Note the inset (in the red box) which shows the general structure for an amino acid in both the (1) un-ionized and (2) zwitterionic forms. For the latter, note the resonance stabilized carboxylate anion in red, the primary ammonium ion in blue, and the variable R group in green.

$$\ldots NH{-}CH(R){-}C(=O){-}NH{-}CH(R){-}C(=O){-}NH{-}CH(R){-}C(=O)\ldots$$

peptide bonds

$$2\ NH_2{-}CH(R){-}CO_2H \underset{\text{hydrolysis}}{\overset{\text{condensation}}{\rightleftharpoons}} NH_2{-}CH(R){-}C(=O){-}NH{-}CH(R){-}C(=O){-}OH + H_2O$$

Helpful Mnemonics for One-Letter Amino Acid Abbreviations:

Alanine, aRginine, asparagiNe, asparDic acid [aspartic acid], Cysteine, Qutamine [glutamine], glutamEc acid [glutamic acid], Glycine, Histidine, Isoleucine, Leucine, Kysine [lysine], Methionine, Fenylalanine [phenylalanine], Proline, Serine, Threonine, tWyptophan [tryptophan], tYrosine, Valine

Nonpolar Amino Acids = G A P V W L I M F or Gap V.W. Lymph

(lymph is important in fatty acid transport . . . think fatty acid tails are nonpolar)

Polar Uncharged Amino Acids = S T Y C N Q or Stick Nick

(stick like a "pole" . . . think polar)

Electric Amino Acids = D E H K R or Dee Hicker

(dee hicker like deelectric . . . think electric)

To be more precise, for the Polar Charged Amino Acids:

Dee Negative, Hicker Positive, D(-) E(-) H(+) K(+) R(+)

General Principles of Proteins

- Primary structure
  - Sequence of amino acids encoded by DNA and linked to each other through covalent bonds (including disulfide bonds)
- Secondary structure
  - Orderly inter- or intramolecular hydrogen bonding of the protein chain
  - Usually organized in a stable α-helix or a β-pleated sheet
- Tertiary structure
  - Further folding of the protein molecule onto itself
  - 3D shape (spatial organization) of an entire protein molecule
- Quaternary structure
  - 2 or more protein chains bonded together by noncovalent bonds

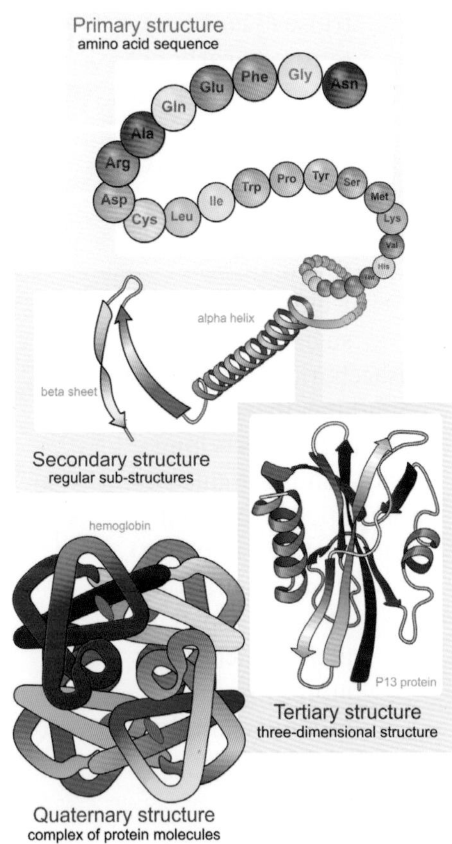

Levels of Protein Organization

- Isoelectric point (pI)
  - pH at which a given amino acid will be neutral (have no net charge)
  - Average of the 2 pK_a values of an amino acid (depending on the dissociated group)
  - Both amino acids and proteins are least soluble at their isoelectric points

$$\text{isoelectric point} = pI = (pK_{a1} + pK_{a2})/2$$

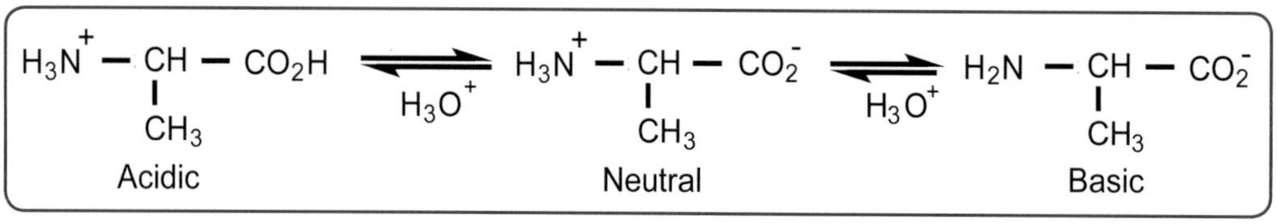

$$H_3N^+-CH(CH_3)-CO_2H \underset{H_3O^+}{\rightleftharpoons} H_3N^+-CH(CH_3)-CO_2^- \underset{H_3O^+}{\rightleftharpoons} H_2N-CH(CH_3)-CO_2^-$$

Acidic — Neutral — Basic

MCAT Biochemistry Macromolecules: Summary II - Carbohydrates

- Compounds consisting of aldehydes and ketones with general formula $C_m(H_2O)_n$
- Monosaccharides = simplest carbohydrate unit
  - Can be named according to number of carbons it contains
  - Common names: triose (3 carbons), tetrose (4 carbons), pentose (5 carbons), hexose (6 carbons)
  - Note: '-ose' suffix denotes sugar
  - Aldose = aldehyde sugar
  - Ketose = ketone sugar
- Disaccharides = two sugars bound together
- Polysaccharides = long sugar chains for glucose storage (i.e. glycogen in animals, starch in plants)
- Absolute configuration
  - Describes spatial arrangement of atoms or groups around a chiral molecule

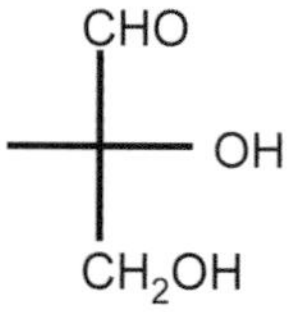

CHO, OH, CH_2OH

D, R-glyceraldehyde

α anomer; condensation; hydrolysis; + H_2O; α - 1,4 glycosidic linkage

D - Glucose
(an aldose hexose)

Haworth projections: Carbons-1 and 2 are intended to be nearer to you.

α - D - Glucose

β - D - Glucose

(axial)

(equatorial)

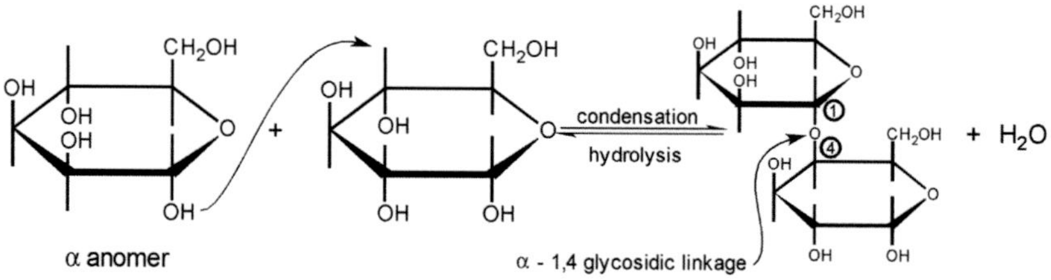

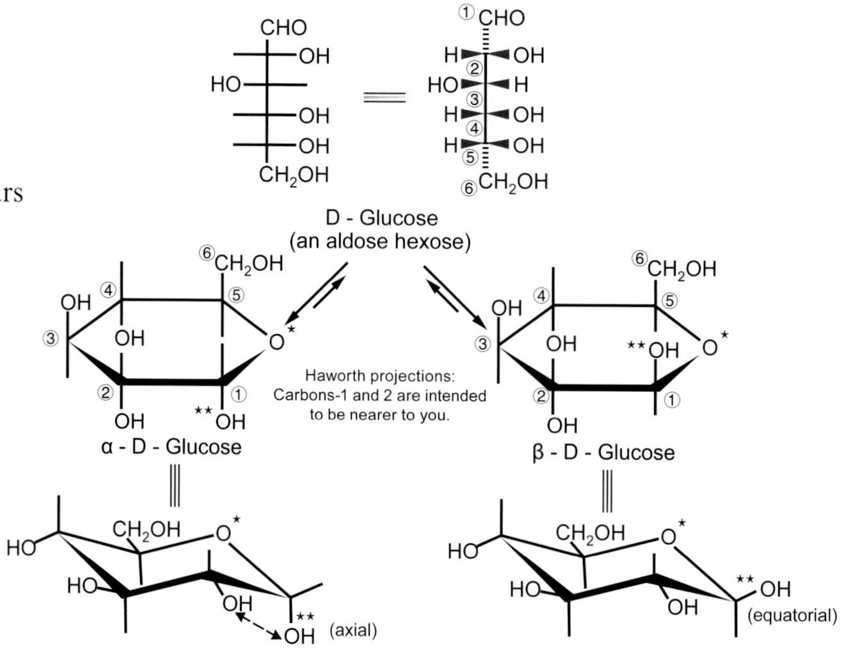

36% at equilibrium (max e^- shell repulsion)

64% at equilibrium

- Assign priority to substituents of the chiral carbon
    - The higher the atomic number, the higher the priority
    - Orient the molecule with the lowest priority substituent in the back
    - If the priorities increase in a clockwise direction = R
    - If the priorities decrease in a clockwise direction = S

- Cyclic structure
    - Monosaccharides can undergo intramolecular reactions to form ring structures
    - Cyclic sugars are stable in solution and can form two types of rings:
        - Six-membered rings (6 carbons in ring) = pyranose
        - Five-membered rings (5 carbons in ring) = furanose
- Glycosidic linkages
    - Covalent bonds between monosaccharides and alcohols
    - When alcohol is another monosaccharide, produces a disaccharide
        - i.e. sucrose, lactose, maltose, cellobiose
    - Linkage between C1 on the first sugar and C2 on the second sugar = 1,2 linkage
    - Linkage between C1 on the first sugar and C4 on the second sugar = 1,4 linkage
    - Linkage between C1 on the first sugar and C6 on the second sugar = 1,6 linkage
    - May also be classified as alpha (α) or beta (β):
        - Hydroxyl group on C1 oriented up = beta (βirds fly in the sky)
        - Hydroxyl group on C1 oriented down = alpha (α - fish - swim in the sea)
- Epimers vs. Anomers
    - Epimers - differ in absolute configuration at only one carbon (R or S)
    - Anomers - differ in configuration at the hemiacetal/acetal (= anomeric) carbon
        - Note: Conversion between anomers = mutarotation

MCAT Biochemistry Macromolecules: Summary III - Fatty Acids

- Amphipathic molecules possessing a polar carboxylate-head group and nonpolar hydrocarbon tail
- Saturated fatty acids
    - Maximum hydrogens - stack together
    - No double bonds
    - Solids at room temperature (= fats; example: butter)
    - Higher melting point, boiling point, and Van der Waals
- Unsaturated fatty acids
    - 1 or more double bonds - bent or kinked structure
    - Liquids at room temperature (= oils; example: olive oil)

$CH_2O-C(=O)-(CH_2)_{14}CH_3$
$CHO-C(=O)-(CH_2)_{14}CH_3$
$CH_2O-C(=O)-(CH_2)_{14}CH_3$

a triglyceride (a fat) $\xrightarrow{3NaOH}$ $CH_2OH-CHOH-CH_2OH$ (glycerol) + $3\,CH_3(CH_2)_{14}CO_2^-Na^+$ (salt of the fatty acid)

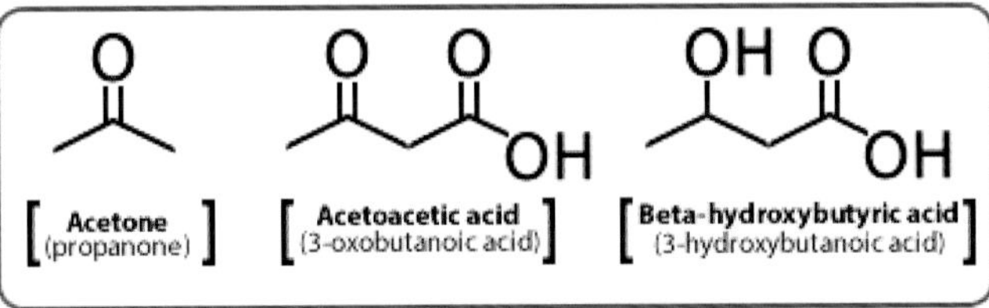

The Three Ketone Bodies

- Exist in body in 3 common forms:
    1. Triglycerides (also known as triacylglycerols)
        - 3 fatty acids esterified to glycerol
        - Nonpolar tails - used for energy storage
        - Digested by lipase
        - With low food intake, broken down by liver to form ketone bodies

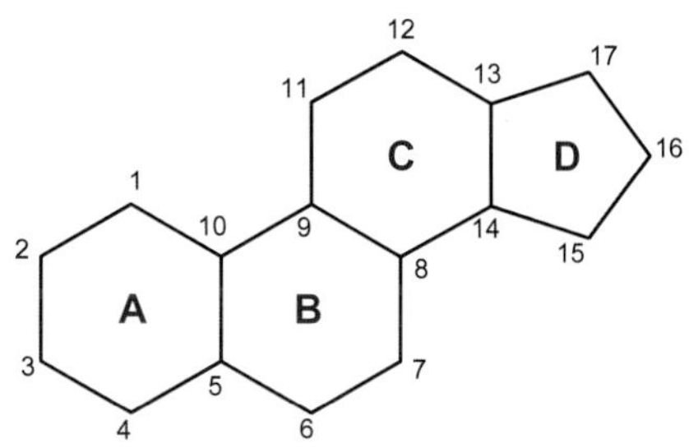

Basic Ring Structure of Steroids

    2. Phospholipids
        - Fatty acids bound to glycerol, phosphate, and other groups
        - Amphipathic (hydrophilic + hydrophobic components) - used for cell membranes
    3. Cholesterol
        - Fatty acids in ring form [isoprene units derived from acetyl-CoA cyclize to form a four-ringed structure]
        - Cholesterol is amphipathic. The ring is nonpolar and the OH-head group is polar.
        - Used for steroid hormones, bile, membrane fluidity

MCAT Biochemistry Macromolecules: Summary IV - Nucleic Acids

- Nucleotides (also known as nucleoside phosphates)
    - are composed of a 5-carbon sugar, a nitrogenous base, and an inorganic phosphate (a glycosidic bond links the nitrogenous base to the sugar)
    - are attached in sequence via phosphodiester bonds to form nucleic acids
    - form the sugar phosphate (negatively-charged) backbone of nucleic acids

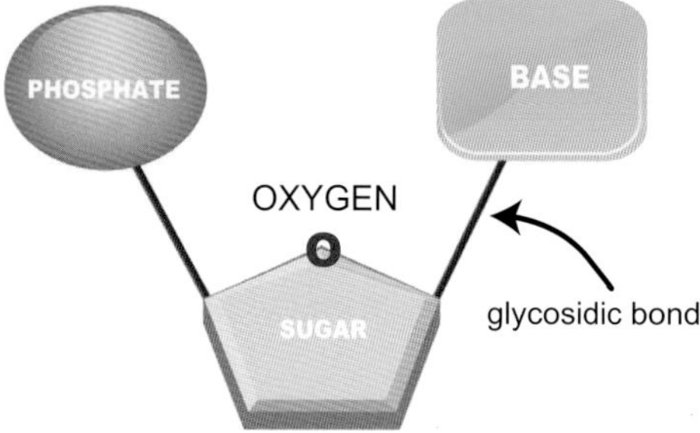

- Nucleosides
    - are composed of a nitrogenous base and a 5-carbon sugar
    - are attached to an inorganic phosphate to form nucleotides
- Nitrogenous Bases
    - Purines
        - 2 rings - adenine (A) and guanine (G) - mnemonic: Pure As Gold
    - Pyrimidines
        - 1 ring - cytosine (C), uracil (U), thymine (T) - mnemonic: CUT the Py

Note that: Pyrimidines are monocyclic (a pie - 'Py' - looks like one ring); as noted above, purines are bicyclic.

Note the direction of hydrogen bonding in the diagram below:

Adenine (A): Purine

Guanine (G): Purine

Cytosine (C): Pyrimidine

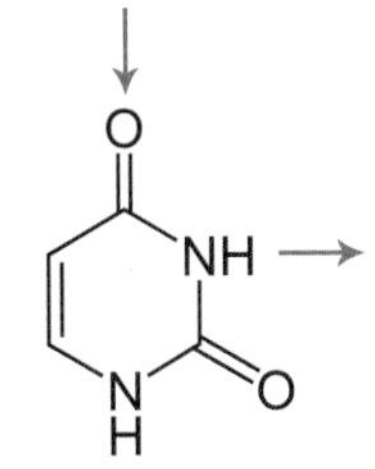

Uracil (U): Pyrimidine

Thymine (T): Pyrimidine

- Watson–Crick model of DNA
  - Double helical structure composed of 2 complementary and anti-parallel DNA strands held together by hydrogen bonds between nitrogenous base pairs
    - A binds T with 2 hydrogen bonds; C binds G with 3 hydrogen bonds
    - Mnemonic: All Tigers and Cats Growl
  - Nitrogenous bases project to center of double helix to hydrogen bond with each other (think of double helix as a winding staircase - each stair represents a nitrogenous base pair keeping the helix shape intact)

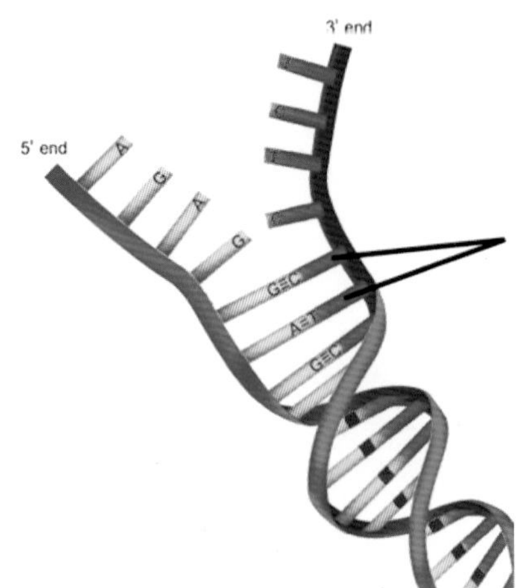

Deoxyribonucleic Acid (DNA)	Ribonucleic Acid (RNA)
Contains the genetic information of the cell - transfers that genetic information	Helps DNA transfer genetic information for creation of proteins
Made from deoxyribose	Made from ribose
Double-stranded	Mostly single-stranded
Adenine binds Thymine Cytosine binds Guanine	Adenine binds Uracil Cytosine binds Guanine
Found in nucleus and mitochondria	Found in nucleus, cytoplasm, and ribosomes
Replicated by DNA polymerases	Transcribed from DNA

- DNA Denaturation
  - Separation of DNA strands due to high temperatures, chemicals (i.e. urea), or UV radiation
  - Occurs when hydrogen bonds between base pairs are broken
  - Separated strands are still complementary
- DNA Reannealing (also known as hybridization)
  - Single, complementary strands stick tightly and reform double-stranded DNA
  - Single strands of DNA can only hybridize with each other if they are complementary

MCAT Biochemistry Macromolecules: Summary V - Metabolism & Nomenclature

Metabolism Summary

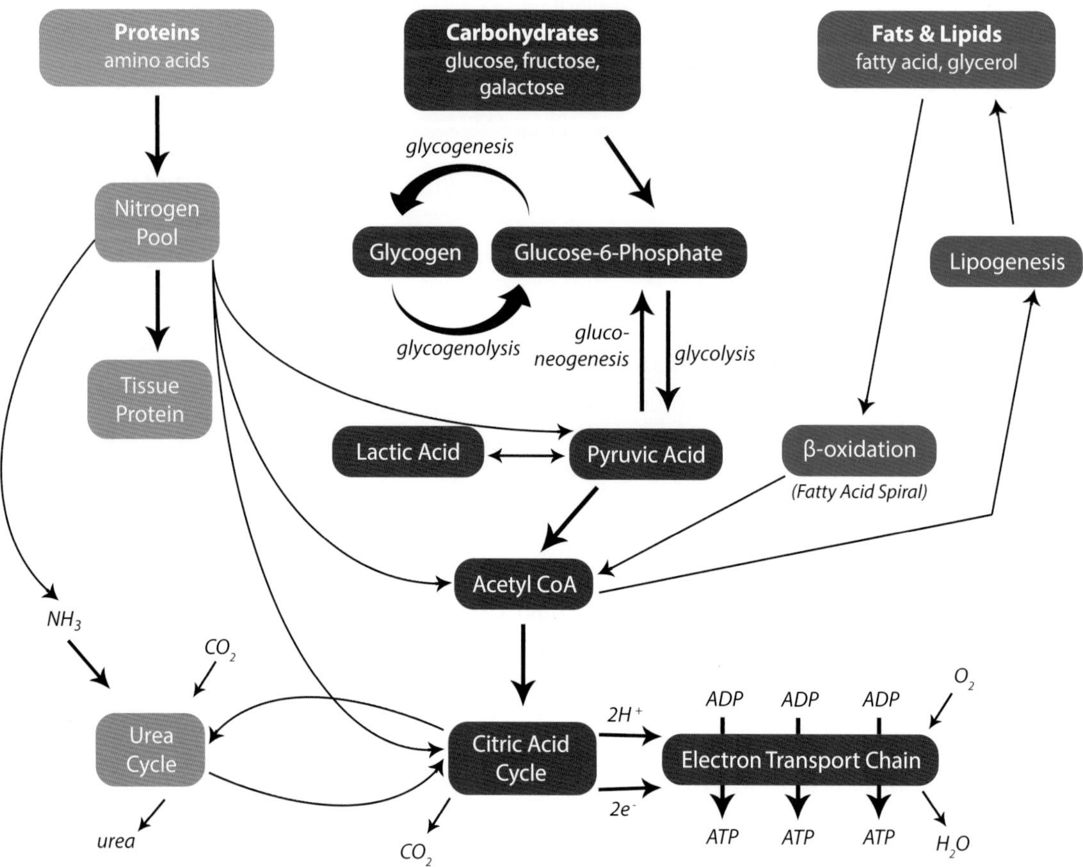

MCAT Biochemistry Kinetics: Summary I

- Kinetics tell how fast a reaction will occur
- Catalysts
    - speed up reactions by speeding up the rate-determining step or providing a different route to the products; lower the energy of activation
    - remain unchanged at the end of the reaction
    - are not included in the overall reaction equation

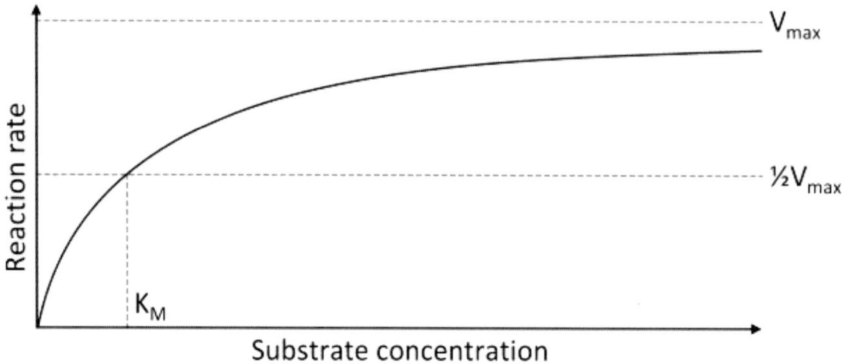

- Michaelis-Menten
  - $V_1 = \frac{V_{max}[S]}{K_m + [S]}$
  - V_0 = initial velocity (reaction rate)
  - V_{max} = maximum reaction rate
  - [S] = concentration of substrate
  - K_m = amount of substrate needed for enzyme to obtain half of its maximum rate of reaction (Michaelis-Menten constant)
    - Low K_m = high affinity for substrate
    - High K_m = low affinity for substrate
    - K_a = association constant of the enzyme-substrate complex
      - Low K_a = low affinity for substrate (enzyme-substrate complex is less stable)
      - High K_a = high affinity for substrate (enzyme-substrate complex is more stable)
    - K_d = dissociation constant of the enzyme-substrate complex
      - Low K_d = high affinity for substrate (enzyme-substrate complex is more stable)
      - High K_d = low affinity for substrate (enzyme-substrate complex is less stable)
    - k_{cat} = number of substrate molecules each enzyme converts to product per unit time (turnover number)
      - Low k_{cat} = enzyme-substrate complex converts less of substrate it binds into product
      - High k_{cat} = enzyme-substrate complex converts more of substrate it binds into product
- Feedback Regulation
  - Positive Feedback - promotes or enhances reactions
  - Negative Feedback - inhibits or reduces reactions
- Cooperativity (also known as positive or negative cooperative binding)
  - Occurs when binding of Substrate B to Substrate A increases (positive) or decreases (negative) activity of Substrate A
  - Michaelis-Menten kinetics do not apply to enzymes engaging in cooperative binding

MCAT Biochemistry Kinetics: Summary II - Enzymes

- Competitive Inhibitors
  - Compete with the substrate in binding to the enzyme's active site
  - Are structurally similar to the substrate
  - Bind to free enzyme (= E) only forming an unreactive enzyme-inhibitor complex (= EI)
  - Cannot bind to the enzyme at the same time as the substrate
  - Can only bind if the substrate has not bound
  - Are reversible with increasing [S]
  - Increase K_m and have no effect on V_{max}
- Uncompetitive Inhibitors
  - Bind to the enzyme-substrate complex (= ES) only forming an unreactive enzyme-inhibitor-substrate complex (= EIS)
  - Can only bind if the substrate has bound
  - Are reversible with decreasing [S]
  - Decrease K_m and decrease V_{max}

- Mixed Inhibitors
  - Bind to the enzyme at a site other than the active site
  - Bind to free enzyme (= E) or the enzyme-substrate complex (= ES) forming an unreactive enzyme-inhibitor complex (= EI) or enzyme-inhibitor-substrate complex (= EIS), respectively
  - Can bind whether or not the substrate has bound
  - Produce a conformational change in the enzyme - binding of the inhibitor reduces the substrate's affinity for the active site
  - Are reduced, but not reversible with increasing [S]
  - Increase or decrease K_m and decrease V_{max}
- Noncompetitive Inhibitors
  - Do not compete with the substrate in binding to the enzyme's active site
  - Bind to the enzyme at a site other than the active site
  - Bind to free enzyme (= E) or the enzyme-substrate complex (= ES) forming an unreactive enzyme-inhibitor complex (= EI) or enzyme-inhibitor-substrate complex (= EIS), respectively
  - Can bind whether or not the substrate has bound
  - Are not reduced or reversible with increasing [S] - must remove inhibitor
  - Decrease V_{max} and have no effect on K_m

Note: Noncompetitive inhibition is sometimes considered a special case of mixed inhibition. Noncompetitive inhibitors have the same affinity for free enzyme (= E) and the enzyme-substrate complex (= ES) whereas mixed inhibitors tend to have a higher affinity for either free enzyme (= E) or the enzyme-substrate complex (= ES).

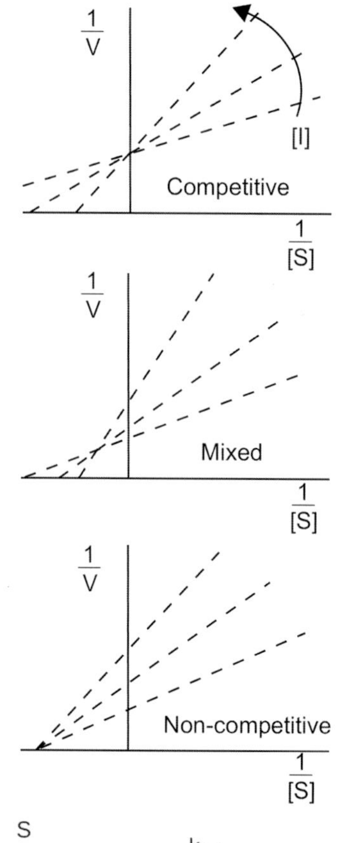

competitive inhibition

E + S ⇌ ES (K_s) → E + P (k_{cat})
E + I ⇌ EI (K_i)

uncompetitive inhibition

E + S ⇌ ES (K_s) → E + P (k_{cat})
ES + I ⇌ EIS (K_{ii})

non-competitive inhibition

E + S ⇌ ES (K_s) → E + P (k_{cat})
E + I ⇌ EI (K_i)
ES + I ⇌ EIS (K_{ii})
EI + S ⇌ EIS (K_{ss})

mixed inhibition

E + S ⇌ ES (K_s) → E + P (k_{cat})
E + I ⇌ EI (K_i)
ES + I ⇌ EIS (K_{ii})
EI + S ⇌ EIS (K_{ss})
EIS → EI + P (k_o)

Six Basic Types of Enzymes	
Class of Enzymes	***What They Catalyze***
Oxidoreductases	Redox Reactions
Transferases	The transfer of groups of atoms
Hydrolases	Hydrolysis
Lyases	Additions to a double bond, or the formation of a double bond
Isomerases	The isomerization of molecules
Ligases or synthetases	The joining of two molecules

Inhibitor	Binds	Reversible?	Effect
Competitive	Free enzyme (E)	Yes with ↑[S]	Increases K_m
Uncompetitive	Enzyme-substrate complex (ES)	Yes with ↓[S]	Decreases K_m and V_{max}
Mixed	Free enzyme (E) or enzyme-substrate complex (ES)	Reduced with ↑[S]	Increases or decreases K_m and decreases V_{max}
Noncompetitive	Free enzyme (E) or enzyme-substrate complex (ES)	Yes with removal of inhibitor	Decreases V_{max}

Ko**M**petitive **IN**hibition = **KM IN**crease (Vmax is unchanged)

NOn-**K**o**M**petitive **IN**hibition = **NO KM IN**crease (but Vmax is decrease)

Uncompetitive Inhibition = BOTH Km and Vmax decrease

- K_i = binding affinity of the inhibitor
  - $K_i > 1$ - inhibitor has higher affinity for enzyme than substrate
  - $K_i < 1$ - inhibitor has lower affinity for enzyme than substrate
- IC_{50} = half-maximal inhibitory concentration
  - Tells how much of a drug is needed to inhibit a biological process by 50%
- Allosteric enzymes have 2 configurations:
  - Active state - catalyzes reactions
  - Inactive state - cannot catalyze reactions
  - Zymogens are inactive enzymes that must be cleaved to become active

MCAT Biochemistry Thermodynamics: Summary

- Thermodynamics tell if a reaction will occur
- Gibbs Free Energy (ΔG) - tells nothing about rate of reaction, only its spontaneity
  - $\Delta G = \Delta H - T\Delta S$
  - Negative ΔG = exergonic = spontaneous
  - $\Delta G = 0$ = equilibrium
  - Positive ΔG = endergonic = nonspontaneous

ΔH	ΔS	...ΔG	Reaction Spontaneity
-	+	-	Spontaneous at all temperatures
-	-	- or +	Spontaneous at low temperatures where ΔH outweighs TΔS Nonspontaneous at high temperatures where TΔS outweighs ΔH
+	-	+	Nonspontaneous at all temperatures
+	+	- or +	Spontaneous at high temperatures where TΔS outweighs ΔH Nonspontaneous at low temperatures where ΔH outweighs TΔS

- Equilibrium constant (K_{eq})
  - K_{eq} = products/reactants = $\frac{[C]^c[D]^d}{[A]^a[B]^b}$ for a reaction A + B → C + D
    - Note: a, b, c, and d are stoichiometries of the substrates and products, respectively
  - $K_{eq} > 1$ - reaction favors products
  - $K_{eq} < 1$ - reaction favors reactants
- Gibbs Free Energy at standard state (ΔG°) = 298K (25°C), 1 atm, pure solids/liquids, 1M solutions
  - $\Delta G° < 0$ and $K_{eq} > 1$ . . . products are favored
  - $\Delta G° = 0$ and $K_{eq} = 1$ . . . products are approx. equal to reactants
  - $\Delta G° > 0$ and $K_{eq} < 1$ . . . reactants are favored
- Le Chatelier's Principle
  - Reaction in equilibrium will change direction according to applied stress
  - Stress could be a change in concentration, pressure, temperature, or volume
- Enthalpy
  - Measure of heat energy absorbed or released when bonds are broken or formed, respectively, during a reaction run at constant pressure
  - Negative ΔH - exothermic - bond(s) formed - energy released
  - Positive ΔH - endothermic - bond(s) broken - energy absorbed

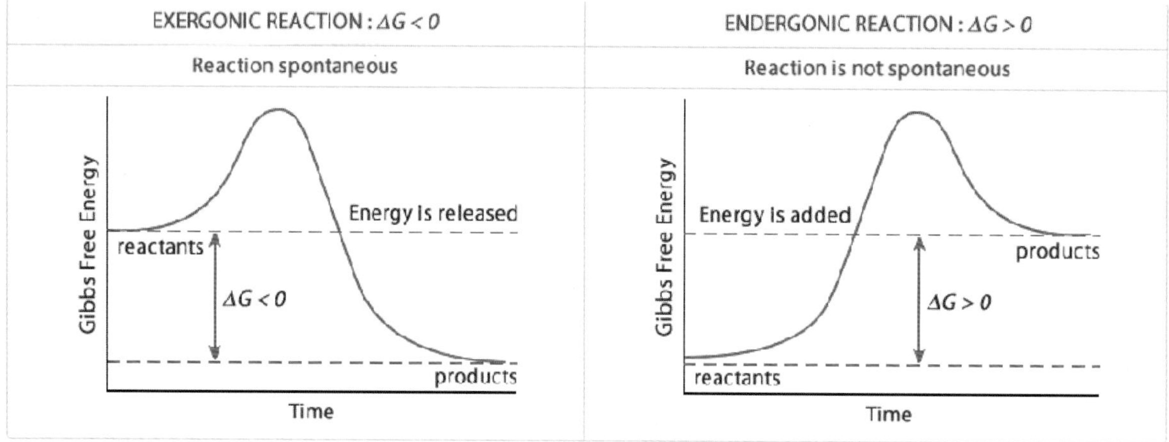

MCAT Biochemistry Plasma Membrane: Summary I

- A phospholipid bilayer that encloses cells
- Outer region - hydrophilic, polar, phosphoric acids (= heads)
- Inner region - hydrophobic, nonpolar, fatty acids (= tails)
- Cholesterol found within membrane for structural support and as a fluidity buffer

- Transmembrane proteins assist in solute transport across membranes

Process (solute type)	Concentration Gradient	Requires Protein?	Requires Energy?
Diffusion (small nonpolar)	High to Low	No	No - passive
Osmosis (water only)	High to Low	No	No - passive
Facilitated Transport (large nonpolar)	High to Low	Yes	No - passive
Active Transport (polar/ions)	Low to High	Yes	Yes - active (ATP)

Note: Difference in polarity between (+) outside and (-) inside along with solute transport creates a membrane potential across the cell membrane.

Osmotic pressure = pressure required to resist movement of water through a semipermeable membrane due to concentration gradient

MCAT Biochemistry Plasma Membrane: Summary II

- Exocytosis
  - Vesicle inside cell fuses with cell membrane and releases contents to outside
- Endocytosis
  - Cell membrane bends inward to form vesicle around particles or liquids
    - If large particles = phagocytosis
    - If small particles or liquids = pinocytosis
- Note: Contents never cross cell membrane in either process
- Biosignaling
  - Ion Channels - allow for passive or active transport of ions; two types:
    - Voltage-gated - transmembrane proteins activated by changes in membrane potential
    - Ligand-gated - transmembrane proteins activated by binding of a specific ligand
- Receptor enzymes (also known as enzyme-linked receptors)
  - Transmembrane proteins
  - Binding of ligand on extracellular side produces activity on the intracellular side
- G protein-coupled receptors
  - Integral membrane proteins
  - Sensing of molecules outside cell activates response inside cell

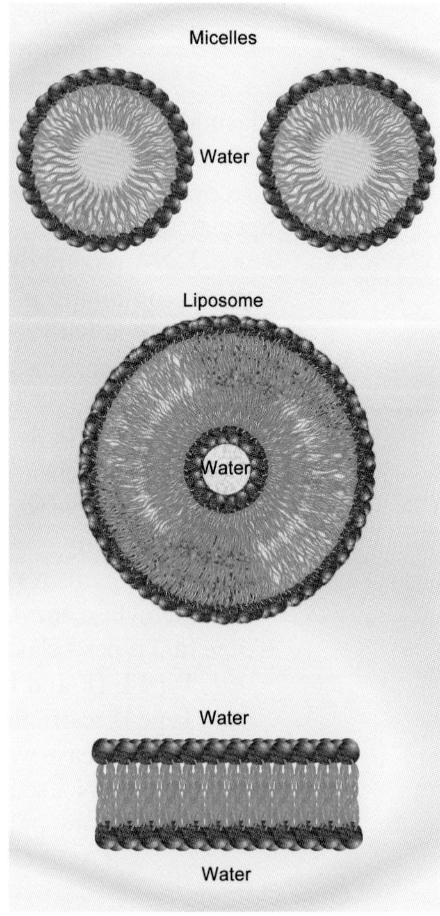

Amphipathic molecules arranged in micelles, a liposome and a bilipid layer [= plasma membrane]

MCAT Biochemistry Biotechnology: Summary I

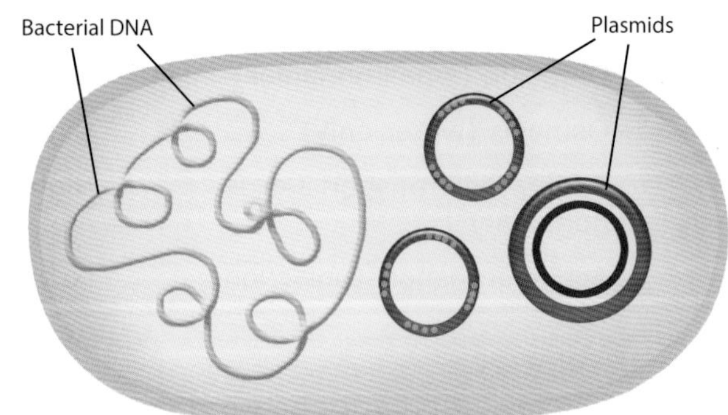

- DNA recombination
  - Involves combining DNA segments or genes from different sources
  - Foreign DNA can come from another DNA molecule, a chromosome, or a complete organism
  - Uses restriction enzymes from bacteria that cut pieces of DNA at specific recognition sites (= nucleotide sequences) along the DNA strand
  - When a double-stranded DNA segment is cut, sticky ends are produced
    - Sticky ends = unpaired, single-strand extensions of DNA that are ready to bind with complementary codons (= sequence of 3 adjacent nucleotides)
    - The cut pieces of DNA = restriction fragments
  - Restriction fragments are then inserted into plasmids
    - Plasmids (also known as replicons)
      - Circular pieces of DNA that replicate independently of chromosomal DNA
      - Cut with the same restriction enzymes as the restriction fragment to generate the same sticky ends
  - Plasmids are introduced into the bacteria via transformation
  - Restriction fragments and linearized plasmids are joined together by DNA ligase to form a recombinant plasmid
  - Special application
    - DNA recombination makes it possible for bacteria to make many copies of recombinant plasmids and produce proteins that are not native to its species (e.g. bacteria with recombinant DNA producing insulin to treat diabetes)
- More on restriction enzymes (also known as restriction endonucleases - endo = internal; nuclease = cut DNA)
  - Naturally found in bacteria and archaea
  - Serve as the organism's own natural defense mechanism
    - Enzymes cleave foreign DNA at specific recognition sites when it enters a bacterium
    - The organism's own DNA is protected by selective methylation at these sites via methylase enzymes
  - Come in 3 types - classified by their structure and how they cleave their DNA substrate
    - Type I, II, and III – Type II is the most common
    - Type II restriction enzymes
      - Cleave within or near specific recognition sites (short, specific, palindromic DNA sequences where cleavage occurs under the right conditions)
      - Note: palindromic sequences read the same forward or backward (e.g. RACE CAR)
- Gene cloning
  - Involves the use of a cloning vector (e.g. plasmid, bacteriophage, virus, etc.)
  - All cloning vectors must contain at least one unique cloning site
  - That cloning site must be cleavable by a restriction enzyme as well as a place where a gene of interest can be inserted

- Multiple Cloning Site
  - An artificially-engineered region of several cloning sites lumped together
  - Found in many commercial and artificially modified cloning vectors
  - Allows the researcher to pick restriction sites that:
    - are unique to the vector
    - ensure that translocation occurs in-frame
- Origin of replication (ori) = allows cloning vectors to self-replicate
- Special applications
  - Cloning vectors are often modified to carry genes that provide resistance to antibiotics, like ampicillin or kanamycin, which allows vectors to be used for selecting certain bacteria
  - Bacteriophage vectors have high transfection (= introduction of nucleic acids into cells) rates and are easy to screen which makes them useful for large-scale applications (e.g. genomic DNA screening)

- DNA libraries
  - are collections of recombinant DNA
  - can consist of (1) genomic DNA or (2) cDNA
  - Genomic DNA library
    - Contains recombinant DNA that represents the entire genome of an organism
    - How it is generated:
      - Partially digest genomic DNA with restriction enzymes to ensure representation of all genes
      - Digests bacteriophage vector with the same enzyme
      - Ligate digested genomic DNA with vector - pack both into bacteriophages
      - Infect densely populated E.coli with bacteriophages
      - Isolate cleared areas of lysed cells (= plaques)
  - cDNA (= complementary DNA) library
    - Contains double-stranded (= dsDNA) that is reverse transcribed from messenger RNA (= mRNA)
    - How it is generated (in eukaryotes):
      - Purify mRNA by applying it to an oligodeoxythymidylate (oligo dT) cellulose filter which binds the mRNA's poly A-tail
      - Synthesize cDNA using oligo dT as a primer
      - Cut mRNA with RNA-nicking RNase H and DNA polymerase I uses the fragments as primers to synthesize cDNA
      - Digest resulting double-stranded cDNA and insert it into vectors
      - Create phage library as discussed for genomic DNA library
    - Unlike genomic DNA libraries, an advantage of cDNA libraries is that they do not include introns or flanking sequences
  - Locating a gene of interest
    - Use a hybridization probe
      - A molecule that recognizes a specific DNA sequence or protein product labeled with a compound that allows for easy detection (e.g. radioactive isotope, reactive enzyme that produces color, or fluorescent dye)
    - Hybridize the probe and the DNA library
      - The sensitivity or stringency of the hybridization reaction can be increased or decreased by changing experimental variables (e.g. salt concentration, temperature)
    - Isolate detected positive hits from phage plates
    - Identify and isolate the gene of interest
    - Amplify the gene using polymerase chain reaction (PCR)

- Polymerase Chain Reaction (PCR)
  - Allows for the rapid amplification of any DNA fragment without purification
  - DNA primers flank the specific sequence to be amplified
  - Primers are then extended to the end of the DNA molecule with the use of a heat-resistant DNA polymerase
  - Newly synthesized DNA strand is then used as the template to undergo another round of replication
  - Technique:
    - Melt target DNA into two single strands by heating the reaction mixture to approximately 94 °C
    - Cool the mixture rapidly to anneal the primers to their specific locations
      - Note: anneal = the sticking together of complementary single strands via the formation of hydrogen bonding between base pairs
    - Raise the temperature to 72°C to allow DNA polymerase to add nucleotides until the entire complementary strand of the template is completed
    - Repeat the cycle to make more copies
  - Special applications:
    - Sex determination
      - Requires amplification of intron 1 of amelogenin gene
      - Amelogenin gene, found on X-Y homologous chromosomes, contains a 184 base pair deletion on the Y homologue
      - That deletion allows females to be distinguished from males in that males will have two different sizes of amplified DNA whereas females will have one unique size
    - Introduce specific mutations into genes for research purposes such as:
      - Deleting entire fragments
      - Changing specific amino acids
      - Adding peptide tags (= peptide sequences tagged onto a protein)

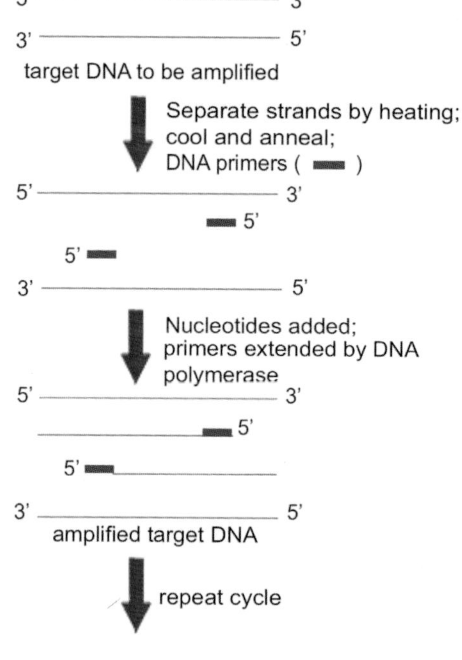

- DNA Sequencing
  - Method by which to ensure that the gene insert of interest does not contain any mistakes
  - Sanger method of DNA sequencing
    - Most commonly used sequencing technique
    - Makes four preparations of DNA
    - Each preparation is incubated with a labeled sequencing primer, DNA polymerase, all 4 DNA triphosphates, and 1 of the nucleotides in its dideoxy form (e.g. ddATP, ddCTP, ddGTP, or ddTTP)
  - Technique:
    - New strands of DNA are synthesized using PCR beginning at the primer and continuing on until a dideoxynucleotide (ddNTP) is inserted at random
    - This results in a mixture of DNA fragments with varying lengths that must be separated by gel electrophoresis and read one nucleotide at a time

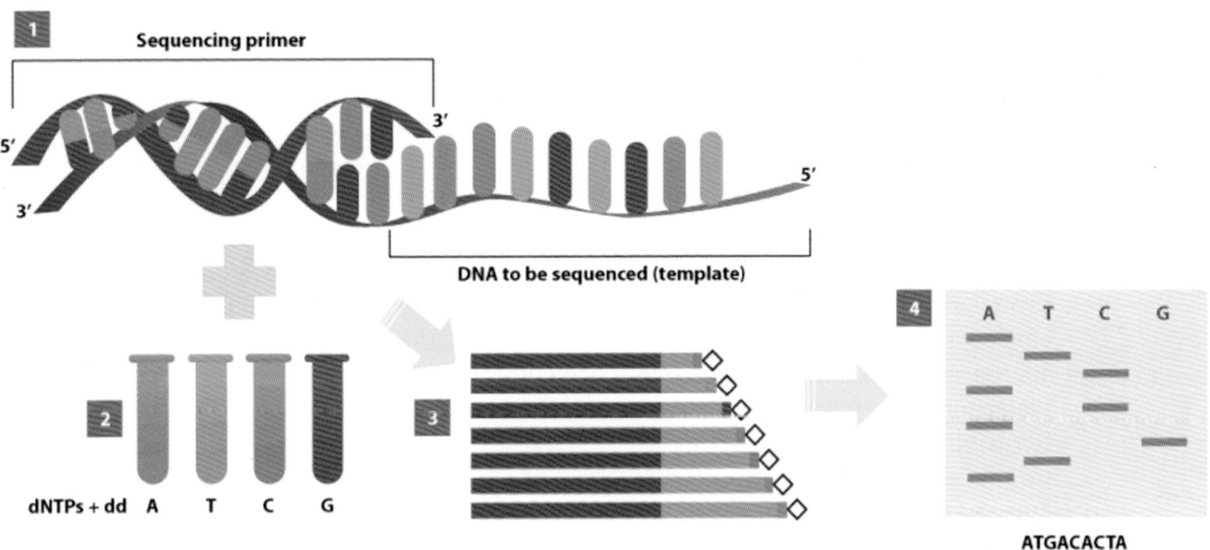

MCAT Biochemistry Biotechnology: Summary II

- Gel electrophoresis
  - Method of separating DNA fragments of differing lengths based on their size
  - Technique:
    - DNA fragments are passed through an electrically-charged agarose gel
    - Since DNA is negatively charged, it moves towards the anode (= positive electrode)
    - Shorter fragments move faster than the longer fragments and can be visualized as a banding pattern using autoradiography techniques

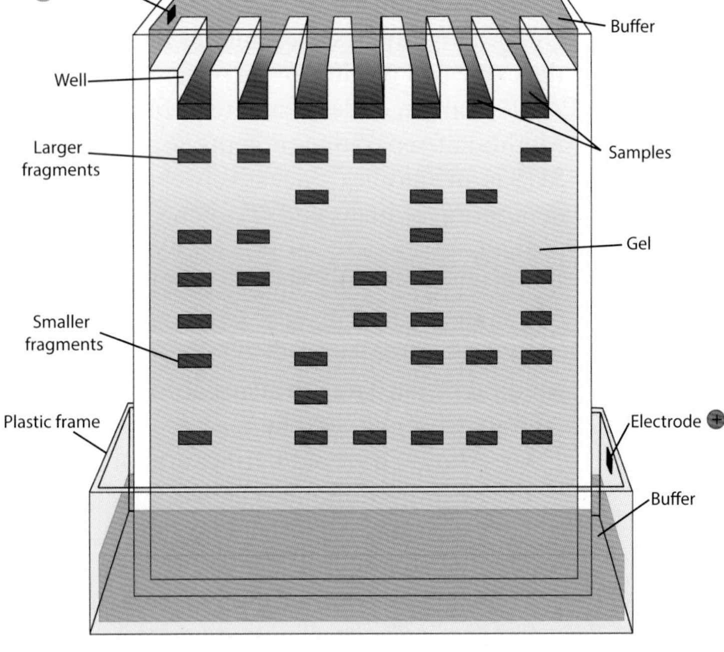

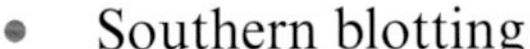

- Southern blotting
  - Method of transferring DNA fragments from the electrophoresis agarose gel onto filter paper where they are identified with probes
  - Technique:
    - DNA is digested in a mixture with restriction endonucleases to cut out specific pieces of DNA
    - The DNA fragments are then subjected to gel electrophoresis

SNOW	DROP
Southern	DNA
Northern	RNA
O	O
Western	Protein

Mnemonic for Remembering the Blotting Techniques

    - Separated fragments are bathed in an alkaline solution where they immediately begin to denature
    - Fragments are then blotted onto nitrocellulose paper and incubated with a specific probe whose location can be visualized with autoradiography

- Northern blotting
  - Method of detecting specific sequences of RNA by hybridization with cDNA
- Western blotting
  - Method used to identify specific amino acid sequences in proteins
  - Proteins are separated by gel electrophoresis on an SDS-PAGE gel and detected using labeled antibodies specific to the protein or part of the protein
- DNA microarrays (= DNA chip or biochip or "laboratory-on-a-chip")
  - Determine which genes are active or inactive in different cell types
  - Evolved from Southern blotting
  - Can be used to genotype multiple regions of a genome
  - Created by robotic machines that arrange small amounts of hundreds of thousands of gene sequences on a single microscope slide
  - Sequences can be a short section of a gene or other DNA element that is used to hybridize a cDNA or cRNA (also called antisense RNA) sample
  - Hybridization is usually observed and quantified by the detection of a fluorescent tag
- Protein Quantification
  - Quantitative analysis techniques allow researchers to determine basic information about the expressed product (e.g. concentration, amount, size)
- SDS-PAGE (sodium dodecyl sulfate polyacrylamide gel electrophoresis)
  - Method of separating proteins according to their electrophoretic mobility
  - SDS is an anionic (= negatively charged) detergent with the following effects: (1) denaturing proteins and (2) giving an additional negative charge to the now-linearized proteins
  - In most proteins, the binding of SDS to the polypeptide chain gives an even distribution of charge per unit mass, thus fractionation will approximate size during electrophoresis
- Column Chromatography
  - Method of purifying proteins according to their size, charge, hydrophobicity, and more
  - Affinity Chromatography
    - Allows the rapid purification of biological molecules based on certain affinities
    - Examples: affinities between antigen and antibody, enzyme and substrate, or genetically engineered protein tags and specific matrices
  - Ion Chromatography
    - Allows the purification of biological molecules based on overall charge:
      - Cation Chromatography - selectively binds positively-charged molecules
      - Anion Chromatography - selectively binds negatively-charged molecules
    - Proteins are removed by washing (= eluting) using increasing concentrations of salt
  - Size-Exclusion Chromatography (SEC) (also known as gel filtration)
    - Allows the purification of biological molecules based on size
    - A mixed protein solution is applied to the top of a long column packed with porous polymer beads
    - As the solution filters through the beads, smaller molecules are slowed down by the pores in the beads while larger molecules are allowed to flowed through at a faster rate - thus, larger molecules are eluted first